THE SPECIALTY PRACTICE OF
REHABILITATION NURSING

A Core Curriculum
Sixth Edition

Cynthia S. Jacelon, PhD RN-BC CRRN FAAN, *Editor*

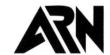

Association of Rehabilitation Nurses
Promoting Excellence in Professional Rehabilitation Nursing Practice

THE SPECIALTY PRACTICE OF
REHABILITATION NURSING

A Core Curriculum
Sixth Edition

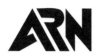

ARN Staff

Executive Director
Karen Nason, CAE

Editorial Director
Clay Baznik

Managing Editor
Rachel Frank

Associate Editor
Amy Hastings

Assistant Editor
Monica Piotrowski

Senior Graphic Designer
Sonya L. Jones

Cover Design
Miku Ishii Kinnear

ISBN 978-1-884278-01-3

Note. As new scientific information becomes available through basic and clinical research, recommended treatments and drug therapies undergo changes. The authors, editors, reviewers, and publisher have done everything possible to make this book accurate, up to date, and in accord with standards accepted at the time of publication. The authors, editors, reviewers, and publisher are not responsible for errors or omissions or for consequences from application of the book and make no warranty, expressed or implied, in regard to the contents of the book. Any practice described in this book should be applied by the healthcare practitioner in accordance with professional standards of care and used in regard to the unique circumstances that may apply in each situation. The reader is advised always to check product information (package inserts) for changes and new information regarding dose and contraindications before administering any drug. Caution is especially urged when using new or infrequently ordered drugs or treatments.

This volume contains many references and resources utilizing Internet addresses. Although these sites were current at the time of research, writing, and/or publication, many Internet postings are volatile and subject to expiration or deletion over time. Therefore, ARN cannot guarantee currency of electronic references. (Readers who wish to pursue the latest information on a cited topic are likely to find new or updated posting via online search engines.)

Contents

Foreword

"Let us each and all realizing the importance of our influence on others—stand shoulder to shoulder— and not alone, in good cause."
—Florence Nightingale

I am honored to provide the foreword for the sixth edition of the Association of Rehabilitation Nurses' (ARN's) *Specialty Practice of Rehabilitation Nursing: A Core Curriculum*. Each edition of the *Core Curriculum* reflects the evolving nature of rehabilitation nursing and the changing context of health care. This *Core*, like each previously published during the past 30 years, is a reflection of all who have contributed to earlier editions. This edition of the *Core*, edited by Cynthia Jacelon and with contributions from 78 authors and reviewers, will serve as the guide to rehabilitation nursing practice in a time that is characterized by both challenge and change.

The words of Florence Nightingale in the opening quote speak to several critical elements of rehabilitation nursing—most obviously our powerful influence on the lives of others as we help individuals affected by chronic and disabling conditions adapt to disabilities, achieve their potential, and work toward productive and independent lives. The second theme of this quote is the importance of working together with others—the patient or client, families, and other members of the healthcare team—to achieve the "good cause" of rehabilitation.

Fulfilling the promise of the good cause of rehabilitation for our clients depends on our ability to be creative and go beyond the routine practice of nursing. In *The Unconscious Conspiracy: Why Leaders Can't Lead* (1976) Warren Bennis cautions that routine work drives out nonroutine work and smothers opportunities for creative planning and change. As rehabilitation nurses practicing in diverse roles and settings, we are all aware that there is much routine work; although it is important, we must make sure that it does not consume us. To accomplish the good but immensely challenging cause of rehabilitation we must use the knowledge and skills outlined in this *Core Curriculum* and blend them with the key personal qualities exhibited by leaders of change: integrity, dedication, generosity of spirit, openness, and creativity (Bennis, 1976).

Integrity encompasses the standards of moral and intellectual honesty that we use as the basis for our individual conduct and nursing practice. There are many pressures—both internal and external—in today's healthcare settings that challenge our integrity. People of integrity strengthen society. They strengthen every organization that they are part of in multiple ways and they are the essence of the nursing profession. Helping clients adapt to a change in health status, whether it is sudden and traumatic or slow and degenerative, requires dedication and a passionate and intense conviction to support the goals of rehabilitation nursing that are reflected in the *Core Curriculum*.

The work of rehabilitation nursing brings us in close contact with many individuals (clients, families, and coworkers) from diverse backgrounds and experiences who may have very different values and behaviors. Although it is easier and unfortunately common today to dismiss the validity of a person's perspective by labeling them in a way we personally oppose, such labels and assumptions eliminate the potential for important opportunities for us to learn from one another. Rehabilitation nurses practicing the art of understanding diverse perspectives exemplify the personal quality of generosity of spirit.

Openness and creativity are essential if we are to meet ARN's mission to promote and advance professional rehabilitation nursing practice through education, advocacy, collaboration, and research and enhance the quality of life of those affected by disability and chronic illness. Openness—being willing to listen to new ideas or suggestions—will allow us to most effectively help individuals affected by chronic illness or physical disability adapt to their disabilities, reach their maximum potential, and work toward productivity and independence. As we seek to influence the good cause of rehabilitation, we must constantly strive to renew our personal creativity to see things in new ways and from new perspectives. We must creatively nurture the generalist aspects of our work as well as carefully attend to the specialty area of practice. It is the generalist perspective that highlights our common and shared humanity with our patients, our colleagues, and especially those who are leading efforts to enhance our organizations and our health care.

This sixth edition of the *Core Curriculum* provides the essential knowledge and information for the specialty practice of rehabilitation nursing. As a reader, carefully review the four sections, starting with the history of rehabilitation nursing and concluding with significant aspects of the current healthcare environment. This comprehensive guide for practice is an essential resource for rehabilitation nursing professionals called to use their knowledge, skills, and leadership to adapt practice for their clients' changing health and wellness needs as well as important emerging changes in the environments of healthcare practice.

Alexa K. Stuifbergen, PhD RN FAAN
July 2011

Reference

Bennis, W. G. (1976). *The unconscious conspiracy: Why leaders can't lead.* New York: AMACOM.

Preface

The sixth edition of the Association of Rehabilitation Nurses' (ARN's) *The Specialty Practice of Rehabilitation Nursing: Core Curriculum* continues to be a comprehensive guide to the practice of rehabilitation nurses wherever and with whomever they practice. In this edition of the *Core*, we have continued to include advanced practice content and have added information related to middle-range nursing theory and the nursing process. We have maintained the emphasis on evidence-based practice and included research findings whenever possible.

In this edition we have revised and updated the *Core* while retaining the format. I am often asked about the format of the *Core*. Core curriculums are produced in an outline format because they are curriculums. A core curriculum is the outline of the essential content of a discipline. With this in mind, the content includes pathophysiology for common rehabilitation diagnoses, application of the nursing process, and a lifespan perspective.

The sixth edition builds on the excellent foundation of previous editions of the *Core*. In the 5th edition Dr. Kristen Mauk led a team of more than 40 authors and 45 reviewers to provide a text with the most current knowledge in rehabilitation available. In the current edition, our team is a bit smaller, including 38 authors and 40 reviewers. The authors share their expertise from diverse settings, including acute rehabilitation, postacute care, community settings, case management, research, consulting, academia, and clinics. Most authors are certified rehabilitation registered nurses (CRRN) and many have graduate degrees. The diverse experience and expertise of the authors and reviewers provides a rich resource for creating a text with the most up-to-date information in the specialty.

The conceptual framework of the sixth edition is new. It is based loosely on the metaparadigm of nursing (nurse, health, client, environment). The content is divided into four sections: the first is focused on the rehabilitation nurse, the second on functional health patterns and rehabilitation nursing practice to promote health, the third section provides information on common disorders experienced by rehabilitation clients and lifespan issues, and the fourth section addresses the environment of care.

Section I is focused on the specialty practice of rehabilitation nursing. The history of rehabilitation and, more specifically, the history of rehabilitation nursing are outlined in the first two chapters. These chapters include the American healthcare system as the context for rehabilitation nursing practice. Chapter three has been revised and updated and addresses the ethical, moral, and legal issues related to our field. The last two chapters in Section I address the role of research and evidence-based practice in rehabilitation nursing and the subspecialty of case management.

Section II is focused on functional health patterns related to rehabilitation nursing. The content has been reorganized into chapters focused on health maintenance, physical healthcare patterns, and psychosocial healthcare patterns. Each chapter includes assessment, diagnoses, planning, interventions, and evaluation.

Section III includes information on common diagnoses for rehabilitation clients and rehabilitation across the lifespan. Content is provided on neuroanatomy, neurological diseases, cerebrovascular accidents, and traumatic injuries of the head and spinal cord. Other common rehabilitation diagnoses such as musculoskeletal problems, cardiac and respiratory disease, and pain are included. There is also a chapter on the issues of clients with less common diagnoses such as genetic disorders, cancer, and burns.

Section IV, "The Environment of Care," addresses topics such as economics, health policy, outcome measurement, and performance improvement. There is also a chapter dedicated to the settings in which rehabilitation nurses work.

Overall, the sixth edition of the *Core Curriculum* provides an outline of the most current knowledge of our profession. The *Core* will be useful for both new and experienced individuals who are learning or teaching rehabilitation nursing and as a resource for preparing for the CRRN examination.

Cynthia S. Jacelon, PhD RN-BC CRRN FAAN

Acknowledgments

I would like thank the 2009 ARN Board of Directors for inviting me to be the editor of the sixth edition of the *Specialty Practice of Rehabilitation Nursing: Core Curriculum*. I also want to thank all of the authors and reviewers of the sixth edition of the *Core Curriculum*, without whose contributions we could not have created a book of such high quality. I would especially like to acknowledge and thank two individuals: Rachel Frank, who has done an excellent job as managing editor, and Marilyn TerMaat, who graciously agreed to review the entire *Core Curriculum* before publication.

Dedication

I would like to dedicate this book to individuals with disabilities and chronic illness. I hope the contents of this text will help rehabilitation nurses effectively serve this population.

Cynthia S. Jacelon, PhD RN-BC CRRN FAAN

Authors

Chapter 1
Cynthia S. Jacelon, PhD RN-BC CRRN FAAN

Chapter 2
Donna Williams, MSN RN CRRN

Chapter 3
Angela Stone Schmidt, PhD MNSc RNP RN; Marian Baxter, MS MA RN GCNS-BC CRRN

Chapter 4
Linda L. Pierce, PhD RN CNS CRRN FAHA FAAN; Pamala D. Larsen, PhD RN CRRN FNGNA

Chapter 5
Donna Williams, MSN RN CRRN; Kathryn Doeschot, MSN RN CRRN

Chapter 6
Karen S. Reed, MSN DHSc RN CRRN CNL

Chapter 7
Cynthia D. Anderson, MSN RN CRRN; Donald D. Kautz, PhD RN CRRN CNE; Sharon Bryant, MPH BSN RN CRRN; Norma Clanin, MS CNS RN CRRN

Chapter 8
Cynthia S. Jacelon, PhD RN-BC CRRN FAAN

Chapter 9
Cynthia K. Fine, MSN CRRN

Chapter 10
Joan P. Alverzo, PhD CRRN; Michele Russell Ward, BS CRRN

Chapter 11
Paddy Garvin-Higgins, MN CNS RN CRRN; Delilah Hall-Towarnicke, MSN CNS RN CRRN; Carla J. Howard, ACNP-BC CRRN

Chapter 12
Paula Martinkewiz, MS RN CRRN; Betty J. Furr, PhD RN CRRN; Catharine Farnan, MS CRRN CBIS; Patricia G. Martinez, BSN RN CRRN

Chapter 13
Cheryl A. Lehman, PhD RN CNS-BC RN-BC CRRN; Ann Gutierrez, MSN RN CRRN CBIS

Chapter 14
Holly Evans Madison, PhD RN

Chapter 15
Diane B. Monsivais, PhD CRRN

Chapter 16
Joan K. McMahon, MSA BSN CRRN

Chapter 17
Mindi Miller, PhD MSN MA RN CRRN

Chapter 18
Dalice Hertzberg, MSN RN FNP-C; Lyn Sapp, MN RN CRRN

Chapter 19
Kristen L. Mauk, PhD DNP RN CRRN GCNS-BC GNP-BC FAAN; Usha K. Patel, APN MSN RN CRRN CWOCN

Chapter 20
Pamala D. Larsen, PhD CRRN FNGNA

Chapter 21
Anne Deutsch, PhD RN CRRN

Chapter 22
Terrie Black, MBA BSN RN BC CRRN; Michele Cournan, DNP RN CRRN ANP-BC FNP

Reviewers

Chapter 1
Teresa L. Thompson, PhD RN CRRN

Chapter 2
Teresa L. Thompson, PhD RN CRRN

Chapter 3
Sherry L. Liske, MS RN CRRN

Chapter 4
Elaine L. Miller, PhD RN CRRN FAHA FAAN

Chapter 5
Karen Preston, MS CRRN FIALCP PHN

Chapter 6
Diane Dudas Sheehan, ND CNP APN; Leslie Neal-Boylan, PhD CRRN APRN-BC FNP

Chapter 7
Carolyn A. Sorensen, MSN RN CRRN CWOCN; Marcia Grandstaff, MSN RN CRRN

Chapter 8
Paddy Garvin-Higgins, MN CNS RN CRRN; Linda R. Stones, MS BSN BS RN CRRN

Chapter 9
Kathleen L. Dunn, MS RN CRRN CNS-BC; Betty Clark, BSN MEd RN CRRN

Chapter 10
Cheryl A. Lehman, PhD RN CNS-BC RN-BC CRRN

Chapter 11
Janice L. Hinkle, PhD RN CNRN; Laura Ferber, MN RN CNRN CRRN; Stephanie Vaughn, PhD RN CRRN

Chapter 12
Kathleen L. Dunn, MS RN CRRN CNS-BC; Bonnie Parker, MSN RN CRRN; Linda Dufour, MSN RN CRRN

Chapter 13
Cynthia S. Jacelon, PhD RN-BC CRRN FAAN

Chapter 14
Pamela Farrell, MSN RN CRRN; Tiffany LeCroy, MSN RN CRRN FNP-C

Chapter 15
Donna Williams, MSN RN CRRN; Sherry King, RN CRRN

Chapter 16
Brenda McCall-Russell, MBA IS BSN RN CRRN

Chapter 17
Judith Muraida DiFilippo, MS CRRN

Chapter 18
Patricia A. Edwards, EdD RN NEA-BC ANEF

Chapter 19
Judith Muraida DiFilippo, MS RN CRRN; Ouida Plemons, BC RN CRRN

Chapter 20
Marilyn L. Ter Maat, MSN RN NEC-BC FNGNA CRRN

Chapter 21
Louis Stackler, MS RN

Chapter 22
Joan P. Alverzo, PhD CRRN

The Specialty Practice of Rehabilitation Nursing

CHAPTER 1
Health Care, Rehabilitation, and Rehabilitation Nursing

Cynthia S. Jacelon, PhD RN-BC CRRN FAAN

Rehabilitation is a philosophy of practice and an attitude toward caring for people with disabilities and chronic health problems. During the next few decades two trends will combine to increase the need for rehabilitation. First, advances in health care have enabled people to survive injuries and illnesses and live longer than in the past; therefore, the numbers of people with chronic illness and disability are expected to rise. Second, the number of older adults is increasing rapidly, and with this increase comes an increase in chronic health problems and disability. The overall goals of rehabilitation are to improve quality of life and help people "who [have] a disability or chronic health problem in restoring, maintaining, and promoting his or her maximal health" (Association of Rehabilitation Nurses [ARN], 2008, p. 13). Rehabilitation is contingent on a team approach, and the discipline of nursing is integral to the team. Rehabilitation nursing is a specialty practice that offers a unique, holistic perspective to the care of clients with disabilities and chronic health problems. Furthermore, this unique perspective can be applied across the continuum of care.

The purpose of this chapter is to present rehabilitation philosophy, goals, and processes and examine the role of nursing within the specialty. Nursing science—the relationship between theory, research, and practice—provides a basis for professional rehabilitation nursing. Included in this chapter is a description of the role responsibilities, educational preparation, competencies, certification, professional associations, and resources for the specialty practice of rehabilitation nursing.

The Evolution of Rehabilitation

Advances in health care during the past century have enabled people to live longer and recover from injuries and illnesses that were previously fatal. However, a consequence of saving lives is that clients are sometimes left with disabilities and chronic illnesses that profoundly change the way they live in the world. The field of rehabilitation emerged to help individuals and families integrate the changes associated with disability and chronic health problems into their lives. Rehabilitation is a philosophy, an attitude, and an approach to caring for people with disabilities and chronic health problems that encourages self-management, improves the quality of their lives, and provides a meaningful context in which to live.

The concept of rehabilitation as a philosophy and attitude is important. Attitudes toward people with disability, which arise from a philosophy, determine societal responsibilities and approaches. For example, in ancient Western civilization, disease and disability often were thought to be the result of evil spirits. Consequently, those so "possessed" were feared and shunned. Parents in ancient Rome could legally drown infants with congenital anomalies, and in Sparta such infants were left to die of exposure. This situation did not improve during the Middle Ages. Some people with disabilities were burned as witches, others were used as court jesters, and all who had disabilities were shunned from everyday societal functions. Even in more modern times, those living with disabilities or handicaps in Nazi Germany were considered "flawed" and were among the first people eliminated in the Holocaust. Fortunately, philosophical approaches and attitudes have changed radically over time. (Refer to Chapter 2 for a historical overview of rehabilitation.)

The interdisciplinary healthcare specialty of rehabilitation was a product of 20th century wars. Many soldiers—young men for the most part—survived injury but faced serious disability. As a result, military hospitals established rehabilitation units that focused extensive efforts on returning these young men to society. Dr. Howard Rusk, head of the American Air Force Convalescent Training Program, was a strong leader in organizing rehabilitation programs (Rusk, 1972). Soon, rehabilitation units and hospitals sprang up around the United States and the interdisciplinary specialty of rehabilitation gained importance. By 1974 ARN was formed, and nursing, which had always been involved in rehabilitation, became formally recognized as a rehabilitation specialty.

I. Legislative Initiatives

Legislation in the United States has been important in the development of the specialty of rehabilitation. The result of these legislative acts has been to increase societal acceptance of people with disabilities and provide opportunities for them to maximize their potential. Rehabilitation is a vital component of health care. Although the root causes of disability have changed over time, the need for rehabilitation today is greater than ever before. Rehabilitation has moved from its era of research and development to one of scrutiny by the healthcare finance community. Initially, reimbursement was a given and model systems and programs of research in major rehabilitation settings were common and well funded. Those days are gone. Today, 75% rules, intensity of service, and other insurance requirements result in rehabilitation nurses being very aware of rules and regulations as part of the care they provide.

A. Legislated Acts
 1. The Americans with Disabilities Act (ADA) of 1990 (U.S. Department of Justice, 2006b)
  a. Title I
   1) Prohibits private employers, state and local governments, employment agencies, and labor unions from discriminating against qualified people with disabilities in job application procedures, hiring, firing, advancement, compensation, job training, and other terms, conditions, and privileges of employment
   2) Describes the traits of a person with a disability
    a) A physical or mental impairment that substantially limits one or more major life activities
    b) A record of such an impairment
    c) Regarded as having such an impairment
  b. Title II
   1) Provides comprehensive civil rights for qualified people with disabilities
   2) Addresses public entities and requires that all activities, services, and programs of public entities be covered by the ADA, including activities of state legislatures and courts, town meetings, police and fire departments, motor vehicle licensing, and employment
   3) Directly influences access, program integration, communication, construction, and alterations
  c. Title III
   1) Addresses the public sector
   2) Defines the private entities that must meet ADA requirements
  d. Title IV: Telecommunication
  e. Title V: Miscellaneous provisions to cover legal fees and to prohibit coercion and retaliation
  f. The impact of the ADA
   1) Allows people with disabilities to have equal opportunities, accessibility, and accommodations in employment, transportation, and public access
   2) Has spawned litigation and clarification to further define its implementation and application (U.S. Department of Justice, 2006a)
   3) Has reinforced the advocate role of rehabilitation nurses based on their knowledge of the ADA as they inform clients, encourage ADA enforcement, and obtain resources
 2. Rehabilitation acts (U.S. Department of Justice, 2006b): Foundation for federal funding and contract requirements
  a. Section 501: Affirmative action and nondiscrimination in employment in federal agencies
  b. Section 503: Affirmative action and nondiscrimination in federal contracts and subcontracts
  c. Section 504: Affirmative action and nondiscrimination in programs that receive federal funding
  d. Section 508: Requires that electronic and information technology used by the federal government be accessible
B. Changes in Rehabilitation Reimbursement
 1. Initial impact of diagnosis-related groups
  a. During the mid 1980s, there was an increase in rehabilitation acute units.
  b. During the early 1990s, the overall census in all inpatient settings decreased.
  c. During the 1990s, competition for rehabilitation clients began and the growth of acute rehabilitation subsided.
  d. Internal and external case management of all clients has increased.
  e. Home health care initially increased and later came under prospective payment systems, capping payment.
 2. Balanced Budget Act of 1997 (Esser, 1998)
  a. Called for Medicare spending cuts that affected rehabilitation (Esser, 1998)
  b. Required a prospective payment system (PPS)
  c. Required the use of Resource Utilization Groups (RUGs) as the basis for rehabilitation PPSs: RUGs-III are based on the Minimum Data Set assessment's Resident Assessment Instrument and Resident Assessment Protocols, which must be completed for each client. RUGs group clients into four major categories (Knapp, 1999; Nathenson, 1999).
 3. 75% rule (Centers for Medicare and Medicaid Services [CMS], 2007)
  a. Initiated in 1984
  b. Established 10 diagnostic categories for admission to rehabilitation
  c. CMS increased to 13 diagnoses in 2003.
  d. Began enforcement in 2004 with initial compliance at 50%, with graded increase to 75% of all admissions by 2008 (Cournan, 2006; Zigmod, 2006).

e. Impact is the denial of admissions or payment for services for those not meeting the diagnostic criteria

f. Lobbying efforts to expand the diagnostic categories persist.

4. Capped Medicare Part B payments (CMS, 2011)

a. Rehabilitation therapy for postacute delivery has an annual financial limitation (cap).

b. Combined outpatient physical therapy and speech-language pathology services share the same cap ($1,870 in 2011).

c. Occupational therapy has a $1,870 cap per year.

d. Treatment must be medically necessary.

e. Twenty percent of the Medicare-approved amount is the client's responsibility.

f. No cap applies if therapy is provided at a hospital outpatient therapy department.

g. Medicare-certified beds in skilled nursing facilities have the same cap amounts.

5. Impact on rehabilitation (Cournan, 2006)

a. Decreased access for people with disabilities that do not fit within the defined categories

b. Increased scrutiny of admission by payers

c. Limited outpatient services

d. Addition of nursing roles for admission and PPS coordinators to ensure compliance and reimbursement

e. Decrease in census of inpatient rehabilitation settings

6. Patient Protection and Affordable Care Act (Scott, 2010)

a. Proposes bundled payments for select diagnoses

b. Demonstration projects being planned

c. Not yet implemented

II. **Rehabilitation Philosophy and Goals Across Disciplines**

Rehabilitation is a philosophy that crosses the boundaries of practice disciplines. It has been defined as "a process of helping a person to reach the fullest physical, psychological, social, vocational, avocational, and educational potential consistent with his or her physiologic or anatomic impairment, environmental limitations, and desires and life plans" (DeLisa, Currie, & Martin, 1998, p. 3). It is an inherently collaborative endeavor, and it places the client and family in the center of the healthcare team. Rehabilitation is contingent on a team approach. Indeed, most rehabilitation professionals would agree that the healthcare system would flourish if the ideals of rehabilitation permeated all aspects of health care. These definitions provide a framework and a language that are not just for rehabilitation but for society as well.

A. International Classification of Impairment, Disability, and Handicap: In 1980 the World Health Organization developed the International Classification of Impairment, Disability, and Handicap (cited in Mauk, 2009, pp. 580–582). This classification system has been translated into 13 languages and distinguishes between the following terms:

1. Impairment: A loss or abnormality of a psychological, physiological, or anatomical structure and function. Impairment occurs at the organ level.

2. Disability: A restriction or lack (resulting from an impairment) of ability to perform an activity in the manner or within the range considered normal for a human being. Disability occurs at the level of the individual.

3. Handicap: A disadvantage for a given person resulting from impairment or disability that limits or prevents fulfillment of a role that is normal for that person. Handicap occurs at the societal level.

B. Goal of Rehabilitation: The overall goal of rehabilitation is "restoring, maintaining, and promoting maximal health" (ARN, 2008).

C. Rehabilitation Team Models: The rehabilitation team consists of, first and foremost, the individual and his or her family. Other team members may vary depending on the needs of the person but typically include a physiatrist, rehabilitation nurse, social worker, physical therapist, occupational therapist, and speech-language pathologist. Team members contributing to a person's rehabilitation are varied and cross many disciplines (**Figure 1-1**). Four models for team functioning have been described: medical, multidisciplinary, interdisciplinary, and transdisciplinary (Mauk, 2009). In all models, nursing is an integral part of the rehabilitation team.

1. Medical model: The medical model is a physician-centered model of care in which all care is directed by the physician. This model is not consistent with rehabilitation philosophy or goals and is uncommon in rehabilitation practice.

2. Multidisciplinary model: The multidisciplinary team, which may be seen in rehabilitation, is one in which the professionals work in parallel; each discipline works toward particular client goals, with very little overlap between disciplines. Communication is more vertical than lateral, with the leader controlling team conferences. In a multidisciplinary model, the person working directly with the client does not always participate in team planning; rather, the department managers usually attend team conferences. This model is effective when the team membership is

Figure 1-1. Members of the Rehabilitation Team

Client and family

Nurses

Physiatrists

Other physicians

Physical therapists

Occupational therapists

Speech-language pathologists

Psychologists

Recreational therapists

Vocational therapists

Orthotists

Chaplains

Insurance case managers or representatives

Employers

Teachers

Audiologists

Nutritionists

Home health professionals

not stable (e.g., when there are different team members for different clients).

3. Interdisciplinary model: The interdisciplinary model is a matrix-like model in which lateral communication is predominant. This is an effective model when team membership is stable (e.g., in an inpatient rehabilitation unit). Decisions are determined by the group working directly with the client, which means that mutual trust must be established between team members, and conflict resolution is an important skill used by team members. Team goal setting is an important feature of this model.

4. Transdisciplinary model: A newer team model is the transdisciplinary model, in which the client has a primary provider from the team who is guided by the team in caring for the client. For example, the primary provider may be a nurse, who then provides physical, speech, and occupational therapy based on the advice and counsel he or she receives from team members in those disciplines. Similarly, the primary therapist could be a physical therapist. Mumma and Nelson (1996) noted that this model requires flexibility and receptiveness on the part of team members because individual roles are less distinct. This model also raises many issues regarding licensure and accountability. It may be best suited for situations in

which the client is stable and in need of long-term services.

5. Team function: Regardless of the rehabilitation team model, all team members can increase their effectiveness by understanding collaborative practice, group dynamics, conflict resolution, and team functioning. Components necessary for effective team function include trust, knowledge, shared responsibility, mutual respect, communication, cooperation and coordination, and optimism. Effective teams require a commitment from each member.

6. In the specialty of rehabilitation no single model dominates and several models coexist. For example, a case management system may be operating within a subacute or postacute pediatric day treatment program. As health care continues to evolve, new models of providing services undoubtedly will emerge, and nurses are in an important position to lead the way.

III. Provision of Services

The rehabilitation philosophy can infuse any healthcare setting. Collaboration between team members (through any of the team models) and the individual, family, and community is a vital aspect of rehabilitation. Mumma and Nelson (1996) offered a useful categorization of models for provision of services: client centered, setting centered, provider centered, and collaborative. For the purposes of this chapter, a collaborative model (i.e., a team concept) is assumed in all rehabilitation models.

A. Client-Centered Care: Client-centered models are those serving specialized populations. The focus may be on a specific developmental stage, such as children or older adults, or on a type of impairment, such as spinal cord or head injury. With a population-specific focus, providers can target their resources and gain extensive expertise through experience.

B. Setting-Centered Care: Acute care, long-term care, outpatient care, home care, and community care are the traditional models focusing on settings. Each describes where rehabilitation takes place. The trend away from inpatient care has accelerated in recent years as a result of changing funding practices. A newer category of setting-focused rehabilitation is subacute care. Subacute or postacute care settings provide rehabilitation to people who continue to need substantial medical care and who are slower to progress. For adults, subacute or postacute care units usually are inpatient settings and often are housed in an acute care, traditional rehabilitation unit or a long-term care facility. However, pediatric subacute or postacute rehabilitation is seen more often in day treatment programs, and the children return to home or residential settings at night (Hertzberg & Edwards, 1999).

C. Provider-Centered Care: Provider-centered models reflect how healthcare providers have decided to organize the provision of care. Many models have been used over the years, with the goal of maximizing the use of human resources. Within nursing, functional, team, and primary nursing and, more recently, case management have been the models. In functional nursing, the tasks are divided (e.g., one nurse delivers all the medications). In team nursing, a nurse oversees the care of a group of clients by providers of various skill levels. Primary nursing (not to be confused with primary care) became popular in the 1980s as a means of providing client-centered care. One nurse provides direct total care to a group of clients and is responsible for planning and coordinating that care when he or she is not on duty. This model generated several variations. Primary nursing has coordinated, client-centered care as its goal, similar to case management.

D. Case Management: Case management, though not a new concept in nursing and health care, is a common provider-centered model within rehabilitation. In this model, the goal is to provide high-quality, individualized, cost-effective care through the process of assessing, planning, organizing, coordinating, implementing, monitoring, and evaluating the services and resources needed to respond to an individual's healthcare needs (ARN, n.d.). Because of nursing's holistic focus, nurses are ideal case managers; however, they do not always assume this role. Although theoretically the case manager is the client advocate, it is important to recognize to whom the case manager is accountable (e.g., the insurance company, the hospital).

E. Major Shifts in the Delivery, Environment, and Expectations of Health Care (Issel & Anderson, 1996)
  1. Customer orientation: This shift involved moving from viewing the person as the customer to viewing the population as the customer.
  2. Wellness orientation: With the movement toward focusing on client populations, the emphasis became health promotion, which redefined the health services that were provided and prioritized.
  3. Cost versus revenue: The emphasis is on managed care and capitation, and the responsibility lies with the provider to control costs. Continued evolution of reimbursement policies will affect rehabilitation practice (Baker, Haughton, & Mongoo, 2003).

  4. Approach to care: This shift involved moving from a departmental or an individual professional approach to an integrated, interdependent approach to care.
  5. Shift for clients: Clients are now viewed as consumers of cost and quality, which allows them to identify the types and cost of services needed to maintain wellness.
  6. Continuity of information: Information is now brought to the client across time and discipline boundaries.

IV. Major Milestones in a Changing Environment
  A. Focus on Outcomes
    1. Outcomes, especially as they relate to function, are the most common measures across all levels of rehabilitation programs.
    2. The Inpatient Rehabilitation Facility Patient Assessment Instrument, used to document rehabilitation admission and reimbursement, is based on functional outcomes data.
    3. Outcomes are used to communicate with consumers of rehabilitation services to describe the following:
      a. Comparison
      b. Contracting
      c. Selection of a rehabilitation setting
      d. Marketing and competition for the rehabilitation client
  B. Recognition of a Transcultural Environment
    1. Acknowledges rapidly changing demographics and increased awareness of cultural expectations
    2. Promotes cultural competence (Andrews & Boyle, 2003; Leininger & McFarland, 2002)
    3. Includes cultural self-awareness of values and beliefs
    4. Conscious awareness of the individual, family, and community context
    5. Confronts prejudices, biases, judgments, and generalizations
    6. Promotes culturally sensitive care, which provides for the preservation and maintenance, accommodation and negotiation, and repatterning and restructuring of care to meet clients' cultural and healthcare needs (Leininger, 1997)
  C. Nursing Focus and Core Values: Nursing brings a unique, holistic focus to rehabilitation. Whereas members of other disciplines treat particular aspects of a person, nurses focus on the person as a whole, providing continuity and integrity to the client's rehabilitation experience.
    1. Fawcett (1984) defined the central foci (or the metaparadigm) of nursing as person, health,

environment, and nursing. The individual's philosophical view of these concepts is the foundation for how he or she approaches nursing care. The core values of rehabilitation as an interdisciplinary practice are congruent with those of nursing.

2. As a profession, nursing has stated its ethical foundation in the *Code of Ethics for Nurses* (American Nurses Association [ANA], 2010b).

3. Rehabilitation nursing arises as a specialty practice from the nursing discipline. Values and assumptions for the discipline are provided in *Nursing's Social Policy Statement* (ANA, 2010a, p. 3)
   a. Humans manifest an essential unity of mind, body, and spirit.
   b. Human experience is contextually and culturally defined.
   c. Health and illness are human experiences. The presence of illness does not preclude health, nor does optimal health preclude illness.
   d. The relationship between nurse and patient involves both in the process of care.
   e. The interaction between the nurse and the patient occurs within the context of the values and beliefs of the patient and the nurse.

4. Rehabilitation nursing, as a specialty of the nursing discipline at large, embraces these values and further explicates its core values, which include the following (ARN, 2008, p. 11):
   a. Individuals with functional limitations have intrinsic worth that transcends their disability and/or chronic illness.
   b. Individuals are complex yet unified, whole persons who have the right and the responsibility to make informed decisions about their future.
   c. Individuals may benefit from rehabilitation nursing at any stage of the lifespan.

D. Definition of Rehabilitation Nursing: Rehabilitation nursing is defined as "the diagnosis and treatment of human responses of individuals and groups to actual or potential health problems relative to altered functional ability and lifestyle" (ARN, 2008, p. 13).

1. Rehabilitation nursing interventions, in promoting maximal health, promote the client's quality of life.

2. Essential in achieving this goal is collaboration with the client, his or her significant others, and other healthcare providers.

3. Rehabilitation nursing is client centered, goal oriented, and outcome based.

E. Nursing Science as a Basis for Rehabilitation Nursing Practice: Nursing's body of knowledge—its science—derives from the relationship between practice, theory, and research with respect to the focus of the discipline (i.e., the metaparadigm).

1. Nursing theory to guide rehabilitation nursing practice: Theorists incorporate their knowledge of existing theories with their nursing knowledge and perspectives to create models and theories that are unique to nursing. Whereas nursing is a discipline within the larger community of scientific disciplines in which knowledge is shared, this knowledge is applied in nursing situations with a nursing perspective.
   a. By using nursing models to guide practice, nurses can gain a clear understanding of their discipline and its unique contribution to health care in general and rehabilitation in particular. When nurses have a clear understanding of their discipline, its role, and the differences from other disciplines, they can confidently assume leadership roles in rehabilitation. Practicing nursing from a nursing model perspective provides that clear understanding.
   b. The metaparadigm concepts provide the focus of nursing, and nursing theories provide the context.
   c. Grand theories
      1) In the 1970s and 1980s there was a move to develop nursing theories that could explain the universe of nursing actions.
      2) Some grand theories (e.g., Roy, Orem, Watson, and Rogers) are still used to guide nursing practice (McEwen & Wills, 2011).
      3) These theories, models, or frameworks provide a lens through which nursing phenomena are viewed and reveal how to approach nursing care.
   d. Middle-range theories: In addition to grand theories that guide nursing practice globally, a group of theories are known as middle-range theories. These theories are used to explain particular phenomena and are testable, including a limited number of variables, but are sufficiently general to be useful for practice and research.
      1) Throughout the 6th Edition of this *Core Curriculum,* middle-range theories are explicated.
      2) Professional practice models are a new type of model for nursing practice.
         a) Professional practice models are "the driving force of nursing care; a schematic description of a theory,

phenomenon, or system that depicts how nurses practice, collaborate, communicate, and develop professionally to provide the highest quality care for those served by the organization (e.g., patients, families, community). Professional practice models illustrate the alignment and integration of nursing practice with the mission, vision, and values that nursing has adapted" (American Nurses Credentialing Center, 2008, p. 24).

   b) Professional practice models are middle-range theory that is specific to the agency in which they are developed.

2. Nursing research to guide practice: Research is necessary to provide a scientific foundation and to establish accountability for professional nursing practice. Health care in general, and nursing in particular, is becoming increasingly complex and costly; these trends place increasing demands on nursing care to be validated through systematic study.

   a. ARN's *Standards and Scope of Rehabilitation Nursing Practice* (2008) reinforces the ANA's recommendations for professional rehabilitation nurses.

      1) These standards state that a research attitude (i.e., one of systematic searching) is important in all aspects of care.

      2) Whether by identifying particular problems in rehabilitation, using the research literature to determine practice approaches, or systematically evaluating nursing practices, nurses can use research to play an important role.

      3) Research should be considered an integral aspect of professional decision making.

   b. Research allows nurses to understand phenomena (through qualitative research) and to describe, explain, predict, and ultimately control events (through quantitative research).

   c. Evidence-based practice is an example of research-driven clinical practice.

   d. Nurses in all areas and levels of practice have an important role in research. LoBiondo-Wood and Haber (2009) delineated the levels of nurses' involvement in research.

      1) Nurses with associate degrees (ADs) help identify research problems, assist with data collection, and use findings in practice with supervision.

      2) Nurses who have bachelor of science (BS) degrees must be able to access and evaluate research for use in practice.

      3) Nurses with master of science (MS) degrees create the environment in which research and its use are fostered, collaborate with experienced investigators, and provide the clinical expertise needed for research.

      4) Nurses with a doctorate of nursing practice (DNP) are proficient at research translation, implementing research in clinical settings.

      5) Doctoral (PhD, doctorate of nursing science [DNSc]) and postdoctoral nurses develop nursing knowledge through research and theory development with funded research.

   e. The Rehabilitation Nursing Foundation (RNF, 1995, 2005) has developed the Rehabilitation Nursing Research Agenda (RNRA) to guide research in rehabilitation nursing. The RNRA is an outline of four areas of inquiry:

      1) Nursing and nursing-led interdisciplinary interventions to promote function in people of all ages with disability or chronic health problems

      2) Experience of disability or chronic health problems for individuals and families across the lifespan

      3) Rehabilitation in the changing healthcare system

      4) The rehabilitation nursing profession

F. The Specialty Practice of Rehabilitation Nursing: ARN and ANA both view rehabilitation nursing as a specialty practice. Professional rehabilitation practice is guided by philosophy, theory, and research and therefore can be practiced in any setting. When the client is at the center of care, and the goals are to optimize health (however it is defined) and improve the quality of life for those with disability or chronic disease, the boundaries of the healthcare system become less important.

   1. ARN's standards (2008) outline the scope of practice, standards of care, and standards of professional performance.

   2. RNF (1994) outlined specific competencies in a separate manual.

   3. ARN now offers a Competencies Assessment Tool (ARN-CAT) online that tests knowledge in 14 basic rehabilitation nursing competency areas and also includes both pediatric and geriatric questions.

4. Settings for rehabilitation nursing: Practice settings for rehabilitation nursing may include homes, work settings, insurance companies, community centers, residential centers, day care centers, clinics, skilled care facilities, inpatient rehabilitation centers, subacute or postacute units, and acute care facilities.

G. Educational Preparation, Licensure, and Certification

1. Practical nursing: Licensed practical nurses (LPNs) generally are educated in programs requiring 9–14 months of study. These nurses are taught many skills but do not have the same depth of knowledge as registered nurses (RNs). Under the supervision of an RN and to the extent of their basic and continuing education, LPNs participate in direct and indirect nursing care, health maintenance, teaching, counseling, collaborative planning, and rehabilitation.

2. Professional rehabilitation nursing: RNs are prepared at the AD and BS levels. Although both AD- and BS-prepared nurses are licensed as RNs, the BS has long been recommended as the entry level for professional practice. A BS better prepares practitioners for the high level of flexibility necessary as health care becomes increasingly sophisticated and provides a basis for practitioners to participate in, evaluate, and use research findings as greater evidence is needed to support practice. Therefore, a BS is important for specialty practice.

3. Licensure: All nurses must be licensed by the state in which they practice. People who want to take the licensure exam for LPNs or RNs may do so after they have successfully completed an accredited nursing program. Licensure for advanced practice nurses (APNs) varies from state to state. In general, a person wanting to obtain licensure as an APN must be an RN; have completed an approved educational program of advanced practice leading to an MS, DNP, or other approved degree; and meet the specific guidelines for licensure in the state in which they want to become licensed. Advanced practice licensure often relies on certification as an APN in the desired specialty area.

4. Certification: Certification is professional recognition of skills in a specialty practice. Certification programs are developed and maintained by professional nursing organizations such as ANA or ARN. Certification in rehabilitation nursing is a means of validating specialized knowledge and skills and communicates a sense of accountability to the public. Certification programs exist in many specialties for RNs and APNs. There are fewer certification programs for LPNs.

5. Certified rehabilitation registered nurse (CRRN): At the RN level of practice, ARN has developed and maintains a certification program in rehabilitation nursing.

a. ARN's standards (2008) do not mandate which type of basic, professional nursing preparation (AD or BS) is necessary for generalist practice or certification.

b. The Rehabilitation Nursing Certification Board, a subsidiary of ARN, offered its first certification examination in 1984.

c. Those who meet the criteria and pass the exam earn the CRRN credential. Currently, approximately 10,000 nurses hold the CRRN credential.

H. Clinical Nurse Leader (CNL): The CNL is an advanced generalist clinician with education at the master's or postmaster's level in a formal CNL education program. Graduate education is necessary because the CNL must bring a high level of clinical competence and knowledge to the point of care and serve as a resource for the nursing team. In practice, the CNL oversees the care coordination and integration of care for a distinct group of clients. This clinician puts evidence-based practice into action to ensure that clients benefit from the latest innovations in care delivery. The CNL evaluates client outcomes, assesses cohort risk, and has the decision-making authority to change care plans when necessary. The CNL is a leader and active member of the interdisciplinary healthcare team. The implementation of the CNL role varies across healthcare settings. (American Association of Colleges of Nursing [AACN], n.d.)

I. Advanced Practice Nursing: Advanced practice nursing is defined as "the application of an expanded range of practical, theoretical, and research-based competencies to phenomena experienced by patients within a specialized clinical area of the larger discipline of nursing" (Hamric, 2005, p. 89). There are four recognized types of advanced practice nurses:

- Nurse practitioners (NPs)
- Clinical nurse specialists (CNSs)
- Certified nurse midwives (CNWs)
- Certified nurse anesthetists (CNAs)

1. AACN (1996) identified the essential focus of all APN roles as clinical. Although nurse educators and administrators may be educated at an advanced level, they do not meet the definition of advanced practice nursing because their primary focus is not clinical practice. According to

Hamric (2005), the core competencies of APNs include the following:

    a. Expert guidance and coaching of clients, families, and other care providers

    b. Consultation

    c. Research skills

    d. Clinical and professional leadership, including competence as a change agent

    e. Collaboration

    f. Ethical decision-making skills

2. Rehabilitation nurses in advanced practice usually are educated as CNSs and NPs.

    a. The MS has been the standard degree for the APN for many years.

    b. The DNP (a relatively new degree) has been approved by AACN as the entry level for APNs as of 2015. The approval and subsequent guidelines for this degree are a result of the increasing complexity and required knowledge for APNs (AACN, 2004).

V. Role Responsibilities for Professional Rehabilitation Nursing

AACN (2008) described the following role responsibilities for generalist nursing practice. They are discussed here in relation to rehabilitation nursing practice.

A. Provider of Care: "The nurse uses theory and research-based knowledge in the direct and indirect delivery of care . . . in the formation of partnerships with clients and the interdisciplinary health care team" (p. 16). Particular roles in rehabilitation with these responsibilities include caregiver, client advocate, client educator, counselor, nurse practitioner, expert witness, and researcher.

B. Designer, Manager, and Coordinator of Care: The nurse needs skills such as communication, collaboration, negotiation, delegation, coordination, and evaluation of interdisciplinary work. These are particularly important skills for rehabilitation nurses who are team members or leaders. Rehabilitation roles fulfilling these responsibilities include care manager, case manager, consultant, administrator or manager, and CNS. Designing and coordinating care becomes increasingly important in nursing as healthcare systems use various skilled and semi-skilled workers in direct care. Additionally, nurses are in a key position to provide leadership in the coordination of care across disciplines.

C. Member of a Profession: Professionals have a responsibility to value lifelong learning, identify with the profession's values, and incorporate professionalism into practice. Client advocacy is an important aspect of professional rehabilitation practice, and although this is an integral aspect of everyday practice, advocacy assumes a particularly important role in a larger societal sense. Rehabilitation nurses are responsible for helping shape public policy in such endeavors as dismantling societal barriers to people with disabilities and educating the public to prevent disease and trauma. Although many of these role opportunities already exist, many more roles could be developed by creative and entrepreneurial nurses. In today's dynamic healthcare system, nurses have the opportunity to develop unique nursing roles that will meet the goals of rehabilitation.

D. Rehabilitation Nurse as a Change Agent in Today's Healthcare Environment

1. Change is a central concern for nursing, healthcare, and society.

    a. "Change in the rehabilitation setting can involve change in knowledge, attitude, behavior, or group organization or functioning" (Chin, Finocchiaro, & Rosebrough, 1998, p. 71).

    b. As a change agent the rehabilitation nurse proactively helps the client or is involved in the change process in the organization.

    c. Change parallels the nursing process.

        1) Identify the problem to be addressed.

        2) Define the changes needed.

        3) Identify the purpose of the change.

        4) Gather and use the elements needed to accomplish the change.

        5) Implement actions to accomplish the change.

        6) Evaluate the change.

    d. Change is continuous, and the nursing process is not linear but is continually evolving, necessitating continuous reassessment.

2. The current demands of health care create an environment of profound change.

3. Rehabilitation nurses must have knowledge of change barriers, identify internal and external barriers to openness to change, and make a commitment to change.

    a. Internal demands

        1) Reorganization

        2) Redesign

        3) Reengineering

        4) Continuous quality improvement

        5) Redeployment

    b. External demands

        1) New knowledge

        2) Competition

        3) Regulations

4. Rehabilitation nurses must understand the external forces driving change.
   a. Venue of care
   b. Expanded knowledge
   c. Upgrade of clinical knowledge and skills
   d. Fiscal accountability
5. Rehabilitation nurses must recognize their own attitudes or personality traits related to change. They must know the role that best describes their own positions and learn how to work with people who fall into the other groups.
6. Rogers (1995) described six types of behavioral groups
   a. Innovators: Adventuresome
   b. Early adopters: Respected leaders in the organization
   c. Early majority: Deliberate
   d. Late majority: Skeptical
   e. Laggards: Hang on to traditional ways and ideas
   f. Rejecters
7. Major hurdles to change-ready thinking (Kriegel & Brandt, 1996) include
   a. Fear
   b. Fatigue
   c. Comfort
8. Reasons for taking a proactive approach to change and seeking out opportunities for change include
   a. Improving the quality of care
   b. Improving the cost-effectiveness of care delivery
   c. Making the adaptations needed to maintain change
9. Resilience in facing change
   a. Attitudes and traits that are characteristic of change-resilient people (Conner, 1996; Giordono, 1997; Jacelon, 1997) include
      1) Positive thinking
      2) Sense of control
      3) Resourcefulness
      4) Focus
      5) Self-discipline
      6) Flexibility
      7) Organization
      8) Proactive behavior
   b. Resilience is needed to manage uncertainty (Porter-O'Grady & Malloch, 2003).
   c. Traits that limit resilience to change (Giordono, 1997) include
      1) Cynicism
      2) Distancing
      3) Avoidance

E. Competencies for Rehabilitation Nurses: The specialty practice of rehabilitation nursing has a defined area of competence within nursing. The ARN-CAT is offered free online and assesses basic competencies in the following areas: autonomic dysfunction, bowel and bladder function, communication, disability/adjustment to disability/grieving, dysphagia, gerontology, musculoskeletal/body mechanics/functional transfer techniques, neuropathophysiology and functional neurological assessment, pain, client and family education, pediatrics, rehabilitation, sexuality and disability, and skin and wound care. The ARN-CAT includes multiple-choice questions in each category and provides instant results for scoring along with rationales for correct answers. Competencies provide accountability and standards of practice for the specialty. This online tool can help nurse managers and supervisors evaluate the proficiency of staff nurses.

References

American Association of Colleges of Nursing. (1996). *The essentials of Master's education for advanced practice nursing.* Washington, DC: Author.

American Association of Colleges of Nursing. (2004). *AACN position statement on the practice doctorate in nursing.* Retrieved November 26, 2006, from www.aacn.nche.edu/DNP/pdf/DNP.pdf.

American Association of Colleges of Nursing. (2008). *The essentials of baccalaureate education for professional nursing practice.* Washington, DC: Author.

American Association of Colleges of Nursing. (n.d.). *Clinical nurse leader.* Retrieved August 27, 2010, from www.aacn.nche.edu/CNC/cnlcert.htm.

American Nurses Association. (2010a). *Nursing's social policy statement.* Kansas City, MO: Author.

American Nurses Association. (2010b). *The code of ethics for nurses with interpretive statements.* Washington, DC: Author.

American Nurses Credentialing Center. (2008). *Application manual Magnet recognition program.* Washington, DC: Author.

Andrews, M. M., & Boyle, J. S. (2003). *Transcultural concepts in nursing care* (4th ed.). Philadelphia: Lippincott Williams & Wilkins.

Association of Rehabilitation Nurses. (2008). *Standards and scope of rehabilitation nursing practice* (5th ed.). Glenview, IL: Author.

Association of Rehabilitation Nurses. (n.d.). *Role descriptions: The rehabilitation nurse case manager.* Retrieved August 27, 2010, from www.rehabnurse.org/pubs/role/casemgr.html.

Baker, G., Haughton, J., & Mongoo, P. (2003). *Pay for performance incentive programs in healthcare: Market dynamics and business process.* Retrieved July 19, 2011, from www.leapfroggroup.org/media/file/Leapfrog-Pay_for_Performance_Briefing.pdf.

Centers for Medicare and Medicaid Services. (2007). *Inpatient rehabilitation facility prospective payment system (IRF PPS) final rule for fiscal year (FY) 2007.* Retrieved July 22, 2011, from www.cms.hhs.gov/inpatientrehabfacpps/downloads/cms_1540f.pdf.

Centers for Medicare and Medicaid Services. (2011). *Your Medicare coverage.* Retrieved August 23, 2011, from www.medicare.gov/publications/pubs/pdf/10988.pdf.

Chin, P. A., Finocchiaro, D. N., & Rosebrough, A. (1998). *Rehabilitation nursing practice.* New York: McGraw-Hill.

Conner, D. R. (1996). How can you survive continuous change? *Medical Economics, 73*(8), 109–114.

Cournan, M. C. (2006). The 75% rule: What rehabilitation nurses need to know. *ARN Network, 23*(5), 11.

DeLisa, J. A., Currie, D. M., & Martin, G. M. (1998). *Rehabilitation medicine: Past, present, and future.* In J. A. DeLisa & B. M. Gans (Eds.), *Physical rehabilitation medicine: Principles and practice* (pp. 3–32). Philadelphia: Lippincott-Raven.

Esser, C. (1998). Sorting out the Balanced Budget Act of 1997. *ARN Network, 14*(3), 1–2.

Fawcett, J. (1984). The metaparadigm of nursing: Current status and future refinements. *Image: The Journal of Nursing Scholarship, 16,* 84–87.

Giordono, B. P. (1997). Resilience: A survival tool for the nineties. *AORN Journal, 65*(6), 1032–1034.

Hamric, A. (2005). A definition of advanced practice nursing. In A. B. Hamric, J. A. Spross, & C. M. Hanson (Eds.), *Advanced practice nursing: An integrative approach* (3rd ed., pp. 85–108). Philadelphia: Elsevier Saunders.

Hertzberg, D., & Edwards, P. A. (1999). Introduction to pediatric rehabilitation nursing. In P. A. Edwards, D. L. Hertzberg, S. R. Hays, & N. M. Youngblood (Eds.), *Pediatric rehabilitation nursing* (pp. 3–19). Philadelphia: W. B. Saunders.

Issel, L. M., & Anderson, R. A. (1996). Take charge: Managing six transformations in health care delivery. *Nursing Economics, 14*(2), 78–85.

Jacelon, C. S. (1997). The trait and process of resilience. *Journal of Advanced Nursing, 25,* 123–139.

Knapp, M. T. (1999). Nurse's basic guide to understanding the Medicare PPS. *Nursing Management, 30*(5), 14–15.

Kriegel, R., & Brandt, D. (1996). *Sacred cows make the best burgers: Developing change-ready people and organizations.* New York: Warner Books.

Leininger, M. (1997). Overview of the theory of culture care with the ethnonursing research method. *Transcultural Nursing, 8*(2), 32–52.

Leininger, M., & McFarland, M. R. (2002). *Transcultural nursing: Concepts, research and practice.* New York: McGraw-Hill.

LoBiondo-Wood, G., & Haber, J. (2009). *Nursing research: Methods and critical appraisal for evidence-based practice* (7th ed.). St. Louis: Mosby.

Mauk, K. L. (2009). Rehabilitation. In P. D. Larsen & M. Lubkin (Eds.), *Chronic illness: Impact and intervention* (7th ed., pp. 577–610). Sudbury, MA: Jones & Bartlett.

McEwen, M., & Wills, E. M. (2011). *Theoretical basis for nursing* (3rd ed.). Philadelphia: Lippincott Williams & Wilkins.

Mumma, C. M., & Nelson, A. (1996). Models for theory-based practice of rehabilitation nursing. In S. P. Hoeman (Ed.), *Rehabilitation nursing. Process and application* (2nd ed., pp. 21–31). St. Louis: Mosby.

Nathenson, P. (Ed.). (1999). *Integrating rehabilitation and restorative nursing concepts into the MDS.* Glenview, IL: Association of Rehabilitation Nurses.

Porter-O'Grady, T., & Malloch, K. (2003). *Quantum leadership: A textbook of new leadership.* Boston: Jones & Bartlett.

Rehabilitation Nursing Foundation. (1994). *Basic competencies for rehabilitation nursing practice.* Glenview, IL: Author.

Rehabilitation Nursing Foundation. (1995). *A research agenda for rehabilitation nursing.* Glenview, IL: Author.

Rehabiltation Nursing Foundation. (2005). *The rehabilitation nursing research agenda* (2nd ed.). Glenview, IL: Author.

Rogers, E. (1995). *Diffusion of innovation* (4th ed.). New York: Free Press.

Rusk, H. (1972). *A world to care for: The autobiography of Howard Rusk.* New York: Random House.

Scott, J. R. (2010). *Two new pilot programs stem from healthcare bill.* Retrieved August 23, 2011, from www.rehabnurse.org/enews/11junjuly/11junjulyadvocacy.html.

U.S. Department of Justice. (2006a). *A guide to disability rights laws.* U.S. Department of Justice Civil Rights Division, Disability Rights Section. Retrieved October 25, 2006, from www.usdoj.gov/crt/ada/cguide.htm.

U.S. Department of Justice. (2006b). ADA home page. Retrieved October 25, 2006, from www.usdoj.gov/crt/ada/adahom1.htm.

Zigmod, J. (2006). Adjusting to new rules. *Modern Healthcare, 36*(22), 24–26, 28.

Suggested Resources

Kessler Medical Rehabilitation Research and Education Corporation: www.rehabtrials.org

Leskowitz, E. (2006). *Complementary and alternative medicine in rehabilitation.* Philadelphia: Churchill Livingstone/Elsevier.

National Institutes of Health ClinicalTrials.gov: www.clinicaltrials.gov/ct

Samdup, D. Z., Smith, R. G., & Song, S. (2006). Use of complementary and alternative medicine in children with chronic medical conditions: Research survey. *American Journal of Physical Medicine & Rehabilitation, 85*(10), 842–846.

CHAPTER 2
Rehabilitation Nursing: Past, Present, and Future

Donna Williams, MSN RN CRRN

The history of rehabilitation dates back to ancient Egypt, during which time there were references to adjustment to disability and adaptive aids such as crutches and artificial limbs. Nursing has its origins in the care of infants and children; the Egyptians first formally used nurses to assist with childbirth (Williams, 2002). Gradually these women evolved into dedicated caregivers who practiced the art of nursing.

Among the Greeks and Romans, it was believed that gods and goddesses influenced healing. There was a deity for almost every human biological function, and Hygeia was the goddess of health. During the Roman Empire, noblewomen cared for sick people. However, in some cultures the care of sick people was not a revered enterprise and was a task delegated to prostitutes.

With the advent of Christianity it became apparent that love and nurturing were not enough to cure disease, and a need emerged for more educated caregivers. With education, nursing started to become more defined. Nurses modeled their practice after the teachings of Christ, caring for the sick, feeding the hungry, and burying the dead.

After the Crusades to the Holy Lands in the early 1300s, the world was ready for social reform. During the 1400s England passed laws that demonstrated concern for people with disabilities. At this time nurses were men and women who cared only for their own sex, and nursing was seen as a function of the church. In 1663 Vincent DePaul founded institutions for crippled children in France. In 1836 the Deaconess Institute at Kaiserswerth, Germany, was established and a small hospital was opened for training deaconesses to provide care (GoNursing Schools, 2010).

Florence Nightingale overcame tremendous social opposition to become a nurse and to care for soldiers during the Crimean War in the 1850s. Her dedication to her profession was responsible for decreasing the death toll among soldiers. Although saving lives was probably the focus, it can easily be imagined that caring for people with disabilities was also part of that service. Nightingale encouraged "allowing patients to do for themselves [as] an important nursing intervention" (Dirstine & Hargrove, 2001, p. 4). Historically, war has placed the greatest demands on nurses.

At the same time, society became focused on children with disabilities, and programs were established that offered restoration and exercise. These programs grew in numbers and content to include a focus on a continuum of care.

During the American Civil War and World War I, the most common operation was extremity amputation, with the majority of those amputations being above the elbow or above the knee. Confederate assistant surgeon Dr. Simon Baruch developed concepts of rehabilitation by using physical agents such as heat, cold, water, and massage (Dirstine & Hargrove, 2001). During World War II and the Vietnam War, below-the-knee amputations were most common. During the Vietnam War the number of multiple-limb amputations started to rise, and we continue to see that trend in today's wars.

Tuberculosis is described in documents dating to 460 BC, but it was not until the 1800s that tuberculosis was treated with good nutrition and fresh air. A study conducted between 1956 and 1963 concluded that an early dynamic physical restoration program for such clients resulted in improved outcomes (Chapman & Hollander, 1964).

Although documentation of polio dates back to the 1700s, it was not until 1911 that Sister Kenny, a nurse, developed a treatment for polio in which moist hot packs were applied to help loosen muscles, relieve pain, and enable limbs to be moved, stretched, and strengthened. The theory of her treatment was muscle "reeducation," the retraining of muscles so that they could function again (Allina Hospitals and Clinics, 2010). In the 1940s she moved to the United States from Australia and shared her techniques. The techniques served as the foundation for physical therapy but were initially performed by nurses in the aftermath of multiple outbreaks of polio.

In 1938 Frank H. Krusen, MD, and a small group of physicians began the struggle to win acceptance of physical medicine and rehabilitation as a medical specialty (Opitz, Folz, Gelman, & Peters, 1997). In 1942 Dr. Howard Rusk introduced the concepts of rehabilitation to the Air Force, working with soldiers who were too well to be considered acute but not well enough to return to combat. Before that time, life expectancy for a person with a spinal cord injury was less than a year (Rusk, 1977). The work of these two physicians was recognized in 1947 with the establishment of the American Board of Physical Medicine and Rehabilitation (American Academy of Physical Medicine and Rehabilitation, 2010). In 1943 Bernard Baruch was successful in appealing for development of comprehensive rehabilitation program that would provide for the "physical, psychological and vocational needs of disabled veterans and facilitate re-socialization" (Cioschi, 1993, p. 8). As the medical specialty of rehabilitation grew, the nursing specialty advanced, and schools of nursing established programs to train rehabilitation nurses, with a focus on bowel and bladder training, crutch walking, and active and passive exercise (Dirstine & Hargrove, 2001).

In 1945 Liberty Mutual hired rehabilitation nurses to conduct comprehensive assessments for insurance purposes. In 1949 Social Security Disability Insurance was receiving serious attention from Congress. By this time the Depression was over and wartime conditions had helped to bring rehabilitation medicine to maturity. As a consequence, the opponents of Social Security Disability Insurance argued that people with disabilities should receive rehabilitation rather than a pension that allowed them to retire from the labor force for life (Social Security Online, 2010).

War has been the driving force behind care techniques and the development of specialized centers of care for victims of war (Meir, 2005). Before World War II there was little emphasis on rehabilitation, but as the ability to treat severely injured soldiers improved, survival rates increased and soldiers needed assistance to return to their communities. Such care spread to the general population as the techniques developed in war were applied to injuries and disabilities in the nonmilitary population. The development of rehabilitation nursing is similarly linked to this history; nurses face a growing population of people with disabilities, advanced age, injuries, and chronic disease.

In the second half of the 20th century people with physical disabilities in the United States began to receive national support for their right to lead normal, satisfying lives despite their physical disabilities. By 2005, 54.4 million Americans reported some form of disability (Brault, 2008). Technological advances continue, and our ability to treat illness, injury, and disability is increasing longevity and the ability to maintain or return to a productive lifestyle. People injured in war are focusing attention on treatment methods that will minimize disability, and both the military and general population will benefit. There is an emphasis on research and evidence-based practice in nursing to provide the highest-quality care and achieve the best outcomes.

The challenges for 21st-century rehabilitation nurses include changing roles and opportunities, the nursing shortage and recruitment problems, changes in practice and care settings, and the continuing healthcare crisis (with increasing limitations on access, equity, and reimbursement; Edwards, 2007). Each rehabilitation nurse is challenged to be responsible for using best practices and advancing rehabilitation nursing knowledge (Miller, 2007). This chapter concludes with possibilities for future rehabilitation nursing practice from rehabilitation nursing leaders and experts in other nursing arenas.

The timelines in this chapter provide a historical overview of rehabilitation and the major events, people, and factors that shaped the healthcare specialty known as rehabilitation nursing. Patricia Edwards, EdD RN CNAA, is acknowledged for providing this historical timeline.

I. Past: A Historical Overview of Rehabilitation
  A. Rehabilitation from Ancient Egypt Through the 18th Century
    1. More than 5,000 years ago, an Egyptian physician recorded an assessment of a client.
    2. 2380 BC: The earliest record of crutches is discovered in hieroglyphics on an Egyptian tomb.
    3. Pre-Christian era: Many biblical references concerned crippled, lame, blind, and afflicted people.
    4. 400–300 BC: Hippocrates, the father of medicine, recorded the use of artificial limbs as an attempt to replace amputated limbs and set forth the basic principle that "exercise strengthens and inactivity wastes."
    5. 200–100 BC: Galen, a Greek physician and writer, described the muscles and bones of the body.
    6. 30 AD: Celsius advocated the use of exercise after a fracture had healed to prevent the loss of function.
    7. 1601: The Poor Relief Act, the first show of responsibility and concern for people with disabilities, was passed in England.
    8. 1633: Vincent DePaul founded institutions for crippled children in France.
    9. 1750: John Hunter, a British physician, focused on the importance of the relationship between the client's will, range of motion, and muscle reeducation.
    10. 1798: Philippe Pinel began practicing psychiatric rehabilitation and occupational and recreational therapies in England (McCourt, 1993).
  B. Rehabilitation in the 19th Century
    1. 1829: The Perkins Institute, the first sheltered workshop for people with disabilities in the United States, was founded by Samuel Gridley Howe. The goal was to train blind people so they could work in the community.
    2. 1836: The Deaconess Institute at Kaiserswerth, Germany, was established and a small hospital was opened that included a training school for deaconesses.
    3. 1854: Florence Nightingale organized professional nursing in England.
    4. 1873: The first U.S. school of nursing was founded in New York at Bellevue Hospital.
    5. 1877: Clara Barton established the American Red Cross.
    6. 1889–1893: The Cleveland Rehabilitation Center began offering services for children, and the first U.S. schools for children with physical disabilities were established (**Figure 2-1**).
    7. Advances in science and medicine increased the potential for survival and physical restoration of people with disabilities.

8. End of the 19th century: Public health departments were established in major cities.

C. Rehabilitation in the 20th Century

1. 1900–1919

    a. Society began to focus on the needs of people with disabilities.

      1) By providing a therapeutic environment for the treatment of specific disabilities

      2) By addressing educational and vocational needs

    b. Certain people promoted occupational and vocational training.

      1) Susan Tracy, a nurse, teacher, and author, pioneered the discipline of occupational therapy by training "occupational nurses."

      2) Eleanor Slagle, a social worker, conducted training courses in occupational therapy.

      3) George Barton, an architect, was interested in the response of the body to occupational therapy.

    c. The Home for Crippled Children was established in Pittsburgh in 1902 to care for children with disabilities.

Figure 2-1. Early Pediatric Rehabilitation Facilities in the United States

1883	The Hospital for Sick Children, Washington, DC
1889	The Cleveland Rehabilitation Center, Cleveland, OH
1892	The Children's Country Home, Westfield, NJ, and The Blythedale Children's Hospital, Valhalia, NY
1893	The Boston Institute School for Crippled and Deformed Children
1895	Health Hill Hospital in Cleveland
1902	The Home for Crippled Children (now The Rehabilitation Institute), Pittsburgh, PA
1919	The Curative Workshop of Milwaukee
1922	Happy Hills Convalescent Center (now Mt. Washington Pediatric Hospital), Baltimore, MD
1930	Elizabethtown Hospital and Rehabilitation Center (now University Hospital Rehabilitation Center for Children and Adults), Elizabethtown, PA
1937	Children's Rehabilitation Institute (now the Kennedy Institute), Baltimore, MD
1940	Alfred I. DuPont Institute, Wilmington, DE (as a hospital for crippled children)
1949	Kennedy Memorial Hospital (now Franciscan Children's Hospital and Rehabilitation Center), Boston, MA
1950	Children's Orthopedic Hospital (now Cardinal Hill Rehabilitation Hospital), Lexington, KY

Edwards, P. A. (1992). The evolution of rehabilitation facilities for children. *Rehabilitation Nursing, 17,* 191–192.

---

d. Electrotherapy was used as a therapeutic modality, and physical therapy modalities were instituted at Massachusetts General Hospital.

e. The need for licensure and definition of the specialty of rehabilitation was identified.

f. The Institute for Crippled and Disabled (established in 1917) and the Curative Workshop of Milwaukee (established in 1919) were pioneering ventures in the area of rehabilitation.

g. World War I had a major impact on physical medicine.

    1) The federal division of specialty hospitals and physical reconstruction at Massachusetts General Hospital was developed in 1917 to treat wounded soldiers and others needing rehabilitation.

    2) Education and vocational rehabilitation was provided through the American Red Cross Institute for Disabled Men.

    3) The first spinal centers incorporated concepts of functional reeducation.

    4) The U.S. Veterans Administration (VA) was created.

2. 1920–1943

    a. 1920

      1) The Vocational Rehabilitation law provided for federal control of vocational rehabilitation.

      2) Congress passed the first Rehabilitation Act and set in motion a focus on the specialty of rehabilitation.

    b. 1921: The Division of Physical Reconstruction and the Federal Board for Vocational Education were established.

    c. Associations for physical and occupational therapists were developed. These organizations began to determine the role, placement, and governance of therapies—the focus points of the emerging specialty of rehabilitation.

    d. 1935: The Social Security Act defined rehabilitation as a process that helped a person with a disability become capable of engaging in a remunerative occupation. The government began providing rehabilitation services beyond the needs of the military and outside hospital walls.

    e. 1938: The American Academy of Physical Medicine and Rehabilitation was founded to set standards and requirements for the practice of rehabilitation medicine.

    f. 1938–1941: In 1938 Dr. Frank Krusen established the hallmarks of physical medicine as controlling disease, relieving suffering, and shortening the period of disability. In 1941 Krusen wrote *Physical Medicine*, the first comprehensive book about treatment methods.

g. 1943

  1) The Sister Kenny Institute was established. Sister Kenny, a nurse, used muscular manipulation, which led to the theory of muscle reeducation. Her techniques pioneered the discipline of physical therapy, and her success with treatment of people with polio advanced the medical specialty of physiatry (McCourt, 1993).

  2) The Vocational Rehabilitation Act was enacted.

    a) Made funds available for professional training and research

    b) Broadened the scope of rehabilitation

    c) Provided a catalyst for the growth of the practice

h. World War II played a tremendous role in the further development of rehabilitation programs.

  1) Dr. Howard A. Rusk dramatically demonstrated the possibilities of rehabilitation when he showed how it could improve the lives of men who had been hospitalized since World War I.

  2) New methods of handling shock and treating infection, along with increasingly sophisticated trauma care, meant more people would survive.

3. 1944–1960

a. The number of industrial-related injuries increased, as did motor vehicle-related accidents and injuries.

b. 1945

  1) Liberty Mutual hired the first rehabilitation nurse in the insurance industry, recognizing the importance of nurses in a rehabilitation role.

  2) The American Paraplegia Association was founded.

  3) World War II was the primary impetus for the clinical nurse specialist (CNS) role. Hildegard Peplau made the first reference to the CNS role in the psychiatric context.

c. 1946

  1) Rehabilitation programs began in U.S. VA hospitals.

  2) The term *physiatrist* was coined to describe a physician with specialized training in rehabilitation medicine.

d. 1947: Dr. Rusk established the first medical rehabilitation services in a U.S. civilian hospital devoted entirely to rehabilitation.

e. Late 1940s: The first board certification exams in physiatry were conducted.

f. 1950s: Barbara Madden, MA RN, contributed significantly to the development of nursing programs for acute and postpolio clients and helped establish regional respiratory centers.

g. 1951: Alice Morrissey, BS RN, wrote the first textbook (*Rehabilitation Nursing*) in the field of rehabilitation nursing.

  1) Principal contributions of nurses in rehabilitative care identified by Morrissey

    a) Basic bedside nursing

    b) Clinical teaching and rehabilitation nursing service management

    c) An emphasis on the importance of nutrition and activities of daily living

  2) The principal message of Morrissey's textbook was "Each sick person is regarded not as a patient with a disease but as a person with a future."

  3) Nurses working at the time reported that client care included baths, linen changes, back rubs, passive exercise, and assistance with ambulation. Only clients with severe strokes came to the unit, and most of them died, as did those with severe head injuries. People with fractured hips and legs were treated with traction. People with mild stroke were sent directly home. There were no policies or procedures, and rehabilitation nursing was not recognized as a specialty. The evening and night shifts were staffed with student nurses (J. Reeves, personal communication, July 24, 2010).

h. 1956–1969: Lena Plaisted, MS RN, founded the first graduate rehabilitation nursing program at Boston University in 1956. She described the role in *The Clinical Specialist in Rehabilitation* in 1969.

i. Important strides were made in technology, and greater emphasis was placed on the needs of those with disabilities and on rehabilitation.

j. The realm of rehabilitation was expanded to include treatment for people with stroke, cardiac conditions, arthritis, orthopedic injuries, and brain injuries.

k. Mary Ann Mikulic was one of the first rehabilitation nursing clinical specialists appointed by the VA.

4. 1960–1989
   a. These 3 decades marked a period of increased recognition of the specialty practice of rehabilitation nursing. As one nurse said, "When starting my rehabilitation career in the '60s, I was frustrated that no one else in other specialty areas seemed to understand what we did in rehabilitation. My mentor acknowledged my frustration and said, 'Barbara, our day will come.' The day did come when I found others calling me about patient education, measuring outcomes, and discharge planning. Nurses in critical care wanted to know about autonomic hyperreflexia and how to talk to patients about sexuality. Finally, I felt that what we did and what we knew were acknowledged and appreciated" (B. Warner, personal communication, July 7, 1999).
   b. The Korean and Vietnam wars influenced continued progress in rehabilitation, in part through the ability to treat wounded people more effectively on the battlefield and the availability of improved transport to medical treatment services, which led to a decrease in mortality rates (McCourt, 1993).
   c. Improved medical technology, institution-based trauma care, and paramedics led to an increased survival rate from injury and focused on the further need for rehabilitation programs and services (McCourt, 1993).
   d. The scope of rehabilitation broadened to include and meet the needs of the following groups:
      1) People with chronic diseases
      2) An aging population
      3) People reentering the workforce after traumatic injury or disease
   e. 1962: Medicare legislation stimulated an increased demand for rehabilitation, and more rehabilitation nurses were hired by insurance companies (McCourt, 1993).
   f. 1965
      1) The Workers' Compensation and Rehabilitation law passed, placing an emphasis on the workplace.
      2) The American Nurses Association (ANA) published *Guidelines for the Practice of Nursing on the Rehabilitation Team: An Answer to a Growing Need*.
      3) The nurse practitioner role was originated by Loretta Ford, PhD RN, and Henry Silver, MD, in response to inequities in the accessibility to health care exacerbated by a physician shortage.
   g. 1966: The Commission on Accreditation of Rehabilitation Facilities was established to provide a consultative accrediting process in the rehabilitation industry.
   h. 1967: Amendments to the Vocational Rehabilitation Act focused on improving workforce reentry for people with disabilities.
   i. Early 1970s: Regional health care became a focal point in rehabilitation services.
   j. In some areas, the physical program was delayed by the need to keep clients immobilized in halos, on Stryker frames or circle electric beds, or in body casts. Orientation was brief, and the nursing focus was on skin care, bowel and bladder management, positioning, and medications. Length of stay was extensive. It was rare to have clients on intravenous medication or oxygen (C. Gender, personal communication, August 14, 2010).
   k. 1973: The Rehabilitation Act was passed, demonstrating increased public awareness of the needs of people with disabilities. The act included guidelines for nondiscrimination in employment and promoted community access by reducing or eliminating physical barriers.
   l. 1974: The Association of Rehabilitation Nurses (ARN) was established under the leadership of Susan Novak. In 1975 four chapters, representing California, Illinois, and New York were chartered. Dagny Engle was the first executive director of the association.
   m. 1975: *ARN Journal* was developed, with Dagny Engle serving as the first editor. The introduction of the journal was a professional milestone for ARN and its members (**Table 2-1**). In 1981 the journal's name was changed to *Rehabilitation Nursing*, and it became a refereed journal. The first annual educational conference was held in Minneapolis, MN.
   n. 1976
      1) ARN was recognized by the nursing profession as a specialty organization and the Rehabilitation Nursing Institute (RNI) was established.
      2) ARN developed and published *The Standards and Scope of Rehabilitation Nursing Practice*.
   o. 1978: Independent living programs helped change societal views of the dependency of people with catastrophic injuries (McCourt, 1993).

Table 2-1. ARN Journal Editors

1975–1977:	Dagny Engle
1977–1980:	Mary Ann Mikulic
1980–1985:	Barbara McHugh
1985–1987:	Glee Walquist
1987:	Susan Novak
1988–1998:	Belinda Puetz
1998–2003:	Susan Dean-Baar
2003–present:	Elaine Miller

p. 1980: Publication of *Rehabilitation Nursing and Related Readings,* a useful resource compiled by Rita Boucher and Sharon Dittmar.

q. 1981: The International Year of the Disabled Person

   1) The needs of people with disabilities became more prominent as a social issue.

   2) The first edition of ARN's core curriculum, the body of knowledge for rehabilitation nursing, was published under the title *Rehabilitation Nursing: Concepts and Practice—A Core Curriculum.* The editor in chief was Shannon Sayles.

   3) A credentialing committee was created, with Jessie Drew as chair, to develop a plan for certification; this became the Rehabilitation Nursing Certification Board.

   4) The continuing education application review subcommittee was established.

   5) The first distinguished service award was presented to Sue Novak.

   6) The seminar "Application of Rehabilitation Concepts to Nursing Practice" was developed to prepare nurses for certification.

   7) In the early 1980s clients were admitted with more acute injuries than previously seen.

r. 1984

   1) ARN developed a formal definition, philosophy, and conceptual framework of rehabilitation nursing and the association.

   2) The first certification examination for the certified rehabilitation registered nurse (CRRN) credential was held, and 965 nurses sat for the exam.

s. 1986

   1) The RNI changed its name to the Rehabilitation Nursing Foundation (RNF), which more clearly represented the entity's goals and purpose to the outside world.

   2) ARN revised and updated *The Standards and Scope of Rehabilitation Nursing Practice.*

   3) The membership campaign "Each One Reach One" was initiated.

   4) The *Rehabilitation Nursing* journal had a new look under the editorial leadership of Glee Walquist.

t. 1987

   1) ARN published the second edition of the core curriculum, with Christina Mumma as the editor, and focused on data collection (assessment) nursing diagnosis, returning clients to the community, and professional development of the rehabilitation nurse.

   2) ARN formally implemented Special Interest Councils (currently called Special Interest Groups [SIGs]) in nine areas: administrators; CNSs; educators and researchers; gerontology; home health care; pain; pediatrics; rehabilitation nurse consultants, insurance, and private practice; and staff nurses.

   3) The Nurse-in-Washington program began.

   4) The basic rehabilitation nursing course called "Rehabilitation Nursing: Directions for Practice" was developed.

u. 1989: RNF funded its first research grant and the first job analysis was conducted.

v. Rehabilitation techniques became more widely used in a variety of settings

   1) Nursing homes

   2) Extended care facilities

   3) Inpatient rehabilitation units

   4) Home care programs

   5) Outpatient programs

   6) Private practice

5. 1990s: A decade of healthcare reform and rehabilitation nursing initiatives

a. Healthcare reform

   1) The 1990s were marked by increasing survival rates from traumatic injury and longer life expectancy, which increased the need for rehabilitation services and rehabilitation nurses.

     a) In critical and acute care settings

     b) As case managers for complex, multifaceted problems

THE SPECIALTY PRACTICE OF REHABILITATION NURSING

2) 1990: The Americans with Disabilities Act increased accessibility options and opportunities for people with disabilities in community, employment, education, and healthcare arenas.

3) Geriatric rehabilitation demanded greater attention, with an increased need for rehabilitation nurses and an increased emphasis on restorative care and prevention of disability.

4) The intensity of care increased at all points in the continuum, and care delivery expanded to outpatient and home care.

5) Early interventions and intense technological treatment increased.

6) Lifelong care planning issues arose because of longer life expectancy for those with injuries and chronic disease.

7) New roles emerged for nurses and the concept of case management was developed.

8) Rehabilitation nurses influenced the standards set for rehabilitation facilities and participated in quality-improvement and program-evaluation activities.

b. Rehabilitation nursing initiatives by ARN

1) 1990: The first role description for case managers was written by an ARN SIG, with many other role descriptions to follow.

2) 1992–1996: ARN published the journal *Rehabilitation Nursing Research.*

3) ARN initiated research to determine interventions and outcomes of specific nursing diagnoses.

4) 1993: ARN published the third edition of its core curriculum with a new title, *The Specialty Practice of Rehabilitation Nursing: A Core Curriculum,* with Ann McCourt as editor.

c. There were increased demands and challenges for rehabilitation nurses.

1) Increased need for services

2) Changes in practice settings

3) Greater demand for client and family education

4) Increased recruitment problems and need for further education of nurses

5) Increased insistence on CRRN certification

6) Expansion of professional activities into consultation and research

7) Need to ensure a unified voice for the specialty

8) Promotion of awareness of rehabilitation and its benefits to individuals and society

d. Changes in healthcare coverage became more apparent.

1) Managed care

2) Cost containment

3) Legislative involvement and client activity

4) Advanced technology

5) Ethical issues

6. 1994

a. ARN updated *The Standards and Scope of Rehabilitation Practice.*

b. ARN published *Basic Competencies for Rehabilitation Nursing Practice.*

7. 1995: ARN published *21 Rehabilitation Nursing Diagnoses: A Guide to Interventions and Outcomes.*

8. 1996: ARN published *The Scope and Standards of Advanced Clinical Practice in Rehabilitation Nursing.* Anne Cordes replaced Dagny Engle as executive director.

9. 1997

a. ARN published *Advanced Practice Nursing in Rehabilitation: A Core Curriculum* with Kelly Johnson as editor.

b. The certified rehabilitation registered nurse–advanced (CRRN-A) credential was introduced, and the first exam was held.

10. 1998: ARN published *Rehabilitation Nursing in the Home Health Setting.*

11. 1999

a. ARN published *Integrating Rehabilitation and Restorative Nursing Concepts into the MDS.*

b. ARN published *Restorative Nursing: A Training Manual for Nursing Assistants.*

c. The *Rehabilitation Nursing* journal, with Susan Dean-Baar as editor, took on a new look with the redesign of the cover and layout and two new columns: "Current Issues" and "Perspectives."

12. 2000: ARN published the fourth edition of its core curriculum, with Patricia Edwards as editor. It included the areas of future challenges listed in **Table 2-2.**

13. 2002

a. A CRRN preparation CD-ROM was developed with test questions based on the new content outline of the certification exam.

b. A professional rehabilitation nursing course was implemented.

Table 2-2. Comparison of Future Challenges in ARN's Core Curricula

Rehabilitation Nursing: Concepts and Practice (2nd ed., 1987)	The Specialty Practice of Rehabilitation Nursing: A Core Curriculum (3rd ed., 1993)	The Specialty Practice of Rehabilitation Nursing: A Core Curriculum (4th ed., 2000)
Insurance issues	Managed care	Healthcare crisis: Access, equity, reimbursement
Increased impact and influence of rehabilitation	Cost containment	Changing role of rehabilitation nurses at both the basic and advanced practice levels
Increased knowledge and education	Increased demand for rehabilitation nursing	Roles include case manager and expert rehabilitation clinical nurse specialist
Increased awareness of cost-effectiveness of rehabilitation	Increased need for services	Nursing shortage and recruitment and education issues
Clearly defined and available levels of rehabilitative care	Increased recruitment and further education of nurses	Value of rehabilitation across the continuum of care
	Increased insistence on certification	Changes in practice and care settings: Hospital is more acute and rehabilitation units are changing; more clients are cared for in the home and community
	Greater awareness of rehabilitation and its benefit to individuals and society	
	Alteration in practice settings	

14. 2003
    a. The ARN website, www.rehabnurse.org, got a new look and a "Members Only" area.
    b. The Advanced Practice in Rehabilitation Nursing certification examination was discontinued.
    c. The ARN board appointed Elaine Miller as editor of *Rehabilitation Nursing*.

15. 2004: ARN led a collaboration with the American Physical Therapy Association and the American Occupational Therapy Association to publish a white paper of strategies to improve client and healthcare provider safety. In addition, with the help of these two organizations, ARN established a Web-based resource for safe client handling in rehabilitation.

16. 2005
    a. A position statement on the rehabilitation nurse as case manager was developed. It indicated that "rehabilitation nurses are the most qualified healthcare professionals to perform the case management function because they have the education, background and expertise needed to coordinate patients' healthcare services from the onset of injury or illness to safe return to work or assimilation into the community as productive members of society" (K. Cervizzi, personal communication, October 25, 2006).
    b. ARN created the Competencies Assessment Tool, with 12 basic rehabilitation nursing competency areas, to be used online.
    c. Anne Cordes stepped down from the executive director position after almost 10 years and was replaced by Karen Nason.

    d. A new rehabilitation nursing research agenda with 19 statements of research priorities was formulated, intended to drive rehabilitation nursing research for the next 10 years.
    e. The Rehabilitation Institute of Chicago became the first rehabilitation hospital to be awarded Magnet status by the American Nurses Credentialing Center, recognizing excellence in nursing services. Craig Hospital became the second Magnet rehabilitation hospital.

17. 2006
    a. *Evidence-Based Rehabilitation: Common Challenges and Interventions*, an updated version of *21 Rehabilitation Nursing Diagnoses*, was published.
    b. The Rehabilitation Nursing Certification Board (RNCB) celebrated its 25th anniversary. As of 2007, there are nearly 10,000 CRRNs. Certification in rehabilitation nursing shows employers, colleagues, clients, and the public that the nurse is committed to excellence in caring for people with physical disabilities and chronic illnesses. It indicates that she or he is an experienced rehabilitation or restorative nurse who has achieved a level of knowledge in this practice area and can lead to increased professional credibility, recognition of expertise, greater impact as a job candidate, and a heightened sense of personal achievement.
    c. As of 2010, there have been 36 presidents of ARN and 21 RNF chairs (**Tables 2-3** and **2-4**).

18. 2007
    a. The 2007 Strategic Plan included core organization values of leadership, professionalism, community, and client care. Goals were

Table 2-3. ARN Presidents

1974–76: Susan Novak	1993–94 Karen Preston
1976–77: Virginia Wright	1994–95 Susan Dean-Baar
1977–78: Albinia Doll	1995–96 Catherine Tracey
1978–79: Barbara McHugh	1996–97: Judy Hartman
1979–80: Rosemarian Berni	1997–98: Lois Schaetzle
1980–81: Patricia Rizio	1998–99: Marilyn Ter Maat
1981–82: Shannon Sayles	1999–00: Cynthia Jacelon
1982–83: Carol Ann Imhoff	2000–01: Judy DiFilippo
1983–84: Diane Burgher	2001–02: Donna Williams
1984–85: Marilyn Pires	2002–03: Paul Nathanson
1985–86: Renee Steele Rosomoff	2003–04: Terrie Black
1986–87: Phyllis Commeree	2004–05: Joanne Ebert
1987–88: Patricia McCollom	2005–06: Stephanie Davis Burnett
1988–89: Teresa Cervantez Thompson	2006–07: Terri Patterson
1989–90: Beth Budny	2007–08: Karen Cervizzi
1990–91: Malcolm Maloff	2008–09: Donna Jernigan
1991–92: Aloma "Cookie" Gender	2009–10: Linda Pierce
1992–93: Kathleen Stevens	2010–11: Kathy Doeschot

established in the areas of leadership, research, government relations, professional development, and the continuum of care.

  b. The fifth edition of the core curriculum was published with Kris Mauk as editor.

  c. ARN became active in influencing healthcare legislation and established the Capitol Hill Gang, members who could respond quickly to the need to be in Washington, DC, to address rehabilitation concerns. Legislative agendas are set for each year.

  d. ARN publishes a position statement: *Role of the Nurse in the Rehabilitation Team.*

19. 2008

  a. *The Standards and Scope of Rehabilitation Nursing Practice* was updated.

  b. ARN published a position statement: *Rehabilitation Nursing Criteria for Determination and Documentation of Medical Necessity in an Inpatient Rehabilitation Facility.*

20. 2009

  a. The ARN membership voted to eliminate regional directors and elect directors-at-large to better establish a board of directors who could meet the goals of the organization and strategic plan.

  b. ARN continued to be active in advocating for appropriate health care for those with chronic diseases and disability.

Table 2-4. RNF Chairs

1977–1978: Marie Sadlick Walker
1978–1979: Angela Walsh-Quintero
1979–1980: Barbara McHugh
1980–1981: Rosemarian Berni
1981–1982: Phyllis Commeree
1982–1983: Phyllis Commeree
1983–1984: Aloma "Cookie" Gender
1984–1985: Beth Budny
1985–1987: Kathryn Barry
1987–1988: Janet LaMantia
1988–1990: Cynthia Bachman Susong
1990–1992: Susan Dean-Baar
1992–1994: Christina Mumma
1994–1996: Audrey Nelson
1996–1998: Teresa Thompson
1998–2000: Kathleen Sawin
2000–2002: Alexa Stuifbergen
2002–2004: Carole Ann Bach
2004–2006: Cynthia Jacelon
2006–2008: Linda L. Pierce
2008–2010: Pamala D. Larsen
2010–Present: Barbara Lutz

c. The CRRN-A was discontinued.

21. 2010
   a. The ARN board of directors approved an updated joint position with the Oncology Nursing Society: *Rehabilitation of People with Cancer*.
   b. ARN asked Congress and the White House to do the following:
      1) Bolster the nation's nursing workforce to safeguard public health
      2) Support rehabilitation research and education
      3) Support continued funding of the Traumatic Brain Injury Act
      4) Support the passage of the Prosthetic and Custom Orthotic Parity Act

II. Present: The 21st Century

A. The Practice of Rehabilitation Nursing in the 21st Century
   1. Rehabilitation nursing continues to be a prominent specialty, and increasing client acuity is changing the basic scope of practice.
   2. The value of rehabilitation nurses continues to increase as the healthcare system recognizes the impact of rehabilitation principles across the continuum of care. Nurses must be involved in efforts to raise public awareness of the value of rehabilitation nursing and be prepared to care for clients with higher levels of acuity.
   3. Rehabilitation nurses continue to define their practice, conduct and use research in everyday work, ensure that rehabilitation nurses have adequate preparation, and support ARN so that it remains a strong voice for rehabilitation nurses in the healthcare community.
   4. Clients continue to be more complex in their needs and require more technologically based, advanced treatment and services as advancing age affects the population.
   5. Rehabilitation nurses with advanced degrees, including doctorates, act in many capacities.
      a. As experts in research and evidence-based practice
      b. As advocates and managers for large populations needing restorative care
      c. As promoters of public policy for people with disabilities at the local and national levels
      d. As independent practitioners in offices, clinics, and other facilities
      e. As educators for the present and future nursing workforce

B. The Effect of Changing Demographics on the Demand for Rehabilitation Nurses and Practice Settings
   1. As the population continues to age, the need for professional nurses who have the skills to treat chronic illnesses and their effects on function, quality of life, and access to care has grown significantly.
   2. Rehabilitation nurses have seen a shift in the distribution of illness from acute to chronic and a shift in the kinds of injuries, especially in survivors of war.
   3. Rehabilitation nurses, who are particularly suited to case management, market their approach and philosophy to a variety of employers, insurance companies, inpatient settings, physicians, private individuals, and other community-based services.
   4. The hospital is more acute, and the rehabilitation unit (acute and subacute) has changed as more clients are cared for in their homes, retirement centers, and other living arrangements in the community. "Practice has expanded to schools, nurse managed clinics in the community, independent nursing practices and more rural and inner urban areas" (T. Patterson, personal communication, October 25, 2006).
   5. "The expertise of case management and life care planning are roles that continue to grow" (T. Thompson, personal communication, October 25, 2006).

C. The Nursing Shortage and Recruitment Issues
   1. A large number of nurses, both direct caregivers and educators, are reaching retirement age. This decrease in the workforce comes at a time when there is also declining enrollment in nursing schools and declining interest among young people in the nursing profession. Because of the shortage of educators in colleges and universities, there is a waiting list for those interested in entering the profession. Keeping nurses in the workforce into their retirement years at healthcare facilities and schools of nursing with flexible job descriptions, schedules, and benefits will be essential.
   2. "Anything the rehabilitation healthcare organization can do to retain, motivate, and keep nurses safe and healthy will be key for the future; consider ergonomics and the environment and safe patient-handling equipment" (K. Cervizzi, personal communication, October 25, 2006).
   3. Yearly educational conferences provide new and timely topics and networking opportunities. Printed educational resources and other conferences sponsored by ARN, as well as the work of

RNF, have all advanced the practice of rehabilitation nursing. Certification has elevated the standard of practice and demonstrates that a certified nurse has the knowledge needed to practice in the field (C. Gender, personal communication, August 14, 2010).

D. The Healthcare Crisis: Access, Equity, and Reimbursement Issues

1. Cost and access to care continue to be of concern as reimbursement continues to change. "Inpatient rehabilitation facilities have become increasingly constrained in the type of patient they can accept for inpatient rehabilitation due to the changes in qualifying conditions found in the 75% rule and medical necessity criteria" (K. Cervizzi, personal communication, October 25, 2006).

2. Health care continues to be at a crisis level, and the lack of funding and other resources has severely changed the landscape of the delivery system and allowed fiscal intermediaries to determine admission and length of stay.

3. Problems with environmental, financial, and geographic access to services and the availability of practitioners who understand the needs of clients who are older, chronically ill, and disabled are important issues.

4. "Reimbursement is tied to the Inpatient Rehabilitation Facility Patient Assessment Instrument and the RIC classification. Today's rehabilitation requires that there is someone who is dedicated to the documentation of need" (T. Thompson, personal communication, October 25, 2006).

5. "Attempts to limit the role of the [advanced practice registered nurse] and other care providers will affect access to those most in need: poor, rural areas, inner cities" (S. Burnett, personal communication, October 20, 2006).

E. Ethical Issues and Dilemmas

1. Nurses increasingly face the challenge of working with people who choose to end their own life and have considered their positions on laws dealing with clients' rights and choices.

2. Nurses have had to assess their own feelings and attitudes related to ethical issues and dilemmas such as cloning, organ transplantation, and assisted suicide.

3. Nurses have to face the dilemma of providing lesser services than are needed to the population because of financial constraints.

III. Future: Nurses' Perspectives on Health Care

A. Integration of Information Technology into Rehabilitation Nursing Practice

1. Advances in technology and telemedicine will link healthcare providers with clients across a greater distance (K. Cervizzi, personal communication to Patricia Edwards, October 25, 2006).

2. Electronic medical records will continue to evolve, resulting in increased use of the computer for all documentation (K. Cervizzi, personal communication to Patricia Edwards, October 25, 2006) and an increase in access to medical records.

3. The information explosion in a high-technology world will continue to expand rehabilitation nursing research beyond national borders; an international collaborative research effort with colleagues across the globe is already occurring. Opportunities to design and carry out collaborative studies through the World Wide Web have become a reality (L. Pierce, personal communication to Patricia Edwards, October 25, 2006).

4. Technology, including computerized documentation systems, will make our work more efficient, and preventive care will reduce the number of people experiencing catastrophic illness and injury. Diagnostic imaging will also change our practice greatly as neural plasticity has already shown us that progress can be made to restore function (Saver, 2006). Scientific advances in stem cell therapy and genetics will be used to treat spinal cord injuries more effectively. Harvesting of body parts, cells, and limbs could make prosthetics obsolete. Robotic, microscopic surgeries will prevent strokes and make repairs more effective. Brain injuries will not be as common, with helmets being required for sports participation. Surgical interventions for traumatic brain injury will be more precise and cause less swelling, reducing recovery time (G. Sims, personal communication, August 15, 2010).

B. Emphasis on Research and Evidence-Based Practice

1. "Research is needed to address new ideas but also to validate old practices" (S. Burnett, personal communication to Patricia Edwards, October 20, 2006).

2. ARN moved from a nursing diagnosis focus to evidence-based practice with its new publication *Evidence-Based Rehabilitation: Common Challenges and Interventions.*

3. "The emphasis on research will continue to grow and will require more data. Rehabilitation hospitals seeking Magnet status will be looking at ways to increase their participation in this part of the process" (T. Thompson, personal communication to Patricia Edwards, October 25, 2006).

C. Magnet Recognition Program for Nursing Excellence (ANA, 2010)
   1. "As more rehabilitation healthcare organizations seek Magnet recognition, the desire for CRRN certification, continuing education programs, and advanced education will increase" (K. Cervizzi, personal communication to Patricia Edwards, October 25, 2006).
   2. The five components of the Magnet Recognition Model may be used as guides to strengthen rehabilitation nursing services and programs.
      a. Transformational leadership
      b. Structural empowerment
      c. Exemplary professional practice
      d. New knowledge, innovations, and improvements
      e. Empirical quality results
   3. The program may be cost prohibitive for some rehabilitation hospitals and long-term care facilities.
D. Recruitment and Education Issues
   1. "The nursing shortage will continue to be issues as baby boomers begin to retire. Ways must be found to continue to attract nurses into the field of rehabilitation across all practice settings" (M. Ter Maat, personal communication to Patricia Edwards, October 25, 2006).
   2. "Future efforts will be aimed at recruiting and retaining aging nurses with incentives and flexibility to motivate them to stay in the workforce well into their retirement years for leading, precepting, mentoring, education, and direct patient care" (K. Cervizzi, personal communication to Patricia Edwards, October 25, 2006).
   3. With people aging and living longer with chronic disease, rehabilitation nursing should become a core requirement in every school of nursing (T. Black, personal communication, August 15, 2010).
   4. Nursing schools will provide practical coursework related to staffing, budgeting, evidence-based research, and quality or outcomes (T. Black, personal communication August 15, 2010).
   5. Jean Watson's caring theory will bring nurses back to the heart of professional nursing practice (G. Sims, personal communication, August 15, 2010).
E. Issues Related to Quality of Life and End-of-Life Decision Making
   1. "Rehabilitation nurses will continue to be involved with these issues and need to be able to support patients' wishes and ensure that they have a comfortable and meaningful period of time while living with disability and experience a good death" (M. Ter Maat, personal communication to Patricia Edwards, October 25, 2006).
   2. "Pain management, alternative therapy, spirituality assessment, and bereavement counseling will have a greater emphasis in the aging population, with more nursing research to develop and implement better therapy options" (K. Cervizzi, personal communication to Patricia Edwards, October 25, 2006).
   3. Rehabilitation principles are of utmost importance to allow clients to live while dying and to help the family make this time productive and meaningful.
   4. Mindfulness will be an essential focus and tool for nurses and an important technique to train patients and families to focus on their recovery. Efforts to make meaning of life's events will be seen in creative expressions of art and music in the lives of patients, families, and healthcare practitioners. Attitudinal barriers will dissolve. *Disability* will be replaced by words such as *life challenges* and *adaptations*. Putting a positive spin on the events that shape our lives will remove stigma from our vocabulary (G. Sims, personal communication, August 15, 2010).
F. Changes in Practice and Care Settings
   1. "Demand for home care and long-term care nurses will increase as the older adult population continues to increase" (M. Ter Maat, personal communication to Patricia Edwards, October 25, 2006).
   2. "Changing health care priorities that reflect ongoing concerns about spiraling healthcare costs, an emphasis on cost-effectiveness, and an outcome-oriented society will continue to change the landscape of rehabilitation nursing" (L. Pierce, personal communication to Patricia Edwards, October 25, 2006).
   3. The team will meet clients where they are for strengthening and functional tasks, providing repetition to maximize the time available with each healthcare provider.
   4. Certified nurses demonstrate a higher level of rehabilitation nursing practice. It shows in the care and education they provide and in their level of confidence. They also tend to do a better job with FIM™ scoring, which is critical for reimbursement (C. Gender, personal communication, August 14, 2010).
   5. Rehabilitation nursing will be incorporated into all areas of health care, especially because rehabilitation is a process and not a place. Most nursing specialties are defined by a practice setting or body system. Rehabilitation nursing's emphasis is on models of wellness, adaptation, and quality of

life (D. Jernigan, personal communication, August 16, 2010).

6. ARN members will embrace education on patient and rehabilitation advocacy provided by ARN and be willing to assume increased responsibilities, taking advantage of opportunities afforded to them (S. Wirt, personal communication, August 17, 2010).

G. Healthcare Reform: Healthcare reform will have a powerful impact on rehabilitation nursing. The most cost-effective method of delivering care will be to not have specialty units but to have specialists, such as certified rehabilitation registered nurses. We will continue to have only clients with the most catastrophic injuries and illnesses using inpatient days, and CRRNs will meet the client at the point of entry to the healthcare system. Clients will not move about from unit to unit to transition between levels of care (G. Sims, personal communication, August 15, 2010).

H. Disaster Preparedness and Education

1. "Disaster education will become more important for rehabilitation nurses and patients in light of the changing world and the risk of natural and human-made disasters" (S. Burnett, personal communication to Patricia Edwards, October 20, 2006).

2. "Many shelters are not wheelchair accessible, and many nurses are not trained in care for the disabled" (S. Burnett, personal communication, October 20, 2006).

3. "ARN will be defining its role in disaster preparedness and education" (T. Patterson, personal communication to Patricia Edwards, October 26, 2006).

I. The Future of ARN

1. ARN's challenge will be to incorporate these new nursing professionals from completion of nursing school into our specialty organization. Our challenge is to continue to find new methods of delivering education and resources to support these nurses in practice (D. Jernigan, personal communication, August 16, 2010).

2. ARN is already a powerful influence in government and legislation, and ARN will emerge as the most powerful nursing organization in the delivery of health care, with the application of rehabilitation nursing practice requested by every other specialty area of healthcare. (G. Sims, personal communication, August 15, 2010).

3. By staying at the forefront of evidence-based practice and keeping current in the field, ARN will help rehabilitation nursing become even more important in helping older adults and those with disabilities stay in their homes (C. Gender, personal communication, August 14, 2010).

4. ARN will be recognized as the leader and preferred partner for all rehabilitation issues, including research, dissemination of information, public policy, and legislative and regulatory issues (S. Wirt, personal communication, August 17, 2010).

J. Thoughts from Nursing Colleagues Outside Rehabilitation Nursing

1. Technology will transform the nursing profession.
   a. Technology will create a global professional community.
   b. Many nursing functions will be automated (e.g., documentation and updating of client records, smart beds to monitor vital signs, bar codes, and automatic medicine carts). As a result of nursing shortages, healthcare facilities will be forced to use their nurses judiciously. Nurses will spend more time at the bedside as educators and care coordinators to refocus on the client (Peters, 2008).

2. Mobility and portability will be the basis for any healthcare delivery model.
   a. There will be growth in nonhospital settings as a result of rising costs and an aging population.
   b. "Technology will extend lives, and healing will take place in the home. Focus on making the transition to home" (Saver, 2006).

3. Evidence-based practice helps nurses get "a handle on what we do that is valuable—what difference it makes. Can we do it again and can we do it even better the next time?" (Saver, 2006).

4. Increasing emphases on quality and safety are trends that have benefited nursing.
   a. The National Database of Nursing Quality Indicators tracks nursing impact on client care outcomes.
   b. Nurses may see more pay for performance: "Nurses must be involved in establishing payment criteria" (Saver, 2006).

5. Nursing workforce issues
   a. The demand for nurses will continue to grow, with only slow increases in supply affected by the availability of educators and those interested in the profession. Some new nurses are second-career nurses.
   b. "Aging nurses need to take the burden out of care; technology can help" (Saver, 2006).
   c. Use of foreign nurses is increasing, and the nursing shortage is recognized worldwide.

d. The physician shortage is increasing the demand for nurse practitioners.

e. The push for staffing ratios and legislation on public reporting continues.

f. "The faculty shortage will worsen; schools are looking for options. Advanced practice nurses will partner in the education of students, and schools will develop certificate programs to develop faculty" (Saver, 2006).

g. Educational delivery and teaching methods will change through the use of distance learning, curriculum restructuring, and simulations.

6. Surviving in the new world

a. Be open to changing demographics and diversity.

b. Emphasize the need for continual learning; recognize that the consumer is increasingly well informed and wants to participate in life's decisions.

c. Alternative or complementary therapies can enhance health and healing and have entered the mainstream of healthcare delivery.

d. Move forward together! Nursing will continue to evolve, but the basics of human caring must remain. Nursing leadership must remain strong, and leaders must model change and mentor future nurse leaders.

e. The Institute of Medicine (IOM) report *The Future of Nursing: Leading Change, Advancing Health* (2010) , released in October 2010, encourages nurses to practice to the full extent of their education and training and achieve higher levels of education, encourages full partnership with physicians and other healthcare professionals, and encourages better data collection. The report recognizes that improving nursing conditions is the responsibility of nurses, professional organizations, government, business, and the insurance industry. ANA notes that this report recognizes that nurses and nursing are essential to the delivery of high-quality, client-focused care. The ANA (2010) offers a full response and recommendations.

"Caring for ourselves and for others is what brought us into this specialty practice. Rehabilitation nurses will be the case managers and nurse educators of the future. The team model of nursing practice will come back as the most cost-effective, efficient delivery of care. Together, the team of experts will support healing and wholeness through the lifespan of those we serve. It has been an exciting adventure to be part of the journey" (G. Sims, personal communication, August 15, 2010).

Acknowledgments

Thanks go to Patricia Edwards, Editor, *Specialty Practice of Rehabilitation Nursing: A Core Curriculum* (4th ed.); Stephanie Burnett, Past President ARN; Karen Cervizzi, Past President ARN; Terri Patterson, Past President ARN; Linda Pierce, Past President ARN; Marilyn Ter Maat, Past President ARN; Teresa Thompson, Past President ARN; Barbara Warner; Cookie Gender, Past President ARN; Donna Jernigan, Past President ARN; Gail Sims, Director at Large ARN; Susan Wirt, President-Elect ARN; and Terrie Black, Past President ARN for sharing their insights on the future of rehabilitation nursing and ARN.

References

Allina Hospitals and Clinics. (2010). *Sister Kenny Rehabilitation Institute*. Retrieved August 11, 2010, from www.allina.com/ahs/ski.nsf/page/history.

American Academy of Physical Medicine and Rehabilitation. (2010). Retrieved August 11, 2010, from www.aapmr.org/academy/historyb.htm.

American Nurses Association. (2010). *Magnet recognition program*. Retrieved January 30, 2011, from www.nursecredentialing.org/Magnet.aspx.

Brault, M. W. (2008). *Current population reports*. Washington, DC: U.S. Department of Commerce Economics and Statistics Administration, U.S. Census Bureau.

Chapman, C., & Hollander, A. (1964). Tuberculosis and rehabilitation: Dynamic physical restoration of patients with active disease. *California Medicine, 100*(2), 88–91.

Cioshi, H. (1993). The history of rehabilitation nursing in the 20th century. In A. E. McCourt (Ed.), *The Specialty Practice of Rehabilitation Nursing: A Core Curriculum* (3rd ed., p. 6). Glenview, IL: Association of Rehabilitation Nurses.

Dirstine, J., & Hargrove, S. (2001). *Comprehensive rehabilitation nursing*. Philadelphia: Saunders.

Edwards, P. (2007). Rehabilitation nursing: Past, present, and future. In K. Mauk (Ed.), *The Specialty Practice of Rehabilitation Nursing: A Core Curriculum* (5th ed., pp 433–465). Glenview, IL : Association of Rehabilitation Nurses.

GoNursingSchools. (2010). *The history of nursing*. Retrieved August 11, 2010, from www.gonursingschools.com/The_History_of_Nursing.htm.

Institute of Medicine. (2010). *The future of nursing: Leading change, advancing health*. Retrieved December 12, 2010, from www.iom.edu/Reports/2010/The-Future-of-Nursing-Leading-Change-Advancing-Health.aspx.

McCourt, A. D. (Ed.) (1993). *The specialty practice of rehabilitation nursing: A core curriculum* (3rd ed.). Skokie IL: The Rehabilitation Nursing Foundation.

Meir, R. H. (2005). *Functional restoration of adults and children with upper extremity amputation*. New York: Demos Medical Publishing.

Miller, E. T. (2007). Research and evidence-based practice. In K. Mauk (Ed.), *The Specialty Practice of Rehabilitation Nursing: A Core Curriculum* (5th ed., pp. 433–447). Glenview, IL: Association of Rehabilitation Nurses.

Opitz, J. L., Folz, T. J., Gelman, R., & Peters, D. J. (1997). *The history of physical medicine and rehabilitation as recorded in the diary of Dr. Frank Krusen: Part 1. Gathering momentum (the years before 1942).* Retrieved August 11, 2010, from http://cat.inist.fr/?aModele=afficheN&cpsidt=2643202.

Peters, S. (2008). *What is the future of nursing careers.* Retrieved August 14, 2010, from www.articlealley.com/article_645644_36.html.

Rusk, H. (1977). *A world to care for: The autobiography of Howard A. Rusk.* New York: Random House.

Saver, C. L. (2006). Nursing—today and beyond. *American Nursing Today, 1*(1). Retreived August 1, 2011, from www.americannursetoday.com/Article.aspx?id=5322&fid=5306.

Social Security Online. (2010). *Social Security history.* Retrieved August 11, 2010, from www.ssa.gov/history/edberkdib.html.

Williams, D. (2002). Today's rehabilitation nursing in America and ARN activities. *Rehabilitation Nursing Research, 3,* 98.

Figure 3-2. Two Models of Ethical Decision Making

Model 1 (Aiken & Catalano, 1994)	Model 2 (Blanchard & Peale, 1988)
1. Collect, analyze, and interpret data.	1. Ask "Is it legal?" If the answer is yes, then stop. If no, go on to Items 2 and 3.
2. State the dilemma clearly.	2. Ask "Is it balanced?" This will help answer issues of fairness vs. giving advantages to one or more parties.
3. Consider choices for action.	
4. Consider and weigh choices	
5. Analyze advantages and disadvantages of each choice.	3. Ask "How will the decision make me feel?" This will help answer issues of personal standards of morality.
6. Make decision from choices.	

Model 1: Adapted with permission of F. A. Davis Company from Aiken, T., & Catalano, J. (1994). *Legal, ethical, and political issues in nursing* (pp. 31–35). Philadelphia: F. A. Davis. Copyright 1994 by F. A. Davis Company. Model 2: Adapted with permission of William Morrow & Company, Inc., from Blanchard, K., & Peale, N. (1988). *The power of ethical management* (pp. 20–27). New York: William Morrow. Copyright 1988 by Blanchard Family Partnership and Norman Vincent Peale by William Morrow & Company, Inc.
Armstrong, M. (Ed.). (1998). *Telecommunications for health professionals: Providing successful distance education and telehealth* (p. 247). New York: Springer.

the nurse has a responsibility to provide competent care in accordance with the nurse practice act or scope of practice for your state. The duty consists of rational respect for fulfilling one's obligations to other human beings (Guido, 2010).

  b. Kant's moral law perspective that the issue of whether free will is possible is foundational in his metaphysical and epistemology ground of ethics in deontology (Morrison, 2008). The test of a good will is whether the person continues to act out of duty and reverence for the moral law even when it has no personal benefit.

   1) Virtue ethics: There is less emphasis on learning rules and regulations and more on the development of good character and habitually performing in this mode. Virtue ethicists' qualities include wisdom, courage, temperance, justice, generosity, self-respect, and sincerity (Guido, 2010). Virtue ethics can be applied in autonomy, beneficence, nonmaleficence, and justice principles (Morrison, 2008).

   2) Duty ethics: Obligations for human beings include duties to God, duties to oneself, and duties to others; duties to self include avoiding wronging others, treating people as equals, and promoting the good of others (Frankena & Granrose,

1974). Ross (2002) considered prima facie duties to include fidelity, reparation, gratitude, justice, beneficence, self-improvement, and nonmaleficence.

   3) Situation ethics: The decision maker acknowledges the unique characteristics of each individual, the caring relationship between the person and the caregiver, and the most humanistic course of action given the circumstances.

  c. Deontology can be subdivided into act and rule deontology (Guido, 2010).

   1) Act deontology is based on the moral values of the person making the ethical decision.

   2) Rule deontology is based on the belief that certain standards for ethical decisions transcend the individual's moral values.

 2. Utilitarianism, consequentialism, and teleology

  a. Utilitarianism, also known as situational ethics (Jeremy Bentham, 1748–1832, and John Stuart Mill, 1806–1873), is based on the assumption that actions should lead to maximizing the overall good; the ends justify the means. Principles or actions can be proven to be good. The best principles or actions are those resulting in good feelings, known as the "happiness theory" (Hinman, 2002; Hoeman, 2008) or teleological theory (Guido, 2010). What makes an action right or wrong is its utility, with useful actions bringing about the greatest happiness, or the least harm and suffering, to an individual.

   1) Rule utilitarianism seeks the greatest happiness for all and appeals to public agreement as a basis for objective judgment about the nature of happiness.

   2) Act utilitarianism seeks to determine which action will bring about the greatest happiness or the least harm and suffering.

  b. Consequentialist moral theories evaluate the morality of actions in terms of progress toward a goal or end and are a version of utilitarianism. Consequentialism is sometimes called teleology, with the goal being the greatest good for the greatest number (Morrison, 2008).

   1) Classical utilitarianism (or act consequentialism): Each act is considered based on its net benefit.

   2) Rule consequentialism: The decision maker develops the rules that will have the greatest net benefit.

 3. Objectivism (St. Thomas Aquinas, 1225–1274): Actions are considered morally right when they are in

accord with our nature, promote good, and avoid evil. *Ethical egoism* is the pursuit of one's own rational self-interest, and one's own happiness is the highest moral purpose of one's life (Morrison, 2008).

4. Applied ethics is the analysis of specific, controversial moral issues such as euthanasia. Resolution of these issues is approached by the use of ethical principles instead of the application of ethical theories.

5. Principalism incorporates various existing ethical principles and attempts to resolve conflicts by applying one or more ethical principles rather than ethical theories (Guido, 2010; McCarthy, 2006).

6. Relational ethics moves decisions into the context of the environment in which these decisions are made and creating a more "practical, action-oriented" ethics (Bergum & Dossetor, 2005; Guido, 2010). There are four components of relational ethics
   a. Engagement
   b. Mutual respect
   c. Embodiment
   d. Environment
   e. There is a shared relationship with obligations and responsibilities to other people, incorporating an understanding of culture and language. Relational ethics in nursing has included mutuality and caring (Gadow, 1999).

7. Normative ethical theories (**Figure 3-3**; Morrison, 2008)
   a. Natural law theories: The right thing to do is that which is in accord with the providentially ordered nature of the world.
   b. Egoistic theories: What is right is that which maximizes a person's self-interest.
   c. Authority-based theories: These may be faith based or purely ideological, with the decision of the right thing to do being based in some authority.
   d. Teleological theories (consequentialism and utilitarianism): The decision depends on the consequences of the action and maximizes the good of a situation.
   e. Deontological theories
   f. Virtue ethics

8. Ethical relativism (Butts & Rich, 2008)
   a. Ethical relativism is the belief that it is acceptable for ethics and morality to differ between people or societies. The two types are ethical subjectivism and cultural relativism.
      1) Ethical subjectivism: Individuals create their own morality, and there are no objective moral truths but only individual opinions.
      2) Cultural relativism: The moral evaluation is rooted in and cannot be separated from

Figure 3-3. Normative Ethical Theories

Normative ethical theories

Natural law theories | Egoistic theories | Authority-based theories | Teleological theories | Virtue ethics

the beliefs and behaviors of a particular culture, and what is wrong in one culture may not be so in another.
   b. Ethical objectivism is the position that universal or objective moral principles exist. Examples include deontology, utilitarianism, and natural law theory.

9. Social equality and justice (John Rawls, 1921–2002): Supports justice and equal rights for all through development of positions that use a "veil of ignorance" so that decisions are not colored by the specific details of those involved, allowing the disadvantaged to receive the same social and economic benefits as others.

10. Ideal observer (Raymond W. Firth, 1901–2002): Decisions should be made by an impartial observer fully informed of the situation and the potential consequences of the decision.

C. Models of Ethical and Moral Decision Making
   1. Process of moral decision making (Hoeman, 2008; **Figure 3-4**): Moral decision making uses ethical principles to guide decision making through a rational course (MacDonald, 2002).
   2. Savage model (Savage & Michalak, 1999) for facilitating ethical decision making (Figure 3-1)
   3. There are four aspects of moral action and interfering factors. Affective (emotion) and cognitive (thought) components are included in moral action and can be applied to direct client care situations (Grace, 2009; Rest, 1982; **Table 3-1**).
   4. Reflective equilibrium as a decision-making model (Morrison, 2008; **Figure 3-5**).
      a. *Healthcare issue at hand* is the middle of the model, containing the basic facts of the situation.
      b. *Considered judgments* or decision-making guides are used for making decisions about what to do.
         1) Intuitions or considered judgments about particular cases
         2) Regarding general moral rules
      c. *Common morality* influences the judgments and intuitions.
      d. *Ethical theory* examines people's motivations.
      e. *Ethical principles* include advancement of liberty, respect for autonomy, and acting out of

beneficence to advance welfare. Also included is the need to ensure that we do nothing to harm others by following the principle of non-maleficence and upholding principles of justice.

5. Josephson Institute of Ethics (Savage & Michalak, 1999) decision-making model
   a. All decisions must take into account and reflect a concern for the interest and well-being of stakeholders.
   b. Ethical values and principles always take precedence over nonethical ones.
   c. It is proper to violate an ethical principle only when it is clearly necessary to advance another true ethical principle, which, according to the decision maker's conscience, will produce the greatest balance of good in the long run.

6. Ethical decision making in difficult situations: Important considerations of ethical decision making in the daily practice of difficult situations requires the exercise of knowledge, experience, and skill, with a continued focus on the good of the client or family, without personal biases (Grace 2009; **Table 3-2**)

7. Proxy decision making: Proxy decision making is the act of deciding which healthcare actions

---

Figure 3-4. Process of Moral Decision Making

A. Recognizing the Moral Dimension
The first step is recognizing the decision as one that has moral importance. Important clues include conflicts between two or more values or ideals.

B. Who Are the Interested Parties? What Are Their Relationships?
Carefully identify who has a stake in the decision. In this regard, be imaginative and sympathetic. Often there are more parties whose interests should be taken into consideration than is immediately obvious.

Look at the relationships between the parties. Look at their relationships with yourself and with each other and with relevant institutions.

C. What Values Are Involved?
Think through the shared values that are at stake in making this decision. Is there a question of trust? Is personal autonomy a consideration? Is there a question of fairness? Is anyone to be harmed or helped?

D. Weigh the Benefits and the Burdens
Benefits—broadly defined—might include such things as the production of goods (physical, emotional, financial, social, etc.) for various parties, the satisfaction of preferences, and acting in accordance with various relevant values (such as fairness).

Burdens might include causing physical or emotional pain to various parties, imposing financial costs, and ignoring relevant values.

E. Look for Analogous Cases
Can you think of other similar decisions? What course of action was taken? Was it a good decision? How is the present case like that one? How is it different?

F. Discuss with Relevant Others
The merits of discussion should not be underestimated. Time permitting, discuss your decision with as many people as have a stake in it. Gather opinions and ask for the reasons behind those opinions. Remember that your ability to discuss topics with others may be limited by the other people's expectations of confidentiality.

G. Does This Decision Accord with Legal and Organizational Rules?
Some decisions are appropriately made based on legal considerations. If one option is illegal, we should at least think very seriously before choosing that option.

Decisions may also be affected by rules set by organizations of which we are members. For example, most professional organizations have codes of ethics that are intended to guide individual decision making. Institutions (hospitals, banks, corporations) may also have policies that limit the options available to us.

Sometimes there are bad laws or bad rules, and sometimes those should be broken. But usually it is ethically important to pay attention to laws and rules.

H. Am I Comfortable with This Decision?
Sometimes your "gut reaction" will tell you if you've missed something.

Questions to be asked in this regard might include:

1. If I carry out this decision, would I be comfortable telling my family about it? My clergy? My mentors?

2. Would I want children to regard my behavior as an example?

3. Is this decision one that a wise, informed, virtuous person would make?

4. Can I live with this decision?

From *Guide to moral decision making*, by C. MacDonald, 2010. Retrieved September 21, 2011, from www.ethicsweb.ca/guide. Copyright 2010 by Chris MacDonald. Reprinted with permission.

Table 3-1. Four Aspects of Moral Action and Interfering Factors

Rest's Processes (1982)	Practical Implications	Interfering Factors
1. Interpretation of the situation	AP's understanding of the inherently ethical nature of any practice situation Assessment of this particular situation and what is needed	Personal troubles Energy level Time available Knowledge level No understanding of the inherently moral nature of practice Lack of connection with the client or inability to engage Perception or sensitivity affected by age and life experiences Lack of self-reflection
2. Discerning the morally ideal action (what should be done)	Using appropriate tools, methods, and resources for decision making Identifying the beneficiary, goal, and appropriate actions	Level of moral development Level of independence Level and types of education Personal values conflict with client's, significant other's, or other professionals' values Lack of reflection on practice
3. Deciding what to do	Deciding between competing courses of action What should be done may not always be possible or consensus may not be reachable	Situational ambiguity Theoretical ambiguity Uncertainty about outcome Lack of institutional or peer support
4. Implementation and perseverance	Envisioning steps and anticipating problems Addressing and overcoming problems and barriers Taking sociopolitical actions to get what is needed Keeping sight of the goal Reminding others of the goal	Too many obstacles Fear of personal consequences, peer or colleague disapproval Fatigue Frustration Lack of resources and supports

From *Nursing ethics and professional responsibility in advanced practice* (pp. 60–62), by P. J. Grace, 2009, Sudbury, MA: Jones & Bartlett. Copyright 2009 by Jones & Bartlett. Reprinted with permission.

Figure 3-5. Reflective Equilibrium at Work

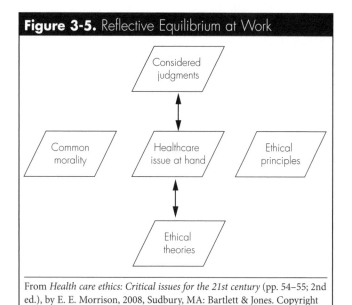

From *Health care ethics: Critical issues for the 21st century* (pp. 54–55; 2nd ed.), by E. E. Morrison, 2008, Sudbury, MA: Bartlett & Jones. Copyright 2008 by Bartlett & Jones. Reprinted with permission.

might be permissible for a person who has lost decision-making capacity, either temporarily or permanently. Proxy decision making may also be applied for a person who has never had decision-making capacity, such as someone with profound cognitive deficits or those lacking maturity to make healthcare decisions, such as children (Grace, 2009; **Table 3-3**).

    D. Resource Allocation
       1. Microallocation
       2. Macroallocation
       3. Cost containment
       4. Individual access to services
       5. Clinical decisions made by for-profit managed care organizations (Habel, 1999)
    E. Issues That Rehabilitation Professionals Must Address
       1. Balancing medical and rehabilitative needs that

Table 3-2. Ethical Decision Making in Difficult Situations: Important Considerations

In the course of daily practice, what is needed for ethical action is the thoughtful exercise of knowledge, experience, and skill together with a constant focus on the good of the client or group in need of services and an understanding of one's own biases.

In more complex situations, where what is good is not so clearly seen, a more in-depth analysis may be needed. This is not necessarily a linear process, nor will all of the following considerations always be pertinent. There are other decision-making models available, but all have similar considerations.

Steps	Questions
Identify the major problem(s); relate them to professional goals.	What are the facts: clinical, social, environmental?
	What implicit assumptions are being made?
	What ethical principles or perspectives are pertinent? Examples: Autonomous decision making is in question, conflict of values between providers and client or significant others, economic versus client good.
	Are there power imbalances? What are these? Who has an interest in maintaining them?
Identify information gaps.	Do you need more information?
	From whom or where might you get this information?
Determine who is involved.	Who is the main focus? Is there more than one important party? Who has (or thinks they have) an interest in the outcome (relatives, staff, other)? Who will be affected by the outcome?
Identify the prevalent values.	Values held by client, staff, institution.
Determine whether an interpreter is necessary (for cultural or language issues).	Are there value conflicts? Interpersonal, interprofessional, personal versus professional, client versus professional.
Who would be the most appropriate interpreter (knowledgeable and neutral)?	Are there cultural perspectives? Who can help with these?
Identify possible courses of action and probable consequences.	Which course of action is likely to be the most beneficial and the least harmful to those involved, including you?
	Can safeguards be put in place in case of unforeseen consequences?
Implement the selected course of action. Conduct an ongoing evaluation.	Does the actual outcome correlate with the anticipated outcome? What was unexpected? Was this foreseeable given more data?
	Do similar problems keep reoccurring? If so, why (may require a look at underlying environmental or societal issues)? Does this point to the need for policy changes or development at the site, institution, or societal level? What further actions might be needed?
	Are there continuing provider education needs related to the issue?
Engage in self-reflection, reflection on practice (individually, in an interdisciplinary group debriefing session, or in a specialty group forum).	Could you have done things differently? What would you have liked to understand better?
	Would a consultation with colleagues or an ethics resource person have changed your understanding of the issue or the course of action taken?
	What valuable insights did you gain that should be shared with others and may be applicable to the approach used for future problems?

From *Nursing ethics and professional responsibility in advanced practice* (pp. 62–64), by P. J. Grace, 2009, Sudbury, MA: Jones & Bartlett. Copyright 2009 by Jones & Bartlett. Reprinted with permission.

present moral quandaries

2. Team contributions to decision making with regard to services for clients and clients' progress and outcomes
3. Definitions of quality-of-life issues
4. Access to rehabilitative services regardless of the client's disability or funding level
5. Legal requirements for providing rehabilitation services
6. Standards and regulations imposed by various entities

7. Client decisions to adhere or not to adhere to recommended regimens as defined by the rehabilitation team
8. Clinical judgment in nursing: Clinical judgment in nursing is a nonlinear process of using knowledge, reasoning, experiential skills, and interpersonal skills to determine probable best actions (Butts & Rich, 2008; Grace, 2009; **Table 3-4**).
9. Nursing process: Identify the problem, gather data, identify options, make a decision, act, and assess (Ellis & Hartley, 2007). The nursing process is a systematic, rational method of planning and providing

Table 3-3. Proxy Decision Making

Type	Explanation
A. Autonomy based: the person's previously expressed wishes	Written: Living will, advance directives Substituted judgment • Durable power of attorney for health care (person appointed to provide information about a client's previous wishes expressed while having decision-making capacity) • Informal (family member, friend, significant other)
B. Best interests	Surrogate determines the "highest net benefit among available options" (Beauchamp & Childress, 2001, p. 192). This is a quality-of-life (QOL) evaluation—it may or may not be based on a person's previously expressed desires. Previous values, beliefs, and wishes are considered to the extent that they give information about what would constitute QOL for the person. This may permit overriding a durable power of attorney's decision that does not seem to further client best interests and when there are no written instructions (from the incapacitated patient) to support the proposed course of action.
C. Reasonable person	A standard used when neither A nor B is applicable. It asks, "What would a reasonable person want?" The typical client was never competent (e.g., a baby or cognitively impaired person) and/or previous wishes cannot be determined. For example • Some permanently unconscious clients who might be said to have no interests and who cannot be "benefited" or "burdened." • Incapacitated, dying clients left on life support to preserve organs for transplantation (Medical College of Georgia, 2000).

From "Ethics in the clinical encounter" (pp. 295–332), by P. J. Grace, 2004. In S. K. Chase (Ed.), *Clinical judgment and communication in nurse practitioner practice*, Philadelphia: F. A. Davis. Copyright 2004 by F. A. Davis. Reprinted with permission.

individualized nursing care. The nursing process is based on a nursing theory developed by Ida Jean Orlando. She developed this theory in the late 1950s as she observed nurses in action.

10. Three-step ACT model (Graham-Eason, 1996)
    a. A: Anticipate obstacles to action.
    b. C: Clarify position related to planning action.
    c. T: Test choice.
11. Moral Ground Model: A virtue-based nursing model (Butts & Rich, 2008)
    a. The Moral Ground Model was adapted from the Eightfold Path and the Four Immeasurable Virtues of Buddhism and was founded in Aristotle's approach to virtue ethics. The commonality is the alleviation of human suffering. As in teleological philosophies, the focus is on human morality moving toward a final purpose or goal (Butts & Rich, 2008; Keown, 2001). The model implies that nurses may start at an uneducated state of moral functioning and move toward moral ground along a path of intellectual and moral virtues.
    b. Intellectual virtues
       1) Insight: Awareness and knowledge of the moral nature of nurses' day-to-day work to transform moral suffering
       2) Practical wisdom: Using deliberative reason to direct actions
    c. Moral virtues

1) Truthfulness: refraining from deception through false communication or self-deception
2) Gentleness: mildness in verbal and non-verbal communication
3) Compassion: the desire to separate others from suffering
4) Loving kindness: the desire to bring happiness and well-being to oneself and others
5) Just generosity: giving and receiving based on need
6) Courage: putting fear aside to act for a purpose that is more important than fear
7) Sympathetic joy: rejoicing in others' happiness
8) Equanimity: an evenness and calmness of being

12. Critical thinking as a decision-making model: Paul and Elder, directors of the Foundation for Critical Thinking, defined *critical thinking* as "the art of analyzing and evaluating thinking with a view to improving it"; it is "self-directed, self-disciplined, self-monitored, and self-corrective thinking [that] requires rigorous standards of excellence and mindful command of their use" (Paul & Elder, 2006, p. 4). They proposed that critical thinkers do the following:
    a. Ask clear, pertinent questions and identify key problems.

THE SPECIALTY PRACTICE OF REHABILITATION NURSING

Table 3-4. Clinical Judgment in Nursing

Definition: *Clinical judgment in nursing* is the nonlinear process of using knowledge, reasoning, tacit (experiential) skills, and interpersonal skills to determine—within the limits of available information—probable best actions given the inevitable existence of uncertainty about the possession of adequate knowledge and outcome of actions.

Components	Categories
Knowledge	The knowledge base of nursing • Nature of the discipline • Purposes and goals • Nature of people and environment • Characteristics of good practitioners • Scope and limits of practice Knowledge derived from other disciplines: philosophical (including ethical theory), physical, social, psychological, spiritual, biological Knowledge related to the situation • Primary subject (who is involved) • Subject's understanding of the situation, values, beliefs, and context • Goals
Experience	Previous experiences • Personal • Professional
Characteristics and skills	Perceptual • Grasp the nature and complexity of issues • Identification of needed and potential resources • Envision resolution • Reflection on practice and self-reflection • Creative, articulate Relational • Interpersonal • Collaborative • Mediation Motivation • Professional responsibility • Emotional engagement

From *Nursing ethics and professional responsibility in advanced practice* (p. 110), by P. J. Grace, 2009, Sudbury, MA: Jones & Bartlett. Copyright 2009 by Jones & Bartlett. Reprinted with permission.

b. Analyze and interpret relevant information by using abstract thinking.

c. Generate reasonable conclusions and solutions that are tested according to sensible criteria and standards.

d. Remain open minded to consider alternative thought systems.

e. Solve complex problems by communicating effectively with other people.

13. Ethics committees generally follow one or a combination of three distinct models or structures

    a. The autonomy model facilitates decision making for the client who has capacity.

    b. The client benefit model uses substituted judgment or best interest and facilitates decision making for the client lacking capacity.

    c. The social justice model considers broad social issues and is accountable to the institution and society.

14. Other ethical decision-making models (see Figure 3-2)

F. Factors Influencing Actions of the Individual Nurse

    1. One's worldview or philosophy concerning what is real; knowledge as fact based on what is experienced versus knowledge as socially constructed or what people agree is knowledge (Gergen, 2009)

    2. Individual beliefs and values

    3. Professional codes of behavior

    4. Institutional policies

    5. Laws

    6. Sensitivity to cultural diversity has broadened the appreciation for and implementation of actions regarding respect for autonomy.

G. Ethical Conflict

    1. Types of ethical conflicts (Fletcher et al., 2005)

a. Conflicts of widely accepted moral duties or obligations
b. Threats to important relationships
c. Collisions of moral principles
d. Collisions of values
e. Conflicts of interest

2. Ethical dilemma is choosing between two equally difficult actions because they are both right, they are both wrong, or both contain uncertainty (Butts & Rich, 2008).

3. Moral distress is the state of being unable to follow the right course of action due to institutional barriers (Jameton, 1984).

4. Moral residue is that which remains when moral distress goes unresolved, increasing job turnover and nurses leaving the workforce (Webster & Baylis, 2000).

H. Ethical Principles and Rights

1. Ethical principles: The relationship of ethical principles to situations encountered in rehabilitation nursing practice or sphere of concern reflects issues common to rehabilitation settings (Hoeman, 2008; **Table 3-5**).

a. Autonomy: Individual actions are independent of the actions and will of others.
b. Nomaleficence: The concept of doing no harm
c. Beneficence: The concept of doing good for another
d. Advocacy: Championing the needs and interests of another
e. Veracity: Responsibility to speak the truth
f. Financial responsibility: Ensuring there is sufficient benefit for the expense provided
g. Care: Providing for and meeting the needs of others for compassion, empathy, and good
h. Sanctity of life: Value of life
i. Quality of life: Correlation between life and participation in activities and interests
j. Consent: Voluntary agreement
k. Confidentiality: Responsibility to keep information private
l. Competence: Ability or legal right to make appropriate decisions
m. Values: Positive qualities held by an object or outcome

2. Rights are the basis of professional, regulatory, and legal codes and judgments; they reflect the things society believes a person is entitled to. Rights can come into conflict with values (Ellis & Hartley, 2007; Masters-Farrell, 2006).

a. Self-determination rights: The Patient Self-Determination Act (1990), or the Danforth

amendment, requires that clients be given an opportunity to decide on life support options on admission to any healthcare service. Organizations must supply documentation and education to support informed choice.

b. Patient rights: The American Hospital Association published *A Patient's Bill of Rights* in 1973, focusing on confidentiality, privacy, and informed consent. Updated in 1992, it began to reflect the responsibilities of healthcare providers and to reinforce the concept of collaborative care. In 2003 the document was rewritten and titled *The Patient Care Partnership*, encouraging clients to get involved in their care and to ask questions. The Joint Commission and the Commission on Accreditation of Rehabilitation Facilities require that clients receive information about their rights. The Joint Commission has expanded these rights to include the right to effective pain management. A federally mandated patient rights program is also under consideration. It includes the following rights:

1) The right to receive considerate and respectful care
2) The right to obtain relevant, current, and understandable information about diagnosis, treatment, and prognosis
3) The right to make decisions about the plan of care
4) The right to have advance directives about treatment
5) The right to privacy in all aspects of care
6) The right to expect that all communication and records will be treated confidentially
7) The right to review records pertaining to care
8) The right to expect reasonable responses to requests for appropriate and medically indicated care and services
9) The right to be informed about business relationships that may influence treatment and care
10) The right to consent to or decline participation in proposed research studies
11) The right to expect reasonable continuity of care
12) The right to be informed about hospital policies and practices that relate to client care, treatment, and responsibility

I. Professional Ethics Codes, Standards, and Statements

Table 3-5. Relationship of Ethical Principles to Situations Encountered in Rehabilitation Nursing Practice or Sphere of Concern

Ethical Principle	Description	Examples
Autonomy	An individual's actions are independent from the actions and the will of others. Individuals have the ability to form their own perspectives on right, wrong, and values.	Rehabilitation nurses must acknowledge that individuals for whom they care have freedom regarding their bodies and actions. Nurses may provide education on wellness and health promotion, but compliance with programs cannot be forced. Clients have autonomy in their healthcare programs.
Nonmaleficence	The concept of doing no harm	Rehabilitation nurses, like all healthcare practitioners, have a duty to do no harm to a client. To intentionally administer a lethal dose of medication to a client is an example of violation of the ethical principle of nonmaleficence. It is unthinkable for a nurse to intentionally harm a client.
Beneficence	The concept of doing good for another.	Nursing care is based on the concept of beneficence. Rehabilitation nurses intend to do good for others. The motivation that drives rehabilitation nurses to go the extra distance in care of their clients is an example of beneficence.
Advocacy	Loyalty: Championing the needs and interests of another	Rehabilitation nurses are in an ideal position to advocate for their clients. Nurses often see clients on a 24-hour basis and have an awareness for and appreciation of clients' abilities and energy levels that other disciplines may not. It is critical that such information be shared with team members in a way to advocate for the best plans for clients.
Veracity	Responsibility to speak the truth	Nurses have an obligation to speak truthfully in all aspects of their role.
Financial responsibility (cost-benefit analysis)	Stewardship: Ensuring there is sufficient benefit for the expense provided	There is an ethical responsibility to meet the client's needs as well as possible while using as few resources as possible. For example, extending lengths of stay in hospitals, home health care, and subacute programs when a client is capable of being discharged to a lesser level of care is not in line with the nurse's financial responsibility of care.
Care	Providing for and meeting the needs of others for compassion, empathy, and good	Care is a component of the rehabilitation nurse's role, regardless of setting.
Sanctity of life	Value of life, right to life	Rehabilitation nurses have an obligation to care for all clients, regardless of the extent of disability or potential for recovery, because all life is of value.
Quality of life	Condition of one's life, based on assessment of correlation between life and participation in valued activities and interests	Quality of life is a frequent question for individuals with devastating disabilities and chronic illnesses. Rehabilitation nurses can assist individuals and families in reframing situations to find quality of life in remaining abilities.
Consent	Voluntary agreement with a procedure, process, or treatment	The role of the rehabilitation nurse in informed consent is key. Because clients often confide in nurses, the rehabilitation nurse is in a position to validate understanding of a procedure, treatment, or course of therapy. As an advocate, the rehabilitation nurse supports the client's abilities to make decisions and participate in his or her plans of care.
Confidentiality	Responsibility to keep information private	Rehabilitation nurses are entrusted with substantial amounts of private information. Such information must be kept confidential, to be shared only as related to the nursing care and needs of the client.
Competence	The ability or legal right to make appropriate decisions	The need for rehabilitation sometimes follows a disability or illness that affects the clarity of the client's decision-making ability. This should not be confused with legal competence.
Values	Worthwhile or positive qualities held by an object or outcome; these should be chosen carefully but freely	The question of the value of life after a disability or chronic illness is sometimes placed in question. Rehabilitation nurses recognize the value of independence and of reframing prior values to achieve higher levels of life satisfaction.

From *Principles of normative ethics*, by D. Ursery, 2005, Austin, TX: St. Edwards University. Copyright 2005 by St. Edwards University. Reprinted with permission.

1. The ethical standard for the profession of nursing is established in the *Code of Ethics for Nurses: Provisions* (ANA, 2006). The ANA *Code of Ethics for Nurses* was developed as a guide for carrying out nursing responsibilities in a manner consistent with quality in nursing care and the ethical obligations of the profession (ANA, 2010). *The Code of Ethics for Nurses with Interpretive Statements* provides a framework for nurses to use in ethical analysis and decision making. The *Code of Ethics* establishes the ethical standard for the profession. It is not negotiable in any setting, nor is it subject to revision or amendment except by formal process of the House of Delegates of the ANA (ANA, 2010).

    a. Provision 1. The nurse, in all professional relationships, practices with compassion and respect for the inherent dignity, worth, and uniqueness of every individual, unrestricted by considerations of social or economic status, personal attributes, or the nature of health problems.

    b. Provision 2. The nurse's primary commitment is to the patient, whether an individual, family, group, or community.

    c. Provision 3. The nurse promotes, advocates for, and strives to protect the health, safety, and rights of the patient.

    d. Provision 4. The nurse is responsible and accountable for individual nursing practice and determines the appropriate delegation of tasks consistent with the nurse's obligation to provide optimum patient care.

    e. Provision 5. The nurse owes the same duties to self as to others, including the responsibility to preserve integrity and safety, to maintain competence, and to continue personal and professional growth.

    f. Provision 6. The nurse participates in establishing, maintaining, and improving healthcare environments and conditions of employment conducive to the provision of quality health care and consistent with the values of the profession through individual and collective action.

    g. Provision 7. The nurse participates in the advancement of the profession through contributions to practice, education, administration, and knowledge development.

    h. Provision 8. The nurse collaborates with other health professionals and the public in promoting community, national, and international efforts to meet health needs.

    i. Provision 9. The profession of nursing, as represented by associations and their members, is responsible for articulating nursing values, for maintaining the integrity of the profession and its practice, and for shaping social policy.

2. ARN (2000, 2008) supported these standards and incorporated them into the *Standards and Scope of Rehabilitation Nursing Practice* (**Figure 3-6**). ARN contributes additional comments about standards of ethical rehabilitation nursing practice in the *ARN Position Statement on Ethical Issues* (Pilkington & Strong, 2003). This statement presents concerns of rehabilitation nurses.

    a. Clients' rights, including the rights of minors. (Minors may or may not be capable of understanding the decisions made in their name by their parents. If a minor was not involved in the decision-making process and does not agree with his or her parents' decision, the minor may have no recourse, which leads to an ethical and legal conflict.)

    b. The use of restraints

    c. Do-not-resuscitate orders

    d. Advance directives, which imply nursing intervention and responsibility regarding living wills and durable power of attorney

    e. Management of clients who are disposed to self-destructive behaviors or suicidal gestures

    f. Issues related to healthcare reform and changes in how health care is allocated and delivered, including providing access to health care and rehabilitation, containing costs, ensuring quality of health care, determining length of stay, defining who meets the criteria for rehabilitation, dealing with clients' noncompliance with treatment and rehabilitation, teaching the client and family in preparation for discharge to home or another level of care, and discharging clients to a care level with appropriate skills for their needs

    g. Confidentiality, security, and privacy related to client care

    h. Substance abuse

    i. Abused clients

    j. The nurse-client relationship (e.g., when does it become too intimate, and when is intimacy between the nurse and the client appropriate?)

3. The International Council of Nurses (ICN) *International Code of Ethics* (2006) is a guide for action based on social values and needs. The code has served as the standard for nurses worldwide since it was adopted in 1953.

    a. According to the ICN *Code of Ethics for Nurses,* nurses have four fundamental responsibilities:

1) To promote health
2) To prevent illness
3) To restore health
4) To alleviate suffering

b. "The need for nursing is universal. Inherent in nursing is respect for human rights, including cultural rights, the right to life and choice, to dignity, and to be treated with respect. Nursing care is respectful of and unrestricted by considerations of age, colour, creed, culture, disability or illness, gender, sexual orientation, nationality, politics, race or social status. Nurses render health services to the individual, the family and the community and coordinate their services with those of related groups" (ICN, 2006, p. 3). Elements of the ICN *Code of Ethics* are
   1) Nurses and people
   2) Nurses and practice
   3) Nurses and the profession
   4) Nurses and coworkers

4. ANA *Scope and Standards of Practice* (2004) acknowledges that the nurse's decisions and actions on behalf of clients are determined in an ethical manner. Standard V: Ethics measurement criteria includes the following:

Figure 3-6. ARN Standards Regarding Ethics

Standard V. Ethics: The rehabilitation nurse's decisions and actions on behalf of clients are determined in an ethical manner.

- The rehabilitation nurse's practice is guided by *Code for Nurses with Interpretive Statements* (ANA, 1985) and ARN's position statement on ethical issues.
- The rehabilitation nurse maintains a client's confidentiality.
- The rehabilitation nurse acts as a client advocate.
- The rehabilitation nurse delivers care in a nonjudgmental and nondiscriminatory manner that is sensitive to clients' diversity.
- The rehabilitation nurse delivers care in a manner that preserves and protects the client's autonomy, dignity, and rights.
- The rehabilitation nurse maintains an awareness of his or her beliefs and value systems and what effect they may have on care he or she provides to the client and client's significant others.
- The rehabilitation nurse supports the client's right to make decisions that may not be congruent with the values of the rehabilitation team.
- The rehabilitation nurse seeks available resources to help formulate ethical decisions.
- The rehabilitation nurse promotes the provision of information and discussion that allows the client to participate fully in decision making.
- The rehabilitation nurse participates in decision making regarding allocation of resources.

Association of Rehabilitation Nurses. (2000). *Standards and scope of rehabilitation nursing practice* (3rd ed.). Glenview, IL: Author.

---

a. The nurse's practice is guided by *The Code for Nurses* and related ANA position statements, such as the *Position Statement on Nurses' Participation in Capital Punishment.*

b. The nurse maintains client confidentiality.

c. The nurse acts as a client advocate.

d. The nurse delivers care in a nonjudgmental and nondiscriminatory manner that is sensitive to client diversity.

e. The nurse delivers care in a manner that preserves and protects client autonomy, dignity, and rights.

f. The nurse seeks available resources to help formulate ethical decisions.

5. The Nuremberg Code specifies 10 basic requirements for medical experimentation (Hoeman, 2008; **Figure 3-7**).

a. The Nuremberg Code was conceptualized and formulated to protect human rights. It codified crucial considerations, important safeguards, and guidelines related to research design, conduct, and human subject protections, including that research results should be likely to benefit humanity in some way, coercion of subjects to participate is forbidden, likely results should justify any risks, and risks should be minimized, including mental or physical suffering, which is not permissible (Grace, 2009).

b. The National Institutes of Health specify the guidelines for clinical research involving human subjects, codified in Title 45, Code of Federal Regulations, Part 46 (National Institutes of Health, 2004).

J. Ethics Committee
1. Definition: An interdisciplinary group of healthcare professionals established specifically to address ethical dilemmas that occur in a particular setting. The group may include members of the community and people with formal ethics education and ethics consultation core competencies (Fletcher et al., 2005).

2. Functions
   a. Provides a forum for ethical dialogue between people with ethical concerns
   b. Ensures the presence of all stakeholders involved in the ethics issue, including client or surrogate
   c. Provides education on ethical options; does not provide second medical opinion or render judgment about what actions should be taken
   d. Is available to all areas of the institution, not just clinical
   e. Reviews requests for ethics help for nonethics-related concerns and assists requester

with appropriate referral, such as legal, compliance, and quality improvement

f. Is available for policy review for ethics content

3. Functions of a nursing ethics subcommittee (Marquis & Huston, 2009)

a. Addresses unique concerns of nursing

b. Helps nurses identify, explore, and resolve ethical issues in practice

c. Provides education and staff development

d. Develops and follows a defined model of critical thinking

e. Reviews department policies related to ethics

II. Legal Issues and Considerations (Ellis & Hartley, 2007)

A. Laws: Laws govern the scope of nursing practice and delivery of care; protect licensure; define specifics of provision, access to services, and reimbursement; and finance education and research. Laws also provide the forum to test ethical issues related to healthcare dilemmas in rehabilitation (Hoeman, 2008).

1. The National Institute on Disability and Rehabilitation Research (Hoeman, 2008) proposed a long-range plan for disability-related funding for 2005–2009 to support people with disabilities.

2. The No Child Left Behind Program and New Freedom Initiative

3. The Office of Special Education Programs offers support in special education, vocational rehabilitation, and research.

4. The Center for National Rehabilitation Research Information and Exchange

5. The Americans with Disabilities Act (ADA; effective July 26, 1992) defined disability as a physical or mental impairment that substantially limits one or more major life activities, a record of such an impairment, or being regarded as having an impairment.

6. The Equal Employment Opportunity Commission issued guidelines for complying with the ADA law.

B. Summaries of Disability Laws (Hoeman, 2008; **Figure 3-8**)

1. Employment

2. State and local government programs and services

3. Housing

4. Education

5. Travel and transportation

6. Technology and telecommunications

C. Other Legal Considerations

1. The Patient Self-Determination Act requires that people receiving medical care be given written information about their right to make decisions about end-of-life issues.

Figure 3-7. Nuremberg Code (Paraphrased)

1. Informed, voluntary consent of the subject is essential.

2. The study must be expected to have a result that will be of benefit to others.

3. The study must be based on an understanding of pathophysiology of the disease or problem or on prior animal studies.

4. Suffering of subjects will be prevented during the study.

5. Death or disability is not expected or predicted as a result of the study.

6. The degree of risk does not outweigh the potential good to be gained.

7. Subjects will be protected and safeguarded against problems that may occur during the study.

8. Researchers will have the appropriate credentials to complete the research.

9. Subjects may withdraw from studies if they cannot continue.

10. Researchers will stop the study if at any time they deem it in the best interests of the subjects to discontinue the study.

From *Rehabilitation nursing: Prevention, intervention, and outcomes* (p. 38), by S. Hoeman, 2008, St. Louis: Mosby Elsevier. Copyright 2008 by Mosby. Reprinted with permission.

2. Living wills and life-prolonging declarations allow people to make their wishes known before hospitalization regarding medical care, illness, or conditions resulting in incompetence.

3. A durable power of attorney enables a competent person to appoint a surrogate decision maker who is empowered to act legally for the client.

4. Guardianship is a position of responsibility granted to a person by the court to make decisions about the incapacitated person's life.

5. Competency is determined by the court based on clinical opinions of the person's mental or cognitive fitness.

6. Informed consent is based on a full description of the risks and consequences of agreeing or refusing to have an operation or procedure.

7. Estate planning involves long-term planning for future care and expenses.

8. Legal death or brain death is based on the legal parameters defining the time at which life ceases.

9. Withholding or withdrawing treatment.

10. Do-not-resuscitate orders allow people to indicate in advance that they do not want to be resuscitated in the event of cardiac or respiratory arrest.

11. Research on human subjects (Macrina, 2005)

a. Basic rules and requirements for research studies can be found in various codes and regulations and focus on issues of informed consent.

b. Participants should understand the purpose

Figure 3-8. Summaries of Disability Law

Employment

Americans with Disabilities Act, Title I: Prohibits discrimination in the workplace against people with disabilities

Section 501, Rehabilitation Act (1973): Requires affirmative action and nondiscrimination in employment by federal agencies of the executive branch

Section 503, Rehabilitation Act: Requires affirmative action and prohibits employment discrimination by federal government contractors and subcontractors with contracts of more than $10,000

Section 188, Workforce Investment Act: Prohibits discrimination against people with disabilities in employment service centers funded by the federal government

State and local government programs and services

Americans with Disabilities Act, Title II: Prohibits discrimination in the provision of public benefits and services (e.g., public education, employment, transportation, recreation, healthcare, social services, courts, voting, and town meetings)

Section 504, Rehabilitation Act: Requires that buildings and facilities that are designed, constructed, or altered with federal funds or leased by a federal agency comply with federal standards for physical accessibility

Housing

Fair Housing Act: Prohibits discrimination in any aspect of selling, renting, or denying housing on the basis of disability. Owners are further required to make reasonable accommodations in their housing policies to afford equal housing opportunities to those with disabilities

Americans with Disabilities Act, Title II: Prohibits discrimination by public housing authorities and other state and local government housing

American with Disabilities Act, Title III: Does not apply to regular privately owned residential dwelling units. However, it does apply to residences that are also public accommodations, such as nursing homes and school dorms. In addition, parts of residential facilities that serve a group of people or the public might be considered public accommodations, such as a swimming pool or a sales and leasing office.

Section 504, Rehabilitation Act: Prohibits discrimination by public housing authorities that receive federal funds, cities and towns that receive Community Development Block Grants or other federal funds, private for-profit or nonprofit housing developers that receive federal funds, and colleges and universities that receive federal funds (student housing)

Architectural Barriers Act: Applies accessibility standards to housing constructed with federal funding

Education

Individuals with Disabilities Education Act (IDEA): Requires public primary and secondary schools to make available to all eligible children with disabilities a free appropriate public education in the least restrictive environment appropriate to their individual needs

Section 504, Rehabilitation Act: Prohibits discrimination against students with disabilities in primary, secondary, or postsecondary schools receiving federal funds

Americans with Disabilities Act, Title II: Prohibits discrimination against students with disabilities in all educational institutions that receive funds from state or local government

Americans with Disabilities Act, Title III: Prohibits discrimination against students with disabilities in private schools

Travel and Transportation

Americans with Disabilities Act, Title II: Prohibits discrimination in transportation provided by state and local government entities such as bus, railway, subway, and other forms of ground transportation

Section 504, Rehabilitation Act: Prohibits discrimination in privately operated transportation services that receive federal funds

Americans with Disabilities Act, Title III: Prohibits discrimination in privately operated transportation such as limousines and hotel shuttle services

Air Carrier Access Act: Prohibits discrimination on the basis of disability in air travel. It applies only to air carriers that provide regularly scheduled services for hire to the public. Requirements address a wide range of issues, including boarding assistance and certain accessibility features in newly built aircraft and new or altered airport facilities.

Technology and Telecommunications

Section 508, Rehabilitation Act: Requires federal agencies to make their electronic and information technology accessible to people with disabilities

Americans with Disabilities Act, Title IV: Requires telephone companies to establish telecommunication relay services for callers with hearing and speech disabilities. Title IV also requires closed captioning of federally funded public service announcements.

Section 255, Telecommunications Act: Requires manufacturers of telecommunication equipment and providers of telecommunication services to ensure that such equipment and services are accessible to and usable by people with disabilities and that people with disabilities have access to a broad range of products and services such as telephones, cell phones, pagers, call waiting, and operator services

From *Rehabilitation nursing: Prevention, intervention, and outcomes* (4th ed., p. 41), by S. Hoeman, 2008, St. Louis: Mosby Elsevier. Copyright 2008 by Mosby. Reprinted with permission.

of the research and what is expected of them.

    c. Participants should be competent to decide to participate.

    d. Participants have the right to have questions answered before participation.

    e. Participants should be free to withdraw from the study at any time without fear of reprisal.

III. **Ethical, Legal, and Moral Issues in Practice (Table 3-6)**

  A. Diagnosis and Prognosis: An Example

    1. Cognition is altered.

    2. The client lacks decision-making capacity and needs a surrogate decision maker.

    3. Cognition may improve, eliminating the need for a surrogate.

  B. Collaborative Decision Making and Effective Communication

    1. Includes the client and family or social support, with the client's permission

    2. Establishes a dialogue to determine cultural and socioeconomic attitudes related to learning, health, and wellness in defining an appropriate level of care

    3. Identifies components of life support systems, policies of the healthcare setting, and support resources

    4. Involves the entire rehabilitation team in communicating with the client and family and discussing their concerns about progress toward rehabilitation goals and treatment

  C. Appropriate Level of Care

    1. Acute care versus long-term care versus outpatient versus home

    2. Involves making decisions based on the client's needs and available resources.

  D. Allocation of Resources

    1. Microallocation: Services are allocated for a specific client's care

    2. Macroallocation: Distribution of available services across a client population

    3. Cost containment

    4. Transparency of allocations

    5. Rationing

    6 Access based on ability to pay and an identified discharge plan

  E. Ethical Rehabilitation

    1. The client or surrogate participates in developing the plan of care.

    2. Independence and wellness are valued.

    3. Improvement in functional status and self-worth are key rehabilitation goals.

    4. Rehabilitation nurses are members of the interdisciplinary rehabilitation team and collaborate with other team members.

    5. The client is assessed for physical pain and pain is treated.

    6. The client is assessed for emotional pain or depression and treatment is provided.

    7. Rehabilitation services are delivered in the most appropriate setting in the shortest amount of time based on the needs of the client and available resources.

  F. Team Issues

    1. The client is a member of the team and at the center of care.

    2. Measurable and objective goals are developed in collaboration with the client or surrogate.

    3. Team members demonstrate respect for each other and for the contribution each member makes.

  G. Ethical Issues Related to Alternative and Complementary Medicine and Therapies

    1. The client's right to choose and request alternative and complementary medicine and therapies

    2. Possible interactions between alternative or complementary medicine and traditional Western medicine

    3. Availability of alternative or complementary medicine and therapies

  H. Ethics of Caring (Gergen, 2009; Gilligan, 1995)

    1. Care and services are delivered and received in the context of relationships.

    2. Relationships are reciprocal and occur in an environment of trust and transparency.

    3. Relationships exist between rehabilitation nurses and other team members, including the client or surrogate and the healthcare institution.

  I. Ethical Foundations of Healthcare Reform (Butts & Rich, 2008; Cerise & Chokshi, 2009)

    1. Universal access: The client has access to health care regardless of the ability to pay.

    2. Comprehensive benefits: Care and services are provided across the healthcare continuum.

    3. Choice: Clients have choices about providers, plans, and treatments. They are informed about the risks and benefits of available treatments and are free to choose between them or refuse treatment according to individual preferences and medical appropriateness.

    4. Equity of care: Care is based on need rather than individual or group characteristics.

    5. Fair distribution of costs: Costs and burdens of care are spread across the entire community, basing the individual contribution on ability to pay.

    6. Personal responsibility: Individuals assume responsibility for protecting and promoting health and contributing to the cost of care based on ability to pay.

Table 3-6. Distinction Between Law and Ethics

Concepts	Law	Ethics
Source	External to oneself; rules and regulations of society	Internal to oneself; values, beliefs, and individual interpretations
Concerns	Conduct and actions; what person did or failed to do	Motives, attitudes, and culture; why one acted as one did
Interests	Society as a whole as opposed to the individual within the society	Good of the individual within society as opposed to all of society
Enforcement	Courts, statutes, and boards of nursing	Ethics committees and professional organizations

7. Age-based distribution: The unique needs of each stage of life are acknowledged, with the benefits and burdens shared fairly across generations.

8. Allocation of resources: The nation should balance prudently the amount it spends on health care against other important national priorities.

9. Effectiveness: The new system should deliver care and innovations that work and are wanted by clients. It should encourage the discovery of better treatments. It should enable the academic community and healthcare providers to exercise their responsibility to evaluate and improve health care by providing resources for the systematic study of healthcare outcomes.

10. Quality: The system should deliver high-quality care and provide people with the information necessary to make informed healthcare choices.

11. Effective management: By encouraging simplification and continuous improvement and making the system easier to use for clients and providers, the healthcare system should focus on care rather than administration.

12. Professional integrity and responsibility: The healthcare system should treat the clinical judgments of professionals with respect and protect the integrity of the provider-client relationship while ensuring that health providers have the resources to fulfill their responsibilities for the effective delivery of high-quality care.

13. Fair procedures: To protect these values and principles, fair and open democratic procedures should underlie decisions about the operation of the healthcare system and the resolution of disputes that arise within it.

14. Local responsibility: The healthcare system should allow states and local communities to design effective, high-quality systems of care that serve all their citizens.

J. End-of-Life Issues
  1. Cardiopulmonary resuscitation and do-not-resuscitate orders
  2. Dying at home
  3. Decisions to limit treatments
  4. Withholding of nutrition and fluids
  5. Palliative care
  6. Euthanasia and assisted suicide

IV. Future Considerations and Directions
  A. Genetic Research
    1. Decoding genes that are responsible for specific diseases
    2. Gene therapy
    3. Genetic engineering
    4. Use of genetic information
    5. Cloning
  B. Beginning-of-Life Issues
    1. Abortion
    2. Newborns with severe defects
    3. Fetal tissue experimentation
    4. Genetic counseling
    5. Genetic manipulation
    6. Surrogacy

References

American Nurses Association. (1985). *Code for nurses with interpretive statemetns.* Washington, DC: Author.

American Nurses Association. (2001). *Code of ethics for nurses with interpretive statements.* Washington, DC: American Nurses Publishing.

American Nurses Association. (2004). *Nursing: Scope and standards of practice.* Silver Spring, MD: Author.

American Nurses Association. (2006). *Code of ethics for nurses: Provisions.* Washington, DC: Author.

American Nurses Association. (2010). *Code of ethics for nurses with interpretive statements.* Silver Spring, MD: Author.

Association of Rehabilitation Nurses. (2000). *Standards and scope of rehabilitation nursing practice* (4th ed.). Glenview, IL: Author.

Association of Rehabilitation Nurses. (2003). *ARN position statement on ethical issues.* Glenview, IL: Author.

Association of Rehabilitation Nurses. (2008). *Standards and scope of rehabilitation nursing practice.* Glenview, IL: Author.

Barrocas, A., Yarbrough, G., Bechnel, P., & Nelson, J. E. (2003). Ethical and legal issues in nutrition support of the geriatric patient: The can, should, and must of nutrition support. *Nutrition in Clinical Practice, 18*(1), 37–47.

Beauchamp, R. L., & Childress, J. F. (2001). *Principles of biomedical ethics* (5th ed.). New York: Oxford University Press.

Bergum, V., & Dossetor, J. (2005). *Relational ethics: The full meaning of respect.* Hagerstown, MD: University Publishing Group.

Blanchard, K., & Peale, N. (1988). *The power of ethical management.* New York: William Morrow.

Brillhart, B. A. (1995). Ethics in rehabilitation nursing. *Rehabilitation Nursing, 20*(1), 44–47.

Butts, J., & Rich, K. (2008). *Nursing ethics: Across the curriculum and into practice* (2nd ed.). Boston: Jones & Bartlett.

Cerise, F., & Chokshi, D. (2009). Orienting health care reform around universal access. *Archives of Internal Medicine, 169,* 1830–1832.

Davis, A., & Aroskar, M. (1991). *Ethical dilemmas and nursing practice.* Englewood Cliffs, NJ: Prentice Hall, Inc.

Derstine, J. B., & Hargrove, S. D. (2001). *Comprehensive rehabilitation nursing.* New York: Saunders.

Eckenhoff, E. (1981). The value of the disabled in life. In N. Martin, N. Holt, & D. Hicks (Eds.), *Comprehensive rehabilitation nursing.* New York: McGraw Hill.

Ellis, J. R., & Hartley, C. L. (2007). *Nursing in today's world: Trends, issues & management* (9th ed.). Philadelphia: Lippincott, Williams & Wilkins.

Fletcher, J., Spencer, E., & Lombardo, P. (Eds.). (2005). *Fletcher's introduction to clinical ethics* (3rd ed.). Hagerstown, MD: University Publishing Group.

Frankena, W. K., & Granrose, J. T. (Eds). (1974). *Introductory readings in ethics.* Englewood Cliffs, NJ:Prentice Hall, Inc.

Gadow, S. (1999). Relational narratives: The post-modern turn in nursing ethics. *Scholarly Inquiry for Nursing Practice, 13*(1), 57–70.

Gergen, K. (2009). *An introduction to social construction* (2nd ed.). Thousand Oaks, CA: Sage.

Gilligan, C. (1995). Hearing the difference: Theorizing connection. *Hypatia, 10,* 120–127.

Grace, P. J. (2004). Ethics in the clinical encounter. In S. K. Chase (Ed.), *Clinical judgment and communication in nurse practitioner practice* (pp. 295–332). Philadelphia: F. A. Davis.

Grace, P. J. (2009). *Nursing ethics and professional responsibility in advanced practice.* Sudbury, MA: Jones & Bartlett.

Graham-Eason, C. (1996). Ethical considerations for rehabilitation nursing. In S. Hoeman (Ed.), *Rehabilitation nursing: Process and application* (2nd ed., pp. 34–46). St. Louis: Mosby.

Guido, G. W. (2010). *Legal and ethical issues in nursing* (5th ed.). Upper Saddle River, NJ: Pearson.

Habel, M. (1999). Bioethics: Strengthening nursing's role. *Nurse Week* [Online]. Retrieved from www.nurseweek.com/ce/ce420a.

Hebert, P. (1996). *Doing right: A practical guide to ethics for medical trainees and physicians.* Toronto, Canada: Oxford University Press.

Hinman, L. (2002). *Ethics: A pluralistic approach to moral theory* (3rd ed.). Belmont, CA: Thomson-Wadsworth.

Hoeman, S. (2008). *Rehabilitation nursing: Prevention, intervention, and outcomes* (4th ed.). St. Louis: Mosby Elsevier.

Hoeman, S. P., & Duchene, P. M. (2002). Ethical matters in rehabilitation. In S. Hoeman (Ed.), *Rehabilitation nursing: Process, application, and outcomes* (3rd ed., pp. 45–55). St. Louis: Mosby.

International Council of Nurses. (2006). *International code of ethics.* Retrieved July 28, 2010, from www.icn.ch/images/stories/documents/about/icncode_english.pdf.

Jacobs, B. B. (2000). Respect for human dignity in nursing: Philosophical and practical perspectives. *Canadian Journal of Nursing Research, 32*(2), 15–23.

Jameton, A. (1984). *Nursing practice: The ethical issues.* Englewood Cliffs, NJ: Prentice Hall.

Kalb, K. A., & O'Conner-Von, S. (2007). Ethics education in advanced practice nursing: Respect for human dignity. *Nursing Education Perspectives, 28*(4), 196–202.

Keown, D. (2001). *Buddhism and bioethics.* New York, NY: Palgrave.

MacDonald, C. (2002). *Guide to moral decision making.* Retrieved September 6, 2011, from www.ethicsweb.ca/guide/.

Macrina, F. (2005). *Scientific integrity: Text and cases in responsible conduct of research* (3rd ed.). Washington, DC: ASM Press.

Marquis, B., & Huston, C. (2009). *Leadership roles and management functions in nursing: Theory and application.* Philadelphia: Wolters Kluwer Health/Lippincott Williams & Wilkins.

Masters-Farrell, P. A. (2006). Ethical/legal principles and issues. In K. L. Mauk (Ed.), *Gerontological nursing competencies for care* (pp. 589–618). Sudbury, MA: Jones & Bartlett.

McCarthy, J. (2006). A pluralist view of nursing ethics. *Nursing Philosophy, 7,* 157–164.

McCourt, A. E. (Ed.). (1993). *The specialty practice of rehabilitation nursing: A core curriculum* (3rd ed.). Skokie, IL: Rehabilitation Nursing Foundation of the Association of Rehabilitation Nurses.

Medical College of Georgia. (2000). Ethics syllabus glossary. Retrieved July 18, 2010, from www.mcg.edu/gpi/ethics/phlsyllabus/bioethic.htm.

Morrison, E. E. (2008). *Health care ethics: Critical issues for the 21st century* (2nd ed.). Sudbury, MA: Jones & Bartlett.

National Institute on Disability and Rehabilitation Research. (2006). Welcome to NIDRR. Retrieved May 17, 2010, from www.ed.gov/about/offices/list/osers/nidrr/index.html.

National Institutes of Health, Office of Human Research Protection. (2004). Title 45 Code of Federal Regulations, Part 46, 102 (d). Retrieved July 22, 2010, fromwww.hhs.gov/ohrp/humansubjects/guidance/.

Online Ethics Center for Engineering and Science. (2005). *The Online Ethics Center for Engineering and Science.* Retrieved May 10, 2010, from www.onlineethics.org/.

Paul, R., & Elder, L. (2006). *The miniature guide to critical thinking concepts and tools* (4th ed.). Dillon Beach, CA: Foundation for Critical Thinking.

Pilkington, D., & Strong, S. (2003). *ARN position statement on ethical issues.* Skokie, IL: Association of Rehabilitation Nurses.

Rest, J. R. (1982). A psychologist looks at the teaching of ethics. *Hastings Center Report, 12*(1), 29–36.

Ross, W. D. (2002). *The right and the good.* Oxford: Oxford University Press.

Savage, T., & Michalak, D. R. (1999). Ethical, legal and moral issues in pediatric rehabilitation. In P. A. Edwards, D. L. Hertzberg, S. R. Hays, & N. M. Youngblood (Eds.), *Pediatric rehabilitation nursing* (pp. 62–83). Philadelphia: W. B. Saunders.

Sliwa, J. A., McPeak, L., Gittler, M., Bodenheimer, C., King, J., Bowen, J., et al. (2002). AAP white paper: Clinical ethics in rehabilitation medicine: Core objectives and algorithm for resident education. *American Journal of Physical Medicine in Rehabilitation, 81*(9), 708–717.

Ursery, D. (2005). *Principles of normative ethics.* Austin, TX: St. Edwards University.

Vincler, L. (2008). *Law and medical ethics.* University of Washington School of Medicine, Attorney General. Retrieved July 29, 2010, from http://depts.washington.edu/bioethx/topics/law.html.

Webster, G., & Baylis, F. (2000). Moral residue. In S. Rubin & L. Zoloft (Eds.), *Margin of error: The ethics of mistakes in the practice of medicine* (pp. 217–230). Hagerstown, MD: University Publishing Group.

Suggested Resources

Aiken, T., & Catalano, J. (1994). *Legal, ethical, and political issues in nursing.* Philadelphia: F. A. Davis.

Andrews, M., Goldberg, K., & Kaplan, H. (2004). *Nurses' legal handbook* (5th ed.). Springhouse, PA: Springhouse.

Armstrong, M. (Ed.). (1998). *Telecommunications for health professionals: Providing successful distance education and tele-health.* New York: Springer.

Aveyard, H. (2005). Informed consent prior to nursing care procedures. *Nursing Ethics, 12*(1), 19–29.

Beauchamp, T. L., & Childress, J. F. (2001). *Principles of biomedical ethics* (5th ed.). New York: Oxford University Press.

Benjamin, M., & Curtis, J. (2010). *Ethics in nursing: Cases, principles, and reasoning* (4th ed.). New York: Oxford University Press.

Butler, K. A. (2004). Ethics paramount when patient lacks capacity. *Nursing Management, 35*(11), 18, 20, 52.

Coverston, D., & Rogers, S. (2000). Winding roads and faded signs: Ethical decision-making in a post-modern world. *Journal of Perinatal & Neonatal Nursing, 14*(2), 1–11.

Ellis, J. R., & Hartley, C. L. (2004). *Nursing in today's world: Trends, issues & management* (8th ed.). Philadelphia: Lippincott, Williams & Wilkins.

Esterhuizen, P. (1996). Is the professional code still the cornerstone of clinical nursing practice? *Journal of Advanced Nursing, 23*(1), 25–31.

Fry, S. T., & Johnstone, M. (2006). *Ethics in nursing practice* (3rd ed.). Englewood Cliffs, NJ: Prentice Hall.

Hall, J. (1996). *Nursing ethics and the law.* Philadelphia: W. B. Saunders.

Lachman, V. D. (2006). *Applied ethics in nursing.* New York: Springer.

Rumbold, G. (1999). *Ethics in nursing practice* (3rd ed.). Philadelphia: W. B. Saunders.

Salladay, S. (1996). Rehabilitation ethics and managed care. *Rehab Management, 9*(6), 38–42.

Scanlon, C., & Fibison, W. (1995). *Managing genetic information: Implications for nursing practice.* Washington, DC: American Nurses Association.

Silva, M. (1995). *Ethical guidelines in the conduct, dissemination, and implementation of nursing research.* Washington, DC: American Nurses Association.

Sletteboe, A. (1997). Dilemma: A concept analysis. *Journal of Advanced Nursing, 26,* 449–454.

Trandel-Korenchuk, D., & Trandel, K. (1997). *Nursing and the law.* Gaithersburg, MD: Aspen.

Westrick, S., & McCormack-Dempski, K. (2009). *Essentials of nursing law and ethics.* Sudbury, MA: Jones & Bartlett.

CHAPTER 4
Empirics in Rehabilitation Nursing: Research and Evidence-Based Practice

Linda L. Pierce, PhD RN CNS CRRN FAHA FAAN • Pamala D. Larsen, PhD RN CRRN FNGNA

The rehabilitation nurse is responsible for using best practices when caring for clients and fostering the advancement of rehabilitation nursing knowledge. Research problems often emerge from nursing practice. According to Burns and Grove (2009), research is a systematic process to validate and refine existing knowledge and generate new knowledge. Evidence-based practice (EBP) is an effort to integrate the best research evidence with the clinician's expertise, the client's values (preferences), and the need to provide high-quality and cost-effective health care (Burns & Grove).

The process of conducting research, publishing the findings, critiquing and synthesizing current knowledge, and applying it to practice is time-consuming. Research shows that very few nurses use research findings when making clinical practice decisions. For example, it may take up to 2 decades for research findings to be translated into nursing practice (Balas & Boren, 2002; Green & Seifert, 2005; Institute of Medicine, 2001). With the explosion of knowledge and the rapid changes that are taking place in health care today, it is imperative that research evidence be translated more quickly into clinical practice. According to Melnyk and Fineout-Overholt (2011), EBP is a way of getting information about the most up-to-date practice into the hands of clinicians.

A major force guiding the blending of the research process with EBP is the 2005 Association of Rehabilitation Nursing (ARN) research agenda (Jacelon, Pierce, & Buhrer, 2007), which identifies four high-priority research areas

- Nursing and nursing-led interdisciplinary interventions to promote function in people of all ages and those with disability or chronic health problems
- Experience of disability or chronic health problems for individuals and families across the lifespan
- Rehabilitation in the changing healthcare system
- The rehabilitation nursing profession

To use research findings in practice and promote ARN's research agenda, rehabilitation nurses need a thorough grounding in the fundamentals of the research process and EBP that together form the foundation for rehabilitation nursing practice. To assist in developing this knowledge and skill, this chapter differentiates research from EBP, describes the importance of EBP to the advancement of rehabilitation nursing, identifies basic sources of research and EBP problems, describes ways to evaluate these problems, distinguishes levels of evidence, identifies ways of locating and then evaluating the literature, and concludes with specific examples of key elements to the application of EBP in rehabilitation nursing practice.

I. **Research and EBP**

Although often used interchangeably, *research* and *EBP* are distinctly different in terms of definitions and associated processes. It is important to recognize that research creates the foundation for EBP.

A. Nursing Research: *Nursing research* is a "scientific process that validates and refines existing knowledge and generates new knowledge that directly and indirectly influences the delivery of evidence-based nursing practice" (Burns & Grove, 2009, p. 3). The research process is orderly and planned, investigates a specific problem, ends with an outcome in the form of results and recommendations, and contributes to the understanding of the phenomenon in question (e.g., pain, anxiety).

1. Major contributions of nursing research to rehabilitation nursing
   a. Builds professionalism that defines the parameters of rehabilitation nursing
   b. Provides accountability (e.g., establishes standards of care, addresses cost containment issues)
   c. Validates the social relevance of nursing and promotes the efficacy of nursing in the changing healthcare arena
   d. Expands the knowledge related to rehabilitation nursing (e.g., education, consultation, administration, theory, the basis for nursing decision making, evaluation of expected outcomes)

2. Paradigms of nursing research: The researcher's worldview (professional perspective) influences what is investigated, the way the research question is stated, and the methods that are selected to generate the knowledge. Two paradigms, worldviews, or frameworks have had an impact on nursing and other disciplines: the empirical paradigm and the naturalistic paradigm.
   a. The empirical paradigm, or quantitative perspective, purports that there is an objective, ordered, and nonrandom reality.

b. The naturalistic paradigm, or qualitative perspective, holds that reality is subjective, mentally constructed by those participating in the research, and variable.

c. Neither viewpoint is better than the other; however, the paradigm that the researcher selects determines how the research is conducted.

3. Purposes of nursing research (Burns & Grove, 2009)

a. Description: Depicts the characteristics of individuals, groups, situations, and health states

b. Exploration: Investigates the dimensions of a phenomenon and helps to develop and refine research hypotheses

c. Explanation: Attempts to understand the underpinnings of phenomena and their interrelationships

d. Prediction and control: Forecasts how combinations of variables will operate in different circumstances involving different people

4. Limitations of research

a. General limitations such as inevitable study flaws (e.g., in design, sampling techniques, data collection and analysis methods, measurement of variables)

b. Moral and ethical constraints, such as those related to informed consent, risks and benefits, freedom from harm or exploitation, the right to privacy, and fair treatment

c. Complexity of human beings

d. Measurement and data collection difficulties, such as concerns about how to capture the phenomenon that is the focus of the research

e. Obstacles to having complete control in the research situation, such as extraneous variables (they can compete with the independent variable as an explanation for the dependent variable) and the dynamic nature of the study phenomena (Burns & Grove, 2009)

B. EBP

1. EBP is a problem-solving approach that informs clinical practice. It integrates

a. A systematic search and critical appraisal of the most relevant evidence to answer clinical questions

b. One's own clinical experience

c. Client values and preferences (Burns & Grove, 2009; Melnyk & Fineout-Overholt, 2011).

2. Client situations are not static, diagnoses may be imprecise, the pathophysiology may be unclear, and client responses to interventions may vary.

a. Evidence is used to either support current practice or guide changes in practice.

b. EBP is broader than research-based practice or research use because the evidence comes not only from research and other sources such as expert opinions but also incorporates the clinical expertise of the care provider along with client preferences (Porter-O'Grady, 2006).

c. EBP is the result of obtaining comprehensive information pertaining to a specific topic, critically evaluating the evidence, and synthesizing the evidence to make conclusions about the knowledge of a topic (Burns & Grove, 2009).

d. Clinical judgment demands a precise and critical examination of the most current science and application of this evidence only when it is relevant to a particular client's condition.

e. Two aspects must be present when one uses evidence or current science to make a clinical decision (Melnyk & Fineout-Overholt, 2011).

1) Validity (level and rigor or strength) of the evidence

2) Applicability to the specific situation: Research evidence does not always have a linear relationship to practice. Client characteristics, study circumstances, and measurement factors can dramatically affect the applicability of findings to another practice situation.

C. Terminology Related to Research and EBP

1. Clinical nursing research: Research designed by nurses and other interdisciplinary professionals to generate knowledge to guide nursing practice and improve the health and quality of life of nurses' clients

2. Phenomena: Observable facts or events that reflect concepts (e.g., observation of a high prevalence of falls on a unit leads one to identify related concepts such as fatigue, vision changes, and environmental factors such as slippery floors)

3. Qualitative research: "The systematic, interactive subjective approach used to describe life-experiences and give them meaning" (Burns & Grove, 2009, p. 717)

4. Quantitative research: "The formal, objective, systematic study process to describe and test relationships and to examine cause-and-effect interactions among variables" (Burns & Grove, 2009, p. 717)

5. Descriptive research: "Research that has as its main objective the accurate portrayal of the characteristics of persons, situations, or groups, or the frequency with which certain phenomena occur" (Polit & Beck, 2008, p. 752)

6. Experimental research: Objective, systematic, controlled study to test the effects of an intervention or treatment on selected outcomes (Burns & Grove, 2009; Melnyk & Fineout-Overholt, 2011). "This is the strongest design for testing cause-and-effect relationships" (Melnyk & Fineout-Overholt, p. 575)

7. Randomized clinical trial: A full experimental test of an intervention involving random assignment (an equal opportunity to be selected for either group); "Phase III of a full clinical trial" (Polit & Beck, 2008, p. 764)

8. Quasi-experimental research: "A type of experimental design that tests the effects of an intervention or treatment but lacks one or more characteristics of a true experiment (e.g., random assignment, a control or comparison group)" (Melnyk & Fineout-Overholt, 2011, p. 580)

9. Evidence-based theory: A theory that has been tested and supported through the accumulation of research findings

10. Opinion leaders: People in an organization who are most likely to influence change because they are usually highly knowledgeable and well respected (Melnyk & Fineout-Overholt, 2011)

11. Research application: Use of the evidence or findings (research knowledge) in clinical practice settings, often based on a single study (Melnyk & Fineout-Overholt, 2011)

12. Terms that are often confused with EBP are *best evidence* and *best practice*. Research involving clinical trials generally is equated with best evidence, whereas best practice is practice that results in the best possible client outcomes (Melnyk & Fineout-Overholt, 2011).

D. Importance of EBP to Rehabilitation Nursing: Rehabilitation nurses function in a dynamic healthcare setting that demands constant decision making in complex circumstances. EBP promotes the use of the best current evidence in these important day-to-day client care decisions. For nurses who function at the highest professional level and strive for the best client outcomes, EBP is a cornerstone of practice. EBP has four components essential to the advancement of rehabilitation nursing practice (The Joanna Briggs Institute, 2008; Law, 2002).

1. Evidence generation occurs where there is an awareness of the current evidence (preferably from the last 5 years) that forms the foundation of rehabilitation nursing practice.

2. Evidence synthesis involves consultation with the client to choose the care strategy that best fits the client and his or her circumstances. Central to

this behavior are excellent communication skills and the ability to educate and work with the client and family to achieve a positive outcome.

3. Evidence or knowledge transfer: Clinical judgment is essential in ascertaining the quality of the evidence and the applicability of the interventions to the particular client and care situation.

4. Evidence use in which creativity and insight must be coupled with nursing skills to determine how the evidence fits and is implemented in specific practice situations

E. Importance of Research and EBP Dissemination and Use in Rehabilitation Nursing Practice

1. The generation and refinement of nursing knowledge through research, whether quantitative or qualitative, is a complex process requiring a special set of skills and resources. An important and equally time-intensive aspect of the research endeavor is disseminating newly obtained knowledge to other professionals through publication or presentation. Even for very accomplished researchers, dissemination of research and use of it in practice poses a special set of challenges. To provide the foundation for EBP, researchers must consistently disseminate their findings, making the research-generated information available to practitioners for scrutiny and application in their practice settings and available to other researchers for replication. Ideally, the results will be published in refereed journals such as *Rehabilitation Nursing, Western Journal of Nursing Research, Nursing Research,* or other professional journals that are widely recognized nationally or internationally.

2. Unfortunately, the literature suggests that the time between generation and implementation of research findings can be lengthy. A classic example is in the case of research evidence indicating that aspirin could reduce the likelihood of myocardial infarction and stroke; it took almost 17 years for the U.S. Food and Drug Administration to approve this preventive use (Marwick, 1997).

F. Barriers to Research

1. Research findings may not address current clinical problems.

2. Findings are not communicated in a form that practitioners can readily understand.

3. There is resistance to change in the agency.

4. Practitioners do not feel confident in reading research reports and articles and mentors are not available to assist them in critically analyzing materials.

5. Practitioners do not know how to apply research findings to practice.

6. There is a lack of administrative support for research and research use (Estabrooks, Floyd, Scott-Findlay, O'Leary, & Gushta, 2003; Grol & Wensing, 2004; Newhouse, Dearholt, Poe, Pugh, & White, 2005).
7. These barriers can be reframed as opportunities and can facilitate practice using the best available evidence to achieve the best possible outcomes. A variety of models exist that describe how research dissemination and use should occur.
   a. Rogers's (1995) theory of diffusion of innovations
   b. Havelock's (1973) linker systems, describing how innovation connects to the user
   c. Stetler's (1994) model of research use
   d. Rosswurm and Larrabee's (1999) model for change to EBP

G. Specific Ways Rehabilitation Nurses Can Participate in Research
1. Communicate and use the findings of nursing research from publications (journals, newsletters), posters, paper presentations, nursing grand rounds, and e-mails featuring research abstracts.
2. Read and critique research articles to determine strengths, limitations, and applicability to your practice situation.
3. Start or participate in a journal club.
4. Participate in a research team consisting of nurse researchers and clinicians and other healthcare team members.
5. Replicate a study already reported in the literature.
6. Promote excitement and a research-friendly atmosphere that encourages use of research and EBP.
7. Form nursing committees to discuss the current state of research and EBP related to a common client problem and, if needed, ways to overcome barriers to use of current knowledge and practice guidelines.

H. Common Sources of Research Problems
1. Personal experiences and everyday rehabilitation nursing practice
2. Unanswered questions in the literature
3. Research priorities or agendas set by various organizations
4. Outside sources such as agencies, clients, families, or other healthcare professionals who express concerns related to quality of care (Pierce, 2009)
5. Theories or conceptual frameworks that stimulate questions: Once a problem has been identified that sparks the researcher's interest, the topic is transformed into a list of questions that can be converted into researchable problem statements.

The difficulty for most researchers is that the questions or hypotheses (relationship statements of concepts) are too broad and not researchable. Therefore, developing precise questions that people passionately want answered is a vital step in the research process. In addition, after the problem is stated succinctly, it must be evaluated to determine whether the next step in terms of performing the research is appropriate (Pierce, 2009).

I. Determining the Significance of the Problem and Its Relevance to Rehabilitation Nursing
1. Using current literature (preferably from the last 5 years) and other forms of available knowledge, determine whether this problem is worth investigating further.
2. Determine whether the problem will expand or improve rehabilitation nursing practice.

J. Assessing the Researchability of the Problem
1. Avoid questions based on values because these questions are not researchable (e.g., "Do nurse practitioners provide better care than physicians?").
2. Determine whether it is possible to obtain the data needed to examine the questions emerging from the problem within a quantitative or qualitative framework.
3. Determine the feasibility of the research by giving early consideration to factors such as time, place, space, and resource materials, which can help identify practical problems such as financial constraints, theoretical problems, control of extraneous variables, or ethical issues that influence the researcher's decision about conducting the study.
4. Assess the availability of subjects (e.g., access and willingness of people to participate).
5. Determine the participation from others (e.g., institutions and agencies, permission of the study population or their guardians or parents) that is needed.
6. Determine the facilities and equipment that are needed (e.g., availability of office or interview space, computers, printers).
7. Estimate financial resources, including funding from public or private, international, national, regional, and local sources.
8. Assess the experience of the researchers, including knowledge about and experience in executing all aspects of the investigation.
9. Address ethical considerations related to working with human subjects, including informed consent, freedom from harm, privacy, anonymity, confidentiality, and voluntary participation.

a. The principal investigator is responsible for ensuring that human rights are not violated.

b. All people involved in the research, such as the data collectors, have the same ethical responsibilities as the principal investigator.

II. **Quantitative and Qualitative Research Designs That Build the Foundation for EBP**

Quantitative and qualitative research and mixed methods that incorporate both approaches create the scientific knowledge to expand and refine practice and form the foundation of EBP. This section is a brief overview of major distinctions between the two research paradigms and key elements to consider when examining the quality of the evidence generated and its generalizability or transferability to your practice situation. Even well-designed research targeted at a different client population may not be transferable to your practice setting. Nurses must evaluate both the strengths and the limitations of the study or studies pertaining to their topic of interest. This critique is a pivotal aspect of EBP, along with consideration of the clinician's expertise and the client's preferences and values.

A. Quantitative Research Designs: **Table 4-1** describes the most common quantitative research designs (Burns & Grove, 2009; Polit & Beck, 2008).

B. Evaluating Quantitative Studies: The focus of this section is a general approach to evaluating quantitative research.

1. Quantitative research reports can be evaluated on several criteria (Burns & Grove, 2009; Polit & Beck, 2008; Rempher & Silkman, 2007).

a. Problem statement, research question, and study purpose

1) Is the problem statement identified and clear?

2) Are key study concepts identified?

3) Does the research question fill a void in nursing knowledge or a theory or model?

4) Does the research problem clearly flow from the stated research purpose?

5) Are *who, what, where, when,* and *why* clearly presented in the research question?

Table 4-1. Types of Quantitative Research Designs

Type of Design	Description	Strengths	Limitations	Examples
Experimental research	A type of research that predicts and controls phenomena, examining causality At least one variable is manipulated. Control exists over the experimental situation. Random assignment.	The most effective way to test hypotheses The most powerful and best-controlled research	Not all variables can be manipulated. Manipulation can create ethical problems. Artificiality is problematic. Generalizability can be limited.	Pretest-posttest design Solomon four-group design Factorial design Repeated-measures design
Quasi-experimental research	One independent variable is manipulated. Lacks at least one of the other two properties that characterize a true experiment.	Practical Feasible Generalizable	Control is lacking, so other hypotheses may exist.	Nonequivalent control group (no randomization) Time series One-group, pretest-posttest design
Nonexperimental research	Researcher collects data without introducing any treatment or changes.			Ex post facto Descriptive research Retrospective and prospective studies Survey research Evaluation research Need assessments Meta-analysis Delphi survey Methodological research Content analysis study

6) Do the research problem and question flow coherently from the stated purpose of the study?

7) Does the purpose statement indicate the study population and the dependent and independent variables? (The dependent variable is the outcome variable or the variable of "effect"; the independent variable is the "cause," or the variable that is presumed to influence the dependent variable or is the treatment or intervention in a study.)

8) Is the research hypothesis (relationship between variables or concepts) measurable and justifiable?

b. Literature review and conceptual or theoretical framework

1) Does the literature give the reader an orientation to what is already known about the topic?

2) Is the literature current and does it include classic studies on the topic? The majority of the reported studies should be less than 5 years old. In addition, current literature should be related to historical research.

3) How does the current literature address knowledge gaps or reflect an improvement in how data are collected or consideration of other variables not studied in the past that could affect study outcomes?

4) Is the significance of the problem being studied thoroughly explained?

5) Is it clear what must be done to fill the void in current literature?

6) If the researcher has provided a conceptual model or theory to guide the study design and data interpretation, does it coherently fit the problem and question under investigation?

7) Are the research variables thoroughly defined?

c. Sample selection, methods, and design

1) Is it clear what method was used to select the sample?

2) Was the process of subject recruitment described?

3) Is it clear what the inclusion and exclusion criteria were for subject selection?

4) Is the sample size appropriate and representative of the population of interest?

5) Is the research design the most rigorous design to address the hypothesis or research questions?

6) Did the researcher provide a rationale for the choice of design?

7) Is the sample size appropriate to address the hypothesis or research question?

8) Was a power analysis used to determine the sample size and does it appear justified?

9) Does the data collection procedure avoid bias?

10) If there was an intervention, was enough detail given to replicate the study?

11) Are the appropriate statistical procedures used to address the hypotheses?

12) Is a rationale provided for the use of the selected statistical tests?

d. Human rights protection

1) Was information included that addressed the protection of human subjects?

2) Was a human subject review of some kind conducted?

3) Is it clear that the study benefits outweighed the potential participant risk?

e. Results, discussion, and limitations

1) Is it clear how the statistical findings relate to the research questions or hypotheses and to the conceptual or theoretical framework?

2) Were tables used to organize large amounts of data?

3) Were limitations to the study discussed?

4) Were important results discussed?

5) Were the data interpretations consistent with the reported results?

6) Did the researcher describe the implications for practice and future research?

2. Approaches to critiquing research literature vary. Evans and Shreve (2000) suggested using the ASK model to critique quantitative studies.

a. **A:** Applicability of the study to nursing practice is assessed (e.g., are the materials relevant to the reader's practice; are the findings significant; do the potential benefits to the client, one's practice, or the agency outweigh the risks of implementing the intervention; is the change cost effective [e.g., time, money, equipment]; and is the outcome for the client or agency worth the effort needed to implement the change?).

b. **S:** Science of the study is judged, including a statement of the problem, purpose, research question or hypothesis, theoretical framework, method, and data analysis.

c. **K:** Knowledge generated from the study is appraised (e.g., do the results fit the existing knowledge base or are they opposite to what is known, and what does the reader need to know before the use of the results could be rejected?).

3. A simpler approach to evaluating quantitative research studies includes the following three questions, identified by O'Rourke and Booth (2000):
   a. Are the study results valid? This refers to whether the results of the study were obtained from rigorous methods and not compromised by bias, anything that would distort the findings, confounding variables, or some unknown variable not investigated (Melnyk & Fineout-Overholt, 2011).
   b. Are the results of the study reliable? This pertains to "whether or not the effects of a study have sufficient influence on practice, clinically and statistically; that is, the results can be counted on to make a difference when clinicians apply them to their practices (Melnyk & Fineout-Overholt, 2011).
   c. Will the results help locally? Are the problems dealt with in the study sufficiently comparable to the present setting to extrapolate the findings?

C. Characteristics of Qualitative Research Studies
   1. Are descriptive or theory building, can be used to develop hypotheses, and can be used to study phenomena about which little is known
   2. Consist of a design that emerges from the data (i.e., questions may change or the focus may be refined during data collection); see **Table 4-2** for different design methods
   3. Have a purposive sample: Participants are selected because they have some characteristic in common.
   4. Allow collection of data to occur in the natural or field setting: Data are collected in the participant's home or natural context.
   5. Involve the researcher closely with the participants
      a. The researcher is immersed in the data.
      b. The researcher's goal is an in-depth understanding of the phenomena under study.
   6. Entail holistic data collection (e.g., interviews, observation, focus groups, observation of participants)
   7. Use inductive data analysis, which proceeds from the specific to the general
   8. Use a narrative approach to report research outcomes: Lengthy, rich descriptions of the data are reported.

D. Evaluating Qualitative Research Reports: The focus of this section is a general narrative literature approach to evaluation. It is not representative of a systematic review, integrative review, or meta-analysis, but identifies key questions to assess the overall quality of a

Table 4-2. Types of Qualitative Research

Type	Description
Grounded theory	Develops theories and theoretical propositions that are based on real-world observations; focuses on process
Ethnography	Focuses on the culture of the people being studied
Phenomenology	Considers the lived experience of the people being studied
Historical research	Explores the past and applies findings to present and future
Case studies	In-depth studies on one particular case
Field studies	Examine people and how they function in real life

qualitative study (Burns & Grove, 2009; Cohen & Crabtree, 2008; Ryan, Coughlan, & Cronin, 2007).

1. Statement of the phenomenon of interest
   a. Is the phenomenon of interest clearly identified?
   b. Has the researcher identified why the phenomenon requires qualitative methods?
   c. Are the philosophical underpinnings of the research described?
2. Purpose
   a. Is the purpose of conducting the research made explicit?
   b. Does the researcher describe the projected significance of the work to nursing?
3. Method
   a. Is the method used to collect data compatible with the purpose of the research?
   b. Is the method adequate to address the phenomenon of interest?
4. Sampling
   a. Does the researcher describe the selection of participants?
   b. Is purposive sampling used?
   c. Are the informants who were chosen appropriate to inform research?
5. Data collection
   a. Is data collection focused on human experience?
   b. Does the researcher describe data collection strategies (e.g., interview, observation, field notes)?
   c. Is protection of human subjects addressed?
   d. Is saturation of the data described?
   e. Are the procedures for collecting data made explicit?
6. Data analysis

a. Does the researcher describe the strategies used to analyze the data?

b. Has the researcher remained true to the data?

c. Does the reader understand the procedures used to analyze the data?

d. Does the researcher address the credibility, auditability, and fittingness of the data?

   1) Credibility: Do the participants recognize the experience as their own?

   2) Auditability: Can the reader follow the thinking of the researcher? Does the researcher document the research process?

   3) Fittingness: Can the findings be applied outside the study situation? Are the results meaningful to people not involved in the research?

e. Is the strategy used for analysis compatible with the purpose of the study?

7. Findings

a. Are the findings presented within a context?

b. Is the reader able to apprehend the essence of the experience from the report of the findings?

c. Are the researcher's conceptualizations true to the data?

d. Does the researcher place the report in the context of what is already known about the phenomenon?

8. Conclusions, implications, and recommendations

a. Do the conclusions, implications, and recommendations give the reader a context in which to use the findings?

b. Do the conclusions accurately reflect the findings of the study?

III. Levels of Evidence

The evidence on which EBP is based must be the result of sound, well-conducted studies using the appropriate design (whether quantitative or qualitative) that provides high-quality data to answer the research questions or hypotheses. It is imperative for the nurse to be able to critically evaluate research when performing a literature review on a specific topic.

A. Evidence Levels: In the literature there are a variety of descriptions of how to label levels of evidence. Burns and Grove (2009, p. 29) describe levels of evidence from strongest or the best evidence to weakest research evidence; this chatper uses those descriptions to categorize levels of evidence.

1. "Systematic review of experimental studies (well designed randomized controlled trials [RCTs])

2. Meta-analyses of experimental (RCT) and quasi-experimental studies

3. Integrative reviews of experimental (RCT) and

quasi-experimental studies

4. Single experimental study (RCT)

5. Single quasi-experimental study

6. Meta-analysis of correlational studies

7. Integrative reviews of correlational and descriptive studies

8. Qualitative research metasynthesis and metasummaries

9. Single correlational study

10. Single qualitative or descriptive study

11. Opinions of respected authorities based upon clinical evidence, reports of expert committees."

B. Melnyk and Fineout-Overholt's Seven Critical Steps of the EBP Process: Other models can be used to examine the evidence, such as the Iowa Model of Evidence-Based Practice and Research Utilization and the ACE Star Model from the University of Texas at San Antonio.

1. Develop a spirit of inquiry.

2. Ask the burning clinical questions (PICOT components).

a. **P:** Patient population of interest

b. **I:** Intervention or issue of interest

c. **C:** Comparison of interest

d. **O:** Outcome of interest

e. **T:** Time it takes for the intervention to achieve the outcome

3. Seek and collect the most relevant and best evidence.

4. Critically appraise the evidence.

a. What were the study results?

b. Are the study results valid (sound scientific methods used)?

c. Will the study findings facilitate care?

5. Integrate the best evidence: Can the study evidence be incorporated into the clinician's practice given the clinician's expertise, the clinical resources available, and the client's preferences?

6. Evaluate the outcomes or the effectiveness of the evidence-based interventions for a particular client or care situation.

7. Communicate and disseminate the outcomes of the EBP changes and decision (Melnyk & Fineout-Overholt, 2011).

IV. Locating the Evidence

There are many resources for searching for evidence on a topic. More information is becoming available online, and it is important to evaluate online evidence as thoroughly as evidence in print.

A. Searching for the Evidence

1. Traditional sources of evidence such as peer-reviewed journals, books, and non–peer

reviewed professional magazines make up scholarly publications. Conversely, the World Wide Web, available 24 hours a day, is made up of interconnected documents that are available through the Internet (e.g., PubMed). Published articles, program descriptions, personal opinions, government documents, and information on businesses, organizations, and agencies are posted to websites. Once traditional and electronic publications are retrieved, scientific publications must be evaluated (Pierce, 2007).

2. Essential steps of a search strategy:
   a. Step 1: Formulate a clear, well-built clinical question without jargon or ambiguity.
   b. Step 2: Determine the type of database that is appropriate for the question. Examples of electronic bibliographic databases that rehabilitation nurses may find useful are presented in **Table 4-3**.
   c. Step 3: Decide which type of study design would best answer the question.
   d. Step 4: Enter a subject heading or text word search guided by the PICOT components of the question.
   e. Step 5: Start combining searches to find relevant evidence.
   f. Step 6: Further restrict combined searches for study design, methods, indicators of clinical meaningfulness, or other appropriate, available limits. Consider limiting the search to English language and human subjects depending on the question and the searcher.
   g. Step 7: Apply a priori inclusion and exclusion criteria to studies gathered in the search to

find the best available evidence (Melnyk & Fineout-Overholt, 2011). A librarian may be helpful in choosing search terms that aid in narrowing the topic (Pierce, 2009).

3. Indexes and other sources
   a. The CINAHL index is "in nursing the most relevant print database which contains citations of nursing literature published after 1955" (Burns & Grove, 2009, p. 94). The CINAHL database is available at www.ebscohost.com/cinahl.
   b. The Cochrane Central Register of Controlled Trials contains published articles from bibliographic databases such as MEDLINE (The Cochrane Library, 2010).
   c. The Cochrane Database of Methodology Reviews is prepared by the Cochrane Collaboration and includes full texts of systematic reviews of empirical methodological studies (The Cochrane Library, 2010).
   d. The Cochrane Database of Systematic Reviews is prepared by the Cochrane Review Groups in the Cochrane Collaboration; each review is highly structured and systematic, with evidence included or excluded on the basis of explicit quality criteria to minimize bias (The Cochrane Library, 2010; Melnyk & Fineout-Overholt, 2011).
   e. The Cochrane Methodology Register is a bibliography of publications (e.g., books, journal articles, and conference proceedings) that report on methods used in the conduct of controlled trials (The Cochrane Library, 2010).

Table 4-3. Examples of Electronic Bibliographic Databases

Name	Purpose
AgeLine	AgeLine focuses on publications related to older adults and aging.
CancerLit	CancerLit contains citations and abstracts for cancer literature.
CANE	Clearinghouse on Abuse and Neglect of the Elderly is the nation's largest computerized collection of elder abuse resources and materials.
CINAHL	Cumulative Index to Nursing and Allied Health Literature contains publications from nursing and allied health professionals.
CDSR	Cochrane Database of Systematic Review contains full-text summaries of randomized trials for the effects of treatments and, when appropriate, the results of other research on a particular topic.
ERIC	Education Resources Information Center displays materials from the field of education.
MEDLINE	MEDLINE (National Library of Medicine) is a compilation of medical and biomedical publications.
MedlinePlus	MedlinePlus presents health information from the National Library of Medicine and has extensive information from the National Institutes of Health and other trusted sources.
PubMed	PubMed is a service of the U.S. National Library of Medicine and is composed of more than 20 million citations for biomedical literature from MEDLINE, life science journals, and online books.

f. Clinical practice guidelines: The classic and accepted definition from the Institute of Medicine is "systematically developed statements to assist practitioner and patient decisions about appropriate health care for specific clinical circumstances" (Field & Lohr, 1990, p. 38).

g. MEDLINE is the bibliographic database covering the fields of medicine, nursing, dentistry, veterinary medicine, the healthcare system, and the preclinical sciences from the National Library of Medicine (U.S. National Library of Medicine, 2010), available at www.ncbi.nlm.nih.gov/sites/entrez.

h. The National Guideline Clearinghouse includes summaries of evidence-based clinical practice guidelines and related documents (National Guideline Clearinghouse, 2010). A condensed version of the guideline and a link to the full clinical practice guideline are available at www.guideline.gov.

i. PsycINFO: This database contains literature in behavioral and social sciences and mental health (American Psychological Association, 2010) and is available at www.apa.org/pubs/databases/psycinfo/index.aspx.

B. Outcomes of the Search: One of the most difficult decisions for the researcher is deciding when enough literature is enough.

1. Use the most current literature in the search. Begin with the last 5 years.

2. Incorporate the classic research literature related to a topic. If you see a researcher's name in all the studies you read and many studies refer to the seminal work by a certain author, then it is important to include that author in the literature you are using. For example, anyone working on the concept of locus of control would have to include Rotter, who conducted the seminal work on locus of control in 1966. If you did not refer to that body of knowledge, then your review would be incomplete.

V. **Assessing the Evidence for EBP**

A. Four Types of Literature Reviews

1. Narrative review

a. Summarizes different primary studies that support an author's point of view from which conclusions are drawn based on the reviewer's interpretation; presents a general background discussion for a particular issue or topic (Melnyk & Fineout-Overholt, 2011)

b. Not systematic in its approach to identifying articles and papers.

2. Systematic review: "A summary of evidence typically conducted by an expert or expert panel on a particular topic, that uses a rigorous process (to minimize bias) for identifying, appraising, and synthesizing studies to answer a specific clinical question and draw conclusions about the data gathered" (Melnyk & Fineout-Overholt, 2011, p. 582).

3. Meta-analysis: "A statistical pooling of the results from several previous studies into a single quantitative analysis that provides one of the highest levels of evidence for an intervention's efficacy" (Burns & Grove, 2009, p. 708). A meta-analysis provides a single effect measure of all the summarized study results (Melnyk & Fineout-Overholt, 2011).

4. Meta-synthesis: "The grand narratives or interpretive translations produced from the integration or comparison of findings from qualitative studies" (Polit & Beck, 2008, p. 758). A meta-synthesis is not a literature review, nor is it a concept analysis (Polit & Beck).

B. Systematic Reviews: These identify, appraise, and synthesize research evidence based on a strict protocol that can be made available to clinicians, policy decision makers, and clients. Systematic reviews are a rigorous approach to minimize bias and compile many studies and relate them to a specific research question (Burns & Grove, 2009; Melnyk & Fineout-Overholt, 2011).

1. Questions for the critical appraisal of the quality of a systematic review (Craig & Smyth, 2007)

a. Does the review include a purpose statement (objectives) and research question that are clear?

b. Was a systematic and comprehensive search strategy identified for relevant studies?

c. Were the inclusion and exclusion criteria for the studies plainly stated and appropriate?

d. Is the quality of the studies gauged appropriately?

e. For the reviewed studies, are the results combined systematically and appropriately?

f. Are the conclusions supported by the data?

2. Phases of a systematic review (Melnyk & Fineout-Overholt, 2011)

a. Phase 1: Deciding what clinical question to propose and the most appropriate research design to answer it

b. Phase 2: Developing inclusion and exclusion criteria for the studies to be included and excluded in the analysis

c. Phase 3: Seeking out and retrieving published and unpublished literature related to the

study question and answering the critical appraisal questions
  d. Phases 4 and 5: Assessing the quality and validity of the studies
  e. Phase 6: Extracting the data from individual studies
  f. Phase 7: Providing an overview evaluation of the studies
3. Example of a systematic review in the literature: The citation for this systematic review is Pearson et al. (2006). What follows is a description of how the various phases of this approach pertain to Pearson's article, which represents a review of a topic with many facets. All phases are applicable to any systematic review.
  a. Phase 1: Deciding what clinical question to propose. Question: What is the best available evidence on the effect of team characteristics, processes, structure, and composition in the context of collaborative practice among nursing teams to create a healthy work environment?
  b. Phase 2: Developing inclusion and exclusion criteria. The search strategy was to find published and unpublished studies in the English language. Inclusion and exclusion criteria were described in terms of type of studies (qualitative and quantitative), type of participants, type of interventions (nursing staff outcomes, client outcomes, and organizational and system outcomes).
  c. Phase 3: Seeking out and retrieving published and unpublished literature. A three-step search approach was used.
    1) Initial limited search of MEDLINE and CINAHL databases to identify search terms, followed by an analysis of text words contained in the title and abstract to describe the article
    2) More extensive search using all the identified keywords and index terms
      a) Search of the reference list led to the identification of more studies.
      b) The databases searched included CINAHL (1982–2005), MEDLINE, other nonindexed citations and Ovid, Cochrane Library, Database of Abstracts of Reviews of Effectiveness, PsycINFO, Embase, Sociological Abstracts, Econ Lit, ABI/Inform, ERIC, and PubMed.
  d. Phases 4 and 5: Assessing quality and validity of the studies. Studies that met the inclusion criteria were identified and grouped into the

following categories: experimental studies, descriptive, descriptive-correlational, interpretive and clinical research, cost minimization studies, and textual and opinion papers. All results were assessed by two independent reviewers for methodological quality, and the review was completed by the System for the Unified Management of the Review and Assessment of Information (SUMARI) package. The two independent reviewers determined that the examined studies fit the identified inclusion and exclusion criteria.
  e. Phase 6: Extracting the data from individual studies. Results of the methodological assessment indicated quantitative and qualitative data. The quantitative data were extracted using a work based on the Cochrane Collaboration and Center for Reviews and Dissemination (Pearson et al., 2006, pp. 154–157), and qualitative data were extracted using the SUMARI package (Pearson et al., pp. 158–159).
  f. Phase 7: Providing an overview evaluation of the studies. Peer review was done by two independent reviewers. Data were synthesized quantitatively and qualitatively through the use of several instruments and software packages that were clearly described (Pearson et al., 2006, pp. 121–122).
4. Additional resources and examples of systematic reviews
  a. Houde (2009; resource)
  b. Windle (2010; resource)
  c. Johnston and Chu (2010; example)
  d. Poslawsky, Schuurmans, Lindeman, and Hafsteinsdottir (2010; example)
C. Meta-Analysis: A *meta-analysis* is a "technique for quantitatively integrating the result of multiple similar studies addressing the same research question" (Polit & Beck, 2008, p. 758). A meta-analysis is an analysis of several analyses and therefore contributes to building evidence. Although a meta-analysis provides a simple and precise estimate of the benefit and harm of the interventions examined, it should be used with caution. In addition, sources of bias and differences may exist between the various clinical research trials, and the conclusions recommended as describing the "average" or "usual" client may actually be unhelpful in clinical practice (Burns & Grove, 2009; Law, 2002; Melnyk & Fineout-Overholt, 2011). The following example of a meta-analysis is from Hodgkinson, Koch, Nay, and Kim (2006):

1. Purpose: To present the best available evidence for strategies to prevent or reduce the frequency of medication errors associated with prescribing, dispensing, and administering medications in older adults (65 and older) who are in acute, subacute, and residential settings
2. Search strategy: PubMed, Embase, Current Contents, Cochrane Library
3. Selection criteria: Systematic reviews, RCTs, other research methods such as nonrandom controlled trials, longitudinal studies, cohort or case-control studies, descriptive studies evaluating strategies to reduce medication errors
4. Data collection and analysis: Tabulated relative risks, odds ratios, mean differences, and associated 95% confidence intervals calculated from comparative studies. All other information is provided in a summary format.
5. Results of the meta-analysis: Most common medication errors occurred in hospitals and were medication ordering, dispensing, administration, and medication recording errors. Contributing factors associated with these hospital errors are largely unreported. In the community improper drugs were ordered, administration errors occurred, and incorrect doses were ordered.
6. The evidence from this meta-analysis revealed common medication errors, but the assumption cannot be made that this always happens.

D. Limitations of Systematic Reviews and Meta-Analyses
1. A disadvantage of systematic reviews is the information cannot be generalized. A systematic review is so detailed that it can be applied only to the specific clinical question that was proposed.
2. A meta-analysis may be detrimental when the studies are too different to combine in a statistically meaningful way (Melnyk & Fineout-Overholt, 2011).

VI. **Using the Evidence: Translating Research into Practice**
Although EBP will advance the quality of care for clients and the practice of rehabilitation nursing, the use of EBP has lagged far behind expectations. Unfortunately, on average it takes 2 decades for new knowledge generated by RCTs, the highest level of evidence, to be incorporated into clinical practice, and even then its application is highly irregular (Balas & Boren, 2002; Institute of Medicine, 2001). Additional research involving countries such as the United States and the Netherlands indicates that in all practice settings at least 30% of clients do not receive care according to current scientific evidence, and another 20% or more of the provided care is not needed or is potentially harmful (Grol & Grimshaw, 2003). New

strategies and models must be developed and implemented to increase the speed with which scientific evidence is instituted in clinical settings. In addition, rehabilitation nurses and researchers need to remain aware of ARN's research agenda (Jacelon et al., 2007), which identifies focus areas to be developed in our specialty.

A. Translating Research into Practice and Policy (TRIPP): Cosponsored by the Agency of Healthcare Research and Quality and the National Cancer Institute, TRIPP (2006) was formed to close the gap between knowledge and practice (between what we know and what we do) and to ensure continued improvement of health care. TRIPP's overriding purpose is to facilitate the translation of research findings into sustainable improvements in health outcomes, quality, effectiveness, efficiency, and cost effectiveness of care.

B. Approach: Although there is no uniform consensus on how to translate evidence into clinical practice, the following steps capture the essence of a suggested approach.
1. Assess the need for change in practice.
2. Link the problem with interventions and outcomes.
3. Synthesize the best evidence.
4. Design a change in practice.
5. Implement and evaluate practice.
6. Integrate and maintain the practice change.

C. Development of EBP in Rehabilitation Nursing
1. EBP has been identified as critical to the present and future practice of rehabilitation nursing. This commitment to EBP is reflected in ARN's publications and practice standards. Although great strides in knowledge have occurred, many areas of EBP in rehabilitation nursing are in their infancy. According to the Rehabilitation Nursing Research Agenda, additional evidence is needed for nursing and nursing-led interdisciplinary interventions to promote function in people of all ages with disability or chronic health problems, experience of disability or chronic health problems for individuals and families across the lifespan, rehabilitation in the changing healthcare system, and the rehabilitation nursing profession (Rehabilitation Nursing Foundation, 2005).
2. Rehabilitation nurses must become EBP practitioners. Whether they are expert rehabilitation nurses or new nurses in this specialty area, all should strive to identify and evaluate current scientific information that can affect practice. Also, EBP practitioners need to foster adoption and sustainability of EBP and educate other nurses

and health professionals about its value. A key component of successful EBP outcomes is the recognition and initiation of interventions at the individual and organizational level that begin to consider the interaction between the individual, social, organizational, and economic factors that affect EBP.

VII. Key Factors Affecting Implementation and Adoption of EBP

A. Implementation: The key factors to implementing EBP are similar to those associated with implementing research.
   1. Change in practice is difficult for the agency, individual units, and healthcare providers.
   2. Practitioners and agencies do not know how to apply the evidence to practice.
   3. Administration is unsupportive of the evidence.

B. Examples of How EBP Can Be Used in Practice: In health care there are a number of guidelines that in the past may have been titled "best practice." The following guidelines for clinical practice can be supported with EBP.
   1. Clinical practice guidelines (CPGs) are systematically developed statements that assist practitioner and client in formulating decisions about appropriate health care. They my be based on expert opinion or consensus or evidence-based practice as identified by research (Burns & Grove, 2009; Melnyk & Fineout-Overholt, 2011). Examples clinical practice guidelines can be found at www.guideline.gov/.
   2. Algorithms are "written guidelines to stepwise evaluation and management strategies that require observations to be made, decisions to be considered, actions to be taken, and basically CPGs arranged in a decision-tree format" (Law, 2002, p. 201). A good example of algorithms can be found in the Inpatient Rehabilitation Facility Patient Assessment Instrument manual and scoring of the FIM™ instrument.
   3. A clinical pathway is a framework or guide based on previous research, agency data, or clinical experience to define expected care actions and outcomes in a particular care situation (Burns & Grove, 2009). Interventions commonly included in a clinical pathway are consultations and referrals; assessments and observations; tests, treatments, measurements, and diagnostics; nutrition, medications, activity, and mobility; safety; client and family education or teaching; and discharge planning and follow-up.

   4. Healthcare policies and laws are derived from evidence. Legislators cannot propose legislation without having the necessary substantiation, based on various sources of evidence (Melnyk & Fineout-Overholt, 2011).

C. Concluding Thoughts
   1. Research is a systematic investigation to validate and refine existing knowledge and generate new knowledge.
   2. Nursing research is part of that planned systematic investigation that collects data to answer questions and collect evidence.
   3. Evidence-based practice is a systematic process that includes using research findings to improve practice.
   4. Moderated by expert clinical opinions and client circumstances and preferences, the evidence is then applied by nurses and other interdisciplinary professionals to improve judgments made in the delivery of care and to facilitate cost-effective care.
   5. The vision for nursing in the 21st century is to narrow the gap between research and practice by helping nurses base their decisions and practice strategies on the best available evidence, thereby improving nursing care and outcomes.
   6. Research is essential to creating best practices that include protocols and procedures as well as evidence-based guidelines.

References

American Psychological Association. (2010). *PsycINFO*. Retrieved July 22, 2011, from www.apa.org/pubs/databases/psycinfo/index.aspx.

Balas, E. A., & Boren, S. A. (2002). Managing clinical knowledge for health care improvement. In J. Bemmel, A. T. McCray (Eds.), *Yearbook of medical informatics* (pp. 65–70). Bethesda, MD: National Library of Medicine.

Burns, N., & Grove, S. (2009). *The practice of nursing research: Appraisal, synthesis, and generation of evidence* (6th ed.). St. Louis: Elsevier Saunders.

The Cochrane Library. (2010). *About the Cochrane collection*. Retrieved July 22, 2011, from www.thecochranelibrary.com/view/0/AboutTheCochraneLibrary.html#CENTRAL.

Cohen, D., & Crabtree, B. (2008). Research in health care: Controversies and recommendations. *Annals of Family Medicine, 6*(4), 331–339.

Craig, J., & Smyth, R. (2007). *The evidence-based practice manual for nurses* (2nd ed.). Edinburgh, Scotland: Churchill Livingstone.

Estabrooks, C. A., Floyd, J. A., Scott-Findlay, S., O'Leary, K. A., & Gushta, M. (2003). Individual determinants of research utilization: A systematic review. *Journal of Advanced Nursing, 43*(5), 506–520.

Evans, J., & Shreve, W. (2000). The ASK model: A bare bones approach to the critique of nursing research for use in practice. *Journal of Trauma Nursing, 7*(4), 83–90.

Field, M., & Lohr, K. (Eds.). (1990). *Clinical practice guidelines: Directions for a new program.* Washington, DC: National Academy Press.

Green, L., & Seifert, C. (2005). Translation of research into practice: Why we can't "just do it." *The Journal of the American Board of Family Practice, 18,* 541–545.

Grol, R., & Grimshaw, J. (2003). From the evidence to best practice: Effective implementation of change in patient's care. *Lancet, 362,* 1225–1230.

Grol, R., & Wensing, M. (2004). What drives changes? Barriers to and incentives for achieving evidence-based practice. *Medical Journal of Australia, 180,* 557–560.

Havelock, R. G. (1973). *The change agent's guide to innovation in education.* Englewood Cliffs, NJ: Educational Technology in Education.

Hodgkinson, B., Koch, S., Nay, R., & Kim, N. (2006). Strategies to reduce medication errors with reference to older adults. *International Journal of Evidence-Based Healthcare, 4*(1), 2–41.

Houde, S. C. (2009). The systematic review of the literature. *Journal of Gerontological Nursing, 35*(9), 9–13.

Institute of Medicine. (2001). *Crossing the quality chasm.* Washington, DC: National Academies Press.

Jacelon, C. S., Pierce, L. L., & Buhrer, R. (2007). Revision of the rehabilitation nursing research agenda. *Rehabilitation Nursing, 32*(1), 23–30.

Johnston, M., & Chu, E. (2010). Does attendance at a multidisciplinary outpatient rehabilitation program for people with Parkinson's disease produce quantitative short term or long term improvements? A systematic review. *NeuroRehabilitation, 26*(4), 375–383.

The Joanna Briggs Institute. (2008). *The JBI approach to evidence-based practice.* Retrieved July 22, 2011, from www. joannabriggs.edu.au/.

Law, M. (2002). *Evidence-based rehabilitation: A guide to practice.* Thorofare, NJ: SLACK Incorporated.

Marwick, C. (1997). Aspirin's role in prevention now official. *Journal of the American Medical Association, 277*(9), 701–702.

Melnyk, B. M., & Fineout-Overholt, E. (2011). *Evidence-based practice in nursing & healthcare: A guide to best practice* (2nd ed.). Philadelphia: Lippincott Williams & Wilkins.

National Guideline Clearinghouse. (2010). *About NGC.* Retrieved July 22, 2011, from www.guideline.gov/about/index.aspx.

Newhouse, R., Dearholt, S., Poe, S., Pugh, L. C., & White, K. M. (2005). Evidence-based practice: A practical approach to implementation. *Journal of Nursing Administration, 35*(1), 35–40.

Pearson, A., Porritt, A., Doran, D., Vincent, L., Craig, D., Tucker, D., et al. (2006). A comprehensive systematic review of the evidence on the structure, process, characteristics and composition of a nursing team that fosters a healthy work environment. *International Journal of Evidence Based Healthcare, 4,* 118–159.

Pierce, L. (2007). Evidence-based practice in rehabilitation nursing. *Rehabilitation Nursing, 32*(5), 203–209.

Pierce, L. (2009). Twelve steps for success in the nursing research journey. *Journal of Continuing Education in Nursing, 40*(4), 154–162.

Polit, D. F., & Beck, C. T. (2008). *Nursing research: Generating and assessing evidence for nursing practice* (8th ed.). Philadelphia: Lippincott Williams & Wilkins.

Porter-O'Grady, T. (2006). A new age for practice: Creating the framework for evidence. In K. Malloch & T. Porter-O'Grady (Eds.), *Introduction to evidence-based practice* (pp. 1–27). Sudbury, MA: Jones & Bartlett.

Poslawsky, I. E., Schuurmans, M. J., Lindeman, E., & Hafsteinsdottir, T. B. (2010). A systematic review of nursing rehabilitation of stroke patients with aphasia. *Journal of Clinical Nursing, 19*(1–2), 17–32.

Rehabilitation Nursing Foundation. (2005). *Rehabilitation nursing research agenda* (2nd ed.). Retrieved July 22, 2011, from www.rehabnurse.org/pdf/ResearchAgendaFlyer.pdf.

Rempher, K. J., & Silkman, C. (2007). How to appraise quantitative research articles. *American Nurse Today, 2*(1), 26–28.

Rogers, E. M. (1995). *Diffusion of innovations* (4th ed.). New York: Free Press.

Rosswurm, M. A., & Larrabee, J. H. (1999). A model for change to evidence-based practice. *Image: Journal of Nursing Scholarship, 31*(4), 317–322.

Rotter, J. (1966). Generalized expectancies for internal versus external control of reinforcements. *Psychological Monographs, 80,* Whole No. 609.

Ryan, F., Coughlan, M., & Cronin, P. (2007). Step-by-step guide to critiquing research. Part 2: Qualitative research. *British Journal of Nursing, 16*(12), 738–744.

Stetler, C. B. (1994). Refinement of the Stetler/Marram model of application of research findings to practice. *Nursing Outlook, 42*(1), 15–25.

Translating Research into Practice and Policy. (2006). Retrieved July 22, 2011, from www.academyhealth.org/files/2006/abstracts/PartII/TranslatingResearchIntoPolicyPractice.pdf.

U.S. National Library of Medicine. (2010). *MEDLINE fact sheet.* Retrieved July 22, 2011, from www.nlm.nih.gov/pubs/factsheets/medline.html.

Windle, P. E. (2010). The systematic review process: An overview. *Journal of PeriAnesthesia Nursing, 25*(1), 40–42.

CHAPTER 5
Rehabilitation Nursing and Case Management

Donna Williams, MSN RN CRRN • Kathryn Doeschot, MSN RN CRRN

Case management is a model of care delivery that has been shown to be a key strategy and innovative approach to managing healthcare services and improving client care. It is comprehensive and client centered and it promotes continuity of care across all settings. Our rapidly changing healthcare system demands financial and clinical outcomes within an appropriate timeframe and with appropriate use of resources. Case management provides a framework for assessing, planning, implementing, and evaluating care and is an effective process for working in the increasingly complex, fragmented, and constrained system of healthcare delivery.

Clients of all ages are served by rehabilitation nurse case managers. In assigning a nurse case manager, consideration should be given to the client's age, diagnosis, and severity of the illness or injury because specialized knowledge may be an important factor in achieving goals.

The objectives of this chapter are to define case management and describe the role of the nurse case manager and the scope of case management. Models, functions, and the processes that affect the quality and cost-effectiveness of healthcare services will be identified. The rehabilitation nurse is in a unique position to serve as a case manager because of his or her specialized knowledge, experience, and holistic approach.

I. **Historical Perspectives on Case Management**
   A. Early 1900s: Social and Legislative Changes
      1. 1920: The Smith-Fess Act, the beginning of public rehabilitation programs, provided funds for vocational guidance, training, occupational adjustment, prosthetics, and placement services.
      2. 1943: The Vocational Rehabilitation Act updated the Smith-Fess Act and included physical restoration and services to people with mental and psychiatric disabilities. It required states to submit a written state plan to the federal government.
      3. 1945: Liberty Mutual hired nurses to coordinate care for their insured.
      4. 1965: Workers' Compensation Rehabilitation Law placed an emphasis on the workplace.
      5. 1965: Medicare and Medicaid were established and required discharge planning.
      6. In the 1970s the Insurance Company of North America began as the first private sector rehabilitation company.
      7. 1973: Public awareness of the needs of the disabled increased and the Vocational Rehabilitation

Act was renamed to the Rehabilitation Act, the foundation for the Americans with Disabilities Act. An Individual Written Rehabilitation Program ensured the involvement of the consumer in developing a rehabilitation plan of action.
   B. Insurance Industry
      1. 1970: Nurses and vocational rehabilitation counselors coordinated care and created long-term plans for people with disabilities.
      2. Entrepreneurs began independent practice in the 1970s, mostly for workers' compensation.
      3. 1993: Boston Consulting Group coined the term *disease management,* an approach to managing specific diseases and client populations.
   C. Facility-Based Case Management
      1. 1980s: Case management was developed in facilities to avoid duplication of services, evaluate care, and contain costs while improving the effectiveness of care (Cohen & Cesta, 2005).
      2. Roots in primary nursing
   D. Government Case Management Programs
      1. 1973: The Health Maintenance Organization Act focused on prevention, wellness, and case management of costs.
      2. 1983: The Social Security Act, amended to include diagnosis-related groups (DRGs), propelled case management into acute settings as hospitals were reimbursed a fixed DRG-specific amount for each client treated.
      3. 1980s: The Department of Veterans Affairs and TRICARE, health insurance for military dependents and retirees, established the use of case management to optimize services and achieve high-quality care.

II. **Definitions of Case Management**
   A. The Association of Rehabilitation Nurses: The process of assessing, planning, organizing, coordinating, implementing, monitoring, and evaluating the services and resources needed to respond to a person's healthcare needs (ARN, 2010).
   B. Case Management Society of America (CMSA): A collaborative process of assessment, planning, facilitation, care coordination, evaluation, and advocacy for options and services that meet an individual's and family's comprehensive health needs through

communication and available resources to promote high-quality, cost-effective outcomes (CMSA, 2010).

C. American Nurses Association (ANA): A dynamic and systematic collaborative approach to provide and coordinate healthcare services to a defined population. It is a participative process to identify and facilitate options and services for meeting people's health needs while decreasing fragmentation and duplication of care and improving cost-effective clinical outcomes. The framework for nursing case management includes five essential functions: assessment, planning, implementation, evaluation, and interaction (ANA, 2007).

III. **Standards of Practice**

A. ARN: Standards were developed in 1994 and updated in 2008. Rehabilitation nursing is viewed as a specialty practice guided by philosophy, theory, and research.
1. Scope of practice
2. Standards of care
3. Standards of professional performance
4. Case manager role description

B. CMSA: Standards were developed in 1995 and updated in 2010. Standards provide a parameter for knowledge, skill, behavior, and practice.
1. Voluntary practice guidelines
2. Define practice settings, roles, and functions
3. Identify standards and how they are demonstrated
4. Encourage use of evidence-based practice

C. ANA: *Standards of Practice* were updated in 2010 and articulate the who, what, when, where, and how of practice. *Code of Ethics for Nurses,* updated in 2010, establishes guidelines for carrying out nursing responsibilities in a manner consistent with quality in nursing care and the ethical obligations of the profession (see www.nursingworld.org).

D. International Academy of Life Care Planners (IALCP): Standards of practice for this subspecialty role were developed in 2002 and revised in 2006.
1. Standards of practice
2. Philosophical overview and goals
3. Roles and functions
4. Standards of performance

IV. **Goals of Case Management**
The goal of case management is the provision of high-quality, cost-effective health and social services. The nurse case manager realizes this goal by organizing rehabilitation and other necessary healthcare services to promote outcomes that will encourage the highest possible level of independence and quality of life for the client (ARN, 2010).

A. Improve Quality Through Appropriate and Timely Use of Services and Resources
1. Meets expected outcomes; promotes optimal functioning and independence in the least restrictive environment
2. Reduces risk of complications by facilitating communication between team members and ensuring that needed services are provided in a timely manner
3. Improves coping with injury, illness, or disability
4. Facilitates successful return to work, school, and community by identifying and including all appropriate team members

B. Facilitate Outcomes of Case Management
1. Coordinates care by ensuring access to healthcare services and monitoring all health care provided to the client.
2. Promotes collaborative practice through ongoing communication with the identified team in each practice setting on the continuum.
3. Educates or promotes the education of clients about their health status and prevention of complications or further disability. Emphasis is placed on self-management and responsibility for healthcare needs.
4. Advocates for the client's optimal functioning and independence in the community by providing the tools necessary to achieve that level of functioning.

V. **Models of Case Management**
Models of case management can be determined by a number of factors. A facility or company may determine its own model or process of how case management is completed. Case management is determined in part by the setting and factors that may include whether the case management is episodic or for an illness, injury, disease, or event.

A. Setting: Case management services are provided in institutional, residential, outpatient, and community settings. These settings may include acute care facilities, rehabilitation facilities, outpatient facilities, skilled nursing facilities or nursing homes, residential facilities, daycare agencies, private residences, or the workplace.

B. Employment: Case managers may be employees, contractors, or private practitioners. Many organizations develop their individual model, or process, of case management.
1. Facility- or agency-based case manager: A case manager employed by a healthcare facility, government or private agency, or healthcare provider. This case manager is responsible for quality and cost-effectiveness of care delivery from

admission to discharge. Research has shown that case management promotes organizational success by reducing length of stay and improving reimbursement.

2. Insurance-based case manager: A case manager employed by a third-party payer (e.g., an insurance company)
   a. The case manager may be responsible for managing acute or chronic disease or incident-based injury or illness. Disease management manages specific diseases across the continuum and promotes aggressive prevention of complications and treatment of chronic conditions.
   b. In workers' compensation the case manager is responsible for coordinating the medical care with a goal of return to work and the file may close after return to work or at the time of settlement.

3. Employer-based case manager: A case manager retained by an employer to provide case management services directly to employees
   a. The case manager may be involved in industrial illness or injury.
   b. The case manager may be responsible for coordinating medical benefits provided by the employer and for promoting wellness.

4. Independent case manager: A private case manager whose services are retained by a third-party payer, facility, attorney, agency, or individual or family. Responsibilities may include all those of other case manager types, depending on the referral source.

VI. **Role Functions and Processes**

A. Client Identification: Early identification of clients who would benefit from case management is essential to successful achievement of outcomes and should occur at the onset of injury or diagnosis of chronic illness.

1. Facility-based case managers, inpatient and outpatient, typically serve all admitted clients and initiate services upon admission.

2. External case managers may receive referrals from insurance carriers; other third-party payers; attorneys; physicians; or concerned parties such as family members, agencies, or protective services. Individual clients may also self-identify and self-refer. Case managers can help referral sources establish appropriate criteria for identifying those who would benefit from case management.

3. Insurance case managers may identify potential recipients of case management by diagnosis of chronic diseases or catastrophic injury. Insurance companies often establish triggers for case management referral, such as high-dollar cases, excessive or inappropriate use of resources, or presence of comorbidities.

B. Data Collection and Assessment

1. Obtains all necessary authorizations to contact the client and family for an initial interview and assessment

2. Reviews and analyzes referral information in consultation with the client, health team members, employers, family, legal representatives, and claims and insurance personnel as indicated

3. Reviews and assesses the client's personal, social, economic, and environmental information and medical history, current status, diagnosis, prognosis, current treatment plan, and care provider's level of knowledge. For catastrophic injuries or illness, an on-site assessment of the client and anticipated or actual provider is highly recommended to determine whether the provider will be able to meet the client's needs.

4. Assesses the client's learning needs related to the medical diagnosis and prognosis, treatment providers, treatment options, financial resources (including specifics of insurance coverage), psychosocial adjustment and coping mechanisms, and vocational rehabilitation needs and potential

5. Assesses the family's knowledge, health status, expectations, and the potential for or actuality of a family member acting as the primary caregiver if necessary

6. Identifies the team members appropriate for each client

C. Data Analysis and Problem Identification

1. Identifies temporary or permanent alterations in function that have resulted from the injury or illness

2. Identifies potential challenges or complications of physiological or psychosocial function

3. Identifies potential challenges in community reintegration where appropriate

4. Identifies the learning needs of the client and significant others

5. Considers the vocational and history prognosis for re-entering or entering the workforce when appropriate

D. Establishment of Goals and Plan of Care

1. Establishes realistic goals to achieve optimal outcomes for the client within available resources; this is done in collaboration with the client and family and the interdisciplinary team

2. Helps the client, family, and team identify the variables that may influence the accomplishment of goals (**Figure 5-1**)
3. Develops a comprehensive plan that includes short- and long-term goals and preventive treatment measures for potential complications and health maintenance; identifies alternatives for the client's treatment when appropriate, including consideration of options of treatment site and potential use of resources, both private and public.
4. Establishes target dates for achievement of goals.
5. Includes evidenced-based practice

E. Implementation and Coordination
1. Uses rehabilitation principles to plan an individualized program for maximizing function to promote identification of optimal outcomes for the client
2. Provides ongoing assessment of the progress of the client and the participation and educational needs of the client, family, and caregivers to evaluate the effectiveness of the treatment plan
3. Coordinates access to accelerated or alternative care options when appropriate
4. Coordinates access to appropriate government and community programs and resources
5. Coordinates and evaluates in a quality-conscious, cost-effective manner the client's and family's use of medical equipment, supplies, medications, and the full spectrum of services
6. Provides instruction to the client and family based on identified learning needs
7. Coordinates referrals for instruction or counseling for the client and family based on identified learning needs

8. Provides education, guidance, and recommendations to the payer about alternatives for care and services where appropriate
9. Intervenes promptly when necessary to promote optimal functioning and prevention or treatment of complications
10. Facilitates and collaborates with the healthcare team for timely discharge planning to an alternative level of care or return to the community when appropriate
11. Coordinates the discharge plan with the healthcare team and providers
12. Educates the client and family on care options and choices, allowing informed decisions even when the decisions are suboptimal or different from the case manager's recommendations

F. Monitoring
1. Ongoing assessment to promote awareness of potential or real complications and the need for plan revision
2. Adherence to the plan
3. Achievement of benchmarks

G. Evaluation
1. Goals and outcomes are monitored continuously.
2. Progress toward goals is evaluated and modified if necessary.

H. Quality Management: A method for assessing how the case manager changes the structure and process of care. Identifies which clinical, administrative, physiological, and client outcomes are influenced by those changes. The goal is to ensure that case management activities are effective and efficient.

I. Outcomes
1. Outcome measurement is a systematic method of assessing the extent to which a program has achieved its intended result and provides professionals with feedback that helps them improve achievement of goals. Measurements may vary depending on the information sought, but a standard tool that includes treatment trends, history, clinical decisions, and results of treatment allows review and alterations of or options for the treatment plan.
2. Categories of measurement of client outcomes include physiological, psychosocial, functional, behavioral, knowledge, home functioning, family strain, safety, symptom control, quality of life, goal attainment, client satisfaction, use of services, and nursing diagnosis resolution (Cohen & Cesta, 2005). Case management practitioners can apply these categories to clarify and specify the results of intervention for individuals and groups.

Figure 5-1. Case Management Variables in Achieving Optimal Outcomes

THE SPECIALTY PRACTICE OF REHABILITATION NURSING

J. Cost Management: The case manager's role in cost management depends on the setting, expected function, and situation. Case managers may recommend and arrange for the purchase of services and supplies and negotiate and coordinate care and services, resulting in effective use of resources. This results in an opportunity for creativity and development of nontraditional options to meet individual client needs.

VII. Certification
  A. Certified Rehabilitation Registered Nurse (CRRN): First offered in 1984 by ARN; requires 2 years of experience as a registered nurse in rehabilitation nursing
  B. Certified Case Manager (CCM): First offered in 1993 by the Commission for Case Manager Certification; requires licensure in professional healthcare and 2 years of experience in case management
  C. ANCC: First offered in 1998 by the American Nurses Credentialing Center. Focused on facility-based practice, the application criteria include licensure as a registered nurse with a minimum of 2 years' full-time work and 2,000 hours of practice.

VIII. Accreditation and Regulation
  A. The Joint Commission determined measures for meeting discharge planning criteria, including documentation of a formal plan of care with expected client outcomes, in 1996. Case managers may be assigned responsibility for discharge planning.
  B. The Commission on Accreditation of Rehabilitation Facilities (CARF) developed standards for medical rehabilitation case management that were implemented July 1, 1999. CARF believes that case management is an integral part of rehabilitation care. Coordination, communication, and advocacy are primary themes in the CARF standards.
  C. The American Health Care Commission/Utilization Review Accreditation Commission developed a process in 1998 to accredit case management programs in organizations including hospitals, health maintenance organizations, preferred provider organizations, and third-party administrators that promote innovation and best practice in the case management industry.

IX. Life Care Plans
  Life care plans were introduced into rehabilitation and the legal literature in 1981 as part of a rehabilitation evaluation to project the impact of catastrophic injury on a person's future. A life care plan was distinguished from a discharge plan by its projection of costs of medical and associated care over a person's lifetime. The life care planner may be a nurse, case manager, physician, or other allied health professional. The case manager may also be involved in overseeing the implementation of the plan.

A. Definition of Life Care Plan: The IALCP defines a life care plan as a dynamic document based on published standards, a comprehensive assessment, data analysis, and research. It provides an organized, concise plan for current and future needs with associated costs for people who have sustained catastrophic injury or have chronic healthcare needs (IALCP, 2006).
  1. Uses of life care plans
    a. Identification of future care needs and costs for attorneys working on personal injury cases
    b. Identification of potential costs ("reserves") for insurance or reinsurance companies to specify damages resulting from injury
    c. Guide case management activities for catastrophic injuries and illnesses
    d. Tool for clients of any age and their families to anticipate and self-monitor care
    e. Tool for expenditures from group healthcare plans and special needs trusts in catastrophic injury or illness
  2. Principles of life care planning
    a. Must be consistent with the clinical needs of the client and should reflect strategies to minimize potential complications
    b. Must include healthcare needs (e.g., evaluations and treatment, medications, supplies, equipment, and attendant or nursing care) and quality of life needs (e.g., recreation, housing, transportation)
    c. Comprehensive plans prepared by assessment of all medical records and other data that might affect the plan (e.g., school and employment records), interview or observation of the client and care provider, and collaboration with treating professionals
  3. Certificate training programs: Programs include University of Florida, Kaplan University, and Capital University Law School.
  4. Certifications
    a. Certified Life Care Planner (CLCP): Administered through the International Commission on Health Care Certification
    b. Certified Nurse Life Care Planner (CNLCP): Offered through the American Association of Nurse Life Care Planners
B. Medicare Set-Asides: Regulated by the Centers for Medicare and Medicaid Services (CMS). A Medicare set-aside (MSA) is a fund to protect Medicare's interests in workers' compensation case settlements and in personal injury cases for people on Medicare or expected to enroll in Medicare within 30 months of settlement. The MSA allocates a portion of the settlement for future medical expenses related to the

injury that would otherwise be funded by Medicare. MSAs may require submission to and approval by the CMS, dependent on the amount of the settlement and on whether the client is already on Medicare.

X. **Advanced Practice**
   A. ANA has recognized advanced practice as a specialization, expansion of practice and knowledge, and graduate-level course of study, although there is active dialogue between ANA and advanced practice nurses about the definition of the advanced practice nurse. Nurses with master's degrees, certified and noncertified, working in the field of case management have expanded responsibilities in that arena. It is recognized that these nurses conduct comprehensive assessments and function autonomously, have advanced skill in leadership and education, and show expert skill in the diagnosis and treatment of complex responses to actual or potential health problems resulting from an altered functional ability and altered lifestyle secondary to a physical disability or chronic illness.
   B. Expanded Nurse Case Manager Functions
      1. Clinician: Uses advanced assessment skills to determine healthcare needs, establish the plan of care, and monitor the progress and outcomes
      2. Educator: Provides information about the plan of care to team members and information on the diagnosis and plan of care to the client
      3. Manager: Manages, assigns, and delegates tasks to team members in a cost-effective manner; organizes appropriate treatments
      4. Consultant: Addresses factors affecting outcomes, ensures quality of care, and acts as a resource
      5. Collaborates with physicians and other healthcare professionals using effective communication styles
      6. Develops and coordinates the plan of care throughout the continuum of care
      7. Researcher: Redesigns plans of care based on outcomes and evidence-based practice and monitors the quality of each plan
      8. Fiscal responsibility: Is familiar with pertinent financial, regulatory, and accreditation issues in whatever setting practice occurs

XI. **Issues**
   A. Multistate Licensure: Nurse licensure rules and regulations were initially formed when nursing was practiced primarily within the boundaries of one state and usually within a facility or agency. As access to health care, the mobility of the population, and coverage by insurance companies change, nurses may find themselves providing services to clients who travel across multiple state lines. Many state nursing licenses are not recognized by other states. This is problematic for case managers providing telephonic services across state lines or on-site services that may cross state lines for border areas. The following are issues for case managers in multistate practice:
      1. There may be additional costs for licensure.
      2. Nurses may be more vulnerable to lacking malpractice insurance. This may affect the employer as well.
      3. As of June 2010, 24 state boards of nursing have joined to form a Nurse Compact in which states mutually recognize nurse licenses from other states.
      4. A CMSA position paper revised in 2006 addresses the problem and may be found at http://CMSA.org.
   B. Education and Certification: The process of case management continues to develop as healthcare systems change, definitions are refined, job functions evolve, and the needs of the consumer and payer grow. Requirements for basic education and continued education will continue to change. Confusion about eligibility for the roles and certification must be addressed because there are trends toward increasing legislation, rules, and regulations in case management practice (Huber, 2006).

XII. **Implications for Practice**
   A. Leadership
      1. Case managers are in a prime leadership position. The case manager assumes responsibility for communication, collaboration, negotiation, and resolution of conflict between team members while identifying and coordinating the treatment plan. Conflict can arise from difficulty in fulfilling the plan because of economic, time, or other resource limitations or lack of client or family understanding. In complex cases multiple providers can be treating the client and may be unaware of the work of other providers. The case manager may be instrumental in identifying all current providers, establishing communication between them, and leading them through the process of coordinated care.
      2. Review of leadership theory and processes may be useful to the nurse seeking case management positions.
   B. Potential Ethical Conflicts in Case Management
      1. Interdisciplinary teamwork involves collaboration, typically through team meetings. Members work together and share resources to arrive at a

decision or position that balances ethical and cost concerns. Through this synergistic process the team model provides support, expertise, and guidance that would not otherwise be available to individual professionals. Many managed care organizations are structured to allow this type of professional interaction.

2. Interdisciplinary teams present potential for ethical conflicts between members because they are
   a. Holistic (addressing medical, social, and functional needs)
   b. Comprehensive in their analysis of cases
   c. Diverse in experience, cultural background, skills, and perspectives
3. Characteristics of case management that may present barriers to ethically appropriate care
   a. Accountability for cost of care: When a physician or medical center is held financially accountable for a client's costs of care, the client-physician relationship may be significantly affected by attempts to contain costs at the expense of client health and well-being. The case manager may feel pressure to prioritize financial goals above care outcome goals.
   b. Proactive care planning: Consideration must be given to future needs. Professionals may be conflicted by their loyalty and commitment to provide necessary care and the need to promote individual autonomy or respect of the client's right to self-determination.
   c. Outpatient services: Such services, whether provided in the clinic or home, help to avoid more costly hospitalizations. Comprehensive assessments must be completed to ensure that care plan recommendations are practical and within the ability of the client and family to perform. Conflict may arise if there is disagreement about the ability to participate in a home or clinic setting.
   d. Interventions for the general population: Most managed care plans exclude inefficient or costly approaches or those that have not been shown in research studies to have sufficient efficacy. Therefore, treatments that may benefit clients with particular conditions may not be covered by managed care organizations. Many payers are experimenting with various guidelines for treatment as they consider approval for plans of care.
4. Factors influencing the effectiveness of an interdisciplinary team

a. One of the most basic barriers to the effectiveness of interdisciplinary team planning is related to autonomy and the goals and desires of the client and her or his family. When these goals and desires are at odds with those presumed by the team, recommendations are likely to bring little improvement.
b. Some cases may be more difficult for a team care approach. The overall effectiveness of a team may be compromised by the lack of clear and concise goals.
c. The means of measuring and demonstrating savings are inadequate when a team approach is used to plan for high-risk clients, particularly older adults. Although it has been very difficult to evaluate outcomes in older adults with debilitating conditions or comorbidities by using existing measures, multiple studies and evidence-based programs for seniors are finding some success in keeping seniors healthier and in their own homes. Challenges include financial viability and sustainability.
d. Because the team process is time consuming and costly, team members often are pressured to demonstrate that the approach meets clients' needs in a cost-effective manner.
5. Principles to promote organizational ethics
   a. Build on an organization's existing resources.
   b. Understand that initially all ethics programs experience growing pains and may meet resistance.
   c. Establish a high level of ethical behavior and accountability.
   d. Encourage and support professionals' efforts toward spiritual growth.
6. Ethical concepts
   a. Elements of ethical competence
      1) Commitment to client well-being: Case managers must ensure that client-centered care and services are provided.
      2) Responsibility and accountability: Through coordination activities, case managers monitor the effectiveness of the plan and can reinforce the accountability of others who are responsible for achieving specific goals or performing specific tasks within the plan.
      3) Ability to act as an effective advocate: With access to and knowledge of the healthcare system, the case manager acts as an advocate for clients within the system and coordinates community-based services.

4) Ability to mediate ethical conflicts: Case managers are in a position to identify ethical conflicts and seek resolution through ethics consultations and other means.

5) Ability to recognize ethical dimensions of practice: Skill in identifying potential ethical dilemmas is derived from an ability to analyze situations from multiple perspectives.

6) Ability to critique the potential to influence a person's well-being: With the availability of new healthcare technologies, case managers must analyze the potential of various interventions (both positive and negative).

b. Ethical approaches

1) Generally, the *principle-based approach* consists of traditional principles of autonomy, beneficence, nonmaleficence, and justice. Ethical dilemmas arise when the case manager cannot uphold one or more of these principles. Case managers may be seen as both a client advocate for care and the gatekeeper of services.

2) The *care-based approach* is based on the professional–client relationship and focuses on the totality of the client's life. It attends to the client's needs and interests while attempting to resolve ethical conflicts by improving relationships between the client, professional, and family.

3) The *shared decision-making model* recognizes the importance of considering the expertise and opinion of both the client and the professional when making a decision. Professionals give the client the information, skills, data, and other support necessary to make an informed decision. The client and the professional are active participants in the discussion leading to a decision. Each voices his or her thoughts and can consider the perspective of the other before making a decision.

4) Criteria to identify the appropriate ethical approach

   a) The client's ability to comprehend information that is relevant to the decision to be made

   b) His or her ability to deliberate using a consistent set of values and goals

   c) His or her ability to communicate preferences

C. Legal Issues in Case Management Based on Changes in Healthcare Delivery

1. More knowledge and access to information through technology such as the Internet may result in clients feeling denied care they see as a right.

2. Clients' expectations of service providers may increase because of their greater knowledge and access to health information. Recommendations of the case manager that result in suboptimal outcomes may place the case manager at risk.

3. Case managers can be exposed to lawsuits as they assume more responsibility, and, if the focus is on cost containment, clients may view the case manager as preventing access to care to save money.

4. Increased caseloads of case management professionals as healthcare organizations downsize necessitate greater attention to the details of diagnosis, treatment plans, goals, placement, and timeframes.

5. Increased autonomy of case managers and other healthcare professionals in their practices necessitates an adherence to standards of practice.

D. Risk Factors in Case Management

1. Case managers are responsible for integrating care and services, advocating for clients and their families, and acting as risk managers. Case managers may reduce the risk of litigation by performing their duties as defined by established standards and relevant scope of practice.

2. Case managers have a responsibility to communicate with the client, the family, and the treatment team in a timely manner. This is particularly true when the condition of the client changes significantly and warrants immediate attention. Case managers must ensure that the treatment plan remains accurate and relevant to the changing needs of the client.

3. Case managers have a responsibility to integrate services. In doing so, they develop relationships with clients, family, service providers, and others involved in the care and rehabilitation processes. Ethical and liability issues arise when the professional cannot integrate necessary care and services because of conflicting obligations (e.g., client advocacy versus contractual obligations to the employer).

4. Case management is a specialty practice with providers held to professional standards of practice. The elements of proof remain the same as in any professional malpractice case (e.g., duty, breach), but for a finding of malpractice, evidence must go beyond the reasonable man standard and establish that the professional did not meet the necessary standards of care.

5. The role and functions of case management according to relevant nurse practice acts, certification standards, standards of professional organizations, and other sources are well documented. The jury compares those standards with the actions of the professional and uses them as guides in the decision-making process in a court setting.

E. Future of Case Management: Illness, injury, chronic diseases, aging, increases in population and use of resources, and increased healthcare costs are all part of the future. If the healthcare reform of 2010 remains in effect, the number of insured will rise. If not, uninsured clients will still need services. Regardless, hospitals, insurance companies, and other providers will be under pressure to provide health care efficiently. The demand for high-quality care and improved outcomes will continue.

1. Case managers will need to continue research for evidence that case management practice provides high-quality, effective, and cost-efficient care.

2. Case managers will need to advocate for themselves and negotiate for job descriptions and roles or models that will be most effective for the system they are working in.

3. Case managers will need to continue the fine art of collaboration with the identified team and learn to delegate tasks that can be done by others.

4. Case managers should be assigned early and be on site to promote the most efficient use of healthcare resources.

5. The population is aging, and older adults will benefit from the care coordination that case management provides as they strive to stay independently in their own homes.

References

American Nurses Association. (2007). *Nursing: Scope and standards of practice.* Washington, DC: American Nursing Publishing.

Association of Rehabilitation Nurses. (2010). *The rehabilitation nurse case manager: Role description.* Glenview, IL: Author.

Case Management Society of America. (2010). *Standards of practice for case management.* Little Rock, AR: Author.

Cohen, E., & Cesta, T. (2005). Nursing case management from essentials to advanced practice applications (4th ed.). St. Louis: Elsevier.

Huber, D. L. (2006). *Leadership and nursing care management* (3rd ed.). St. Louis: Elsevier.

International Academy of Life Care Planners. (2006). *Standards of practice.* Glenview, IL: International Association of Rehabilitation Professionals.

Suggested Resources

Allen, J. (2009). Building a group into a team. *Internet Journal of Healthcare Administration, 6*(1), 15312933.

American Nurses Association NursingWorld: www.nursingworld.org

Association of Rehabilitation Nurses: www.rehabnurse.org

Association of Rehabilitation Nurses. (2008). *Standards and scope of rehabilitation nursing practice.* Glenview, IL: Author.

Blackwell, T. L., Kraus, J. S., Winkler, T., & Steins, S. A. (2001). *Spinal cord injury desk reference: Guidelines for life care planning and case management.* New York: Demos.

Blank, A. E. (2001). Linking the restructuring of nursing care with outcomes: Conceptualizing the effects of nursing case management. In E. Cohen & T. Cesta (Eds.), *Nursing case management: From essentials to advanced practice application* (3rd ed.). St. Louis: Mosby.

The Care Planner Network: www.careplanners.net

Carter, J. (2009). Finding our place at the discussion table: Case management and healthcare reform. *Professional Case Management, 14*(4) 165–166.

Case Management Society of America: http://CMSA.org

Commission on Accreditation of Rehabilitation Facilities: www.CARF.org

Gutbezahl, C., & Mullahy, C. (2010). Case management role is likely to expand under healthcare reform. *Hospital Case Management, 18*(6), 81–84.

Johnson, K. M. (Ed.). (1997). *Advanced practice nursing in rehabilitation: A core curriculum.* Glenview, IL: Association of Rehabilitation Nurses.

The Joint Commission: http://jointcommission.org

Riddick-Grisham, S. (2004). *Pediatric life care planning and case management.* New York: CRC Press.

Rossi, P. A. (2003). *Case management in health care* (2nd ed.). Philadelphia: Elsevier Science.

Skeet, J., & Perry, A. (2008). Exploring the implementation and use of outcome measurement in practice: A qualitative study. *International Journal of Language and Communication Disorders, 43*(2), 110–125.

Stock, R., Reece, D., & Cesario, L. (2004). Developing a comprehensive interdisciplinary senior healthcare practice. *Journal of the American Geriatrics Society, 52*, 2128–2133.

Tahan, H., & Campgana, V. (2010). Case management roles and functions across various settings and professional disciplines. *Professional Case Management, 15*(5), 245–277.

Thomas, P. (2009). Case management delivery models: The impact of indirect care givers on organizational outcomes. *Journal of Nursing Administration, 39*(1), 30–37.

Weed, R. O. (2010). *Life care planning and case management handbook* (3rd ed.). New York: CRC Press.

SECTION II
Functional Health Patterns and the Rehabilitation Client

CHAPTER 6

Health Maintenance and Management of Therapeutic Regimens

Karen S. Reed, MSN DHSc RN CRRN CNL

The purpose of this chapter is to provide the rehabilitation nurse with the theoretical structure necessary to develop and implement a family-centered plan of care so that a person with a disability can successfully maintain and manage his or her therapeutic regimens in the community.

"Rehabilitation nurses help individuals affected by chronic illness or physical disability to achieve their greatest potential, adapt to their disabilities, and work toward productive, independent lives. They take a holistic approach to meeting patients' medical, vocational, educational, environmental, and spiritual needs" (Association of Rehabilitation Nurses, 2005, p. 1). Rehabilitation clients must use effective health management strategies to achieve and maintain an optimal quality of life. People with disabilities are living longer and need long-term health promotion interventions. Maintenance of optimal health includes both the prevention of further loss of function and the prevention of secondary conditions such as cardiovascular, cardiopulmonary, and psychosocial disorders. In addition, the impact of falls and injuries on both clients and their families exacerbates the challenge of successful health maintenance and management. Successful rehabilitation nursing includes the transfer of knowledge and accountability for healthcare needs from nurses to clients and their families and significant others in a manner that promotes health and wellness for the person with a disability (Viggiani, 2000). Strategies are best conceived when developed in a nursing theory framework that provides education and training to address weaknesses and maximize strengths to meet the needs of clients and families and to promote health in the community.

I. Background

A. The Current Status of Disabilities in the United States: *The 2008 Disability Status Report* (Erickson & Von Schrader, 2010) provides the rehabilitation nursing community with a summary of the most recent demographic and economic statistics on noninstitutionalized people with disabilities. This report focuses primarily on the working-age population because "employment is a key factor in the social integration and economic self-sufficiency of working-age people with disabilities" (Erickson & Von Schrader, p. 1). In addition, the results of the 2010 U.S. Census report are not immediately available, making prior U.S. Census data of limited value in the current rehabilitation practice setting. The statistics selected were chosen based on their value in the development of a home-and community-based plan of care. An overall description of the state of disability in the United States is represented by the following statistics (Erickson & Von Schrader, 2010):

1. Age. In the United States in 2008, the prevalence of disability across the lifespan was
   a. 12.1% for people of all ages
   b. 0.7% for people age 4 and younger
   c. 5.1% for people age 5–15
   d. 5.6% for people age 16–20
   e. 10.4% for people age 21–64
   f. 26.6% for people age 65–74
   g. 51.5% for people age 75 and older

2. Race. In the United States in 2008, the prevalence of disability for working-age people (age 21–64) was
   a. 10.2% among Whites
   b. 14.3% among African Americans
   c. 4.6% among Asians
   d. 18.8% among Native Americans
   e. 9.8% among people of other races

3. Education. In the United States in 2008, the percentage of working-age people with disabilities
   a. With only a high school diploma or equivalent was 34.0%
   b. With only some college or an associate degree was 29.7%
   c. With a bachelor's degree or more was 12.3%

4. Employment, poverty, education, and health insurance coverage. In 2008, the employment rate of working-age people (ages 21–64) with disabilities in the United States was 39.5%, with another 8.7% looking for work. The poverty rate for working-age people with disabilities was 25.3%, and 81.8% of working-age people with disabilities had health insurance.

5. Legislation. The Americans with Disabilities Act (ADA; ADA, 2010) protects the 54 million Americans with physical or mental impairments that substantially limit daily activities. These activities include working, walking, talking, seeing, hearing, or caring for oneself. Its five titles oversee legislation in the areas of employment (Title I), public services (Title II), public accommodations and services operated by private entities (Title III),

telecommunications (Title IV), and miscellaneous provision (Title V).

II. Conceptual Framework

The use of a conceptual framework provides structure within which to organize thinking, provide rationales for chosen interventions, and explain choices and options to others. Rehabilitation nurses create conceptual frameworks using nursing theories, various viewpoints of health, and knowledge of community settings to create a family-centered plan of care.

A. Use of Nursing Theories: In broad terms, a nursing theory is a body of knowledge used for nursing practice. Barnum (1998) divided theories into those that describe and those that explain nursing phenomena. Nursing theories may be classified as grand theory (the most abstract), middle-range theory, or practice theory (the most narrow in scope and practice). Each type of theory has a specific use within the application of nursing principles.

1. Grand theories. "Grand theories provide the broadest scope and present general concepts and propositions" (Parker, 2005, p. 7). Though useful for predicting and providing insight into nursing practice, they are not designed for empirical testing. Examples of grand theories include the following (Nursingtheory.net):
   a. Imogene King: Open Systems Theory
   b. Patricia Benner: Humanistic Model
   c. Dorothy Johnson: Behavioral Systems Model

2. Middle-range theories. Middle-range theories bridge the divide between grand theories and nursing practice theories. "They offer concepts and propositions at a lesser level of abstraction" (Parker, 2005, p. 7), and nursing journals reflect increased usage of these theories in the development of clinical practice and health promotion strategies. Examples of middle-range theories include the following (Nursingtheory.net):
   a. Smith and colleauges: Caregiver Effectiveness Model
   b. Hildebrandt and Persily: Community Empowerment
   c. Lobiondo-Wood: Family Stress and Adaptation
   d. Pender: Health Promotion Model
      1) The Health Promotion Model (HPM) is a middle-range nursing theory by Dr. Nola Pender.
      2) HPM assumes that people seek to regulate their own behavior, and health professionals play an influential role throughout their clients' lifespan (Pender, Murdaugh, & Parsons, 2011).
      3) The personal belief in one's own capacity to control life events is a tenet of the health-promotion model (Scrof & Velsor-Friedrich, 2006).
      4) "Families, peers, and health care providers are important sources of interpersonal influence that can increase or decrease commitment to and engagement in health-promoting behavior" (Pender, Murdaugh, & Parsons, 2011, p. 64).
      5) There are five core self-management concepts around which outcomes and interventions are developed to promote self-efficacy: problem solving, decision making, resource use, collaboration, and action (Lorig & Holman, 2003).

3. Nursing practice theories. This type of theory uses a conceptual framework to predict outcomes that affect nursing practice (Parker, 2005, p. 7). Rehabilitation nurses use nursing practice theories to develop measurable objectives and then craft the interventions that will allow the client or family to meet the objectives.

B. Viewpoints of Health

1. Health. "Health is a state of complete physical, mental and social well-being and not merely the absence of disease or infirmity" (World Health Organization, 1948). "Optimal health is a dynamic balance of physical, emotional, social, spiritual, and intellectual health" (O'Donnell, 2009, p. iv).

2. Wellness
   a. "Wellness is a journey that each of us takes in our quest for well-being of body, mind, and spirit. Key components of wellness include personal responsibility, balance through all phases of health, body-mind-spirit connectedness, and relationships with self, others, and the environment" (Miller, 2008, p. 4).
   b. "Wellness is first and foremost a choice to assume responsibility for the quality of your life. It begins with a conscious decision to shape a healthy lifestyle. Wellness is a mind set, a predisposition to adopt a series of key principles in varied life areas that lead to high levels of well-being and life satisfaction" (Don Ardell, n.d.).

3. Health promotion
   a. "Health promotion is the process of enabling people to increase control over, and to improve, their health. To reach a state of complete physical, mental and social well-being, an individual or group must be able to identify and to realize aspirations, to satisfy needs,

and to change or cope with the environment. Health is, therefore, seen as a resource for everyday life, not the objective of living. Health is a positive concept emphasizing social and personal resources, as well as physical capacities. Therefore, health promotion is not just the responsibility of the health sector, but goes beyond healthy life-styles to well-being" (World Health Organization, 1986).

    b. "Health promotion is the art and science of helping people discover the synergies between their core passions and optimal health, enhancing their motivation to strive for optimal health, and supporting them in changing their lifestyle to move toward a state of optimal health" (O'Donnell, 2009, p. iv).

C. Settings and Models of Community-Based Care: The settings for the provision of community-based rehabilitation nursing concepts include residential institutions, such as long-term care facilities and subacute care centers, outpatient programs, community and faith-based organizations, and private homes (**Table 6-1**).

Table 6-1. Settings, Models, and Programs Where Community-Based Rehabilitation Is Used

Setting	Purpose	Types of Clients	Delivery System	Nursing Roles
Home health care	To provide health care to individuals and families in their place of residence for the purpose of prompting or restoring health, maximizing independence, and minimizing the effects of disability (Hankwitz, 1993)	All age levels Common conditions: • Fractures • Degenerative joint disease • Multiple sclerosis • Parkinson's disease • Cancer • Alterations in function secondary to neuropathy or myopathy • Amputations • Burns	Primary care Case management	Partner Teacher Resource manager Clinician (Neal, 1998)
Subacute care	To serve clients whose medical treatment does not allow for participation in acute rehabilitation programs or who are classified as slow to progress or who cannot qualify for a standard rehabilitation program (Mumma & Nelson, 1996)	Typically older than age 16, although specialty pediatric facilities are available Common conditions • Closed-head injury with quadriparesis • Anoxic encephalopathy secondary to cardiac arrest • Strokes • Aneurysms	Team nursing Primary care delivered by nursing assistants; licensed vocational nurses (LVNs) provide unit supervision and treatments; RNs serve in the case management and coordination role	Planner Coordinator Evaluator of client outcomes Client advocate
Long-term care	To serve clients who are unable to live independently and meet their self-care needs	Primarily the geriatric population, as well as an unknown number of younger people with chronic disabilities Common conditions • Joint fractures • Strokes • Closed-head injury • Anoxia • Rheumatoid arthritis	Team nursing Primary care delivered by LVNs and nursing assistants with RNs serving the case coordination and management role	Planner Coordinator Evaluator of client outcomes Client advocate
Independent living	To serve individuals who want to take control of their lives, participate in decision making, and achieve the highest level of independence possible	Primarily adults Common conditions • Spinal cord injury • Closed-head injury	Care provided by personal care attendants RN serves as care manager	Partner Educator Client advocate

1. Outpatient rehabilitation clinics. Nurses in outpatient rehabilitation clinics focus on integrating rehabilitation principles into the community.
2. Assisted living. Nurses in assisted living environments focus on promoting health in a structured community living setting that is accessible for people with disabilities.
3. Home. Home healthcare nurses provide hands-on nursing care in the client's home.
4. School. School nurses provide education, counseling, and referral services for health promotion and disease prevention and for meeting the needs of children with disabilities.
5. Congregation. Parish nurses act as health counselors, educators, and referral sources; use a holistic focus with a foundation based on spiritual health; and usually provide care within a faith community.
6. Case managers. Case managers act as liaisons, health educators, health promoters, and referral sources. They facilitate return to work for workers with injuries and integrate workers with catastrophic injuries back into the community.

D. Roles of Rehabilitation Nurses in Health Maintenance and Health Restoration Activities

1. Partner or physical caregiver. Clients and families have become more educated as consumers and take responsibility for making healthcare choices, resulting in a shift of the nurse-client relationship to one of partnership. The client assumes primary responsibility for setting the goals, and the nurse's role varies depending on the client's degree of independence.

2. Teacher
   a. The most important goal of teaching in community-based rehabilitation is to help the client and family achieve the following possible outcomes:
      1) Improvements in care
      2) Facilitation of health promotion
      3) Reduction of complications
      4) Resumption of functional activities
   b. Sharing knowledge about health care improves client and family satisfaction (Kim & Moon, 2007). Education increases the client's and family's sense of control by encouraging mutual participation in care planning (**Figure 6-1**).

3. Resource or care manager. In this role, the nurse maintains responsibility for tracking and directing the client's care and progress throughout the healthcare system. The nurse oversees the client's primary needs; he or she
   a. Assesses the client appropriately

Figure 6-1. Benefits of Client Education

Better Outcomes for Client and Family
- Improved care
- Reduction of complications
- Development of self-care skills
- Achievement of highest possible level of independence
- Provision for personal needs
- Resumption of functional activities

Improved Client and Family Satisfaction
- Acquisition of knowledge
- Acquisition of confidence
- Sense of control through participation
- Individual decision making

Improved Staff Satisfaction
- Satisfaction regarding safety to move through different types of healthcare services
- Positive results from discharge
- Client successfully manages care

Continuity of Care
- Identical plans and actions by all professionals
- Movement through different types of healthcare services that does not disrupt treatment

Cost Containment
- Efficient use of resources
- Prevention strategies incorporated into care

Hunt, R., & Zurek, E. (1997). *Introduction to community-based nursing.* Philadelphia: Lippincott.

---

   b. Establishes the plan of care
   c. Delegates specific nursing care tasks to other qualified personnel
   d. Initiates interventions
   e. Coordinates and collaborates with the healthcare team
   f. Evaluates outcomes
      Collaboration and coordination are vital to the implementation of this role because rehabilitation clients and families interact with many healthcare professionals who have different areas of expertise and training. The care manager facilitates the client's treatment plan to ensure that it is consistent with the client's needs and is achieved in a timely manner. In addition, the nurse in this role must have an effective understanding of the cultural norms of the client's community and their influence on the client's behavior.

4. Advocate
   a. An advocate defends the cause of another person. In nursing, advocacy involves empowering clients, families, and client populations through knowledge (**Figure 6-2**).
   b. Works to change the system, collaborating with other professionals, role modeling, and maximizing the use of community resources

Figure 6-2. Keys to Developing Advocacy Skills

Understanding and Knowledge of Self Personally and Professionally
- Knowledge of oneself: Awareness of personal goals and how these goals affect relationships with clients
- Realistic self-concept: Awareness of own limitations and abilities that will affect client care
- Value clarification: Awareness of personal bias and prejudices, moral and ethical values; knowledge of personal perceptions concerning what is fair and acceptable and how these perceptions may affect relationships with clients

Knowledge of Treatment and Intervention Options
- Development of a strong knowledge base about interventions and outcomes
- Awareness of rationale for interventions

Knowledge of the Healthcare System
- Awareness of how the healthcare system relates to clients, families, and the community
- Awareness of specific aspects of community (e.g., politics, economy) and how these factors affect the healthcare system

Knowledge of How to Put Advocacy into Action
- Assessment
  - What does the client identify as the problem?
  - What support or resources does the client already have?
  - What knowledge does the client have about health services and treatment options?
  - In what areas does the client feel a need for more personal control?
- Planning: Mobilizing resources, consulting, collaborating with the healthcare team
- Implementation: Educating and empowering the client (the nurse helps the client assert control over variables affecting the client's life)

c. Coordinates referrals to not-for-profit and private home care agencies

d. Identifies agencies that provide free care or sliding-scale fees for services based on income and the duration of needed services

e. Arranges for social work services to help gain access to community systems that can provide subsidized housing, Medicaid applications, Supplemental Security Income and Social Security Disability Insurance, counseling services, advocacy assistance, equipment, and transportation and that can help find organizations that provide services

f. Contacts the local department of human services about services available for rehabilitation care

g. Contacts legislators to support funding for transferring clients to independent living centers and for training care attendants and supplemental funding that allows people with disabilities to work without a drastic reduction in or termination of medical benefits

h. Attends public hearings on issues that affect people with disabilities

i. Acts as a community advocate to increase environmental accessibility, decrease architectural barriers, increase access to public transportation, decrease cost of services to older adults on fixed incomes, and increase access to healthcare services

j. Makes referrals to rehabilitation counselors, peer counselors, and those providing psychological services

k. Contacts state disability offices, commissions, or departments for assistance

l. Promotes the education of healthcare providers and caregivers within facilities and the community

m. Provides in-service education

n. Consults one-on-one with providers regarding healthcare issues, ways to manage individual clients' healthcare needs, and ways to promote access to healthcare services

o. Encourages family involvement early in the rehabilitation process and teaches family members about equipment, procedures, medications, and ways to manage emergencies

p. Coordinates a home visit by the rehabilitation team to evaluate the need for modifications, equipment, and safety improvements

q. Promotes interagency communication about rehabilitation needs, follow-up teaching needs, and previous nursing interventions in the event of a transfer to a different environment

r. Periodically reassesses and evaluates the client's ability to perform activities of daily living, changes in levels of independence, healthcare needs, and barriers to necessary services

s. Contacts healthcare providers in the community to determine access to buildings, cost of services, insurance coverage, ways to modify the office environment, and availability of transportation

t. Speaks at service club meetings

u. Actively participates in professional organizations that support legislation and advocacy activities for people with disabilities

v. Promotes the appointment of people with disabilities to public office and commissions and to private-sector industry and business boards

w. Helps clients with disabilities prepare testimony for legislative hearings

x. Participates in health planning endeavors and advocate for services that meet the needs of children and adults

III. Nursing Challenges: Ineffective Health Maintenance

A higher percentage of adults with disabilities (40%) report fair or poor health than do adults without disabilities (10%). Among adults with disabilities, African Americans, Hispanics, and Native Americans report fair or poor health at disproportionately higher rates than Whites and Asian Americans. Finally, adults with disabilities are more likely than adults without disabilities to smoke, to be obese, and to be physically inactive (Centers for Disease Control and Prevention [CDC], n.d.).

A. Definition of Problem: The North American Nursing Diagnosis Association (NANDA) defined ineffective health maintenance as the "inability to identify, manage, and/or seek out help to maintain help" (Ackley & Ladwig, 2008, p. 412).

B. Defining Characteristics
   1. Demonstrated lack of adaptive behaviors to environmental changes
   2. Demonstrated lack of knowledge about basic health practices
   3. Lack of expressed interest in improving health behaviors
   4. Impairment of personal support systems
   4. Inability to take responsibility for meeting basic health practices (Ackley & Ladwig, 2008).

C. Causes or Related Factors
   1. Impaired cognition
   2. Impaired judgment
   3. Impaired gross or fine motor movement
   4. Spiritual or emotional distress
   5. Lack of financial resources
   6. Ineffective family coping

D. Nursing Outcomes Classification (NOC)
   1. Suggested outcomes include improving health-seeking behavior and supporting health promotion behaviors.

E. Assessment
   1. Client's self-management abilities and knowledge
      a. What is the client's coping status regarding responsibility for and access to health care?
      b. What was the client's health and lifestyle before the injury or illness?
      c. Does the client's health insurance plan cover ongoing telephone disease management by nurses?
      d. Is the client interested in a health management program?
      e. What is the client's ability and motivation to take responsibility for health, including knowledge of nutritional needs?
      f. What is the client's access to and availability of healthcare providers and facilities?
      g. What is the client's knowledge of prescribed medications and their effects?
      h. What is the client's knowledge of his or her medical status and related treatment program such as written action plans developed collaboratively by the client and primary care practitioner (physician, nurse practitioner, physician assistant, and clinical specialist)?
   2. Client's emotional and spiritual state
      a. What stage of grief is the patient experiencing related to the injury or disease?
      b. What methods of coping does the client use?
      c. Is there evidence of chemical dependency? Self-neglect? Self-mutilation?
      d. What are the client's sources of hope and strength?
      e. Does the client believe in God or another deity?
      f. What is the client's perceived relationship between spiritual beliefs and health?
      g. Does the client observe religious practices?
   3. Client's social support system. Five categories of caregivers can make up a client's social support system: family, friends, social service organizations or churches, agencies, and private pay services. What is the frequency, amount, kind, and level of support provided to the client by each category? Who are the contacts within each category? How does the client manage this information? Is there a plan in place in case support from one or more sources is temporarily or permanently unavailable?

F. Nursing Interventions Classifications (NIC)
   1. Educate the client at his or her learning level using age-specific adult learning principles to facilitate health maintenance.
   2. Determine readiness to learn.
   3. Controlled stimulation may be needed to help the client focus on the learning task.
   4. Use teaching tools (e.g., written materials, audiotapes or videotapes, lectures, models).
   5. Use demonstrations and return demonstrations.
   6. Use memory aids (e.g., written reminders [large print when necessary], medication dispensers, and consistent location of supplies).
   7. Provide progressive sequential learning experiences that build on skills without overwhelming the learner (e.g., help the client take on progressive responsibility for bladder management).
   8. Design a physical environment that minimizes dependency and the sick role by maximizing all opportunities to create a feeling of home.
   9. Encourage the client and healthcare providers to wear street clothes.

THE SPECIALTY PRACTICE OF REHABILITATION NURSING

10. Encourage the client to eat meals with others and follow the family's pattern of eating as much as possible.
11. Help the client identify and begin to resume family role responsibilities.
12. Provide privacy when the client is performing physical care and interacting with others and allow time for the client to be alone.
13. Introduce the client to role models (e.g., other clients who competently manage their health and wellness).
14. Encourage the client to set realistic and achievable goals with the help of healthcare providers.
15. Encourage the client to become involved in all phases of care planning; promote the client's control of the process.
16. Negotiate to simplify or alter client behaviors and outcomes; adapt program methods or schedules to the client's preferred routine.
17. Avoid assuming a "powerful other" role that reinforces eternal control.
18. Create a contract with the client to define agreed-upon responsibilities, conditions, and goals for program participation.
19. Help the client and caregivers manage desired health practices and promote wellness.
20. Provide anticipatory guidance to maintain and manage effective health practices during periods of wellness.
21. Identify adaptation strategies to use when progressive illness or long-term health problems occur.
22. Monitor adherence to a prescribed medical regimen.
23. Help the client and family develop stress management skills.
24. Identify ways to adapt an exercise program to meet the client's changing needs, abilities, and environmental concerns.

IV. Nursing Challenges: Ineffective Family Therapeutic Regimen Management

A. Definition of Problem: NANDA defined ineffective family therapeutic regimen management as a "pattern of regulating and integrating into family processes a program for treatment of illness and sequelae of illness that is unsatisfactory for meeting specific health goals" (Ackley & Ladwig, 2008, p. 826).
B. Defining Characteristics
1. Acceleration of illness symptoms of a family member

2. Failure to take actions to reduce risk factors
3. Inappropriate family activities for meeting health goals
4. Lack of attention to illness
5. Verbalizes difficulty with therapeutic regimen (Ackley & Ladwig, 2008)
C. Causes or Related Factors
1. Complexity of the healthcare system
2. Complexity of the therapeutic regimen
3. Decisional conflicts
4. Economic difficulties
5. Excessive demands
6. Family conflict
D. NOC
1. The middle-range theory of caregiver stress was developed from Roy's Adaptation Model. There are four assumptions in the caregiver stress theory:
   a. Caregivers can respond to environmental change.
   b. Caregivers' perceptions determine how caregivers respond to environmental stimuli.
   c. Caregivers' adaption is a function of their environmental stimuli and adaptation level.
   d. Caregivers' effectors (e.g., physical function, self-esteem and mastery, role enjoyment, and marital satisfaction) are results of chronic caregiving" (Tsai, 2003).
2. Hanks, Rapport, and Vangel (2007) found a modest to strong relationship between caregivers' perceived social support and caregiver assessment of family functioning.
3. Health-seeking behavior
4. Knowledge of treatment regimen
5. Participation in healthcare decisions
E. NIC
1. Determine the types of equipment, supplies, and services that are lacking for an adequate health state to be maintained safely.
2. Identify who in the client's support system is willing to develop the strategies necessary to improve management of the therapeutic regimen.
3. Foster the client's advocate as he or she assumes responsibility in promoting the client's wellness and health management.
4. Encourage the client's advocate to use reliable electronic sources when searching for health-related information (**Table 6-2**).
5. Educate the client and the client's primary advocate on their learning level using age-specific adult learning principles to facilitate health maintenance.

Table 6-2. Use of Websites for Health Information

Accuracy	Is the information accurate, reliable, and free from error?
Authority	Is the author identified? Are the author's credentials presented? Is the publisher identified? Is contact information, such as a phone number or e-mail address, provided? What is the domain (.gov, .edu, .com, .org)?
Objectivity	What is the goal of the site? Is there bias? Is the information trying to sway opinion?
Currency	Is a date provided for publication or updates? Is the site updated regularly?
Coverage	Is a special browser or payment of a fee required for complete viewing? Are the topics explored in depth? Are the links relevant?

V. **Nursing Challenge: Ineffective Community Therapeutic Regimen Management**

NANDA defined ineffective community therapeutic regimen management as a "pattern of regulating and integrating into community processes programs for treatment of illness and the sequelae of illness that are unsatisfactory for meeting health-related goals" (Ackley & Ladwig, 2008, p. 822).

A. Defining Characteristics
   1. Deficits of advocates for the aggregates
   2. Deficits in community activities for prevention
   3. Insufficient healthcare resources (Ackley & Ladwig, 2008)

B. NOC
   1. Community competence
   2. Community health status
   3. Community risk control: Chronic disease

C. NIC: Accessibility means more than transportation (**Figure 6-3**). There are more than 40 million Americans with disabilities who need care associated with their disability as well as primary care services (U.S. Census Bureau, 2006). Are there the outpatient and community services available that the client needs? Are there funding sources available in adequate amounts to support acquisition of the services? Can the client get in and out of his or her home? In addition, accessibility related to transportation means more than transportation to healthcare services or access to social services. Transportation is necessary for grocery shopping, filling prescriptions, or simply enjoying the pleasures of a public park. One can become easily overwhelmed by the potential multitude of community barriers. However, it is essential for the rehabilitation team to be familiar with the limitations of the home and community setting to which the client is returning because that setting may not be an appropriate option for discharge. Additionally, one aspect of the rehabilitation nursing role is to facilitate the health and wellness of the community, and identifying accessibility deficits is a first step in helping the community develop a corrective plan of action.

   1. Transportation. Adults with disabilities are twice as likely as those without disabilities to have inadequate transportation (31% versus 13%; CDC, n.d.). Determine the availability and the costs of clients accessing transportation services, including the following:
      a. Service to clients living in rural areas
      b. Vehicle modifications or purchase of a modified vehicle
      c. Designated parking
      d. Private transportation services
      e. Reduced-rate bus passes
      f. Paratransit services
      g. Parking stickers
   2. Funding for attendant care. Funding is typically tied to eligibility for income assistance and the waiting period can be as long as 2 years. Challenges include minimal reimbursement for care attendants, which makes it difficult to recruit and retain qualified people. Funding levels fluctuate by age group, so the adolescent who is able to procure services at 17 may have to compete at age 18 for a sharply reduced pot of funds as a member of a broader age range (e.g., 18–55).
   3. Funding for independent living arrangements (residential and nonresidential models). Although funding is mandated by the Rehabilitation, Comprehensive Services, and Developmental Disabilities Amendments of 1978, the amendment is not formula driven but rather funded based on voted amounts. States may be able to provide some attendant assistance and community support services through Medicaid Title XIX funding. Most states provide an Internet database identifying licensed residential and nonresidential service providers by county. These government websites are valuable resources for identifying legitimate providers for home- and community-based services, healthcare services, medical care, and long-term and day care.
   4. Barriers to medical services.

Figure 6-3. Gaining Access to Community Resources

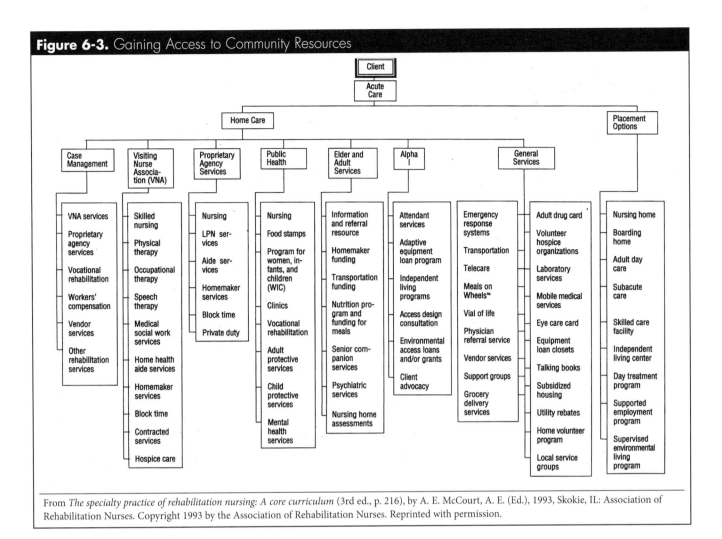

From *The specialty practice of rehabilitation nursing: A core curriculum* (3rd ed., p. 216), by A. E. McCourt, A. E. (Ed.), 1993, Skokie, IL: Association of Rehabilitation Nurses. Copyright 1993 by the Association of Rehabilitation Nurses. Reprinted with permission.

a. Harrington, Hirsch, Hammond, Norton, and Bockenek (2009) conducted an assessment of people with disabilities and their perceived barriers to primary care services. Results revealed that most people participating in the survey have a primary care physician and receive routine screening and health maintenance examination. The prevalent barrier was lack of primary care physician knowledge related to the disability rather than physical barriers to care. The physical barriers reported included examination rooms too small to negotiate in a wheelchair, lack of transfer assistance to an examination table, and the inability of women with a disability to maintain correct positioning for Pap smears and mammograms. The sample was made up of people receiving treatment at a rehabilitation clinic; therefore, the viewpoint of people who lack transportation or are homebound were not captured.

b. A study of the barriers to mammography by women with disabilities (Barr, Giannotti, Van Hoof, Mongoven, & Curry, 2008) revealed difficulty accessing care sites, lack of transportation, nonadjustable equipment, communication challenges, and fears, both of the examination and of being touched by strangers.

5. Funding for consumable and durable medical supplies. Assess a client's ability to obtain needed equipment, supplies, and medications. This assessment should include availability of delivery, availability of all necessary medications, delivery costs, deductibles, and coverage limits.

6. Accessible housing

a. Architectural modification of a client's living environment takes time, and projects often are completed long after discharge. Determine whether the client's home is accessible, taking into consideration the equipment needed after discharge. Checklists are available from a variety of academic and government sources that rehabilitation teams and families can use to assess the appropriateness of the home environment (**Figure 6-4**).

b. If a client wants to modify his or her home, is there technical assistance available for the development, design, and building of the modifications? Are there building loans available for the specialized modifications? Federal programs are available for housing modification.

c. The U.S. Department of Veterans Affairs Specially Adapting Housing Grant provides not more than 50% of the costs, up to $50,000 maximum. Eligible veterans have a service-connected disability due to military service and have lost at least one lower extremity and

---

Figure 6-4. Safe Home Environment

Domain-Health Knowledge and Behavior   Care Recipient:

Class-Risk Control and Safety (T)   Data Source:

Scales(s): Not adequate to Totally adequate (f)

Definition: Physical arrangements to minimize environmental factors that might cause physical harm or injury in the home

Outcome Target Rating: Maintain at_____Increase to _____

Safe Home Environment Overall Rating	Not adequate 1	Slightly adequate 2	Moderately adequate 3	Substantially adequate 4	Totally adequate 5	
Indicators:						
191001 Provision of lighting	1	2	3	4	5	NA
191002 Placement of handrails	1	2	3	4	5	NA
191023 Carbon monoxide detector maintenance	1	2	3	4	5	NA
191003 Smoke detector maintenance	1	2	3	4	5	NA
191004 Use of personal alarm system	1	2	3	4	5	NA
191005 Provision of accessible telephone	1	2	3	4	5	NA
191006 Placement of appropriate hazard warning labels	1	2	3	4	5	NA
191024 Safe storage of medication to prevent accidental use	1	2	3	4	5	NA
191007 Disposal of unused medications	1	2	3	4	5	NA
191008 Provision of assistive devices in accessible location	1	2	3	4	5	NA
191009 Provision of equipment that meets safety standards	1	2	3	4	5	NA
191010 Safe storage of firearms to prevent accidents	1	2	3	4	5	NA
191011 Safe storage of hazardous materials to prevent injury	1	2	3	4	5	NA
191012 Safe disposal of hazardous materials	1	2	3	4	5	NA
191025 Safe storage of matches/lighters	1	2	3	4	5	NA
191013 Arrangement of furniture to reduce risks	1	2	3	4	5	NA
191014 Provision of a safe play area	1	2	3	4	5	NA
191015 Removal of unused refrigerator and freezer doors	1	2	3	4	5	NA
191016 Correction of lead hazard risks	1	2	3	4	5	NA
191017 Provision of age-appropriate toys	1	2	3	4	5	NA
191018 Use of electrical outlet covers	1	2	3	4	5	NA
191019 Room temperature regulation	1	2	3	4	5	NA
191020 Elimination of harmful noise levels	1	2	3	4	5	NA
191021 Placement of window guards as needed	1	2	3	4	5	NA

From *Nursing outcomes classification (NOC)*, by S. Moorhead, M. Johnson, and M. Maas, 2004, St. Louis: Mosby. Copyright 2004 by Mosby. Reprinted with permission.

have other disabilities. The grant will not modify vehicles, and any veteran 18 and older may qualify. There is no time limit for use of the grant monies. Veterans should contact a local VA office, and more information is available at www.benefits.va.gov/homeloans/sah.asp.

d. The U.S. Department of Agriculture (USDA) provides grants (maximum $7,500) and loans ($20,000) to help very-low-income applicants remove health and safety hazards or repair their homes. The applicants must be in a rural area with a population of 10,000 or less and the loan homeowner must be 18 years of age or older and the grant homeowner 62 years of age or older. The monies may not be used to modify vehicles. Interested applicants should contact the local USDA office, and more information is available at www.rurdev.usda.gov/rhs/common/indiv_intro.htm.

7. Employment. Three times as many adults with disabilities live in poverty, with annual household incomes below $15,000 (26% versus 9%; CDC, n.d.). Federal legislation prohibits discriminatory hiring, compensation, and training practices. The U.S. Equal Employment Opportunity Commission enforces the federal laws related to employment discrimination against a person with a disability.

   a. Title I and Title V of the ADA of 1990, as amended, prohibit employment discrimination against qualified people with disabilities in the private sector and in state and local governments.

   b. Sections 501 and 505 of the Rehabilitation Act of 1973 prohibit discrimination against qualified people with disabilities who work in the federal government.

   c. Title VII of the Civil Rights Act of 1964 (Title VII) prohibits employment discrimination based on race, color, religion, sex, or national origin.

   d. The National AgrAbility Project was created to assist people with disabilities employed in agriculture. The project links the cooperative extension services at a land grant university with a private nonprofit disability service organization to provide practical education and assistance that promotes independence in agricultural production and rural living. The AgrAbility Project assists people involved in production agriculture who work on both small and large operations. State projects may be located at www.agrabilityproject.org.

   e. The Job Accommodation Network (2009) has conducted an ongoing study since 2004 of 1,182 employers. The study results have consistently shown that employers want to provide accommodations so they can retain valued and qualified employees. The majority of employers, 56%, reported that the accommodations cost nothing, another 37% experienced a one-time cost, and only 5% stated that the accommodation resulted in an ongoing, annual cost. The typical one-time expenditure was $600.

   f. Employers are expected to make reasonable accommodations for employees with disabilities. The costs associated with those accommodations are often nominal. The Job Accommodation Network conducted a survey that found 71% of accommodations made by small businesses cost less than $500.

   g. Employers may want to offer employment to people with disabilities but need financial assistance to make the necessary accommodations. The IRS offers tax incentives to businesses that hire people with disabilities and incentives for businesses that must make accommodations. Examples include the Disabled Access Credit, Barrier Removal Tax Deduction, and Work Opportunity Credit. Information on the Tax Incentives Packet of the ADA may be located at www.irs.gov/businesses/small/article/0,,id=185704,00.html.

8. Recreation. Recreation activities and sports inspire confidence and restore dignity as well as help people with disabilities deal with challenge and change (Disabled Sports USA, n.d.)

   a. The U.S. National Park Service offers free lifetime park passes to people with disabilities. The ADA published guidelines for accessibility to recreation facilities in the Federal Register on September 3, 2002; however, they have not been incorporated into the Department of Justice accessibility standards and are therefore unenforceable (Disability.gov, n.d.).

   b. Disability.gov refers readers seeking information on disability travel and recreation resources to www.makoa.org, which is maintained by a man with quadriplegia who is ventilator dependent. The website includes travel planning, travel companies, and destinations. Many parks and recreation divisions across the United States have information on their websites on special programs and activities and their level of accessibility and available equipment.

9. Resources. The federal website Disability.gov has a plethora of Web links and information for professionals, consumers, and family members on a wide number of subjects. Topics are easy to navigate on one side of the page and include employment, housing, recreation, emergency preparedness, and technology, to name a few. A primary advantage to using federal and state websites and databases is that the sites are frequently updated and maintained by reputable sources. Because not all websites contain accurate information or are from reputable sources, rehabilitation nurses, clients, and family members should assess websites before using their contents (see Table 6-2).

VI. **Nursing Challenges: Risk for Injury**
   A. Injury Prevention
      1. Public health experts and epidemiologists identify three levels of injury prevention that are defined by the timing of an injury. For every injury event, there is a primary (pre-event), secondary (event), and tertiary (postevent) period. Another way to present the three levels of injury prevention is to consider injury as the result of disease or a negative health state.
      2. Primary prevention consists of activities that decrease the opportunity for illness or injury. Secondary prevention includes early diagnosis and treatment of a condition to lessen its severity, and tertiary prevention is the restoration to one's optimum function (Murray, Zentner, Pangman, & Pangman, 2006).
      3. When a rehabilitation nurse is planning prevention strategies for a particular type of injury occurrence, the strategy should include actions that can be taken at all three levels (Indian Health Services, n.d.).
   B. Secondary Conditions
      1. Adults with physical disabilities are at risk for a variety of secondary conditions that may reduce their health and independence. The American Association on Health and Disability (2009) defined secondary conditions as "a condition that results from a specific type of primary disability, birth defect or medical condition. Examples of secondary conditions are pressure sores, bowel/bladder challenges, depression."
      2. A secondary condition differs from a comorbidity in that a comorbidity is an additional disease that occurs after diagnosis of the primary disabling condition.
      3. The term *secondary conditions* adds three dimensions not captured by the term *comorbidity:*

nonmedical events (such as isolation), conditions that affect the general population (such as obesity), and problems that arise at any time during the lifespan.
      4. The public health goal is to prevent and reduce secondary conditions associated with unnecessary activity limitations, health costs, lost wages, reduced participation, and reduced quality of life (CDC, 2004).
      5. Strategies or interventions that will improve the factors that influence secondary conditions include the following:
         a. Available and accessible medical facilities, private offices, fitness centers, shelters, mobile units, and transportation
         b. Modified equipment in those facilities
         c. Websites with approved accessibility features
         d. Policies that facilitate postsecondary education, hiring, and purchase of the best technology (CDC, 2004).
   C. Definition: NANDA defined risk for injury as "a result of the interaction of environmental conditions interacting with the individual's adaptive and defensive resources" (Ackley & Ladwig, 2008).
   D. Risk Factors: This is a broad label that includes both external and internal risk factors. This nursing diagnosis should be used only for people who are at unusually high risk for this problem because most people are at some degree of risk for injury and should take precautions.
      1. External: Biological (e.g., the percentage of the community vaccinated for influenza), chemical (e.g., exposure to contaminated water, foods), human (e.g., hospital-acquired infections), mode of transport, nutritional, physical
      2. Internal: Abnormal blood profile; developmental age; autoimmune dysfunction; physical, psychological, sensory dysfunction, malnutrition (Ackley & Ladwig, 2008)
   E. NOC
      1. Risk control: Actions that will eliminate or reduce actual, personal, and modifiable health threats, including the following:
         a. Monitoring environmental and personal behavior risk factors
         b. Developing and following selected risk-control strategies
         c. Modifying lifestyle to reduce risk
      2. Safety behavior: Client or caregiver actions to minimize environmental factors that might cause physical harm or injury in the home (**Table 6-3**).
      3. Clients and caregivers manipulate the physical environment to promote safety.

4. Safety behavior: Client or caregiver efforts to control behaviors that might cause physical injury, such as the following:
  a. Identify risks that increase susceptibility to injury.
  b. Avoid physical injury.
5. Safety status: Fall occurrence (number of falls in the past week)
6. Safety status: Physical injury (severity of injuries from accidents and trauma)

F. NIC
  1. Assessment
    a. Identify factors that affect safety needs, such as changes in mental status, fatigue, medications, and motor or sensory deficits (e.g., with gait, balance).
    b. Identify environmental factors that create risk for falls.
    c. Check the client for presence of constrictive clothing, cuts, burns, or bruises.
  2. Exemplars: People with disabilities are susceptible to physical conditions and injuries. Collaboration with professionals in sports medicine, recreation therapy, and physical therapy provides rehabilitation nurses with valuable insight on a client's risk for injury because people with disabilities increasingly participate in recreational and competitive sports.
    a. People with cerebral palsy are at high risk for orthopedic conditions such as contractures, physical deformities, and hip dislocations, which can develop over time and decrease the person's range of motion, cause pain, negatively affect posture, and increase the risk of overuse injuries (Naugle, Stopka, & Brennan, 2006a). In addition, people with cerebral palsy commonly experience incontinence and drooling, which can lead to dehydration during activities if not monitored and treated.
    b. People born with spina bifida are predisposed to hip dislocation and fracture, which they may not notice because of the lack of sensation in the lower extremities (Naugle, Stopka, & Brennan, 2007).
    c. There are 300,000–500,000 people living in the United States with an amputation, either congenital or acquired. Many of these people participate in athletics. They are susceptible to blisters, pressure ulcers, "choke syndrome" (i.e., tissue swelling caused by an obstruction in the venous outflow due to constriction in the prosthetic socket), dermatitis, folliculitis,

and muscle contractures (Naugle, Stopka, & Brennan, 2006b).
    d. Hyperthermia and hypothermia are potential problems for people with spinal cord injuries participating in recreation events. There is impaired sweating below the lesion level and lack of heat loss by convection and radiation because of venous pooling in the lower limbs (Patel & Greydanus, 2010). In addition, because they do not shiver below the level of injury, people participating in water sports such as swimming are at higher risk for hypothermia. People with spinal cord injuries using a wheelchair are at higher risk for skin breakdown because their knees often are higher than their buttocks, placing additional pressure over the sacrum (Patel & Greydanus).
  3. Interventions
    a. Specify the techniques the client and family must learn to prevent injury after discharge.
    b. Use heating devices with caution to prevent burns in clients with sensory deficit.
    c. If appropriate, use an alarm to alert the caregiver when a client is getting out of bed or leaving the room.
    d. Place a bell or call light within reach of dependent clients at all times.
    e. Instruct clients to call for assistance with movement, as appropriate.
    f. Remove environmental hazards.
    g. Make no unnecessary changes in the physical environment.
    h. Refer to interventions for fall prevention as appropriate.

VII. Nursing Challenge: Risk for Falls
  NANDA defines risk for falls as "increased susceptibility to falling that may cause physical harm" (Ackley & Ladwig, 2008).
  A. Risk Factors
    1. Age: Adults age 65 and older
    2. History of falls
    3. Lower limb prosthesis
    4. Use of assistive devices
    5. Impaired sensation or perception, which may increase the risk of falls: temperature (neuropathies), touch (neuropathies), positive sense (proprioception), vision, and hearing
    6. Unmet elimination need or urinary incontinence
    7. Use of chemical or physical restraints
    8. Environmental hazards
    9. Lack of knowledge related to safety
    10. Impaired mobility

Table 6-3. Home Safety Checklist

Entry to the Home

Lighting: Is there adequate lighting in the following areas?

Y	N	Driveway
Y	N	Garage
Y	N	Walkways
Y	N	At all doors
Y	N	Near the trash area
Y	N	Any other areas of the yard that are used after dark

Driveway

Y	N	Is the driveway smooth and evenly paved?
Y	N	Is the transition between the driveway and surrounding surfaces (e.g., the yard) smooth and even, free of ruts and other things (rocks) that could cause tripping?
Y	N	Is the slope of the driveway low enough that it does not cause a problem?

Walkways

Y	N	Are walkways smooth and level (no cracks, gaps, or other tripping hazards)?
Y	N	Are steps along walkways clearly visible?
Y	N	Do they have handrails?
Y	N	Are transitions between different surfaces (e.g., a patio and sidewalk, concrete and asphalt, walkway and grass) even and level?
Y	N	If there are steeply inclined walkways, do they have sturdy, easy-to-grasp handrails?
Y	N	Are shrubs, bushes, and grass trimmed back or removed so that they do not infringe on or obstruct the walkway (potential tripping hazard)?

Steps to the Doors

Y	N	Do all steps (even single steps) have sturdy, easy-to-grasp (cylindrical) rails on both sides?
Y	N	Are the risers on stairs and multiple steps of equal height?
Y	N	Are the stair treads sturdy, level, and in good condition?
Y	N	Have small single steps (that could cause tripping) been mini-ramped?

Garage

Y	N	Are there adequate overhead lights in the garage?
Y	N	Is there a clear pathway to walk through?
Y	N	Do entry stairs or ramps to the house have railings?

Ramps (If Applicable)

Y	N	Are ramps rising at a minimum slope of 12:1? (12 inches of ramp length for every 1 inch of height is standard. However, 16:1 is recommended.)
Y	N	Do ramps have sturdy rails on both sides?
Y	N	Are the rails cylindrical for easy grasping?
Y	N	Do ramps have smooth transitions from ramp surface to ground surface?
Y	N	Do ramps have nonskid surfaces, or have nonskid strips been added?
Y	N	Do ramp railings extend beyond the ramp to help people transition off the ramp?
Y	N	Do ramps have sufficient width of at least 36 inches between handrails?

continued

THE SPECIALTY PRACTICE OF REHABILITATION NURSING

Table 6-3. Home Safety Checklist *continued*

Entry Landings

Front		Rear		
Y	N	Y	N	Have all potential tripping hazards been removed?
Y	N	Y	N	Is the landing wide and deep enough to safely open the door?
Y	N	Y	N	Is there a clearly visible, easily reachable doorbell?
Y	N	Y	N	Do porches and decks have railings or barriers to prevent someone from stepping or falling off? (Are the railings secure?)
Y	N	Y	N	Does the decking have secure, even floorboards with no protruding nails?
Y	N	Y	N	Is there a nonskid surface on the porch, deck, or landing?
Y	N	Y	N	Do doormats have nonskid backing with no upturned corners?

Exterior Doors

Front		Rear		
Y	N	Y	N	If necessary, are doorways wide enough to accommodate wheelchairs?
Y	N	Y	N	Are locks in good working order and easy to use?
Y	N	Y	N	Are latches and door handles in good condition and easy to use?
Y	N	Y	N	If someone has trouble turning a doorknob, are there lever handles?
Y	N	Y	N	Do the doors open and close easily without sticking?
Y	N	Y	N	Do doors on springs close slowly enough (so they do not close on someone going through the door)?
Y	N	Y	N	Is the threshold at the door less than 1 inch high?
Y	N	Y	N	Do glass sliding doors have decals at eye level?

Other Outdoor Area Concerns

Y	N	
Y	N	If there is a patio or deck, is it level, smoothly surfaced, and free of tripping hazards?
Y	N	Are walkways around the house smooth and free of obstacles and overgrown shrubbery, grass, and weeds that could cause tripping?
Y	N	Are garbage and recycling areas well lighted?
Y	N	Do these areas have safe, accessible stairs and railings?

Inside the Home

Entryways and Vestibules

Front		Rear		
Y	N	Y	N	Have throw rugs (potential tripping hazards) been removed?
Y	N	Y	N	Is there a clear pathway (devoid of clutter) through the entry hall?
Y	N	Y	N	Are all cords and wires out of the pathway?
Y	N	Y	N	Are thresholds low enough so someone does not trip over them?
Y	N	Y	N	Is there adequate lighting?
Y	N	Y	N	Is the light switch at the entrance to the room?
Y	N	Y	N	If necessary, is the entryway wide enough for a wheelchair or walker?

continued

Table 6-3. Home Safety Checklist *continued*

Hallways

#1		#2		#3		
Y	N	Y	N	Y	N	Are there handrails along the hall?
Y	N	Y	N	Y	N	Are halls free of clutter and other tripping obstacles?
Y	N	Y	N	Y	N	Are carpet runners tacked down or have antiskid backing?
Y	N	Y	N	Y	N	Are thresholds less than 1 inch high so they are not tripping hazards?
Y	N	Y	N	Y	N	If necessary, are halls wide enough for a wheelchair or walker?
Y	N	Y	N	Y	N	Is there adequate lighting?
Y	N	Y	N	Y	N	Is there a light switch at both ends of the hall?

Doors and Doorways

Y	N	Do all doors open easily?
Y	N	Are thresholds less than 1 inch high?

Interior Stairs

2nd Floor		Basement		Other		
Y	N	Y	N	Y	N	Do stairs have sturdy rails on both sides?
Y	N	Y	N	Y	N	Do rails continue onto the landings?
Y	N	Y	N	Y	N	Are the stair treads sturdy, not deteriorating or broken?
Y	N	Y	N	Y	N	Are edges of stair treads clearly visible (no dark, busy patterns)?
Y	N	Y	N	Y	N	Are stair pads in good repair (tacked down, in one piece)?
Y	N	Y	N	Y	N	(If bare wood) Are stair treads slip-resistant?
Y	N	Y	N	Y	N	(If carpeted) Is carpet securely attached, not worn or frayed?
Y	N	Y	N	Y	N	Are top and bottom steps highlighted?
Y	N	Y	N	Y	N	Are stairs free of clutter?
Y	N	Y	N	Y	N	If stairs have a low, overhanging beam that people could bump their heads on, has it been padded?
Y	N	Y	N	Y	N	Are stairs and landings well lit, with light switches at both top and bottom?

Living, Dining, Family, and Other Rooms

LR		DR		FR		Other		
Y	N	Y	N	Y	N	Y	N	Is the lighting adequate?
Y	N	Y	N	Y	N	Y	N	Is there a light switch at the entrance to the room?
Y	N	Y	N	Y	N	Y	N	Is there a clear, unobstructed path through the room (no clutter, cords, wires, baskets, and other things to trip over)?
Y	N	Y	N	Y	N	Y	N	Are thresholds minimal and carpet binders tacked down?
Y	N	Y	N	Y	N	Y	N	Are carpets in good condition (not frayed or turned up, torn, or with worn spots that someone could trip over)?
Y	N	Y	N	Y	N	Y	N	Are plastic runners or carpet protectors tacked down (not folded or turned up at edges)?
Y	N	Y	N	Y	N	Y	N	Do throw rugs have antiskid backing and no upturned corners?
Y	N	Y	N	Y	N	Y	N	Is tile or linoleum free of chips or tears and not slippery?
Y	N	Y	N	Y	N	Y	N	Are bare wood floors slip resistant?
Y	N	Y	N	Y	N	Y	N	Is there at least one comfortable chair people can get in and out of safely and easily?
Y	N	Y	N	Y	N	Y	N	Do tables have rounded edges that are clearly visible (no sharp edges or made of glass)?
Y	N	Y	N	Y	N	Y	N	Do windows open easily?
Y	N	Y	N	Y	N	Y	N	Are shades and blinds easy to open?
Y	N	Y	N	Y	N	Y	N	Are they securely attached?

continued

Table 6-3. Home Safety Checklist *continued*

Bathrooms

Family Considerations

Bath 1		Bath 2		
Y	N	Y	N	Is there a light switch at the entry?
Y	N	Y	N	Is there adequate lighting overall?
Y	N	Y	N	At the sink?
Y	N	Y	N	Over the tub or shower?
Y	N	Y	N	Is there a night light?
Y	N	Y	N	Is the door threshold less than 1 inch high?
Y	N	Y	N	Is the room free of clutter and tripping hazards?
Y	N	Y	N	Is the flooring nonslip or nonskid (including throw rugs)?
Y	N	Y	N	Are there grab bars in other areas of the room as needed?
Y	N	Y	N	Is the room kept warm during bathing (e.g., heat lamp, towel warmers)?

Sinks

Bath 1		Bath 2		
Y	N	Y	N	Are sink faucets easy to reach and read?
Y	N	Y	N	Is it easy to determine where the hot and cold areas of the faucet are?
Y	N	Y	N	Is it easy to mix the temperature?
Y	N	Y	N	If necessary, have antiscald devices been installed?
Y	N	Y	N	Is the sink wheelchair accessible, or can someone sit at the sink?
Y	N	Y	N	Are mirrors at an appropriate height?

Tub or Shower

Bath 1		Bath 2		
Y	N	Y	N	Are there sturdy grab bars in the tub or shower, if needed?
Y	N	Y	N	Is the shower curtain bottom out of the way so it is not a tripping hazard?
Y	N	Y	N	Are toiletries in the tub easily reached from sitting and standing positions?
Y	N	Y	N	Is there a nonskid bathmat in the bathtub?
Y	N	Y	N	Is there a handheld shower head?
Y	N	Y	N	Are tub or shower faucets easy to use and read (hot and cold clearly marked)?
Y	N	Y	N	If needed, is there a tub or shower seat?

Toilet

Bath 1		Bath 2		
Y	N	Y	N	Are there sturdy grab bars at the toilet (or toilet arms and a raised seat)?
Y	N	Y	N	Is toilet paper easily reachable from the toilet seat?
Y	N	Y	N	Is the toilet seat in good condition and securely fastened?

continued

Table 6-3. Home Safety Checklist *continued*

Kitchen

Y	N	Are frequently used items visible and easily reached (front of pantry and refrigerator)?
Y	N	Are sink faucets easy to reach and read?
Y	N	Is it easy to determine where the hot and cold areas of the faucet are?
Y	N	Is it easy to mix the temperature?
Y	N	If necessary, have antiscald devices been installed or the hot water temperature lowered?
Y	N	If necessary, have timers been installed on the oven and cooktop?
Y	N	Are burners and control knobs clearly labeled and easy to use?
Y	N	Are the controls on the front of the stove, not the back?
Y	N	Is there a close resting place nearby for hot vessels coming out of the oven?
Y	N	Is glass cookware being used so one can see that the food is being cooked thoroughly?
Y	N	Is the microwave easy to read, reach, and operate?

Laundry Room

Y	N	Is there a light switch at the entry?
Y	N	Is there sufficient lighting?
Y	N	Is the route to the laundry room (stairs) safe?
Y	N	Are the appliances at the right height so it is easy to get clothes in and out of the washer and dryer?
Y	N	Are the control knobs easy to reach, read, and operate?
Y	N	Are laundry supplies easy and safe to reach?
Y	N	Is there a nonslip floor surface?
Y	N	Are tripping hazards off the floor (laundry basket or dirty clothes)?

Bedrooms

BR1		BR2		
Y	N	Y	N	Is there a light at the entrance to the room?
Y	N	Y	N	Is a light reachable from the bed?
Y	N	Y	N	Can bureau drawers be reached (height of the drawer) and opened easily?
Y	N	Y	N	Is there a clear, unobstructed path through the room (clutter and furniture are out of the way)?
Y	N	Y	N	Are cords and wires off the floor?
Y	N	Y	N	Do throw and area rugs have nonslip backing and no upturned corners?
Y	N	Y	N	Are wood and linoleum floors nonskid?
Y	N	Y	N	Is carpet smooth (no folds or holes) and tacked down?
Y	N	Y	N	Are curtains and bed coverings off the floor so they are not tripping hazards?
Y	N	Y	N	Is there support for getting in and out of bed, if needed?
Y	N	Y	N	Is there a place to sit and get dressed, if needed?
Y	N	Y	N	Are windows easy to open and close?
Y	N	Y	N	Are window blinds and shades working properly and easy to open?
Y	N	Y	N	Are blinds and shades properly secured?

continued

THE SPECIALTY PRACTICE OF REHABILITATION NURSING

Table 6-3. Home Safety Checklist *continued*

Closets

Clo1		Clo2		
Y	N	Y	N	Are shelves and clothes poles easy to reach?
Y	N	Y	N	Have closet organizers been installed to maximize use of space?
Y	N	Y	N	Are closets organized so clothes are easy to find?
Y	N	Y	N	Are clutter and other tripping hazards off the floor?
Y	N	Y	N	Do closets have lights that are easy to find and reach?
Y	N	Y	N	Are closet doors easy to open?
Y	N	Y	N	If the closet has sliding doors, do they stay on track?

General Home Safety Concerns

Y	N	Can an older person contact someone in an emergency (e.g., Medi-Alert, names and numbers by phone, picture telephone)?
Y	N	Are smoke detectors and carbon monoxide alarms installed and working?
Y	N	Is there a fire extinguisher in the house?
Y	N	Is there a safe place outside to hide a key to the house for emergency entry?

Specific Checklist for Alzheimer's Disease and Other Dementias
If wandering is a problem, complete the following checklist:

Y	N	Is there a safe outdoor area that the person with dementia can use without wandering away (escape-proof porch or deck, fenced-in yard with locked gate)?
Y	N	Have poisonous plants and shrubs or plantings with berries been removed?
Y	N	Are there security locks on all exterior doors (e.g., double key, installed out of sight)?
Y	N	Is a key hidden outside in case the person locks out the caregiver?
Y	N	Are exterior and other doors to off-limit areas alarmed?
Y	N	Is access to stairwells, storage areas, basements, garages, and other off-limit areas controlled (e.g., with locks, secure gates, Dutch doors)?
Y	N	Is access to home offices and computer or home finance areas controlled?
Y	N	If necessary, can all doors to off-limit areas be disguised?
Y	N	Are there eye-level decals on all glass doors and large picture windows?
Y	N	Can all windows be securely locked?
Y	N	Is there a safe, clear pathway through the house where the person can walk or wander safely without tripping or knocking into or damaging something?

If orientation or getting lost in the house is a problem, complete the following checklist:

Y	N	Are there signs, arrows, photographs, and the like pointing to the bathroom, bedroom, and other places the person needs to find?
Y	N	Are doors that the person needs to use highlighted (e.g., signs, color)?
Y	N	Is there a photo or memento on the door to help someone find his or her bedroom?
Y	N	Are there night lights or light strips leading to the bathroom from the bedroom?
Y	N	Is the bathroom door left open when not in use to serve as a visual cue?
Y	N	Are closets, drawers, and cabinets that hold things the person can use labeled?

If hallucinations and misrecognition are problems, complete the following checklist:

Y	N	Are light levels even so that shade and shadows are kept to a minimum?
Y	N	Has ominous-looking artwork been removed (masks, distortions, abstract work)?

If the person gets upset by his or her or another person's image:

Y	N	Are windows covered at night so a person cannot see his or her reflection?
Y	N	Are mirrors covered?
Y	N	Have portraits and large photographs of people been removed or covered?

continued

Table 6-3. Home Safety Checklist *continued*

Bathroom Checklist for Dementia

Bath1		Bath2		
Y	N	Y	N	Have all medicines and nonelectric razors been put away?
Y	N	Y	N	Have all cleaning agents been put away?
Y	N	Y	N	Are other harmful objects removed from the cabinets and fixtures?
Y	N	Y	N	Are sink faucets easy to reach and read?
Y	N	Y	N	Is it easy to determine where the hot and cold areas of the faucet are?
Y	N	Y	N	Is it easy to mix the temperature?
Y	N	Y	N	Have antiscald devices been installed?
Y	N	Y	N	Does the color of the toilet fixture or seat contrast with the wall and floor for easy identification?
Y	N	Y	N	Have all trash cans been removed if the person uses them as a toilet?
Y	N	Y	N	Are there night lights or signs giving directions to the bathroom and fixtures?
Y	N	Y	N	Are instructions posted by the toilet, sink, and shower or tub?

Kitchen Checklist for Dementia

Y	N	Are all drawers and cabinets with safe objects labeled?
Y	N	Are there childproof locks on drawers and cabinets that are, or should be, off limits?
Y	N	Has access to the stove been controlled (knobs removed, lock on oven door, stove connected to hidden circuit breaker or gas valve)?
Y	N	If necessary, has access to the refrigerator and freezer been controlled with a refrigerator lock?
Y	N	Is there a night light in the kitchen (for safe midnight snacking)?
Y	N	Have sharp knives and other dangerous implements been removed or locked up?
Y	N	Has excess clutter been removed from countertops and tables?
Y	N	Have all vitamins, sweeteners, over-the-counter medicines, and prescription drugs been removed (or left out in limited quantities only)?
Y	N	Have all poisonous cleaning agents been removed or locked up?
Y	N	Have all "fake" foodstuffs been removed (wax or ceramic fruit, food-shaped magnets)?
Y	N	If necessary, has the kitchen been closed off?

Bedroom Checklist for Dementia

Y	N	Are there night lights (and signs, if necessary) along the path to the bathroom?
Y	N	Is there a monitor or intercom between the client's and the caregiver's areas?
Y	N	Has clutter and other potentially dangerous items (e.g., cologne, aftershave lotion, deodorant) been removed from dresser tops?
Y	N	Are drawers organized simply and labeled?

General Home Safety Checklist for Dementia

Y	N	If necessary, are childproof plugs in all unused electrical outlets?
Y	N	Are radiators and hot water pipes that the person might touch covered?
Y	N	Are all prescription medications and over-the-counter medicines locked up?
Y	N	Have all poisonous plants been removed (including artificial ones that look real)?
Y	N	Is alcohol out of sight and locked up?
Y	N	Are plastic or dry cleaner's bags out of reach (could cause choking or suffocation)?
Y	N	Are all weapons locked up or removed from the house (e.g., guns, knives)?

From *A Home for Life*, by R. Olsen and B. L. Hutchings, 2006, Center for Building Knowledge, New Jersey Institute of Technology. Copyright 2006 by New Jersey Institute of Technology. Reprinted with permission.

THE SPECIALTY PRACTICE OF REHABILITATION NURSING

11. Cognitive deficits
12. Clutter, inadequate lighting, and safety hazards (e.g., throw rugs, tub mats) in the home (Ackley & Ladwig, 2008)

B. NOC
1. Fall prevention behavior: Personal or family caregiver actions to minimize risk factors that might precipitate falls
2. Fall occurrence: Number of times a client falls (specify number per period of time)
3. Knowledge, personal safety: Extent of client's understanding about prevention of unintentional injuries

C. NIC
1. Falls
   a. In 2002 more than 1.8 million people were treated in emergency departments for fall-related injuries (CDC, 2008). In 2003 falls represented nearly 47% of all safety reports and aggregated events in the VA National Center for Patient Safety's database, and 11% of all Root Cause Analyses occurring in calendar year 2003 were fall related (U.S. Department of Veterans Affairs, 2004).
   b. The consequences of falls are both emotional and physical. They include morbidity and mortality, hip fractures, decreased quality of life, and the emotional fear of a repeat fall, and they can lead clients to self-impose restrictions on independence and mobility (Tennstedt et al., 1998).
   c. The costs associated with fall-related injuries are expected to increase to $240 billion by 2040 (Stevens, Corso, Finkelstein, Miller, 2006).
   d. Fall prevention and management strategies must take a multifactorial approach that includes assessing intrinsic and extrinsic fall risks and developing personalized muscle strengthening and balance retraining and health and environment risk factor screening and intervention (Dite, Connor, & Curtis, 2007; Gates, Fisher, Cooke, Carter, & Lamb, 2008.; Mackintosh, Hill, Dodd, Goldie, & Culham, 2005).

2. Assessment
   a. Monitor gait, balance, and fatigue level with ambulation.
   b. Determine risk or presence of altered gait, orthostatic hypotension, dizziness, or altered mental status associated with prescribed medications.

3. Interventions for use in institutions are listed in **Figure 6-5**. For use in the home and community
   a. Evaluate the degree of risk by using a home safety assessment tool.
   b. Assess the client's and family's knowledge of safety needs and injury prevention and motivation to prevent injury in home, community, and work settings.
   c. Assess socioeconomic status and availability and use of resources.
   d. Identify interventions and safety devices to promote a safe physical environment and individual safety. Make referrals to occupational or physical therapists as appropriate.
   e. If it is covered by the client's health insurance plan, arrange a home safety evaluation by a home health agency. Teach the client and family to monitor environmental hazards and recommend changes to promote the highest level of safety.
   f. Install secured grab bars or handrails.
   g. Use mobility devices.
   h. Unclutter the floors (e.g., get rid of scatter rugs).
   i. Place frequently used items in easily accessible places (e.g., small kitchen appliances, pots, and pans). Ensure adequate lighting, especially at night; most falls occur at night en route to the bathroom.
   j. Place the bed in a low position.
   k. Help the client meet self-care needs until independence can be achieved or until the care attendant or caregiver has received appropriate education.
   l. Teach the client, family, and significant others about the potential side effects of medications and alcohol.
   m. Ensure safety for the client who has deficits in cognitive or thought processes by changing the environment to meet safety needs.
   n. Provide methods to communicate with caregivers.
   o. Establish a toileting program.
   p. Install door locks or an escape alarm.
   q. Provide an organized, consistent, uncluttered environment.
   r. Install a large bell on the door of a room where entrance is restricted; the noise may stop the client and alert others to wandering (Joint Commission on Accreditation of Healthcare Organizations [JCAHO], 2003).
   s. Install bright yellow tape strips on the floor in front of doors (JCAHO, 2003).

Figure 6-5. Fall-Prevention Behavior

Domain: Health Knowledge and Behavior Care Recipient:

Class-Risk Control and Safety (T) Data Source:

Scales(s): Never demonstrated to Consistently demonstrated (m)

Definition: Personal or family caregiver actions to minimize risk factors that might precipitate falls in the personal environment

Outcome Target Rating: Maintain at_____Increase to _____

Fall Prevention Behavior Overall Rating		Never demonstrated 1	Rarely demonstrated 2	Sometimes demonstrated 3	Often demonstrated 4	Consistently demonstrated 5	
Indicators:							
190903	Places barriers to prevent falls	1	2	3	4	5	NA
190905	Uses handrails as needed	1	2	3	4	5	NA
190915	Uses grab bars as needed	1	2	3	4	5	NA
190914	Uses rubber mats in tub/ shower	1	2	3	4	5	NA
190910	Uses well-fitting tied shoes	1	2	3	4	5	NA
190901	Uses assistive devices correctly	1	2	3	4	5	NA
190918	Uses vision-correcting devices	1	2	3	4	5	NA
190902	Provides assistance with mobility	1	2	3	4	5	NA NA
190919	Uses safe transfer procedure	1	2	3	4	5	NA
190922	Provides adequate lighting	1	2	3	4	5	NA
190909	Uses stools/ladders appropriately	1	2	3	4	5	NA
190906	Eliminates clutter, spills, glare from floors	1	2	3	4	5	NA
190907	Removes rugs	1	2	3	4	5	NA
190908	Arranges for removal of snow and ice from walking surfaces	1	2	3	4	5	NA
190911	Adjusts toilet height as needed	1	2	3	4	5	NA
190912	Adjusts chair height as needed	1	2	3	4	5	NA
190913	Adjusts bed height as needed	1	2	3	4	5	NA
190916	Controls agitation and restlessness	1	2	3	4	5	NA
190917	Uses precautions when taking medications that increase risk for falls	1	2	3	4	5	NA

THE SPECIALTY PRACTICE OF REHABILITATION NURSING

t. Place a traffic stop sign on exit doors or restricted areas to prevent wandering and falls (JCAHO, 2003).

u. Teach ways to compensate for sensory-perceptual deficits.

v. Test water before bathing.

w. Use compensatory strategies for visual field deficits.

x. Prevent burns, frostbite, and skin integrity penetrations.

y. Teach the client and family the signs and symptoms of seizure activity and ways to maintain safety during and after a seizure.

z. Teach safety factors associated with transfer techniques, gait training, and mobility devices.

aa. Provide proper, well-maintained footwear with an adequate toe box and keep the client from going barefoot. Ensure that the toileting program is adequate to meet nighttime needs.

bb. Teach the client and family how to decrease the effects of orthostatic hypotension (e.g., sit on the edge of the bed for several seconds before transferring).

cc. Provide appropriate information on community resources (e.g., emergency call devices for outside assistance when the client is alone).

dd. Use distraction, redirection, humor, and quiet areas to decrease agitated behavior and avoid the use of restraints.

ee. If available, put the telephone within easy reach.

D. Restraints

1. The use of restraints in facilities has been declining since they have proven to be counterproductive and lead to falls and injuries (Dunn, 2001).

2. In response to both research results and consumer awareness, regulatory bodies have defined with greater specificity the use of restraints in client care. Centers for Medicare & Medicaid Services (CMS, 2007) implemented revised regulations outlining the use of restraints and seclusion for behavior management. CMS defined a restraint as "any manual method, physical or mechanical device, material or equipment that immobilizes or reduces the ability of a patient to move his or her arms, legs, body or head freely; or a drug or medication when it is used as a restriction to manage the patient's behavior or restrict the patient's freedom of movement and is not a standard treatment or dosage for the patient's condition."

3. The following list of nursing measures, provided by Cindy Gatens, RN CRRN-A (2007), allows the rehabilitation nurse to predict and anticipate behaviors that increase a client's injury risk and individualize the client's plan of care.

a. Avoid medications that can aggravate acute confusion in older adults (e.g., hypnotics, sedatives, antianxiety agents, tricyclic antidepressants, other medications with anticholinergic side effects).

b. Look for other medical conditions that could cause confusion such as infection, dehydration, and pain.

c. Potential restraint-free interventions for managing clients with confusion include maximizing structure and consistency (e.g., memory book, calendar, consistent routines), frequent reorientation, a room near the nursing station, opportunities for exercise and ambulation, toileting schedules, lower bedrails (or use of half rails if ambulatory), implementation of wheelchair and bed exit alarms, discontinuation of lines and tubes if possible, low bed, abdominal binder, and long-sleeved clothing (or knit sleeve to limit access to lines and tubes).

d. Use exit alarms that signal an attempted elopement and continuous observation or recommend family staying with client, if appropriate.

e. Restraint-free interventions for impulsivity include cuing the client to stop, think, and act.

f. Verbally review steps before beginning an activity, have the client rehearse the steps to complete a task, and intervene immediately when impulsive behaviors occur.

g. Review and rehearse how to appropriately engage in a behavior.

h. Complete frequent checks, activating and explaining the bed and wheelchair exit alarms.

i. Use a low bed, if appropriate, place the client in a common area where staff can frequently visualize client and behaviors, arrange for constant observation, or ask the family to stay with the client, if appropriate.

j. Document activities and behaviors that may trigger agitation and aggression.

k. Modify behavior by moving and speaking quietly, slowly, and directly; staying relaxed; safely positioning self; redirecting the client to a less stimulating or frustrating activity; discontinuing an activity; not arguing with a client about behavior; being flexible; and modifying treatment interventions.

l. Modify the environment to minimize stimulation (e.g., lights, noise, visitors).

m. Maximize consistency; provide safe motion, activity, and verbalization; provide clear expectations of interactions and treatment; schedule rest periods; facilitate safety by removing items that could cause injury; and arrange for constant observation or involve family (if calming and reassuring to the client).

References

Ackley, B., & Ladwig, G. (2008). *Nursing diagnosis handbook: An evidence-based guide to planning care.* St. Louis: Mosby.

American Association on Health and Disability. (2009). Secondary conditions. Retrieved August 9, 2011, from www.aahd.us/page.php?pname=about.

Americans with Disabilities Act. (2010). ADA National Network: Information, guidance, and training on the Americans with Disabilities Act. Retrieved August 9, 2011, from http://adaanniversary.org/.

Association of Rehabilitation Nurses. (2005). Rehabilitation nurses make a difference. Retrieved August 9, 2011, from www.rehabnurse.org/profresources/makeadiff.pdf.

Ardell, D. (n.d.) Seek wellness. Retrieved August 9, 2011, from www.seekwellness.com/wellness/articles/what_is_wellness.htm.

Barnum, B. (1998). *Nursing theory.* Philadelphia: Lippincott-Raven.

Barr, J., Giannotti, T., Van Hoof, T., Mongoven, J., & Curry, M. (2008). Understanding barriers to participation in mammography by women with disabilities. *The Journal of Health Promotion, 22*(6), 381–385.

Centers for Disease Control and Prevention. (2004). Secondary conditions: Children and adults with disability. Retrieved August 9, 2011, from www.cdc.gov/ncbddd/disabilityandhealth/relatedconditions.html.

Centers for Disease Control and Prevention. (2008). WISQARS (Web-Based Injury Statistics Query and Reporting System). Retrieved July 27, 2011, from www.cdc.gov/injury/wisqars/index.html.

Centers for Disease Control and Prevention. (n.d.). CDC promoting the health of people with disabilities. Retrieved August 9, 2011, from www.cdc.gov/ncbddd/disabilityandhealth/pdf/PromotingHealth508.pdf.

Centers for Medicare & Medicaid Services. (2007). Medicare and Medicaid programs; Hospital conditions of participation: Patients' rights: Final rule. (Federal Register 42 CFR Part 482). Retrieved August 3, 2011, from www.cms.gov/CFCsAndCoPs/downloads/finalpatientrightsrule.pdf.

Disability.gov. (n.d.). Accessibility guidelines for recreation facilities. Retrieved August 9, 2011, from www.disability.gov/clickTrack/confirm/11193673?external=false&parentFolderId=7233&linkId=106001.

Disabled Sports USA. (n.d.). Retrieved August 9, 2011, from www.dsusa.org/about-overview.html.

Dite, W., Connor, H., & Curtis, H. (2007). Clinical identification of multiple fall risk early after unilateral transtibial amputation. *Archives of Physical Medicine Rehabilitation, 88*(1), 109–114.

Dunn, K. (2001). The effects of physical restraints on fall rates in older adults who are institutionalized. *Journal of Gerontological Nursing, 27*(1), 40–48.

Erickson, W., & Von Schrader, S. (2010). *2008 disability status report: The United States.* Ithaca, NY: Cornell University Rehabilitation Research and Training Center on Disability Demographics and Statistics.

Gatens, C. (2007). Restraints and alternatives. *Association for Rehabilitation Nursing Network*, October/November, p. 8.

Gates, S., Fisher, J., Cooke, M., Carter, Y., & Lamb, S. (2008). Multifactorial assessment and targeted intervention for preventing falls and injuries among older people in community and emergency care settings: Systematic review and meta-analysis. *British Medical Journal, 336*(7636), 130–133.

Hanks, R., Rapport, L., & Vangel, S. (2007). Caregiving appraisal after traumatic brain injury: The effects of functional status, coping style, social support and family functioning. *NeuroRehabilitation, 22*(1), 43–52.

Hankwitz, P. E. (1993). Role of the physician in home care. In B. J. May (Ed.) *Home health and rehabilitation concepts of care* (pp. 1–23). Philadelphia: F. A. Davis.

Harrington, A., Hirsch, M., Hammond, F., Norton, H., & Bockenek, W. (2009). Assessment of primary care services and perceived barriers to care in persons with disabilities. *American Journal of Physical Medicine and Rehabilitation, 88*(10), 852–863.

Indian Health Services. (n.d.). The 5 public health principles. Retrieved August 9, 2011, from www.ihs.gov/medicalprograms/portlandinjury/worddocs/getting%20started/publichealthprinciples.pdf.

Joint Commission on Accreditation of Healthcare Organizations. (2003). Alternatives to restraint and seclusion. In *Complying with Joint Commission standards* (Chapter 3). Oak Brook, IL: Joint Commission Resources.

Job Accommodation Network. (2009). Workplace accommodations: Low cost, high impact. Retrieved August 9, 2011, from http://askjan.org/ENews/2009/Enews-V7-I4.htm#5.

Lorig, K., & Holman, H. (2003). Self-management education: History, definition, outcomes and mechanisms. *Annals of Behavioral Medicine, 26*(1), 1–7.

Kim, J. W., & Moon, S. S. (2007). Needs of family caregivers caring for stroke patients: Based on the rehabilitation treatment phase and the treatment setting. *Social Work in Health Care, 45*(1), 81–97.

Mackintosh, S., Hill, K., Dodd, K., Goldie, P., & Culham, E. (2005). Falls and injury prevention should be part of every stroke rehabilitation plan. *Clinical Rehabilitation, 19*(4), 441–451.

McCourt, A. E. (Ed.). (1993). *The specialty practice of rehabilitation nursing: A core curriculum* (3rd ed., p. 216). Skokie, IL: The Rehabilitation Nursing Foundation of the Association of Rehabilitation Nurses.

Miller, C. (2008). *Nurse's toolbook for promoting wellness.* New York: McGraw-Hill Medical.

Moorhead, S., Johnson, M., & Maas, M. (2004). *Nursing outcomes classification (NOC).* St. Louis: Mosby.

Mumma, C., & Nelson, A. (1996). Models for theory-based practice of rehabilitation nursing. In S. P. Hoeman (Ed.) *Rehabilitation nursing: Process and application* (2nd ed., pp. 21–33). St. Louis: Mobsy.

Murray, R., Zentner, J., Pangman, V., & Pangman, C. (2006). *Health promotion strategies through the life span.* Toronto, Canada: Prentice Hall.

Naugle, K., Stopka, C., & Brennan, J. (2006a). Disability and special needs: Medical conditions to know about when working with athletes with cerebral palsy. *Athletic Therapy Today, 11*(5), 44–45.

Naugle, K., Stopka, C., & Brennan, J. (2006b). Medical conditions of athletes with amputations. *Athletic Therapy Today, 11*(4), 39–41.

Naugle, K., Stopka, C., & Brennan, J. (2007). Common medical conditions in athletes with spina bifida. *Athletic Therapy Today, 12*(1), 18–20.

Neal, L. (1998). *Rehabilitation nursing in the home health setting.* Glenview, IL: Association of Rehabilitation Nurses.

O'Donnell, M. (2009). Definition of health promotion: Embracing passion, enhancing motivation, recognizing dynamic balance, and creating opportunities. *American Journal of Health Promotion, 24*(1), iv.

Parker, M. (2005). *Nursing theories and nursing practice.* Philadelphia: F. A. Davis.

Patel, D., & Greydanus, P. (2010). Sport participation by physically and cognitively challenged young athletes. *Pediatric Clinics of North America, 57*(3), 795–813.

Pender, N., Murdaugh, C., & Parsons, M. A. (2011). *Health promotion in nursing practice.* Upper Saddle River, NJ: Prentice Hall.

Scrof, B., & Velsor-Friedrich, B. (2006). Health promotion in adolescents: A review of Pender's health promotion model. *Nursing Science Quarterly, 19*(4), 366–373.

Stevens, J., Corso, P., Finkelstein, E., & Miller, T. (2006). The costs of fatal and non-fatal falls among older adults. *Injury Prevention, 12*(5), 290–295.

Tennstedt, S., Howland, J., Lachman, M., Peterson, E., Kasten, L., & Jette, A. (1998). A randomized, controlled trial of a group intervention to reduce fear of falling and associated activity restriction in older adults. *Journal of Gerontology, 53*(6), 84–92.

Tsai, P. (2003). A middle-range theory of caregiver stress. *Nursing Sciences Quarterly, 16*(2), 137–145.

U.S. Census Bureau. (2006). American community survey 2006. Retrieved August 9, 2011, from www.census.gov/hhes//www/disability/2006acs.html.

U.S. Department of Veterans Affairs. (2004). National Center for Patient Safety 2004 falls kit. Retrieved April 16, 2010, from www.patientsafety.gov/safetytopics/fallstoolkit/index.html.

Viggiani, K. (2000). Health maintenance and management of therapeutic regimen. In P. Edwards (Ed.), *The specialty practice of rehabilitation nursing* (pp. 80–101). Glenview, IL: Association of Rehabilitation Nurses.

World Health Organization. (1948). Preamble to the Constitution of the World Health Organization as adopted by the International Health Conference, New York, 19–22 June, 1946; signed on 22 July 1946 by the representatives of 61 States (Official Records of the World Health Organization, no. 2, p. 100) and entered into force on 7 April 1948. Retrieved August 9, 2011, from www.searo.who.int/EN/Section898/Section1441.htm.

World Health Organization. (1986). The Ottawa Charter for Health Promotion. First International Conference on Health Promotion. Retrieved August 9, 2011, from www.who.int/healthpromotion/conferences/previous/ottawa/en/.

Suggested Resources

Access to Disability Data: www.infouse.com/disabilitydata/home/index.php

American Association on Health and Disability: www.aahd.us/page.php?pname=about

Bureau of Labor Statistics: Employment Status of People with Disabilities: www.bls.gov/cps/cpsdisability.htm

CaregiverNJ: www.state.nj.us/caregivernj/basic/helptools/safety.shtml

Disability.gov: www.disability.gov/search/list?q=recreation&format=html

Disabled Sports USA: www.dsusa.org

Minnesota Safety Council: www.minnesotasafetycouncil.org/seniorsafe/fallcheck.pdf

National Disability Sports Alliance: www.ndsaonline.org

Online Resource for U.S. Disability Statistics: www.ilr.cornell.edu/edi/DisabilityStatistics/

Special Olympics International: www.specialolympics.org

Tax Benefits for Business Who Have Employees with Disabilities: www.irs.gov/businesses/small/article/0,,id=185704,00.html

Temple University Institute on Disabilities: http://disabilities.temple.edu/publications/download.asp

Texas Agrilife Extension Service: AgriLife.org

U.S. Association of Blind Athletes: www.usaba.org

U.S. Census Bureau American Fact Finder: http://factfinder.census.gov/home/saff/main.html?_lang=en

U.S. Census Bureau Disability Statistics Home Page: www.census.gov/hhes/www/disability/disability.html

U.S. Department of Labor: Finding Facts and Figures: Disability Data Resources: www.dol.gov/odep/archives/ek99/resources.htm

United States Paralympics: www.usparalympics.org

USA Deaf Sports Federation: www.usadsf.org

Wheelchair Sports USA: www.wsusa.org

CHAPTER 7
Physical Healthcare Patterns and Nursing Interventions

Cynthia D. Anderson, MSN RN CRRN • Donald D. Kautz, PhD RN CRRN CNE • Sharon Bryant, MPH BSN RN CRRN • Norma Clanin, MS RN CNS CRRN

Changes in the physical patterns of health form the basis of rehabilitation nursing. Nutrition, elimination, sleep, rest, activity, exercise, and sexual and reproductive patterns are all affected by the major illnesses, impairments, and disabilities seen in rehabilitation practice. Rehabilitation nurses must be experts in identifying actual and potential problems resulting from the disruption of these health patterns. In collaboration with clients and their families or caregivers, rehabilitation nurses set realistic, appropriate goals and must be astute when selecting interventions to reach these goals in a timely and cost-effective manner.

Nursing process provides a working framework, functional health patterns provide substance, and the nurse's professional philosophy and emerging evidence-based guidelines all influence current nursing practice. Nursing process begins with an understanding of what the client needs, expects, or wants, followed by a thorough assessment of the client's current health status. When planning care, nurses address identified needs (or nursing diagnoses [NDs]; North American Nursing Diagnosis Association International [NANDA-I], 2009–2011) using thoughtfully selected interventions (from the Nursing Interventions Classification [NIC]; Johnson et al., 2011) in a stepwise fashion as short-term goals are met or not met. The process concludes with ultimate goals (expected outcomes, or nursing outcomes classification [NOC]; Johnson et al., 2011) that promote optimal restoration of client health, independence, family function, interaction with others, and self-actualization. Nurses must integrate nursing practice into the interdisciplinary team's work of restoration and rehabilitation. Although all rehabilitation professionals work together to provide interdisciplinary care, rehabilitation nurses and case managers coordinate care, interact with family and community supports, and advocate for the client across disciplines when services must be added, adapted, or revised.

As the nursing profession evolves toward evidence-based practice, existing facility clinical pathways, protocols, policies, and procedures will be challenged by emerging science. Nursing interventions are now being scrutinized for efficacy, efficiency, and economy. What was once accepted as tried and true is now being put to the test. The electronic age is upon us, and access to resources for international nursing knowledge and science is ever expanding. Evidence-based practice emphasizes conscientious and judicious decision making based on current research and consideration of the client's goals and wishes (Ehrlich-Jones, O'Dwyer, Stevens, & Deutsch, 2008). Combining best evidence with the client's goals and wishes is

the art of rehabilitation nursing (Kautz, 2011). Rehabilitation nurses are stretching beyond their comfort zone to keep current with best practice guidelines and recommendations.

We have focused our efforts to provide the most current clinical guidelines available for each topic included in this chapter to provide a level of evidence (LOE) for the major interventions listed. Nurses are encouraged to obtain these guidelines for more detailed information and to view the original sources. Many studies lacked sufficient numbers of subjects or the scientific rigor needed for meaningful conclusions. Many of the interventions recommended have not been systematically tested for their effectiveness. Rehabilitation nurses need to be at the forefront of research to test the efficacy of these interventions. LOEs are defined as follows:

LOE 1: Evidence obtained from meta-analysis or systematic review of randomized controlled trials

LOE 2: Evidence obtained from controlled studies or randomized controlled trials

LOE 3: Evidence obtained from quasiexperimental or descriptive studies

LOE 4: Evidence obtained from expert committee reports or respected authorities.

I. Nutrition: Eating, Swallowing, and Feeding
   A. Overview
      1. Adequate nutrition is of particular importance for people with disabilities, chronic illness, or developmental difficulties.
      2. Adequate nutrition and hydration provide the energy, strength, and endurance clients need to participate in therapeutic exercises and relearn daily activities.
      3. Inadequate or excessive intake of food or fluid for body demands places the client at significant risk for multiple complications.
      4. Impaired swallowing and risk for aspiration, often seen in people with neurological illness or injury, warrants prompt and accurate identification to minimize the risk of aspiration and its associated complications.
      5. Although a causal effect has not yet been determined, poor oral care has been found in several studies to be associated with systemic diseases, including septicemia, pneumonia, and heart disease (Pear, 2007).
      6. Rehabilitation nurses must assess nutritional adequacy and select appropriate interventions to restore nutritional health.

B. Nutritional Needs

The body needs more than 40 nutrients and micronutrients each day, including carbohydrates, fats, proteins, vitamins, minerals, and water. Dietary preferences vary widely, and cultural food items, medically prescribed diets, and religious restrictions must be respected when helping clients achieve the appropriate balance of nutrients during health and illness. Factors affecting nutritional status may include psychosocial factors, mobility, medication regimens, dietary supplements and herbs, physical disorders, occupation, habits, substance abuse, home environment, education, social support, financial resources, and access. The goal for rehabilitation clients is to have adequate nutritional intake to support healing and meet metabolic demands and to modify the diet as needed during acute and chronic illness or disability.

1. Nursing assessment of nutritional status and adequacy includes the following (Mueller, Compher, Ellen, and the American Society for Parenteral and Enteral Board of Directors, 2011):
   a. Body weight and height
   b. Health history, dentition status, dysphagia, colitis, constipation, and substance abuse or chemical dependency, including recent and remote past
   c. Recent and remote dietary history, preferences, and cultural and religious patterns
   d. Ability to purchase, select, store, and prepare food properly (e.g., mobility and economic, cognitive, and access factors)
   e. Apparent muscle wasting and absence of body fat stores (e.g., as assessed by triceps measurement)
      1) Acute illness
      2) Comorbidities
      3) Depression
      4) Eating disorders (e.g., anorexia, bulimia), malabsorption syndromes
      5) Substance abuse
   f. Presence of excessive body fat stores: The client who is morbidly obese may have severe underlying nutritional deficiencies.
      1) Energy demands of body weight
      2) Inactivity
      3) Greater reliance for energy on fats, simple carbohydrates, and glucose
      4) Lower dietary fiber intake
   g. Diagnostic laboratory data
      1) Serum albumin indicates available protein stores.
      2) Hemoglobin indicates the ability to transport oxygen.
      3) Glycohemoglobin (hemoglobin A1c) indicates average blood glucose during the past 3 months.
      4) Prealbumin level indicates nutritional status, protein synthesis, and catabolism.
   h. Review of home medications, over-the-counter medications, supplements, and herbs for potential nutritional implications and drug interactions (e.g., Ritalin, Adderal, Provigil, steroids)
   i. Aging process
      1) Impaired mastication due to poor dentition or dentures
      2) Decreased esophageal peristalsis
      3) Decreased production of salivary secretions and digestive enzymes

2. NDs related to fluid and nutritional status (NANDA-I, 2009–2011)
   a. Impaired dentition
   b. Risk for electrolyte imbalance
   c. Adult failure to thrive
   d. Readiness for enhanced fluid balance
   e. Deficient (hypertonic or hypotonic) fluid volume
   f. Deficient (isotonic) fluid volume
   g. Excess fluid volume
   h. Risk for deficient fluid volume
   i. Risk for imbalanced fluid volume
   j. Risk for unstable blood glucose
   k. Risk for impaired liver function
   l. Nausea
   m. Imbalanced nutrition, less than body requirements
   n. Imbalanced nutrition, more than body requirements
   o. Imbalanced nutrition, risk for more than body requirements
   p. Readiness for enhanced nutrition
   q. Impaired oral mucous membrane
   r. Impaired swallowing

3. NDs related to eating, dietary choices, and dietary and fluid intake (NANDA-I, 2009–2011)
   a. Fatigue
   b. Anxiety
   c. Disturbed body image
   d. Ineffective coping
   e. Ineffective denial
   f. Grieving
   g. Hopelessness
   h. Disturbed personal identity
   i. Chronic or situational low self-esteem
   j. Bowel incontinence

k. Perceived constipation

l. Diarrhea

m. Dysfunctional gastrointestinal motility

n. Urge urinary incontinence

o. Urinary retention (acute or chronic)

p. Disturbed sensory perception (specify: visual, auditory, kinesthetic, gustatory, tactile, olfactory)

q. Impaired comfort

r. Risk for aspiration

s. Hyperthermia

t. Impaired physical mobility

u. Impaired spontaneous ventilation

v. Impaired verbal communication

w. Dysfunctional family process

x. Deficient knowledge

y. Noncompliance (adherence, ineffective)

z. Ineffective family therapeutic regimen management

4. Nursing interventions (NIC) to promote nutritional adequacy (See the Dietary Guidelines for Americans, 2010; U.S. Department of Health and Human Services and U.S. Department of Agriculture, 2010; LOE 1 and 2.)

a. Teach about daily recommended intake of essential nutrients and help the client select balanced meals.

1) Teach that all food selections should be based on the following two overarching guidelines:

a) Maintain calorie balance over time to achieve and sustain a healthy weight by decreasing calories and increasing physical activity.

b) Focus on consuming nutrient-dense foods and beverages by limiting intake of sodium, solid fats, added sugars, and refined grains and instead eat vegetables, fruits, whole grains, fat-free or low-fat milk and milk products, seafood, lean meats and poultry, eggs, beans, and peas, and nuts and seeds.

2) Select from foods that are available and acceptable and meet nutritional demands. Limit intake of saturated and trans fats, cholesterol (less than 300 mg/day), and saturated fatty acids (less than 10% of calories), avoiding added sugars, salt, and alcohol.

3) Maintain prescribed restrictions and adaptations appropriate to client condition (e.g., calories, carbohydrates, fats, protein, sodium, uric acid, allergies, intolerances, pregnancy, age).

b. Monitor actual intake at meal time for quantity and nutrient value.

c. Pay attention to possible food-drug interactions.

d. Encourage and support efforts to improve intake for desired weight loss, gain, or maintenance.

e. Monitor weight, albumin levels, and hemoglobin levels.

f. Use nutritional supplements, vitamins, and fluids as needed or prescribed.

g. Institute small, frequent meals to meet caloric needs when indicated.

h. Encourage sufficient fiber intake to promote bowel peristalsis.

i. Ensure adequate fluid intake for nutritional balance and elimination. Fluid restrictions may be appropriate for those with heart failure and renal disease.

j. Adjust food consistency for ease of chewing, for client safety, and to compensate for swallowing impairment.

k. Teach the client to read food labels.

l. Teach the client about correct and adequate portion control.

m. Assess the need for medications to stimulate appetite, such as oxandrolone (Oxandrin) or megestrol (Megace).

n. For clients with diabetes, see the Standards for Medical Care in Diabetes (2011) for guidelines on glucose monitoring, A1C, glycemic goals, diabetes self-management, as well as recommendations for nutrition and physical activity.

o. For clients with complex needs, consider referral to a clinical registered dietitian.

p. Provide a pleasant environment with limited distractions.

q. Provide training for professional and family caregivers who are hand-feeding clients. When feeding a client, follow the nursing interventions for dysphagia in section I.E. Dependence for feeding, not dysphagia, is the strongest predictor of aspiration pneumonia (Langmore et al., 1998).

C. Water Protocols for Clients with Dysphagia or While Taking Nothing by Mouth (NPO): Rehabilitation nurses are encouraged to work with speech-language pathologists (SLPs) in their own facility when implementing a water protocol. Information about both protocols can be obtained from the American Speech-Language-Hearing Association's website (www.asha.org).

1. The Frazier Rehabilitation Center (Louisville, KY) developed the Frazier Free Water Protocol, allowing clients with dysphagia or NPO (nil per os) to drink water between meals (Panther, 2008; Suiter, 2005). The rationale is that small amounts of water, even when aspirated, do not contribute to aspiration pneumonia, provided the client practices good oral hygiene. This protocol has been used for more than 20 years at the Frazier Rehabilitation Institute and is gaining popularity across the country. Wagner (2005) discusses the legal and ethical implications of the protocol. The Frazier Protocol balances safety, hydration, and quality of life. Good oral hygiene is the foundation of the protocol. This protocol is described here.

    a. All clients are first screened with 3 ounces of water at the bedside. Videofluoroscopic swallowing evaluation is recommended to identify silent aspirators. Impulsive clients or those with excessive coughing and discomfort are restricted to drinking water only under supervision. The physical stress of coughing may prevent oral intake of water in those with extreme coughing.

    b. For clients on oral diets, water is permitted after oral care before meals and starting 30 minutes after meals, once again after oral care. The 30-minute timeframe allows the client to swallow completely and clear the oral cavity of food residues.

    c. Medications are administered whole or crushed with a spoonful of applesauce, pudding, yogurt, or thickened liquid, never with water.

    d. Staff, clients, and families are educated on the rationale for encouraging water between meals, the guidelines for the intake of free water, and any restrictions. In some facilities, clients on the protocol wear armbands that indicate "no thin liquids except water between meals, after oral care."

    e. In all cases, the recommendations of the speech therapist for safe swallowing in each client should be followed. Additional compensatory measures may be recommended, such as chin tuck, head turn, or fluids by spoon or cup only.

2. Another promising protocol currently under study is the G. F. Strong Water Protocol (G. F. Strong Rehabilitation Centre, Vancouver, BC, Canada), which features different exclusion criteria, use of an algorithm, specific oral care regimens, interdisciplinary team involvement, an interdisciplinary team care plan, and staff supervision (Carlaw & Steele, 2009).

D. Swallowing and Aspiration: Swallowing (deglutition) is a series of complex physiologic activities that require both voluntary and involuntary actions. The cerebral cortex controls voluntary movements, and the brainstem controls involuntary movements needed for swallowing. Several cranial nerves affect nutrition and swallowing (**Table 7-1**).

    1. Normal anatomy and physiology of swallowing (**Figure 7-1**): There are four stages of swallowing, although some texts combine the oral preparatory and oral phases.

        a. Oral preparatory phase
            1) Food is prepared, food is smelled, salivation occurs, food is put into the mouth.
            2) Food is manipulated in the mouth to form a bolus and is pushed posterior toward the oropharynx.
            3) Voluntary event
        b. Oral phase
            1) The tongue is elevated to the roof of the mouth (palate).
            2) Lips close to contain oral contents.
            3) Buccal and facial tone are necessary for chewing.

Table 7-1. Cranial Nerve Functions Related to Swallowing and Nutrition

Cranial Nerve	Major Functions Related to Swallowing and Nutrition
CN I: Olfactory	Transmits sensation of smell to olfactory area of the cerebral cortex
CN V: Trigeminal	Innervates muscles of mastication and facial expression
	Sensory impulses from teeth, gums, and lips
CN VII: Facial	Receives sense of taste from anterior two-thirds of tongue
	Sensation of oropharynx
CN IX: Glossopharyngeal	Motor impulses to the muscles of the pharynx used in swallowing
	Sensory impulses from taste buds of posterior one-third of tongue
CN X: Vagus	Contractions of muscles of pharynx (swallowing) and larynx (phonation)
CN XI: Spinal accessory	Innervates the skeletal muscles of the soft palate, pharynx, and larynx, which contract reflexively during swallowing
CN XII: Hypoglossal	Motor innervations of the muscles of the tongue, allowing for coordinated contraction of the tongue muscles necessary for food manipulation, swallowing, and speech

Figure 7-1. Normal Swallow

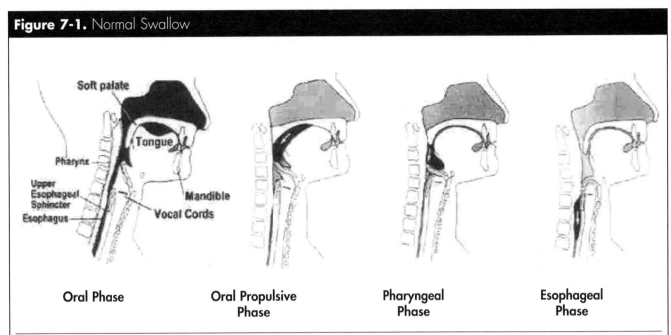

Oral Phase   Oral Propulsive Phase   Pharyngeal Phase   Esophageal Phase

From "Cough and aspiration of foods and liquids due to oral–pharyngeal dysphagia: ACCP evidence-based clinical practice guidelines," by C. A. Smith Hammond and L. Goldstein, 2006, *Chest, 129,* 156S. Copyright 2006 by the American College of Chest Physicians. Reprinted with permission.

4) Voluntary event

c. Pharyngeal phase

1) The bolus is carried by the swallowing reflex through the pharynx.

2) The soft palate and uvula are elevated to close the nasal pharynx.

3) The hyoid and larynx are elevated so food is less likely to enter the trachea.

4) An involuntary event is elicited by stimulation of sensory receptors located at the opening of the oral pharynx. This phase takes less than 1 second.

d. Esophageal phase

1) The bolus enters the stomach via peristalsis and gravity.

2) The lower esophageal sphincter opens.

3) Takes 5–8 seconds for solid foods

4) Involuntary event

2. Dysphagia is the subjective awareness of swallowing difficulty during the passage of a solid or liquid bolus from the mouth to the stomach. This symptom can be caused by functional or structural abnormalities of the oral cavity, pharynx, or esophagus (Scottish Intercollegiate Guidelines Network, 2010).

a. Causes of dysphagia may include radiation treatment, stroke, worsening dementia, myasthenia gravis, and amyotrophic lateral sclerosis.

b. Dysphasia is diagnosed through bedside assessment, videofluoroscopic swallow study, or endoscopic evaluation of swallowing. Other signs of dysphagia include pocketing, leakage of food

from the mouth, delayed or prolonged swallowing, frequent pneumonia, and weight loss.

c. Clinical manifestations that indicate a high risk of aspiration and the need for a swallowing evaluation, preferably by an SLP, include the need for oral pharyngeal suctioning, dysarthria (slurred, slow speech), dysphonia (impairment of the voice), weak voluntary cough, drooling, cough, wet voice or nasal regurgitation after water bolus, presence of a nasogastric tube, tracheal intubation, fever, shortness of breath, reflux, or vomiting (LOE 2).

d. Dysphagia can predispose clients to aspiration and malnutrition. Swallowing disorders may lead to embarrassment and social isolation.

3. Nursing interventions (NIC) for dysphagia: Rehabilitation nurses are encouraged to obtain the Smith Hammond and Goldstein (2006) evidence-based guideline developed by the American College of Chest Physicians Medical Specialty Society. It is current as of June 2010. Unless otherwise noted, LOEs for interventions in this section were determined by Smith Hammond and Goldstein. The guideline is available at www.guideline.gov.

a. Clients with a reduced level of consciousness should not be fed orally until consciousness has improved (LOE 2).

b. Clients with cough and a high risk of aspiration should be observed drinking 3 ounces of water. If the client coughs or shows clinical manifestations of aspiration, refer to an SLP for further evaluation before further oral intake (LOE 2).

c. Clients with dysphagia are best managed by an interdisciplinary team, including an SLP, nurse, physician, dietitian, and physical and occupational therapists (LOE 2).

d. Clients with intractable aspiration may be considered for surgical intervention (e.g., endogastric tube).

e. Abnormal lung radiographs of the right lower lobe, right upper lobe and left lower lobe, and auscultated rales and rhonchi are typical findings in true aspiration pneumonia. Lung assessment before and after a meal is essential in suspected "silent aspiration" (Sievers, 2008).

f. Clients may have difficulty swallowing medications. (See Wright, 2009, for a consensus guideline for these clients.)

g. Seat the client upright, preferably at 90 degrees in a chair with head or neck flexion if possible.

h. Minimize distractions. Provide a quiet environment with no television, and discourage talking during meals.

i. Select foods of appropriate consistency and texture.
   1) Progress over time from pureed to ground to regular food.
   2) With ground food, gradually add food that fragments easily.
   3) Stay with one food and texture at a time.
   4) Do not mix solids and liquids.

j. Progress liquid intake from pudding thick, to applesauce thick, to honey thick, to nectar or syrup thick, to thin. Use a commercial thickener to achieve the appropriate consistency as needed.

k. The speech therapist may recommend placing food on the unaffected side of the mouth and using small mouthfuls; encourage the client to turn his or her head to the unaffected side to bring food into the midline.

l. Teach the client to concentrate fully on chewing each small mouthful, forming a food bolus, and swallowing it before taking another mouthful or speaking.

m. Use the chin-tuck method to protect the airway.
   1) Encourage the client to do a tongue sweep of mouth to self-check for food pocketing.
   2) Use compensatory strategies such as a double swallow between mouthfuls to prevent aspiration.
   3) Instruct the client to take small sips of water between mouthfuls or to alternate liquid and solid mouthfuls as appropriate.

n. Visually inspect the oral cavity for pocketing and use wide-mouth drinking vessels to allow visualization of progress of liquids into the oral cavity.

o. Provide a calm, unhurried atmosphere and appropriate supervision. Do not allow the client to eat unattended or unobserved.
   1) Use adaptive devices for self-feeding and independence.
   2) Give clients with impulsivity one item of food or drink at a time and limit distractions.

p. Give cues for strategies; follow the speech and occupational therapist's recommendations.

q. Ensure the client remains upright for 20–30 minutes after eating a meal.

r. Before discharge, instruct family and caregivers in dysphagia precautions, the current dysphagia diet, use of thickeners if necessary, signs of aspiration, and the Heimlich maneuver. Suggest enrollment in a CPR course (Sievers, 2008).

E. The National Dysphagia Diet (NDD) provides guidelines for progressive diets for those with dysphagia (Garcia & Chambers, 2010). Diets must be individualized and reassessed as the client's condition or skills change.
   1. NDD1: Dysphagia pureed
      a. Pudding-like consistencies
      b. No chunks
      c. Avoid lumpy foods and small pieces.
   2. NDD2: Dysphagia mechanically altered
      a. Soft, moist foods
      b. Ground meats, soft vegetables
      c. No bread, peas, or corn
      d. Avoid skins and seeds.
      e. Mechanical soft (same as above but can have bread, cakes, rice)
   3. NDD3: Dysphagia advanced
      a. Regular foods except very hard, sticky, or crunchy foods
      b. Avoid hard fruits and vegetables, corn, skins, nuts, seeds.
   4. Liquid consistencies (viscosities) are described as spoon thick, honey-like, nectar-like, or thin. Some facilities use the descriptors *pudding, applesauce, honey, syrup,* and *thin.* Several studies have noted variability in the viscosity of thickened liquid consistencies even among SLPs. New studies are emerging with various methods to measure and standardize the interpretation of these terms.

THE SPECIALTY PRACTICE OF REHABILITATION NURSING

F. Administration of Specialized Nutritional Support

1. Rehabilitation nurses may care for clients who need enteral (feeding tube) or parental (intravenous) nutritional support. The American Society for Parenteral and Enteral Nutrition (ASPEN) regularly updates its clinical guidelines for assessing clients in need of specialized nutritional support, access devices, and administration of nutritional supplements through the enteral and parenteral routes (2009). The recommendation for clients with acute traumatic brain injury is to attain full caloric replacement feeding by Day 7 after injury to avoid nitrogen wasting (LOE 2; Brain Trauma Foundation, 2007).

2. Clients are fed by gastrostomy tube to provide temporary or permanent access to the gut when oral intake is not possible. Aspiration pneumonia is a lethal complication of tube feeding.

   a. Ensure adequate fluid intake by frequently assessing hydration status.

   b. Monitor body weight and serum albumin.

   c. Regularly check tube placement and aspirate gastric contents for residual before instillations.

   d. Maintain the head of bed at 30 degrees or higher during feeding and do not lay the client flat for at least 30 minutes after meals (LOE 2). Minimize nighttime feedings. Never add blue dye to enteral formula.

   e. Time feedings to be either continuous or bolus. If caloric needs can be met, bolus is preferred, with a gradual return to normal patterns of intake.

   f. Assess lungs for rales and rhonchi often.

   g. Sterile water is preferred for flushes and hydration purposes in immunocompromised and critically ill clients (LOE 4). Flushes of 30 ml water should be provided every 4 hours during continuous feedings and before and after intermittent feedings, aspirations for residuals, and medication administrations (LOE 2).

   h. Medications should be diluted in water before administration. Each medication should be administered individually to prevent physical and chemical incompatibilities and tube obstruction (LOE 2). Liquid dosage forms are preferred. Do not crush enteric-coated, time-release, or extended-release tablets. Flush with at least 15 ml sterile water between medications. Do not add medications directly into the formula.

   i. Acceptable hang times of enteral formula for adults are 8 hours for open systems using decanted formula and 24–48 hours in closed systems per the manufacturer's guideline. Administration sets for open systems should be changed at least every 24 hours (LOE 2). Maintain aseptic technique with tubing changes.

   j. Use portable equipment to allow participation in the therapy regimen.

   k. Protect the gastrostomy site with skin shields and routine skin cleansing.

   l. Encourage client and family participation in feeding and medication administration as soon as possible. Before discharge with a gastric tube in place, teach auscultation for tube placement, aspiration for gastric contents, skin care at the insertion site, cleansing of equipment, medication preparation and administration, and storage and measurement of formula and water boluses.

3. Clients are fed by hyperalimentation via central intravenous catheters when use of the gut is not possible. All aspects of facility policies and procedures regarding hyperalimentation and central venous access devices should be reviewed annually for compliance with current best practice.

   a. Provide special care for the access site, tubing, and solution.

   b. Ensure adequate caloric intake through periodic use of lipid solutions.

   c. Regularly monitor body chemistries to help in the adjustment of solution electrolytes and lipids.

   d. Gradually introduce oral intake and taper hyperalimentation.

G. Expected Outcomes (NOC)

1. The client achieves and maintains a healthful weight (body mass index 18.5–24.9).

2. Laboratory measures of albumin, prealbumin, hemoglobin A1c, hemoglobin, hematocrit, blood urea nitrogen, protein, and creatinine are all within normal limits.

3. The client experiences no complications related to dysphagia, parenteral alimentation, or hyperalimentation.

II. **Skin Integrity, Impairments, and Interventions**

A. Overview

1. Rehabilitation clients present with multiple risk factors for skin injury and breakdown. Clients at highest risk are those who have been hospitalized longer than 1 week, those who have been residents of long-term care facilities for longer than 4 weeks, clients older than 65 years of age, children

younger than age 5, neonates, and those with spinal cord injury. "Adult inpatient hospital stays with a diagnosis of pressure ulcers totaled $11.0 billion in 2006" (Wound, Ostomy and Continence Nurses Society [WOCN], 2010, p. 1). Pressure ulcers significantly increase the length of hospital stay from the usual 3–5 days to 13 or 14 days, and clients are three times more likely to be discharged to long-term care facilities (WOCN).

2. Client and family education about prevention of skin breakdown is extremely important during care and must be a component of the interdisciplinary plan of care.

3. Several groups have published practice guidelines based on extensive critiques of research literature and expert reviews on the prevention and treatment of pressure ulcers. The major resources and guidelines for this section are from the WOCN (2010), the National Pressure Ulcer Advisory Panel and European Pressure Ulcer Advisory Panel (NPUAP & EPUAP, 2009), and the Registered Nurses Association of Ontario (RNAO, 2005). The RNAO guideline was used to provide the LOEs for many of the interventions listed.

4. Rehabilitation nurses need to be skilled in maintaining intact skin and identifying, documenting, and aggressively treating pressure ulcers upon initial discovery. In addition, skillful identification and treatment of vascular ulcers, neuropathic ulcers, surgical incisions, skin tears, and burns is extremely important because these lesions are commonly encountered in rehabilitation practice.

5. Rehabilitation nurses should immediately institute appropriate interventions to prevent, identify, and treat skin breakdown due to maceration (e.g., moisture from incontinence or intertriginous skin folds) and fungal, bacterial, or viral skin infections.

6. The nursing priorities for skin care are to prevent and heal wounds. All wounds should be treated with appropriate techniques and dressings that protect the wound and facilitate healing.

B. Anatomy and Function of the Skin (DuVivier, 1993; Porth & Matfin, 2008)
The major functions of skin are protection, immunity, thermoregulation, sensation, metabolism, and communication. The skin is the largest organ, covering almost 2 square meters in the average adult, weighing about 6 pounds, and receiving one-third of the body's circulating blood. Adult skin varies in thickness from 0.5 mm to 6 mm (Bryant & Nix, 2007; **Figure 7-2**).

1. Epidermis: The outermost layer, made of five thin layers. It lacks a blood supply, contains melanin and keratin to protect deeper layers of the skin, and is constantly being replaced by newer cells from the dermis every 45–75 days, or about every 2 months. Mucous membranes are a modified form of very thin epidermis that lacks tough keratin layers.
   a. Protects against ultraviolet radiation
   b. Protects from environmental antigens
   c. Protects the body from injury
   d. Retains moisture
   e. Excretes waste products
   f. Assists in regulating body temperature

2. Dermal layer: Fibrous connective tissue, thicker than epidermis, contains blood supply, lymphatic vessels, nerves, glands, hair follicles, and nail beds
   a. Allows elasticity of skin
   b. Permits motion
   c. Supports healing
   d. Contains sweat glands, oil glands, and hair follicles
   e. Contains neuron receptors for touch, pain, and vasomotor response
   f. Provides nutritional support, immune surveillance, thermal regulation, hemostasis, and anti-inflammatory responses

3. Subcutaneous layer: Forms a continuous layer of connective tissue over muscles, tendons, ligaments, and bones, sometimes called the fatty insulation layer, with the upper portion being fatty and the lower layer being thin elastic tissue, varies in thickness with little or no tissue at heels, bridge of nose, scalp, and behind ears

4. Fascia: The fibrous connective tissue membrane that covers and separates muscles, ligaments, and tendons
   a. Contains fat, collagen, sweat glands, and tissue fluids
   b. Varies in thickness and composition depending on body location

5. Circulation
   a. Provides nutrients, oxygenation, and moisture
   b. Promotes healing through increased blood supply, phagocytosis, and tissue rebuilding
   c. Provides support and healing in response to tissue load damage

6. Nerve supply: Provides response to environment and supports homeostasis

C. Normal Skin Changes with Aging
   1. Epidermis and dermis become thinner, fat in subcutaneous layer decreases, fine hair on limbs and face decreases, and cohesion of the dermal and

Figure 7-2. Normal Skin

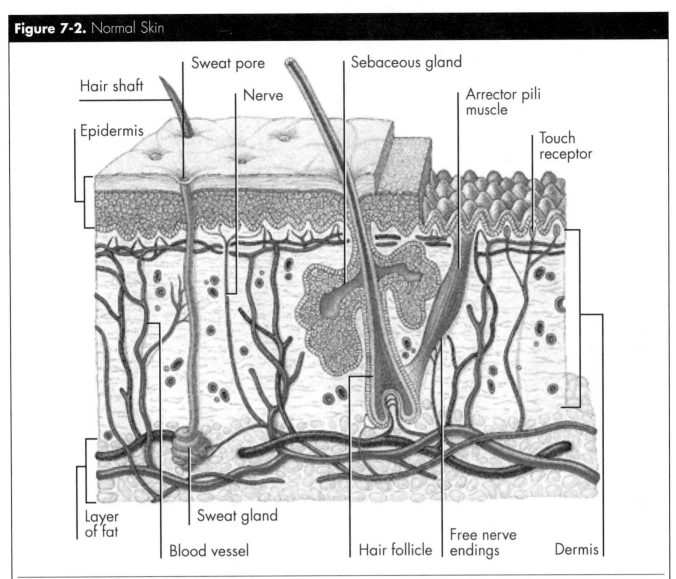

From *Acute and chronic wounds: Current management concepts* (3rd ed.), by R. A. Bryant and D. P. Nix, 2007, Philadelphia: Mosby. Copyright 2007 by Mosby. Reprinted with permission.

epidermal layers decreases (flattening of the junction layer).

2. Blood vessels become more prominent.
3. Production of basal cells, mast cells, collagen, melanin, elastin, and Langerhans cells decreases.
4. Physiologic functions such as hair and nail growth, glandular secretions, immune surveillance, vascular supply, vitamin D synthesis, inflammatory response, and tissue repair decrease.
5. Surface becomes pale, wrinkled, dry, and less stretchable; brownish spots appear on the face and hands.
6. Reduced sensation, especially pain receptors
7. Itching is common.
8. Sensitivity to fabrics, soaps, deodorants, and cosmetics increases.
9. Difficulty regulating body temperature due to reduced fatty insulation of the subcutaneous layer, more prone to hypothermia and heat stroke
10. Increased vulnerability to minor trauma (e.g., skin tears, hematomas, bruises, abrasions, and lacerations)

D. Risk Factors for Loss of Skin Integrity
1. Physiological factors
   a. Altered metabolic states that increase the body's need for nutrients, indicated by low serum protein, albumin, prealbumin, and hemoglobin, which impair the body's cellular rebuilding ability
   b. Underlying acute or chronic medical conditions (e.g., diabetes, cardiopulmonary or renal disease) or disease treatment (e.g., high-dose steroids after spinal cord injury, radiation)

c. Impaired circulation from peripheral neuropathies, anemia, atherosclerosis, hypertension, or smoking, which causes vasoconstriction and impairs the vascular bed

d. Prolonged pressure and immobility, leading to pressure ulcer formation

e. Neurological injuries that result in impaired sensations of proprioception, temperature, and touch, resulting in the inability to perceive the need to move the body

f. Immunosuppressant medications

g. Poor nutrition, especially inadequate intake of protein, vitamin C, thiamine, and zinc

h. Bladder and bowel incontinence

i. Advanced age: Older adults have less effective skin protection because of changes in the epidermis, diminished glandular secretions and vascular supply, thinning of the dermis, reduced numbers of elastin fibers, reduced tactile sensitivity, and slowed inflammatory response, all contributing to delayed wound healing. Older adults also have a higher incidence of skin disorders (e.g., stasis dermatitis, seborrheic dermatitis and keratoses, comedones, benign tumors, dermatophytosis, xerosis, cherry and spider angiomas, eczema, psoriasis, lichen planus, nevi, skin tags, lentigo, ringworm, rosacea, tinea pedis and cruris, varicosities, and neoplasms) and are more likely to have comorbidities and mobility problems (Balin, 1990).

2. Mechanical factors

a. Sustained pressure: Resting surfaces that are hard and unyielding and maintain constant pressure in one direction, particularly over bony prominences when repositioning is infrequent

b. Shearing: The movement of muscle, subcutaneous, and fat tissues downward and compression against the bony skeleton while the epidermis does not slide (as occurs when the client is sitting up in bed and slides down in response to gravity)

c. Friction: Rubbing of tissue across a rough surface (as occurs with incomplete lifting or dragging of a client to pull him or her up in bed) and ill-fitting prostheses, braces, orthoses, or shoes, especially in the presence of neuropathy

d. Body moisture: Incontinence, diuresis, or sweating, especially in the skin folds of an obese client; drainage associated with stomas (e.g., gastrostomy tube, tracheostomy, colostomy, ileostomy, and urostomy)

3. Psychosocial factors

a. Noncompliance with recommended healthcare practices

b. Substance abuse that impairs judgment, nutrition, mobility, or sensation

c. Impaired cognitive or intellectual ability

d. Depression

e. Social isolation, particularly when the client needs assistance in daily care

E. Assessment of Clients at Risk for Impaired Skin Integrity: Assess all of the following on admission to a rehabilitation facility and daily for those identified as at risk for skin breakdown (LOE 4; RNAO, 2005). Many facilities now require documentation of skin risk assessments every shift.

1. General assessment components

a. Underlying medical conditions

b. Nutritional status: Protein, albumin and prealbumin, hemoglobin, transferrin, and white blood cell count; hemoglobin A1c if diabetic, appetite, and recent unintentional weight loss or gain

c. Hydration status

d. Circulatory support

e. Presence of neurological injury

f. Exposure to moisture: Incontinence of bladder or bowel, body moisture

g. Sensory-perceptual ability

h. Mobility, activity and exercise, body positioning

i. Pressure, shearing, and friction, which may occur in the course of bedside care

j. Age: Older adults are at particular risk for developing pressure ulcers because they are most likely to have problems in all of these categories.

2. Assessment scales: Assessment scales are routinely used in all inpatient care settings. However, only one study from Brazil was located that demonstrated good predictive validity of the Braden Scale in older long-term care facility residents (Tosta de Souza, Conciecao de Gouveia Santos, Iri, & Oguri, 2010). The Braden Scale is the most popular in the United States and internationally. Other assessment scales exist (i.e., Performance Palliation Scale, Karnofsky Performance Scale, Neonatal Skin Risk Assessment Scale, Neonatal Skin Condition Score, and Starkid Skin Scale), but data to support their reliability and validity are limited. Rehabilitation nurses need to gather data to show whether completing a risk assessment scale actually triggers specific interventions that prevent skin breakdown.

a. The Braden Scale was developed in 1987 and is used internationally. Its reliability and validity have been tested with evidence-based interventions. It contains six weighted elements—sensory perception, moisture, activity, mobility, nutrition (each of which is graded from 1 [*very poor or very limited*] to 4 [*excellent, normal*] and friction/shear (which is scored from 1 to 3). Grades are summed across all elements for a total risk status score (**Figure 7-3**). The subscales for activity and friction/shear alone have shown higher predictive value than other subscales on the tool. Scores of 15–18 indicate mild risk, 13–14 indicate moderate risk, 10–12 indicate high risk, and scores of 9 or below are very high risk. The Braden Q Scale was a later development adapted for pediatric populations.

b. Norton scale: Developed in 1961, it contains a simpler list of five weighted elements including physical condition, mental condition, activity, mobility, and incontinence, which are scored from 1 (*immobile or poor*) to 4 (*excellent*) and summed for a total risk status score. Scores of 14 or above indicate mild risk, 13 indicates moderate risk, and 12 or below indicates high risk.

c. For both scoring systems, low scores prompt specific interventions to decrease risk and maintain or restore skin integrity. Skin risk scores over time can be reviewed to demonstrate improvement.

F. Nursing Diagnoses Related to Skin Integrity and Associated Risk Factors (NANDA-I, 2009–2011)
1. Impaired bed and impaired wheelchair mobility
2. Impaired transfer ability
3. Activity intolerance
4. Impaired physical mobility
5. Ineffective peripheral tissue perfusion
6. Acute and chronic pain
7. Posttrauma syndrome
8. Bowel incontinence
9. Diarrhea
10. Urinary incontinence (functional, overflow, reflex, stress, urge)
11. Imbalanced nutrition, less than body requirements
12. Imbalanced nutrition, more than body requirements
13. Impaired oral mucous membrane
14. Impaired swallowing
15. Self-neglect
16. Unilateral neglect
17. Risk for peripheral neurovascular dysfunction
18. Disturbed sensory perception (kinesthetic, tactile)
19. Deficient fluid volume
20. Noncompliance (ineffective adherence) with preventive interventions (e.g., weight shifts, turning in bed, management of incontinence, daily skin checks, disease management, dietary restrictions)
21. Contamination (of lesions, wounds, incisions)
22. Impaired environmental interpretation syndrome
23. Hyperthermia
24. Hypothermia
25. Impaired verbal communication
26. Disturbed personal identity
27. Impaired skin integrity
28. Risk for impaired skin integrity
29. Impaired tissue integrity
30. Ineffective thermoregulation
31. Ineffective health self-management
32. Deficient knowledge (self-care, skin care, hygiene, foot care)
33. Ineffective therapeutic regimen management
34. Ineffective family therapeutic regimen management

G. Nursing Interventions (NIC) to Maintain Skin Integrity: Unless indicated otherwise, the LOE is 4 for all of the following interventions (NPUAP & EPUAP, 2009; RNAO, 2005; WOCN, 2010).
1. Ensure good nutritional support; Use supplements if needed. Protein or calorie malnutrition inhibits wound healing by reducing fibroblast and collagen synthesis.
2. Manage tissue loads.
   a. Turn and reposition the client frequently.
      1) Every 2 hours in bed, even if using a pressure-reducing mattress
      2) Every hour in a chair
      3) Weight shift every 15 minutes in a chair if independent.
   b. Use good lifting, transfer, and turning techniques. Consult an occupational or physical therapist as needed.
   c. Cushion bony prominences.
   d. Protect skin against friction and shearing. Elevate heels off the mattress with pillows or pressure-relieving boots. Use turn sheets to reposition or lift the client. Maintain the head of bed at or below 30 degrees unless contraindicated by the condition; position at 30 degrees or less lateral incline for side-lying.
   e. Position the client with adequate support; avoid placing the client on an existing ulcer.
   f. Increase the client's efforts toward mobility and activity. An overhead trapeze may be appropriate for some clients.
   g. Provide a pressure redistribution mattress

Figure 7-3. Braden Scale for Predicting Pressure Sore Risk

Patient's Name _____   Evaluator's Name _____   Date of Assessment _____

	1.	2.	3.	4.				
SENSORY PERCEPTION Ability to respond meaningfully to pressure-related discomfort	**1. Completely Limited** Unresponsive (does not moan, flinch, or grasp) to painful stimuli due to diminished level of consciousness or sedation. OR Limited ability to feel pain over most of the body	**2. Very Limited** Responds only to painful stimuli; cannot communicate discomfort except by moaning or restlessness OR Has a sensory impairment that limits the ability to feel pain or discomfort over 1/2 of body.	**3. Slightly Limited** Responds to verbal commands but cannot always communicate discomfort or the need to be turned. OR Has some sensory impairment that limits ability to feel pain or discomfort in one or two extremities.	**4. No Impairment** Responds to verbal commands; has no sensory deficit that would limit ability to feel or voice pain or discomfort.				
MOISTURE Degree to which skin is exposed to moisture	**1. Constantly Moist** Skin is kept moist almost constantly by perspiration, urine, etc. Dampness is detected every time a patient is moved or turned.	**2. Very Moist** Skin is often, but not always, moist. Linen must be changed at least once a shift.	**3. Occasionally Moist** Skin is occasionally moist, requiring an extra linen change approximately once a day.	**4. Rarely Moist** Skin is usually dry, linen only requires changing at routine intervals.				
ACTIVITY Degree of physical activity	**1. Bedfast** Confined to bed	**2. Chairfast** Ability to walk is severely limited or nonexistent. Cannot bear own weight and/or must be assisted into a chair or wheelchair.	**3. Walks Occasionally** Walks occasionally during the day but for very short distances, with or without assistance. Spends majority of each shift in bed or chair.	**4. Walks Frequently** Walks outside the room at least twice a day and inside the room at least once every two hours during waking hours				
MOBILITY Ability to change and control body position	**1. Completely Immobile** Does not make even slight changes in body or extremity position without assistance	**2. Very Limited** Makes occasional slight changes in body or extremity position but is unable to make frequent or significant changes independently.	**3. Slightly Limited** Makes frequent though slight changes in body or extremity position independently.	**4. No Limitation** Makes major and frequent changes in position without assistance.				

continued

THE SPECIALTY PRACTICE OF REHABILITATION NURSING

Figure 7-3. Braden Scale for Predicting Pressure Sore Risk *continued*

	1. Very Poor	2. Probably Inadequate	3. Adequate	4. Excellent
NUTRITION Usual food intake pattern	Never eats a complete meal. Rarely eats more than 1/3 of any food offered. Eats two servings or less of protein (meat or dairy products) per day. Takes fluids poorly. Does not take a liquid dietary supplement OR Is NPO and/or maintained on clear liquids or IV for more than 5 days.	Rarely eats a complete meal and generally eats only about 1/2 of any food offered. Protein intake includes only three servings of meat or dairy products per day. Occasionally will take a dietary supplement. OR Receives less than optimum amount of liquid diet or tube feeding	Eats over half of most meals. Eats a total of four servings of protein (meat, dairy products) per day. Occasionally will refuse a meal, but will usually take a supplement when offered OR Is on a tube feeding or total parenteral nutrition regimen which probably meets most of nutritional needs	Eats most of every meal. Never refuses a meal. Usually eats a total of 4 or more servings of meat and dairy products. Occasionally eats between meals. Does not require supplementation.
	1. Problem	**2. Potential Problem**	**3. No Apparent Problem**	
FRICTION AND SHEAR	Requires moderate to maximum assistance in moving. Complete lifting without sliding against sheets is impossible. Frequently slides down in bed or chair, requiring frequent repositioning with maximum assistance. Spasticity, contractures or agitation leads to almost constant friction	Moves feebly or requires minimum assistance. During a move skin probably slides to some extent against sheets, chairs, restraints, or other devices. Maintains relatively good position in a chair or bed most of the time but occasionally slides down.	Moves in bed and in chair independently and has sufficient muscle strength to lift up completely during a move. Maintains good position in a bed or chair.	
				Total Score

(i.e., low-air-loss or air-fluidized mattress for stage III or IV [LOE 1]) and a wheelchair cushion for high-risk clients. Gel or air cushions are more effective than foam in preventing ischial pressure ulcers (LOE 1).

    h. Involve the interdisciplinary team.

    i. Avoid foam rings, donuts, and sheepskin. These may provide temporary comfort but do not provide pressure relief; they transfer pressure to surrounding tissue and may contribute to friction or shear (NPUAP & EPUAP, 2009).

3. Routine daily skin care:

    a. Inspect skin daily and pay special attention to all bony prominences.

    b. Cleanse skin at regular intervals and use a mild cleansing agent to preserve the neutral pH of the skin.

    c. Apply nonsensitizing, pH-balanced emollients to help maintain skin moisture (LOE 3).

    d. Avoid massaging bony prominences to prevent tissue damage (LOE 2).

    e. Minimize exposure to incontinence, perspiration, or wound drainage (LOE 4).

        1) Use wicking materials to draw moisture away from the skin (e.g., underpads, diapers, or briefs).

        2) Use topical agents as protective barriers.

        3) Institute bladder and bowel training regimens for incontinence management. Consider short-term use of indwelling or external catheters while the client is extremely immobile. Consider a pouch or collection device for urine, stool, or draining wounds.

        4) Change wet or soiled absorbent briefs immediately. Cleanse gently and dry the skin thoroughly. Avoid the use of absorbent briefs and propping urinals for long periods through the night. Remove bedpans promptly after use. A bedside commode is preferred over a bedpan at night as soon as the client is able to transfer safely and maintain sitting balance.

4. Teach clients and caregivers about the importance of self-efficacy in nutrition, management of tissue loads, skin inspection, and general skin care (LOE 3).

H. Essential Elements for Planning Wound Care and Expected Client Outcomes (NOC)

1. Nutritional assessment and support: Nutritional support provides sufficient protein to produce serum albumin values of at least 3.5, and the client's weight will be more than 80% of ideal. Several weeks of intensive therapy are needed to increase serum albumin. Prealbumin testing shows a rise in 3–5 days.

2. Management of tissue loads: Resting surfaces and positioning provide adequate protection for tissue load to encourage healing and prevent further breakdown (LOE 4).

3. Wound care: Wound-specific care promotes wound cleansing and healing. Response to treatment may be slow because of underlying vascular damage, comorbidities, and immobility.

I. General Nursing Interventions for Wounds and Pressure Ulcers (NIC)

1. Promote increased protein intake, vitamin supplementation, and adequate hydration. Correct any nutritional deficiencies (LOE 4). Ensure that the client's diet provides 30–40 kcal per kilogram body weight per day and total protein of 1.25–1.5 g protein per kilogram body weight (NPUAP& EPUAP, 2009). Consult a dietitian for appropriate supplementation, especially if a client with a pressure ulcer is underweight or losing weight (NPUAP & EPUAP, 2009). Small studies have demonstrated improved healing rates in high-risk clients given supplemental protein, arginine, zinc, and vitamin C for 3 weeks (WOCN, 2010).

2. Keep the client off the wound as much as possible (LOE 3).

3. Turn and reposition the client at least every 2 hours while in bed, every hour in a chair, using sheets to lift (not drag) the client; if possible, use an over-the-bed trapeze to encourage the client to assist with lifting (LOE 3).

4. Use positioning pillows and blocks to maintain pressure relief; consider using pressure-reducing devices (e.g., air mattresses, specialty foam surfaces, gel pads, low-air-loss mattresses, and wheelchair cushions). Float heels off the bed using pillows, foam, or sheepskin-lined boots or other flotation devices (LOE 3).

5. Manage pain. Encourage mobility (LOE 3).

6. Assess circulatory status. Wounds must receive adequate circulation to heal (LOE 4).

7. Keep the skin clean, dry, and lubricated; do not massage reddened bony prominences because this may cause capillary destruction (LOE 3).

8. Manage incontinence. Initiate toileting and bladder and bowel training programs. Change linens promptly and clean the skin after any episodes of bladder or bowel incontinence; remove wrinkles in linens to prevent further pressure. Apply a moisture barrier (e.g., ointment, paste, lotion, or film-forming spray) to exposed skin for further protection (LOE 3).

9. Provide consistent, timely treatments and document progress (LOE 3). Spray cleanse the wound with isotonic saline, Vulnopur (saline, aloe vera, silver chloride, and decyl glucoside), a commercial wound cleanser, or sterile water. Recent studies found no statistical difference in wound healing when comparing saline with water, but there was a significant improvement for wounds cleansed with Vulnopur (Moore & Cowman, 2005).

10. Focus treatment approaches on the whole person and the environment; pressure ulcers tend to be multivariate in cause (LOE 4).

11. Assess and reassess pressure ulcers using standard staging guidelines. Pressure ulcers are staged according to depth, characteristics of the wound bed, and potential involvement of deep fascia (**Figure 7-4**). In some states, inpatient healthcare facilities are required to report all stage III and stage IV pressure ulcers. Therefore, some facilities allow only specially trained nurses to document the stage of ulcers.

J. Wound-Specific Nursing Interventions for Pressure Ulcers (**Table 7-2**)

K. Phases of Wound Healing
   1. Vascular supply and wound stabilization (i.e., the wound bleeds and then clots)
   2. Inflammation of the tissues with influx of lymphocytes, macrophages, and granulocytes, concurrently while phagocytes remove dead tissue (inflammatory phase)
   3. Proliferation of fibrin and formation of a loose matrix within the wound, which supports additional tissue formation and retention (granulation and epithelialization)
   4. Maturation of the fibrin matrix into intact skin (remodeling)

L. Documentation of Wound Healing (LOE 4)
   1. Stage and document the wound upon first discovery. Describe the location and measure (in centimeters) length (head to toe), width (side to side), and depth of the wound; use transparent grids for accuracy in measurement if needed. Measure wounds each week to determine effectiveness of treatments and healing.
   2. Describe the wound base and tissue type (e.g., color, presence or absence of moisture, epithelialization, granulation, hypergranulation, slough, eschar).
   3. Evaluate undermining or sinus tract or tunneling formation by gently probing the wound with sterile gauze swabs to determine the depth of pockets, tunnels, or tracts. Use the clock method to describe the location of the undermine or tract (e.g., "2-cm tunnel at 2 o'clock").

4. Evaluate the amount and type of drainage. Note any odor from the wound.
5. Evaluate the periwound skin. Note any erythema, maceration, or callus formation. Evaluate for infection (presence or absence) and wound edges (open, attached, closed, or rolled).
6. Note evidence of pain, induration, or inflammation and remember that redness, hardness, or discoloration around pressure areas that have poor blood supply (e.g., heels, sacrum) can mask major tissue necrosis behind apparently intact skin.
7. Include the present and planned treatment regimen.
8. Photograph the wound for baseline reference and repeat at periodic intervals (generally every week) until the wound is healed. This is a helpful visual measure to document the effectiveness of therapy. Obtain written client consent before taking pictures.
9. Document pressure wounds that are healing by retaining the label of the original stage adding the descriptor "healing"; do not revert to lesser staging as the wound heals. Exception: The Minimum Data Set and Inpatient Rehabilitation Facility Patient Assessment Instrument both require staff to revert to lesser staging.

M. Expected Client Outcomes (NOC) Related to Potential or Impaired Skin Integrity
   1. Expect signs of healing within 14 days (LOE 2).
   2. Intact skin
   3. The client performs appropriate self-efficacy measures in the maintenance of skin integrity.
   4. No new areas of skin breakdown

III. Elimination: Bladder and Bowel Function
   A. Overview
      1. The human body eliminates the waste of metabolism through urine and stool.
      2. Requirements for normal function include the following:
         a. Anatomical integrity
         b. Intact neurological components for both voluntary control and synergistic emptying
         c. A predictable pattern of waste production
         d. Physical and mental ability and the willingness to carry out toileting-related tasks
      3. Clients in rehabilitation facilities often need treatment for constipation, urinary or bowel incontinence, or management of neurogenic bowel and bladder.
      4. Bowel and bladder disorders are major barriers to community living, employment, and social activity.
      5. Rehabilitation nurses must be knowledgeable about the normal physiology of bladder and

Figure 7-4. Stages of Pressure Ulcers

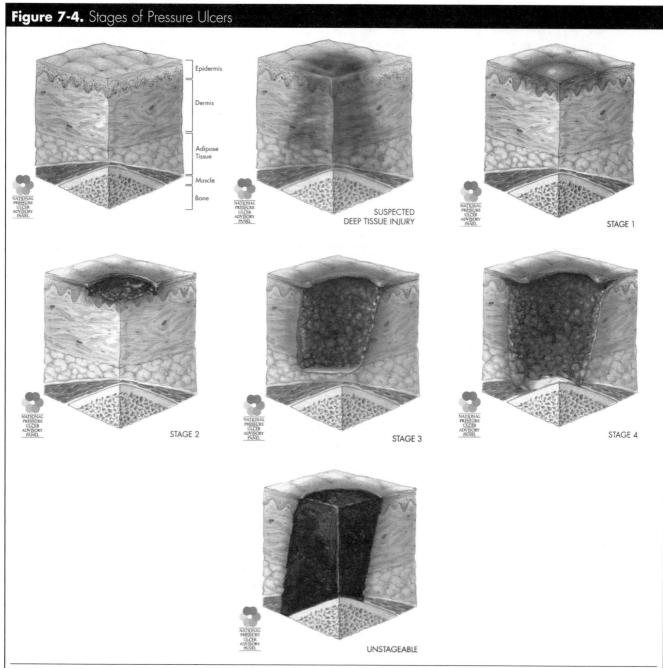

From *Pressure ulcer category/staging illustrations*, by the National Pressure Ulcer Advisory Panel. (n.d.), Retrieved September 21, 2011, from http://npuap.org/resources.htm. Copyright by National Pressure Ulcer Advisory Panel. Reprinted with permission.

bowel function, clinically astute in identifying disruptions that produce incontinence and dysfunction, and expert in selecting interventions that will help the client develop predictable, effective elimination patterns.

6. Management of bowel and bladder function is a key aspect of rehabilitation nursing; however, bowel and bladder goals are best achieved through interdisciplinary team goals because cognitive ability, communication ability, hand function, and level of independence in activities of daily living (ADLs) and transfers are key factors in the choice of appropriate bowel and bladder management strategies.

7. Desired outcomes (NOC) of bladder management are to remain continent, empty the bladder completely, and avoid recurrent urinary tract infections and other complications of bladder dysfunction.

8. Desired outcomes (NOC) of bowel management are to remain continent, have a formed bowel movement on a regular schedule, prevent diarrhea

Table 7-2. Nursing Interventions for Pressure Ulcers

Wound cleansing	Wear gloves, gown, mask, and eyewear or face shield as appropriate to anticipated potential for overspray of contaminated matter.
	Minimize trauma to the wound.
	Cleanse the periwound area and the wound to reduce the bacterial count.
	Appropriate solutions include the following:
	• Water: Tap, distilled or cooled boiled; use sterile water if client is immunosuppressed or if tap water is of poor quality
	• Saline: No statistical benefit over water
	Avoid antiseptics and products designed for use on intact skin or for removal of fecal material because these may be toxic to the wound bed.
Techniques	Irrigation, swabbing, showering, or bathing
	Whirlpool has been shown to have no statistical benefit since 2005
	For heavy exudate, use a commercial wound cleanser containing surfactant.
	Use nonabrasive, light scrubbing with a cloth or sponge, minimizing trauma to the wound bed.
	Use high-pressure irrigation of 4–15 psi to remove slough or necrotic tissue.
	A 35-ml syringe with a 19-gauge needle or angiocatheter yields 8 psi.
Signs of infection or colonization	New or increased pain, delayed healing, friable granulation tissue, discoloration of the wound bed, change in odor, increased serous exudate, induration, pocketing, tunneling, or bridging
	Infection is defined as bacteria $>10^5$ CFU/cm^2 or presence of beta-hemolytic streptococcus (NPUAP & EPUAP, 2009; LOE 3).
Treatments	Topical antibiotics for 14 days for wounds that show poor healing or have had purulent exudate for more than 2 weeks of routine care
	Silver or honey dressings for wounds with multiple organisms on culture, in combination with alginate or foam dressing (WOCN, 2010). Silver dressings speed healing, decrease odor and exudate, and allow longer wear time. Honey dressings have shown increasing evidence of efficacy for chronic wounds taking more than 5 weeks to heal. However, randomized trials are lacking.
	Antiseptics are used in the short term to control bacteria and reduce inflammation in wounds that are not expected to heal.
	Systemic antibiotics are used in the presence of bacteremia, sepsis, advancing cellulitis, or osteomyelitis. These antibiotics do not reach ischemic or granulation tissue. Therefore, topical antibiotics are applied directly to the wound.
Debridement	Surgical is recommended for wounds with extensive tunneling, undermining, or necrosis.
	Conservative sharp.
	Mechanical, as in saline wet-to-dry.
	High-pressure fluid irrigation.
	Ultrasonic mist reduces purulent drainage, but evidence of effectiveness for debridement is insufficient.
	Autolysis, either chemical or enzymatic using collagenase
	Larval using maggots has limited evidence of effectiveness
	Dry eschar must be scored or cross-hatched before application of collagenase.
	Hard, dry eschar on ischemic limbs or feet should *not* be debrided.
Stage I	Keep skin clean and dry. Use barrier lotion or spray to protect from abrasion or maceration.
	Use pressure redistribution devices, padding, or elevation off hard surfaces at sites of reddened, intact skin and bony prominences.
	Keep head of bed at or below 30 degrees, use good turning techniques to prevent friction and shearing.
Stage II	Cleanse wound at each dressing change (see "Wound Cleansing" items).
	If necessary, irrigate gently to remove nonadherent particles.
	Keep wound moist and clean.
	Use foam, hydrocolloids, hydrogels, hydrofiber, or transparent absorbent acrylic dressings.
	Adjust frequency of dressing change to allow assessment, but avoid disturbing fibroblastic action and possible introduction of pathogens. Initially, change dressings every 2–3 days. As healing progresses, reduce frequency.

continued

Table 7-2. Nursing Interventions for Pressure Ulcers *continued*

Stage III	Cleanse and irrigate the wound at each dressing change.
	Assess for slough, exudate, tunnels, and undermining.
	Select dressing type based on appearance of the wound bed.
	For shallow wounds with granulation, use hydrocolloid or transparent absorbent acrylic dressing.
	For wounds with slough, use a targeted enzymatic debridement product and a secondary dressing.
	If tunneling is noted, pack dead spaces with an appropriate absorbent wicking product (e.g., foam, alginate tape) and cover with a secondary dressing (e.g., antimicrobials, gauze, or foam).
	Adjust the frequency of dressing changes according to the amount of drainage.
	Apply a barrier wipe or spray to the periwound intact skin to protect from moisture and provide a surface allowing adhesives to adhere well.
	Vacuum-assisted closure may be appropriate for particular wounds.
	Debridement of eschar and slough as described in "Debridement."
Stage IV	Cleanse as indicated for stage III.
	Vacuum-assisted closure, surgical closure, grafts, or flaps may ultimately be selected after clean margins are established.
	Electrical stimulation may be helpful for stages II, III, and IV.
	Cytokines may be prescribed for use on stage II, III, and IV wounds.

Wound, Ostomy and Continence Nurses Society. (2010). *Guideline for prevention and management of pressure ulcers*. Retrieved September 12, 2011, from www.guideline.gov/content.aspx?id=23868.

National Pressure Ulcer Advisory Panel & European Pressure Ulcer Advisory Panel. (2009). *Prevention and treatment of pressure ulcers: Clinical practice guideline*. Washington, DC: National Pressure Ulcer Advisory Panel,

and constipation, and prevent complications such as hemorrhoids, abdominal distention, autonomic dysreflexia, and fecal impaction.

B. Physiology of Bladder Elimination (Doughty, 2006; Porth & Matfin, 2008)

1. The purpose of the bladder is to store and control the elimination of urine.

2. Urination is a function of the peripheral autonomic nervous system.

3. Inhibition or facilitation of urination is controlled by spinal cord reflex centers, the micturition center in the pons, and cortical and subcortical centers in the brain.

4. Bladder filling control originates in the T10–L2 segments of the spinal cord, which cause the detrusor muscle to relax and the internal sphincter to contract due to sympathetic innervation via the hypogastric nerve plexus (Doughty, 2006).

5. Micturition occurs when the bladder detrusor muscle contracts and the internal sphincter relaxes via parasympathetic signals from S2–S4 via the pelvic plexus. The external urinary sphincter relaxes with somatic voluntary control via the pudendal nerve.

6. Skeletal muscle in the external sphincter and pelvic muscles that support the bladder are controlled by the pudendal nerve, which exits the spinal cord from the S2–S4 segments.

C. Urinary Incontinence: Urinary incontinence is the involuntary loss of urine resulting from pathological,

anatomical, or physiological factors. Postmenopausal women and men with prostatic hyperplasia and those with cognitive dysfunction, neurological movement disorders (e.g., multiple sclerosis, Parkinson's disease), or stroke are at risk for incontinence. Refer all clients who dribble or leak urine for diagnosis and treatment. Treatment decisions are best made after completing a detailed client history, physical exam, and diagnostic tests including a voiding diary; postvoid residual bladder scan measurements; urodynamic testing; and a urologic workup by physicians, advanced practice nurses, or specialty nurses trained to manage urinary incontinence. Content for this section is adapted from Dowling-Castronovo and Bradway (2008) to provide LOEs for assessment items and specific nursing interventions related to type of incontinence.

1. Types of urinary incontinence

   a. Stress: Small losses of urine that occur when intra-abdominal pressure is increased by activities such as coughing, laughing, exercising, or sneezing

   b. Urge: Loss of urine caused by abnormal detrusor contractions and sometimes associated with urinary retention; characterized as a strong urge to void, frequency and nocturia (Doughty, 2006), a major component of "overactive bladder syndrome"

   c. Mixed: Characteristics of both urge and stress incontinence

THE SPECIALTY PRACTICE OF REHABILITATION NURSING

d. Overflow: Loss of urine caused by bladder overdistention or retention; characterized by urgency, frequency, dribbling, and both stress and urge incontinence.

e. Total: Continuous uninhibited loss of urine, even with minimal activity

f. Functional: "Loss of urine and/or stool caused by factors outside the urinary or GI tract that interfere with the ability to respond in a socially appropriate way to the urge to void or defecate. The lower urinary tract and bowel produce normal sensation of urge, and the ability to inhibit urge is intact but other factors precipitate the loss of control. Functional incontinence is often associated with cognitive impairment and/or loss of the ability to perform behaviors needed for independent toileting. The end result is the inability to respond to bladder or bowel urge, which results in varying degrees of incontinence" (Doughty, p.167).

2. Assessment data

a. Premorbid level of function, presence or absence of incontinence on admission (LOE 4)

b. Past voiding habits, use of pads or diapers, awareness of fullness, dribbling, interrupted stream

c. Fluid intake volume and pattern: strict intake and output monitoring for 3 days

d. Age and activity level

e. Prior history of bladder problems: Onset, frequency, urgency, stress incontinence, retention, infections, childbirth, prolapse of uterus or bladder, enlarged prostate, prostate surgery, bladder surgery

f. Mobility impairments, prescribed restrictions, braces, splints, immobilizers

g. Neuromuscular status

h. Communication impairments

i. Sensory and motor status

j. Environment: Accessibility, privacy

k. Adaptive equipment use, current needs

l. Current medications, drug allergies, comorbidities

m. Postvoid residual volumes per ultrasound scan

n. Urine analysis, microscopic examination and culture

o. Presence or absence of indwelling catheter upon admission (LOE 4)

p. Collaborate with other team members to determine if incontinence is transient, established or both, document type and duration (LOE 1)

q. Collaborate with team members to identify and document possible etiologies of incontinence (LOE 1)

3. NDs related to urinary incontinence and neurogenic bladder (NANDA-I, 2009–2011)

a. Impaired urinary elimination

b. Readiness for enhanced urinary elimination

c. Urinary incontinence (functional, overflow, reflex, risk for urge, stress, urge)

d. Urinary retention (acute or chronic)

e. Associated diagnoses: Mobility impairments, ego integrity items, deficient or excess fluid volume, self-care deficit in toileting, self-neglect, disturbed sensory perception, pain, communication impairment, and social isolation

f. Risk for autonomic dysreflexia

4. General bladder training interventions (NIC) for all types of incontinence: The Cochrane Collaboration published an exhaustive review of literature between 1980 and 2005, compiled by Wallace, Roe, Williams, and Palmer (2009), comparing randomized and quasirandomized studies of bladder training with variables labeled no treatment, biofeedback, behavioral treatment (specified), pharmacological treatment (specified), psychological treatment (specified), surgical intervention (specified), and specified medical devices. In addition, combinations of bladder training with these same variables were compared. Both short-and long-term outcomes were examined along with client perception of cure and quality of life. Results and conclusions were disappointing. The authors' conclusions and implications for practice are quoted here.

"There is inconclusive evidence to judge the effects of bladder training in both the short and long term. The results of the trials reviewed tended to favour bladder training (with no evidence of adverse effect) but there were too few data to assess this reliably. The data that were available were from trials of variable quality and small size. There are resource implications but the magnitude of these is not clear from the trials. The data are also too few to provide any guidance on the choice among bladder training, drug treatment, or other conservative approaches, or on whether adding bladder training to another treatment enhances any effect." (Wallace et al., 2009, p. 18)

LOEs for the interventions listed were retrieved from Milne (2008) and Stevens (2008).

a. Adjust fluid intake: Monitor intake and output carefully, ensure that fluid intake is 2,000–2,400 ml/day unless medically restricted, limit fluids after the evening meal to minimize nocturia, consider a scheduled fluid program of 240–300 ml eight times a day, and consider fluid restriction for clients habitually taking large volumes of oral fluids. Evidence related to limiting caffeine is not well supported in the literature, but obesity, smoking, and carbonated beverages are noted as risk factors for overactive bladder with urge incontinence (Milne, 2008).

    b. Toileting self-care assistance: Ensure a clear pathway and assist to toilet. Use a bedside commode at night. Evaluate needs for assistive devices. Modify the environment to facilitate continence (LOE 1).

    c. Bladder training: Initiate a timed (scheduled) toileting program. Help the client sit on the toilet, bedpan, or commode every 2 hours for at least 5 minutes. As continence improves, gradually reduce toileting to every 3 hours, especially before and after meals and before bedtime. Enlist the cooperation and assistance of therapy staff to provide opportunities to toilet between therapies. In addition, teach pelvic floor muscle training (Kegel exercises) to increase success, even for older women in long-term care facilities (Aslan, Komurcu, Beji, & Yalcin, 2008; Milne, 2008; Shimaliyan, Kane, Wyman, & Wilt, 2008).

    d. Assess for urinary retention: Perform at least two postvoid residual bladder scans within 20 minutes after voiding to assess bladder emptying.

    e. Nighttime incontinence care: Initially, disposable diapers may be used day and night. As continence improves, discontinue diapers at night; instead, use absorbent underpads. Consider condom catheters for men who sleep so soundly that they do not awaken with incontinent episodes. Do not prop urinals or leave the client on a bedpan for long periods. Remove bedpans promptly after use. Discontinue bedpans as soon as the client is mobile enough to use a bedside commode at night. Perform a skin check and provide perineal hygiene in conjunction with a timed toileting program.

    f. Avoid indwelling catheters when possible to avoid risk of urinary tract infection (LOE 1).

    g. Immediately cleanse the skin after incontinent episodes and apply barrier ointments to prevent skin breakdown (LOE 1).

5. Specific interventions (NIC) for incontinence (**Table 7-3**). In addition, these LOEs are provided by Dowling-Castronovo and Bradway (2008).

    a. Stress incontinence
      1) Teach pelvic floor muscle (i.e., Kegel) exercises (LOE 1 and 2).
      2) Provide toileting assistance and bladder training (LOE 4).
      3) Refer to other team members for pharmacological or surgical therapy.

    b. Urge incontinence
      1) Implement bladder training (retraining; LOE 1 and 4).
      2) If the client is cognitively intact and motivated, teach urge inhibition (LOE 4).
      3) Combine bladder training with pelvic floor muscle exercises (LOE 3).
      4) Collaborate with prescribing team members if pharmacological therapy is warranted.
      5) Initiate referrals for a further diagnostic workup if the client does not improve.

    c. Overflow incontinence
      1) Allow sufficient time for voiding.
      2) Determine postvoid residual (LOE 4).
      3) Provide the client with education about double-voiding and the Credé maneuver (LOE 4).
      4) If catheterization is needed, sterile intermittent is preferred over indwelling (LOE 2).
      5) Refer clients needing pharmacological or surgical intervention.

    d. Functional incontinence
      1) Provide individualized scheduled or prompted voiding (LOE 1 and 4).
      2) Provide adequate fluid intake.
      3) Refer for occupational and physical therapy as indicated.
      4) Modify the environment to be conducive to maintaining independence with continence (LOE 1 and 4).

6. Department of Health and Human Services, Department of Medicare and Medicaid Services regulations (2005; F315, 483.25d) require that
    a. Residents entering a facility without an indwelling urinary catheter not receive one unless medically necessary.
    b. Residents with urinary incontinence receive appropriate services and treatment to prevent urinary tract infections and restore as much bladder control as possible.

D. Neurogenic Bladder and Neurogenic Bladder Management: The content for this section is adapted from the Consortium for Spinal Cord Medicine (2006). This is an excellent guideline that rehabilitation nurses will find useful.

                                             THE SPECIALTY PRACTICE OF REHABILITATION NURSING

Table 7-3. Management of Bladder Dysfunctions

Impairment	Symptoms	Etiology	Management
Stress incontinence	Small loss of urine occurring with increased abdominal pressure as with coughing, sneezing, laughing, and exercising	Weak external sphincter, weak pelvic floor musculature, and secondary effects of smoking and obesity	Dietary modifications: Avoid caffeine, carbonated beverages, alcohol, chocolate, artificial sweeteners, tomato, citrus, and spicy foods. Adjust fluid intake: Achieve 2,000–3.000 ml daily in increments of 250–300 ml 8–10 times a day. Limit fluids after 8 pm. Kegel exercises: Ten contractions then 30 seconds of rest five times daily. Timed voiding program: Every 2 hours while awake, every 3–4 hours at night; assist as needed. Slowly extend intervals to every 3 or 4 hours. Biofeedback, electronic stimulation
Urge incontinence/overactive bladder	Urgency, frequency, nocturia	Detrusor hyperreflexia, uninhibited bladder contractions, suprapontine lesions	Urge suppression training; Crede; condoms catheter at night; surgery (bladder augmentation, diversion); weight loss; smoking cessation; use of oxybutynin, tolterodine, flavoxate, and imipramine
Spastic bladder	Unable to store urine	Upper motor neuron injury	
Mixed stress and urge incontinence			
Overflow	Frequent small voids	Reflex or neurogenic components, external sphincter dyssynergy, weak detrusor	Pessary, trigger void, double void, Foley or suprapubic catheter followed by bladder retraining, botox injection of sphincter, use of Flomax or alpha blockers, surgery (stent, TURP, sphincterotomy)
Flaccid bladder	Unable to empty urine	Lower motor neuron injury	
Functional incontinence	Incontinence in route to toilet	Mobility, coordination or cognitive impairments interfere with allowing adequate time to get to the toilet	Timed or prompted voiding program with helper assist as need; modify environment to reduce obstacles
Neurogenic-retention	Episodic large voids	Destrusor-sphincter dyssynergia	Intermittent catheterization at 4- or 6-hour intervals for bladder scan volumes greater than 400 ml

1. Classifications of neurogenic bladder disorders
   a. Spastic bladder dysfunction or failure to store urine, often associated with upper motor neuron spinal cord injuries
   b. Flaccid bladder or failure to empty urine, often associated with lower motor neuron spinal cord injuries
   c. Overactive bladder or detrusor hyperreflexia without detrusor sphincter dyssynergia, often seen with suprapontine lesions from other cerebrovascular diseases
2. Specific neurogenic bladder management strategies: The consortium presented the indications, contraindications, advantages, disadvantages, and nursing considerations for the most common bladder management strategies. The consortium noted that there is no strong evidence that one method is superior to another. The goals of any bladder management program are to prevent upper urinary tract damage, minimize lower urinary tract complications (e.g., stones, fistulas, chronic effects of infections), and be compatible with client and caregiver lifestyles. When choosing a management strategy, a urologic evaluation is necessary to detect and manage spinal shock, uninhibited bladder contractions, autonomic dysreflexia, or detrusor-external sphincter dyssynergia during the acute phase of rehabilitation. Head injury may accompany spinal cord injury, complicating bladder function and choice of bladder management strategy.

Currently there is debate in the literature about the use of sterile or clean technique for intermittent self-catheterization during hospitalization.

Small studies have revealed insignificant or minimal increased incidence of urinary tract infection among clients using clean technique for several days before discharge. Some contend that this reduces client and caregiver confusion in the transition to the home environment. Others point out the increased risk for hospital-acquired infection. Large, carefully controlled studies are needed to determine best practice.

a. Intermittent self-catheterization may be effective for those who have sufficient hand skills or a willing caregiver to perform intermittent catheterization (LOE 3).

 1) Paralyzed Veterans of America recommends keeping bladder volumes below 500 ml by catheterizing every 4–6 hours to prevent overdistention of the bladder. The client may need to wake during the night for catheterization. Keeping bladder volumes below 400 ml has been recommended in the past by many sources (LOE 4).

 2) Train the client or caregiver and institute clean intermittent catheterization before discharge (LOE 3). See the ARN website at www.rehabnurse.org for client education materials.

 3) Consider sterile catheterization in those with recurring symptomatic infections (LOE 3).

 4) Treat urine leakage between catheterizations with anticholinergic medication and limit fluid intake (LOE 3). (Note: Botulinum toxin injections have been used experimentally as nerve blocks in the urinary sphincter with good short-term results. However, this is currently an off-label use not approved by the FDA.)

 5) Catheter selection depends on economic considerations and latex sensitivity.

 6) Hands are cleansed with soap and water or aseptic wipes both before and after catheterization.

 7) Ideally, single-use sterile catheter kits are used in the outpatient environment. Many medical supply companies have disposable kits containing sterile catheters of various materials and lengths, with or without urine collection bags.

b. Credé and Valsalva: Applying suprapubic pressure to express urine from the bladder may be effective for those with lower motor neuron injuries and low outlet resistance or those who have had a sphincterotomy (LOE 3).

c. Indwelling catheters: Urethral or suprapubic catheters are used for those with high fluid intake, poor hand skills, cognitive impairment, active substance abuse, elevated detrusor pressures managed with anticholinergic drugs, vesicoureteral reflux, lack of success with less invasive methods, or limited assistance from a caregiver (LOE 3). See ARN's website at www.rehabnurse.org for client education materials.

 1) Suprapubic catheterization has several benefits over urethral catheterization and is especially preferred by those with quadriplegia or complete spinal cord injury. Suprapubic catheters are recommended for those with urethral abnormalities, bladder or urethral trauma, small bladder capacity, recurrent catheter obstruction, urethral incompetence, prostatitis, or epididymitis and those who want improved sexual genital function.

 2) Surveillance for urinary tract infections and bladder stones is recommended.

 3) Urethral catheters (14–16 Fr) with a balloon filled with 5–10 ml sterile water are replaced every 2–4 weeks or weekly in those prone to catheter encrustation or bladder stones.

 4) Suprapubic catheters (22–24 Fr) are changed every 4 weeks by a trained healthcare provider, more often in those with catheter encrustation or stones.

 5) Anchor the catheter with a belt, tape, or other device to the abdomen or thigh. To prevent urethral trauma, alternate legs for the tubing anchor point daily.

 6) Daily irrigation is not recommended. Irrigation is used only to clear clots or obstructions.

 7) If daytime and nighttime collection devices are reused, clean daily with a 1:10 bleach solution or 1:3 vinegar solution.

 8) Maintenance of a closed drainage system has been found to be a key element in prevention of catheter-associated urinary tract infections. Disconnection invites bacterial invasion.

 9) Urine for culture and sensitivity should be obtained only from a newly inserted catheter and drainage bag to avoid culturing the system (i.e., catheter and drainage bag) rather than the urine.

d. Reflex voiding with a condom catheter is appropriate for men who have adequate hand skills, poor compliance with fluid restriction, and small bladder capacity (LOE 4). See ARN's website at www.rehabnurse.org for client educational materials.

1) Apply the condom catheter securely to avoid constriction and leakage for 24 hours.
2) To avoid skin breakdown, wash the glans daily when the condom is changed and air dry skin for the 20–30 minutes. Anchor the tubing on the alternate leg each day to prevent skin breakdown.
3) Clean urinary collection bags and tubing daily with a 1:10 bleach solution.
4) Choose the appropriate size and length self-adhesive condom. Those with allergies to the adhesive can use nonadhesive condoms. Those with latex allergy can use nonlatex condom catheters.

e. Additional management strategies: The consortium guideline outlines recommendations for these additional bladder management strategies and provides advisory information about application in clients who might benefit from each strategy, potential complications, and nursing considerations for each strategy.

1) Alpha blockers
2) Botulinum toxin injection
3) Urethral stents
4) Transurethral sphincterotomy
5) Electrical stimulation and posterior sacral rhizotomy
6) Bladder augmentation
7) Continent urinary diversion
8) Urinary diversion
9) Cutaneous ileovesicostomy

f. Potential long-term complications of indwelling catheters include the following:

1) Bladder stones
2) Kidney stones
3) Urethral erosions
4) Epididymitis
5) Recurrent infection
6) Incontinence
7) Pyelonephritis
8) Hydronephrosis due to fibrosis or thickening of the bladder wall
9) Bladder cancer

E. **FIM™ Scoring: Rehabilitation nurses must enter scores for bladder function on the FIM™ tool daily (Table 7-4).**

F. **Bowel Function**
1. Normal anatomy and physiology of bowel elimination

a. Peristalsis moves the stool along the gut. Haustral contractions roll and mix fecal materials.
b. The small intestine and ascending colon absorb nutrients from liquid stool (chyme).
c. The transverse colon absorbs some of the fluid, and stool begins to be more formed. Mass movements propel stool toward the descending colon, occurs up to three times daily, usually after a meal, and generally last up to 30 minutes.
d. The descending, sigmoid, and rectal portions of the colon absorb additional water and electrolytes. Kidney waste is added. Stool is compacted into a more solid form. Moisture content of stool depends on the length of time stool rested in the distal colon.
e. The internal sphincter retains stool in the rectum.
f. The external sphincter expands to allow the passage of stool from the rectum.
g. Abdominal wall musculature assists with evacuation.
h. Bowel function continues with cerebral or spinal cord impairment.

1) Voluntary and involuntary innervations occur at the reflex, segmental, and cortical levels.
2) Parasympathetic and sympathetic innervations occur from the autonomic nervous system.
3) The enteric nervous system influences the intrinsic neural control of the mobility, absorption, and secretion activities of the gut; it is independent of but influenced by the autonomic nervous system.
4) Like the bladder, the bowel is capable of emptying at a reflex level when stretch fibers in the descending large colon stimulate the reflex arc.

2. Requirements for stool formation and normal bowel function
a. Adequate fiber in the diet to produce bulk and trap water in the stool; adequate solid matter for peristalsis to move the stool and to allow the body to defecate in an organized, effective manner
b. Adequate fluid intake to limit the amount of liquid reabsorbed from the descending colon
c. General activity and mobility to support and enhance peristalsis
d. Upright posture to allow gravity to assist in stool formation and passage

3. Patterns of defecation through the lifespan
a. Infants: The gut functions at the reflex level.

Table 7-4. Functional Independence Measure (FIM™) Scoring—Bladder

Part 1: Level of Assistance

7 = Complete independence—Client does not require helper, assistive device or medication, does not void (dialysis)

6 = Modified independence—Requires assistive device or medications, performs intermittent self-cath, applies/removes condom cath, Foley, ileostomy or suprapubic cath, urinal, bedpan elevated or bedside commode, peripad or adult diaper. Independently manages device and discards urine, changes appliances, empties collection bags. Medications: Detrol, Ditropan, Flomax, Sudafed (pseudoephedrine) urecholine, Cardura. Must score as 6 even if the client uses the toilet during the day and only uses the urinal, commode, or condom cath at night.

5 = Supervision or set-up—Nursing empties the urinal, sets out equipment or supplies, client requires cues to maintain clean or sterile technique or to maintain an intermittent cath or voiding schedule, client discards the peripad or diaper properly.

4 = Minimal assistance—Client participates in >75% of bladder management tasks, requires touching to assist to place equipment in hand.

3 = Moderate assistance—Client participates 50%–75%, performs only one or two tasks, consistently tells helper of urge to void, full bladder, requires assistant to place urinal, bedpan, apply gloves, open packages and hand supplies to client.

2 = Maximum assistance—Client participates in 25%–50% of tasks, inconsistently tells helper of urge to void, bladder fullness, may participate in changing diaper or peripad, may tell helper leg bag needs emptying but cannot participate in the task.

1 = Total assistance—Client participates less than 25%. Helper changes diapers, peripads, maintains Foley or condom cath, performs intermittent cath, cleans patient, and changes clothing and linens after incontinent episodes.

0 = This score is not valid for bladder.

Part 2: Frequency of Accidents

7 = 100% continent, never has accidents, does not void due to dialysis

6 = 100% continent but uses an assistive device or medication to maintain bladder control

5 = 1 episode incontinence, urinal or bedpan spill in the past 7 days AND patient cleans self and soiled linens

4 = 2 episodes incontinence/spills in the past 7 days AND patient cleans self and soiled linens/clothing

3 = 3 episodes incontinence in the past 7 days AND cleans self and linens

2 = 4 episodes incontinence in the past 7 days AND cleans self, linens, changes clothes

1 = 5 episodes or helper must clean patient, linens, and clothing

0 = Not a valid score for bladder.

Note: Admission score includes events of the past 3 days, enter the lowest scores.

Score Part 1, score Part 2, enter lowest score on Uniform Data System Inpatient Rehabilitation Facility Patient Assessment Instrument (UDS IRF-PAI). The form is used by inpatient rehabilitation facilities to submit data to the national data base in Buffalo, NY.

---

b. Children: As the child matures, he or she develops cortical control over the time and place of defecation.

c. Adults: Middle age is a time of intense activity and relative regularity, which may vary slightly with diet changes, infrequent bouts of illness, or activity; however, the bowel generally responds to simple interventions.

d. Older adults
   1) Changes occur in striated and smooth muscle strength.
   2) Activity gradually lessens.
   3) Older adults generally consume less roughage and have poorer dentition.
   4) Self-limiting hydration may be present secondary to concerns about urinary incontinence or nocturia.
   5) Comorbidities may begin, along with increased medication use. These give rise to problems of constipation and help explain the focus on bowel regularity by many older adults.

G. Bowel Impairment (Rye & Mauk, in press)
   1. Constipation: Infrequent, small, hard, dry stool less than three times per week or none at all in several days, accompanied by straining and sensations of abdominal bloating or fullness
      a. Acute constipation: Recent onset of symptoms, a large amount of stool in the rectal ampulla, colon, or rectum
      b. Chronic constipation: Symptoms lasting longer than 3 months, enlarges the descending colon and produces dependency on laxatives, cathartics, or enemas
      c. Severe constipation and impaction cause sympathetic systemic problems (e.g., sweating, nausea, irritability, acute abdominal discomfort, and elevated blood pressure)

THE SPECIALTY PRACTICE OF REHABILITATION NURSING

2. Diarrhea: Highly frequent liquid stool with accompanying cramping
   a. May be explosive, generally related to excessive caffeine ingestion, infection, irritability of the gut, or possibly food poisoning
   b. May be associated with ulcerative colitis if not self-limiting
3. Sensory paralytic (afferent nerve root loss or damage)
   a. Occurs subsequent to diabetes or tabes dorsalis
   b. Produces diminished or absent ability to distinguish the need or time of defecation but rarely produces incontinence because the motor function of the rectum is intact
4. Motor paralytic (efferent nerve root loss or damage)
   a. Occurs subsequent to poliomyelitis, intervertebral disc disease, tumor, or trauma
   b. Results in the inability to assist with defecation
   c. Associated with incontinence only if there is widespread disease due to the innervation of the intestines
5. Colostomies and ileostomies: Artificial openings on the abdominal wall to provide an exit for stool. (To obtain the current guidelines on ostomy care, consult the Wound, Ostomy and Continence Nurses Society at www.wocn.org.)
   a. Used when the colon has become obstructed and the rectum cannot be used (malignant tumors)
   b. Used when the gut is irritated beyond repair (ulcerative colitis)
   c. Used when it is necessary to rest the colon while it repairs (major abdominal resections)
6. Neurogenic bowel disorders associated with spinal cord injury
   a. Reflexic neurogenic bowel (upper motor neuron)
      1) The bowel is capable of reflexive emptying of the rectum without cortical awareness of the need to defecate.
      2) Associated with spinal cord injury above T12–S1 or damage to the cerebral cortex
      3) Because of the innervation of the sympathetic nervous system, the client may be aware of defecation and nervous system activity but have no conscious control over it.
   b. Autonomous, areflexic, flaccid, or atonal bowel (lower motor neuron)
      1) Subsequent to spinal cord damage at or below T12–S1
      2) No cortical control
      3) Lack of tone in the internal and external sphincters with frequent oozing of stool, caused by damage to the reflex arc

H. Nursing Assessment of Bowel Function
   1. Prior level of function, past bowel habits, usual time of day, frequency of stool, past reliance on laxatives, dietary measures, exercise, or other aids
   2. Age and activity level
   3. Usual diet and fluid intake pattern
   4. Prior history of incontinence, frequent diarrhea, constipation, hemorrhoids, diverticulitis, or bowel surgery
   5. Present bowel status and pattern, including time and characteristics of last stool
   6. Oozing or small hard stool alternating with watery discharge, which may indicate impaction
   7. Abdominal palpation to determine abdominal discomfort or palpable obstruction; rectal exam
   8. Medications that may affect bowel function (e.g., sedatives, opioids, diuretics, antihistamines)
   9. Infection, trauma, or stress that may affect stool formation
   10. Malodorous breath, dentition status
   11. Problems that may affect selection of interventions
       a. Neuromuscular dysfunction related to current diagnosis
       b. Cardiac conditions, which would preclude the use of digital stimulation or the Valsalva maneuver
       c. Renal impairment, which would preclude the use of milk of magnesia
       d. Mobility restrictions related to current diagnosis
       e. Communication abilities
       f. Sensory and motor status
       g. Current medications and drug allergies
       h. Tube feeding schedule
       i. Cognitive deficits, dementia, psychosis
I. NDs related to bowel impairments (NANDA-I, 2009–2011)
   1. Activity intolerance
   2. Impaired bed mobility
   3. Impaired transfer ability
   4. Risk for autonomic dysreflexia
   5. Bowel incontinence
   6. Perceived risk for constipation
   7. Diarrhea
   8. Dysfunctional gastrointestinal motility
   9. Nausea
   10. Imbalanced nutrition, less than body requirements
   11. Toileting self-care deficit
   12. Self-neglect
   13. Anorexia
   14. Confusion (acute, chronic)
   15. Pain (acute, chronic)
   16. Impaired comfort
   17. Impaired physical mobility

18. Impaired sensory perception
19. Impaired verbal communication
20. Social isolation
21. Delayed growth and development
J. Nursing Interventions (NIC) for Bowel Impairments: It is possible to use existing neural pathways to establish a regular bowel pattern; therefore, interventions for impaired bowel elimination are similar, although clients may have different clinical pictures.
   1. Prevention of constipation (adapted from Rehabilitation Nursing Foundation [RNF], 2002, and Rye & Mauk, in press): Rehabilitation nurses need to conduct initial trials to determine the true effectiveness of these standards of practice.
      a. Toileting habits include a nurse promptly responding to the client's urge to defecate, providing a consistent time for defecation, and providing privacy (LOE 4).
      b. Use an upright position if possible. If the client is unable to sit, a left-side-lying position is recommended (LOE 4). The left-side-lying position is recommended to receive an enema or suppository because this promotes absorption. Right side lying promotes evacuation of stool. Position the client with knees against the chest to help open the pelvic floor. Abdominal massage right to left may promote evacuation.
      c. Use a toilet or commode with a backrest and siderails for defecation. Avoid use of bedpans (LOE 4).
      d. Provide the client with 20–35 g fiber per day and 2 L fluid per day.
      e. An exercise program should be a component of plans to prevent or treat constipation.
      f. Pharmacological treatment of constipation should be short term. Stool softeners and bulking agents are administered once or twice daily until bowel patterns are reestablished, then only as needed.
   2. Neurogenic bowel management (adapted from Consortium for Spinal Cord Medicine, 2010a, and RNF, 2002). Those with neurogenic bowel also need to follow the guidelines for preventing constipation.
      a. Reflexic bowel: Use an appropriate chemical suppository or mechanical rectal stimulant, a consistent personalized schedule (preferably after a meal), and appropriate adaptive equipment (LOE 4).
      b. Areflexic bowel management includes manual evacuation, a consistent personalized schedule, and appropriate adaptive equipment (LOE 4).

K. Expected Client Outcomes (NOC) Related to Bowel Elimination
   1. Establish a regular bowel regimen with complete emptying of soft stool from the rectum every 1–3 days using the least medication possible.
   2. Maintain a consistent habit and time.
   3. No incontinent episodes
   4. Absence of complications: Hemorrhoids, abdominal distention, autonomic dysreflexia, or fecal impaction
L. FIM™ Scoring: Rehabilitation nurses must enter scores for bowel function on the FIM™ tool daily (**Table 7-5**).

IV. **Sleep and Rest**
   A. Overview
      1. Adequate and restful sleep is essential to maintaining health, strength, endurance, and cognitive functioning.
      2. Illness, particularly neurologic injury, deep pain, the effects of medications such as sedatives and hypnotics, the comorbidities of aging, and recent intensive care hospitalization all affect sleep patterns.
      3. Rehabilitation nurses often care for people who have experienced major illnesses and subsequent disruption of normal sleep cycles.
      4. To promote healing and endurance, rehabilitation nurses should assess disruptions in clients' sleep and apply specific interventions to restore restful sleep patterns.
      5. There is a great need for nursing research to identify level 1 evidence for effective nursing interventions to promote sleep for clients admitted to rehabilitation facilities.
   B. Normal Sleep Patterns (adapted from Porth & Matfin, 2008; normal sleep patterns are a middle-range theory.)
      1. Sleep is part of the sleep-wake cycle. The inactivity of sleep appears to restore mental and physical function. Melatonin, a hormone produced by the pineal gland, is generally believed to have a role in regulating the sleep-wake cycle.
      2. There are two types of sleep: rapid eye movement (REM) and non-REM sleep.
         a. REM sleep is characterized by rapid eye movements, a lack of muscle movement, and vivid dreaming. The person is responding to internal auditory and visual sensory circuits.
         b. Non-REM sleep is characterized as quiet sleep, with a fully regulating brain and fully movable but inactive body. Non-REM sleep is divided into four stages, each deeper than the previous stage.

Table 7-5. Functional Independence Measure (FIM™) Scoring—Bowel

Part I: Level of Assistance

7 = Complete independence—Does not require a helper, medication, or assistive device to maintain a normal stooling pattern.

6 = Modified independence—Requires an assistive device or medication to manage bowel function; is independent in using and maintaining the device or equipment; may use a bedpan, commode, colostomy, ileostomy, suppository, stool softener, or prunes; but client applies, empties, and cleans equipment independently, inserts own suppository and is never incontinent.

5 = Supervision or set-up—Client performs more than 75% of tasks; requires cues, set-up, or supervision from helper; helper hands supplies or a suppository to the client; helper empties the commode or bedpan.

4 = Minimum assistance—Client performs more than 75% of tasks but requires touching assistance, helper disposes of or empties the stool-collection device, client cannot place suppository.

3 = Moderate assistance—Client performs 50%–74% of tasks and requires touching assistance to perform more than one task in bowel management.

2 = Maximum assistance—Client performs 25%–50% of tasks, helper handles most equipment and supplies, client participates in applying or emptying the appliance, but requires touching assistance to do so.

1 = Total assistance—Client performs less than 25% of tasks; is dependent on a helper to apply, maintain, and clean assistive device, empty appliance, and change diaper; helper places suppository, cleans client, changes client clothing and linens after incontinent episodes.

0 = Not a valid score for bowel.

Part 2: Frequency of Accidents

7 = Complete independence—Does not require an assistive device or medication to maintain normal stooling pattern; is never incontinent.

6 = Modified independence—Is never incontinent and uses medication or an assistive device (e.g., elevated toilet, commode, bedpan, colostomy, or ileostomy) but completely manages, maintains, empties, and cleans the appliance or assistive device independently. Client manages medications independently, including stool softeners, suppositories, bowel stimulants, fiber supplements, enemas, or prunes.

5 = 1 accident in the past week and client cleans up independently.

4 = 2 accidents in the past week, cleans up independently.

3 = 3 accidents in the past week, cleans up independently.

2 = 4 accidents in the past week, cleans up independently.

1 = 5 or more accidents in the past week OR helper is required to clean the client, linens, and change the client's clothing following an incontinent episode.

0 = Not a valid score for bowel function.

Admission score includes the events of the past 3 days, enter the lowest score.

Score Part 1, score Part 2, enter the lowest score on the UDS IRF-PAI form.

1) Stage 1: Brief transitional stage, occurs at the onset of sleep. The person appears asleep but is easily aroused and if asked later may deny being asleep.

2) Stage 2: Deeper sleep, lasts 10–25 minutes. Slowed respiration and heart rate, metabolic rate, and muscle tone continue into stages 3 and 4.

3) Stages 3 and 4: Deep sleep. Muscles of the body relax, and gastrointestinal activity is slowed.

3. The sleep-wake cycle is integrated into a 24-hour circadian rhythm, apparently controlled by the hypothalamus.

C. Changes in Sleep Patterns Throughout the Lifespan (adapted from Porth & Matfin, 2008)

1. In the newborn, REM sleep occurs at sleep onset, and periods of sleep and waking are distributed throughout the day.

2. By 8 months of age, an infant sleeps an average of 13 hours a day, and REM is approximately one-third of that time.

3. At 12–15 years of age, sleep is approximately 8 hours a day, with one-quarter in REM sleep.

4. Children usually do not complain of sleep disorders; common complaints of parents about their children include irregular sleep habits, too little or too much sleep, nightmares, sleep terrors, sleepwalking, and bedwetting.

5. Sleep changes in aging include fragmented sleep, shorter duration of stage 3 and 4 sleep, and reduced REM sleep. Older adults are also likely to have health problems and take medications that interfere with sleep.

D. Disruptions in Sleep Patterns Related to Illness and Disability: Managing the clinical manifestations of these illnesses and disabilities will assist in restoring the sleep-wake cycle.
   1. Traumatic brain injury and stroke: Disrupted normal patterns and initial reversal of day-night cycles, usually temporary
   2. Myasthenia gravis: Sleep apnea caused by skeletal muscle weakness
   3. Multiple sclerosis, spinal cord injury, and uremia caused by renal disease: Muscle twitching (clonus) or restless legs syndrome (RLS)
   4. Rheumatoid arthritis: Stiff, aching joints that make comfortable positioning difficult and frequent repositioning necessary
   5. Cardiac disease: Treatment with diuretics, necessitating nighttime toileting and disruption of sleep
   6. Pulmonary disease: Orthopnea, dyspnea, disrupted ability to breathe deeply
   7. Morbid obesity: Potentially partially occluded trachea caused by the compressing effect on the neck and jaw from facial and neck fat when supine
   8. Permanent lifestyle changes resulting from injury and body image disruption: Depression that causes disruption of adequate restful sleep
   9. Medications (particularly sedatives, hypnotics, tranquilizers, and antidepressants): Disrupted normal sleep, primarily through depression of delta wave sleep. Barbiturates depress delta and REM sleep, decrease consolidated sleep, and leave the person feeling less rested.
E. NDs Related to Sleep (NANDA-I, 2009–2011)
   1. Insomnia
   2. Readiness for enhanced sleep
   3. Sleep deprivation
   4. Disturbed sleep pattern

The following sections on sleep are summarized and adapted from Chasens, Williams, and Umlauf (2011).

F. Interdisciplinary Management of Chronic Primary Insomnia or Excessive Sleepiness
   1. Clients in acute rehabilitation settings are likely to have difficulty sleeping because of noise, being woken during the night for procedures, and a loss of usual sleep routines. See Young, Bougeois, Hilty, and Hardin (2009) for strategies to optimize sleep in the hospital. Evidence-based guidelines for promoting sleep of inpatients were not found. This is a key area for rehabilitation nursing research. After the client is discharged home, clinical manifestations of his or her disability or chronic illness may continue to impair sleep. If so, the nursing interventions recommended in section H may be effective if implemented.
   2. If nursing interventions do not correct these sleeping problems, the client may need a comprehensive evaluation by sleep medicine specialists, which includes the following (adapted from Chasens et al., 2011; LOE 1):
      a. Sleep history (LOE 1)
      b. Clinical measures to assess excessive sleepiness
         1) Epworth Sleepiness Scale (LOE 2)
         2) Avidan (2005; LOE 1)
         3) Multivariable Apnea Prediction Index
         4) Functional Outcomes of Sleep Questionnaire
         5) Pittsburgh Sleep Quality Scale
      c. Overnight sleep studies (polysomnography; LOE 1)
      d. Evaluation of the client's knowledge and use of sleep hygiene measures (LOE 1)
      e. Assessment for clinical manifestations of disorders causing excessive sleepiness, including obstructive sleep apnea (OSA), insomnia, RLS, and narcolepsy (LOE 1)
G. Interdisciplinary Interventions (LOE 1)
   1. Adjust medications that cause drowsiness and sleep impairment.
   2. Ensure that positive airway pressure devices are being used appropriately; educate the client and family as needed.
   3. Weight loss, regular exercise, and long-term diabetes control (LOE 1)
H. Nursing Interventions (NIC) to Promote Sleep in Those with Chronic Insomnia or Excessive Sleepiness (adapted from Chasens et al., 2011, and Schutte-Rodin, Broch, Buysse, Dorsey, & Sateia, 2008; LOE 1)
   1. Manage problems that interfere with sleep (see section D).
   2. Refer the client to a sleep specialist for OSA and RLS.
   3. Help the client implement sleep hygiene measures.
I. Sleep Hygiene Measures (LOE 1; adapted from Chasens et al., 2011): Sleep hygiene measures are effective only when OSA, RLS, and other sleep disorders have been treated.
   1. Use the bed and bedroom only for sleeping and sex.
   2. Adopt consistent and rest-promoting bedtime routines, including maintaining the same bedtime and waking time every day.

3. Get out of bed slowly upon awakening.
4. If awakening during the night, avoid looking at the clock because this heightens anxiety and makes sleep onset more difficult. For those with insomnia, remove clocks from the bedroom.
5. Avoid naps entirely or limit naps to 10–15 minutes.
6. Sleep in a quiet, cool, and dark environment. Sleep with earplugs or a mask if necessary.
7. If unable to fall asleep after 15–20 minutes, get up, go to another room, and read or do a quiet activity using dim lighting until sleepy again. Do not watch television, which emits too much bright light. Low-impact activities, including board games and gentle stretching, have been shown to improve daytime performance and sleep quality.
8. Before bedtime avoid the following:
    a. Tobacco, stimulants, caffeine, or alcohol 4–6 hours before bedtime
    b. Large meals or exercise 3–4 hours before bedtime
    c. Emotionally charged, upsetting, unpleasant, or stimulating activities right before bedtime
9. If sleeping with pets or another person contributes to sleeping problems, moving to another bed or couch for a few nights or keeping pets from sharing the bed may be helpful.

J. Short-Term Use of Medications to Treat Insomnia in Clients Admitted to Rehabilitation Units: The following recommendations are based on a review of literature for management of insomnia in hospitalized clients by Young and colleagues (2009). Nurses are encouraged to consult this source.
    1. Nonpharmacologic approaches are the first line of treatment. If they are ineffective, short-term use of the following agents may be effective.
        a. Intermediate-acting benzodiazepines (e.g., estazolam, temazepam) are good first-line agents.
        b. Eszopiclone, zaleplon, zolpidem, and zopiclone
    2. Note that clients taking medications for sleep are at higher risk of falls.

K. Nonpharmacologic Nursing Interventions for Clients Admitted to Rehabilitation Units (These are common practices that cannot cause harm; however, the authors have not identified sources that establish the LOE for these interventions.)
    1. Use aspects of the client's prior bedtime routines (e.g., unwinding, relaxing activities).
    2. Play low music with gentle rhythm patterns (e.g., classical or chamber music).
    3. Provide milk or herbal decaffeinated teas and low-sugar snacks.
    4. Provide skin care or massage, especially using backrubs or lotions.
    5. Ensure toileting before lights out.
    6. Provide warmth (e.g., light blanket, bath blanket, socks).
    7. Use comfort measures (e.g., hand holding, touch therapy, prayer, guided imagery, relaxation).
    8. Ensure a quiet environment.
    9. Ensure low levels of light, sound, and voices during the night.
    10. Provide pain medication if indicated.
    11. Use sleep medication only as a last resort because it produces artificial sleep.
    12. Use available waking time, whenever that occurs, to consolidate nursing activities (e.g., repositioning, toileting, skin care, medications, vital signs) in ways that encourage returning to sleep.
    13. Maintain an unhurried demeanor that calms the client; keep the lights low and voices hushed unless absolutely necessary.
    14. Express confidence that sleep will come if the client rests calmly.

L. Interventions for Common Sleep-Related Problems (NIC; These are common practices that do not cause harm; however, the authors have not identified sources that establish the LOE for these interventions.)
    1. Nightmares and night terrors: Use low lights to reorient the person, offer reassurance, and reestablish sleep-inducing interventions.
    2. Snoring and sleep apnea: Reposition the person to a side-lying position and use pillows to retain that position.
    3. Restlessness and irritability: Provide the person with a quiet, private opportunity to discuss what is troubling him or her, offer comfort and reassurance, and then redirect to sleep.
    4. Sleepwalking: Gently guide the person back to bed; it is not necessary to wake the client.
    5. Loud talking in sleep: Reposition the client; it is not necessary to wake the client.

M. Expected Client Outcomes (NOC) Related to Sleep Patterns
    1. An established pattern that provides high-quality sleep and restoration of energy and comfort
    2. Knowledge of effective sleep-enhancing modalities
    3. NOC: Sleep

V. **Mobility and Immobility**
    A. Overview (Koenig, Teixeira, & Yetzer, in press)
        1. The desire to maximize mobility

---

and independence in ADLs through physical and occupational therapy is the key reason clients are admitted for rehabilitation. Nurses have a key role in ensuring that clients are able to participate in therapy and that they follow through with goals on the inpatient unit and at home.

2. Mobility allows clients to care for themselves, to interact with the environment, and to carry out purposeful activities.

3. Balance, strength, and endurance are all components of mobility.

4. Mobility may be lost suddenly through disease or trauma or more gradually through inactivity or illness.

5. Prolonged immobility produces marked diminution of all body functions and places clients in a life-threatening situation. Adverse effects of immobility include decreased cardiac output; orthostatic hypotension and inability to sit or stand; dehydration; and increased risk of deep vein thrombosis, pneumonia, renal calculi, pressure ulcers, sensory deprivation, and impaired thought processes (Porth & Matfin, 2008).

6. Rehabilitation nurses identify problems of impaired mobility; set realistic goals; and collaborate with clients, families, and therapy team members to achieve these goals.

B. Nursing Assessment for Mobility

1. Assessment of functional mobility traditionally includes four major areas.
   a. Bed mobility
   b. Transfers, including toilet transfers
   c. Wheelchair mobility
   d. Ambulation

2. All interdisciplinary team members evaluate levels of assistance by using rankings and descriptive tools that are reliable and valid. These tools identify the amount of help or supervision needed or a device the person needs to perform a specific activity safely, over the required distance, and in a timely fashion. The FIM™ instrument, for use with adults, and the WeeFIM™, for pediatric populations, are the most common instruments used in rehabilitation facilities. To subscribe to the Uniform Data System for Medical Rehabilitation (UDSMR), FIM™ System, or WeeFIM™ system and for the most current versions of the FIM™ and WeeFIM™, instructions in their use, and other related topics, see www.udsmr.org.
   a. The FIM™ instrument (UDSMR, 1997a) is scored as follows for 18 domains (e.g., eating, grooming, dressing upper, dressing lower, bathing):
      1) 7 = Independent
      2) 6 = Modified independence (device)
      3) 5 = Supervision or setup
      4) 4 = Minimal assistance (patient is able to do 75% or more of task)
      5) 3 = Moderate assistance (patient is able to do 50%–74% of task)
      6) 2 = Maximal assistance (patient is able to do 25%–49% of task)
      7) 1 = Total assistance (patient is able to do less than 25% of task)
   b. The FIM™ is required in acute rehabilitation facilities by Prospective Payment System.
   c. WeeFIM™ (UDSMR, 1997b): The FIM™ instrument, adapted for pediatric populations, is scored as follows for three domains (16 motor, 14 cognitive, 6 behavioral):
      1) 0 = Never
      2) 1 = Rarely
      3) 2 = Sometimes
      4) 3 = Usually
   d. Other functional scales (e.g., Barthel, Katz, NANDA) are available.

3. Nurses assess the components of mobility.
   a. Range of motion (ROM): Evaluate the range of unassisted active motion of both sides (**Figure 7-5**) and distinguish between active, assisted, and passive ROM. Rehabilitation nurses who use these ROM terms will be better able to communicate with physical therapists, occupational therapists, and physiatrists when discussing the client's mobility goals.
   b. Balance: Sitting, standing, moving, amount of assistance needed, and distance involved
   c. Bed mobility: Ability to turn side to side, move up in bed, move to the side of the bed, sit up in the bed, and bridge (i.e., raise hips while in the supine position)
   d. Transfer ability: Ability to move between wheelchair and bed, toilet, bath bench or shower chair, standard seating (or automobile)
   e. Wheelchair mobility
   f. Ambulation
   g. Neuromuscular problems (e.g., spasticity, rigidity, resting tremors, intention tremors, flaccidity)
   h. Coordination and proprioception
   i. Ability to follow and remember instructions
   j. Client's expectations and past level of mobility, both recent and remote
   k. Age-appropriate growth and development and behaviors
   l. Comorbidities and general endurance

C. Expected Patient Outcomes Related to Impaired Mobility

THE SPECIALTY PRACTICE OF REHABILITATION NURSING

Figure 7-5. Range of Motion

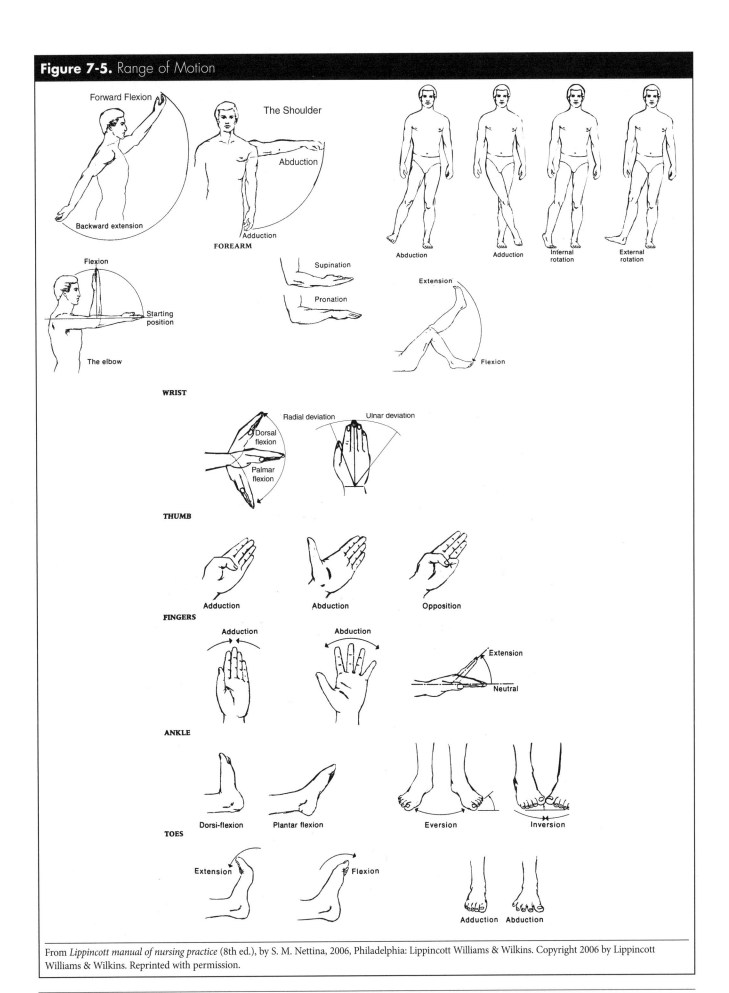

From *Lippincott manual of nursing practice* (8th ed.), by S. M. Nettina, 2006, Philadelphia: Lippincott Williams & Wilkins. Copyright 2006 by Lippincott Williams & Wilkins. Reprinted with permission.

1. Attain optimal functional mobility using the simplest level of assistance possible.
2. Demonstrate the safe use of any needed device.

D. Injury Prevention: Nurses are at risk for injury to themselves when transferring clients, assisting clients with ADLs, and helping clients ambulate. See ARN's five-part safe patient handling toolkit (2008).

E. Nursing Interventions (at the time of publication no guidelines were available to determine LOEs for the following interventions; rehabilitation nurses need to develop evidence-based practice guidelines for all these interventions).

1. For bed mobility
   a. Provide adequate changes in position and encourage the client's active participation.
   b. Use assistive devices (e.g., siderails, trapeze, overhead frame).

2. For transfers
   a. Provide the amount of assistance needed using a consistent approach and verbal cues.
   b. Use assistive devices (e.g., slide board, sit-to-stand lift, total or mechanical lift).
   c. Make adaptations for impaired transfer mobility.
      1) For impaired weight-bearing mobility of one side of the body (e.g., hemiplegia, total hip precautions, fractures of the leg, unilateral leg amputation): The client's physical therapist may make recommendations for helping clients transfer other than these. Follow the therapist's recommendations.
         a) The nurse places the wheelchair on the client's strong or unaffected side (the nearest armrest may need to be removed if the client is unable to come to a standing position), locks the brakes, and moves foot pedals out of the way.
         b) The client comes to a standing position and places the strong or unaffected foot forward toward the chair.
         c) The client places his or her unaffected arm on the armrest of the opposite side of the chair.
         d) The client rotates his or her body on the ball of the unaffected foot so the body is square to the chair.
         e) The client lowers himself or herself into the chair.
         f) When another person helps the client, the nurse explains the planned moves and encourages the client to take sufficient time to complete each move and maintain as much weight over his

or her own feet as possible. The helper should stand in front of the client and use his or her own knees to control the client's descent into the chair seat while keeping one foot in front of the client's feet to guard against slipping.

2) For impaired weight-bearing mobility of both legs (e.g., paraplegia, bilateral amputation)
   a) The nurse places the wheelchair perpendicular to the middle of the bed in the locked position.
   b) The client raises himself or herself to sit on the bed with legs and back to the chair.
   c) The client lifts his or her trunk by pushing down on the mattress and hitching the trunk backward.
   d) The client grasps the arms of the wheelchair and lifts himself or herself into the chair.

3) For impaired weight-bearing mobility due to poor balance or low strength (using a slide board)
   a) The nurse places the wheelchair next to the bed in the locked position and removes the armrest nearest to the bed.
   b) The client comes to a sitting position at the side of the bed.
   c) The nurse places one end of the slide board just under the client's buttocks and the other end on the chair.
   d) The client hitches himself or herself toward the chair along the board by pushing down with the arms and raising the trunk or by pulling on the armrest of the wheelchair. The legs and feet follow.
   e) Once in the chair, the client tilts away from the bed so the slide board can be removed.

4) For impaired weight-bearing mobility due to poor balance or low strength (e.g., sliding board, sit to stand lift, or total or mechanical lift)
   a) The nurse positions slings under the client either in one piece or under the arms and the thighs.
   b) The nurse positions the lift over the client and lowers it so the crossbar is accessible.
   c) The nurse uses the chains to attach the

slings to the crossbar, taking care to have equal length on each side and with the hooks facing away from the client.

    d) With a second person available to guide the legs and torso, the nurse pumps up the lift until the client's body clears the bed.

    e) The nurse slowly moves the lift away from the bed and over the chair, which is in the locked position.

    f) The nurse slowly releases the lift, allowing the client to descend into the chair.

    g) The nurse removes the chains and may leave the slings in place for ease in returning the client to bed.

3. For impaired wheelchair mobility: Wheelchairs may be used as a primary means of locomotion or for energy conservation and may be adapted to meet individual needs.

    a. May be powered manually or electrically with rechargeable batteries

    b. May have frame adaptations for sport participation, pediatric sizes, or body positioning needs

    c. May be controlled by one or two hands, extensions to wheel spokes or brake levers, joysticks, pneumatic (sip and puff) switches, or voice activation

    d. Wheelchair safety requires locking and unlocking brakes, controlling speed, changing direction, and having an appropriate body support and seating surface.

4. For impaired ability to ambulate

    a. Requirements for ambulation: Balance, strength, endurance, and ability to navigate various walking surfaces (e.g., floor, carpet, stairs, grass, pavement, uneven surfaces, hills)

    b. Components of a normal gait: Erect balance, foot lift, push off with alternate foot, heel strike, ride-over, and heel strike of opposite foot; contralateral arms may swing to provide stability and balance

    c. Protective assistance (e.g., gait belt, hands-on supervision, verbal cues)

    d. Quadriceps strengthening exercises for knee and hip strength (e.g., isometric tightening of the knee and gluteus muscles, holding the contraction for 3–5 seconds and then relaxing; repeated in sets of 5–10 and increased in frequency as strength returns), bicep and tricep exercises for crutch weight bearing

    e. Devices used to assist with ambulation

      1) Walkers for help with balance and forward gait: Height can be adjusted so that hands can bear some weight with elbows bent at about 30 degrees; the walker may be fitted with or without wheels; slit tennis balls may be placed over the base of the walker legs to encourage a smooth forward gait and a more normal forward progression.

      2) Hemiwalkers and platform canes for increased balance are used with the platform extending away from the body.

      3) Canes to provide stability and strength to one leg are adjusted for fit so that the wrist can bear some weight with the elbow slightly bent, used by placing ahead of and with the movement of the weak leg. The base tip should have a secure gripping rubber base.

      4) Crutches for protected or partial weight bearing (two- or four-point gait) or for nonweight bearing (three-point gait)

        a) Proper fit for standard crutches should extend from three fingers below the axilla to a point 6–8 in. to the side and out from the heel, with the handpiece allowing a 30-degree bend at the elbow and the wrist to rest on the handpiece.

        b) The base tip should have a secure, wide rubber grip.

        c) Proper gait instruction includes non–weight bearing on the axilla, careful placement of crutch tips, and caution on uneven surfaces, ice, or debris (**Table 7-6**).

        d) Forearm, Canadian, or Lofstrand crutches use the forearm for weight and are used when it is necessary to protect all joints in ambulation.

        e) Specially fitted orthoses, prostheses, and braces for support and protection: It is imperative to do skin checks before and after use.

5. For all clients

    a. Encourage functioning at the maximally independent level that is safe.

    b. Use verbal cues, reinforce learning, provide sufficient rest periods, and encourage adequate nutrition.

F. Disuse: The Hazards of Immobility: In 1967 Olson published a landmark article documenting the hazards of immobility. The following is an update of Olson's work, adapted from Porth (2005).

1. Overview

    a. Research continues to describe the deleterious consequences to all body systems from

Table 7-6. Crutch Walking Gaits

Four-Point Gait: Protected weight bearing on both feet

Right crutch followed by left foot

Left crutch followed by right foot

Repeat the pattern

Two-Point Gait: A faster version of the four-point gait

Right crutch and left foot move forward together

Left crutch and right foot move forward together

Repeat the pattern

Three-Point Gait: Full weight bearing on only one foot

Both crutches and the nonweight-bearing foot move forward together

Full weight bearing on the remaining foot

Repeat the pattern

Swing-Through Gait: A faster version of the three-point gait, also used with weight on both feet

Both crutches move forward together

Both legs are brought up to the crutches

Repeat the pattern

immobility and prolonged bed rest.

    b. Affects all body systems, not just limbs affected by disease

      1) Decreased cardiac output

      2) Orthostatic intolerance

      3) Dehydration

      4) Thrombophlebitis

      5) Muscle atrophy from disuse, especially in quadriceps

      6) Bone demineralization from decreased stress on bones

      7) Pneumonia from lowered tidal volume and decreased ability to clear bronchial secretions

      8) Formation of renal calculi, urinary retention, and urinary reflux

      9) Skin breakdown and the development of pressure ulcers from compromised circulation and pressure

      10) Bowel constipation from lowered peristalsis and inactivity

      11) Sensory deprivation

      12) Impaired thought processes, feelings of isolation, and depression

  2. Expected client outcomes related to actual or potential hazards of immobility

    a. Prevention of as many of the sequelae of immobility as possible

    b. Early identification of impairments related to disuse

    c. Self-advocacy regarding the need to include preventive measures in daily self-care

  3. Nursing interventions to prevent or limit the effects of disuse

    a. Provide frequent turning and skin care to relieve pressure and restore circulation.

    b. Use pressure redistribution surfaces (e.g., air mattresses, seat cushions).

    c. Pay careful attention to skin to ensure early recognition of reddened areas, wash skin gently with neutral pH soap, use lotions to lubricate skin and protect from moisture.

    d. Pay attention to incontinent episodes; provide frequent checks, thorough cleaning, and protective barrier creams; and adjust bowel and bladder training regimens.

    e. Encourage adequate fluid intake by mouth, by gastrostomy tube, or intravenously; monitor regularly for symptoms of dehydration.

    f. Establish an effective bowel program without creating long-term dependence on laxatives, cathartics, or enemas.

    g. Monitor lung sounds and encourage frequent deep breathing and coughing to move and clear bronchial secretions.

    h. Provide regular gentle exercise such as ROM exercises (e.g., quadriceps-setting exercises).

    i. Ensure early identification of venous thrombus (e.g., fever, pain, calf redness or warmth; positive Homans sign often is used as an indication of deep vein thrombosis, although there is no evidence to support its use).

    j. Implement postural hypotension (e.g., quadriceps-setting exercises, elastic stockings, sitting before standing).

    k. Use weight-bearing exercises to encourage retention of calcium in bones (e.g., tilt table, supported transfers).

    l. Use recreational and diversional therapy to stimulate social interaction.

VI. Self-Care and Activities of Daily Living

  A. Overview (Keonig, Teixeira, & Yetzer, in press)

    1. The functional pattern of activity and exercise includes the basic elements of self-care (e.g., feeding, toileting).

      a. ADLs include eating, bathing, dressing, and grooming.

      b. Instrumental activities of daily living (IADLs), or more complex aspects of independence, include meal preparation, household management, finances, transportation, and outdoor and community-based activities.

    2. Payer sources have a major role in determining the extent of services provided and the setting in

which these services are provided.

3. Rehabilitation nurses are the link between therapies, expected outcomes, and the realities of returning to community living.

B. Nursing Assessment of Self-Care Ability

1. Assess ability to independently perform basic ADLs (bathing, dressing, grooming, and eating), IADLs (e.g., meal preparation, shopping, housework), and social activities and determine the assistance needed to accomplish these tasks.

2. Use rating scales to measure the level of independence or burden of care.

a. FIM™ and WeeFIM™ systems.

b. NANDA-I (2009–2010) scores for self-care and mobility: 0 = *fully independent,* 4 = *dependent and unable* (note that scoring is the opposite of FIM™ scoring).

c. Mini-Mental State Exam: A short test of cognitive functions including orientation, registration, recall, calculation, language, and visual constructs

3. Assess specific motor impairments.

a. Spasticity, paralysis, flaccidity, tremors (e.g., constant, resting, intention), rigidity, contractures

b. Energy, endurance, strength, and safety

c. Balance while sitting and standing and the ability to self-correct alone or if pushed gently

4. Assess specific sensory impairments.

a. Visual field and acuity: Diminished or lost visual field and acuity, hemianopia, peripheral field loss, macular degeneration, use of corrective lenses

b. Tactile loss: Paresthesia, proprioception, temperature discrimination (needed for bathing and meal preparation)

c. Hearing: Diminished or lost hearing, use of hearing aids

5. Assess cognitive ability, which can affect the ability to perform ADLs.

6. Assess level of pain, which can interfere with learning and create additional body splinting.

a. Assess location, intensity, and possible causes of pain.

b. Treat pain before planned therapy.

C. Expected Client Outcomes Related to Impaired Self-Care Ability

1. Complete basic self-care activities as safely and independently as possible with or without devices as appropriate.

2. Demonstrate the ability to use and care for assistive devices if appropriate.

3. Perform IADLs as independently as possible.

4. Demonstrate the ability to direct self-care when unable to perform independently.

D. Nursing Interventions for Impaired Self-Care Ability

1. Use general teaching strategies.

a. Use the client's preferred method of learning as much as possible.

b. Begin with simple tasks that are familiar and meaningful to the client.

c. Repeat sequential tasks consistently.

d. Use demonstration, hand-over-hand, verbal, and written instruction.

e. Select the time of day at which the client's attention span and energy are highest.

f. Collaborate in teaching with other disciplines so the client receives consistent, reinforcing instruction.

2. Use available devices for specific losses.

a. Feeding: Plate guards, rocker knives, hand braces for utensils, nonskid placemats for stability, drinking cups with weighted bases and wide mouths

b. Bathing and hygiene: Face cloths, mitts, soap-on-a-rope, long-handled sponges, nailbrushes with suction cups, hand braces for toothbrush, freestanding mirrors, shower mats, grab bars, shower seats

c. Dressing: Long-handled shoe horns, reachers, Velcro closures for clothes, elastic shoelaces, devices that help to don socks

d. Grooming: Long-handled combs, adapted holders for razors, long-handled mirrors for skin inspection

e. Toileting: Raised toilet seats, transfer bars

3. Adapt care to manage impaired energy and endurance.

a. Teach pacing techniques.

b. Provide work simplification strategies.

c. Ensure changes in the workplace environment to accommodate height and sitting needs.

d. Recruit assistance.

e. Gradually increase tasks when the client's skills and strength return.

4. Provide strategies for household management and use of community resources.

VII. Sexuality and Reproduction

In this section the reader is referred to specific evidence-based guidelines for the treatment of some problems of sexuality and reproduction. However, much of the literature on sexuality and reproduction is based on the personal experiences of clients and their partners. What is effective for one couple may not be generalizable to others.

A. Overview
   1. Sexuality and reproduction are important issues for rehabilitation clients.
   2. Disability and major illnesses affect sexual function, self-esteem, body image, and social relationships. It is likely that all clients with new disabilities will have sexual changes. Some will want information on overcoming these changes; others will not care. However, it is best to ask all clients whether they have questions.
   3. Rehabilitation nurses play a major role in educating clients about the effects of injury or illness on sexual function and reproduction.
   4. To promote an atmosphere of permission and acceptance, rehabilitation nurses should separate their own values and attitudes in the area of sexuality to address the issue objectively.
   5. Rehabilitation nurses should know about available methods and aids to enhance sexual expression and conception after disability. A key intervention is to provide clients and their partners with educational materials. To find information for clients and their partners on specific chronic illnesses or disabilities, use a search engine and type in "sex and arthritis" or "sex and head injury," for example. For more information on sex after stroke, see Kautz (2007) and the resources listed in **Table 7-7**.
B. Kaplan's (1990) Stages and Descriptions of Human Sexual Response Cycle: common problems, changes with aging, and recommendations (**Table 7-8**)
C. Normal Physiology of Sexual Response
   1. Men
      a. The penis is innervated by sympathetic (T10–L2), parasympathetic (S2–S4), and somatic (pudendal nerve) fibers.
      b. Erection is under parasympathetic, sympathetic, and somatic control.
      c. Psychogenic response is initiated by cortical input, including visual and tactile senses, and mediated by sympathetic pathways (T10–L2).
      d. Reflex is initiated by internal or external tactile stimulation and mediated by the sacral spinal reflex (S2–S4).
      e. Emission is under sympathetic control (T10–L2), and ejaculation is under sympathetic and somatic control (S2–S4).
      f. Fertility depends on endocrine regulation, ejaculatory ability, and semen quality.
   2. Women
      a. Genitalia are innervated by sympathetic (pudendal nerve and perineal nerve) and parasympathetic (splanchnic nerve) fibers.
      b. Orgasm is thought to be under parasympathetic (S2–S4) and somatic control.
      c. Fertility depends on endocrine regulation of ovulation cycles.
D. Expected Client Outcomes (NOC) Related to Sexual Function
   1. Personal satisfaction with sexual function
   2. Avoidance of sexually transmitted diseases
   3. Pregnancy, if desired and possible; avoidance of pregnancy if not desired
   4. Ability to plan and carry out parenting roles if appropriate
E. PLISSIT Model for Sexual Counseling (Annon, 1976)
   1. *Permission:* Process of allowing questions or fears

Table 7-7. Sex Education Resources for Clients and Their Partners

The Web addresses and publications listed in this table were active and available at the time of publication; however, titles of publications and Web addresses often change.

Resources for Information and Comfortable Positions for Intercourse

Being Close: COPD and Intimacy: Available from http://lungline.njc.org

Chronic Low Back Pain and How It May Affect Sexuality: Available from http://ukhealthcare.uky.edu/patiented/booklets.htm

Sex and Arthritis: Available from www.orthop.washington.edu

Sex After Stroke: Our Guide to Intimacy After Stroke: Available from www.strokeassociation.org

Sex and Cancer (several Web articles by the American Cancer Society): Available from www.cancer.org

Intimacy and Diabetes: Available from www.netdoctor.co.uk

Diabetes and Men's Sexual Health and Diabetes and Women's Sexual Health: Available from www.diabetes.org

Sex Education Websites

The following are professional Web sites that are highly recommended for those with chronic illness and disabilities. These are legitimate sex education Web sites, not pornography sites.

www.womenshealth.org

www.erectile-dysfunction-impotence.org

http://marriage.about.com

www.4woman.gov (sexuality and disability for women)

THE SPECIALTY PRACTICE OF REHABILITATION NURSING

Table 7-8. Stages of Human Sexual Response and Common Sexual Problems

Building on early work by Masters and Johnson, Kaplan (1990) identified a triphasic model of human sexual response. The three phases are desire, excitement, and orgasm. Kaplan's model is more useful to the rehabilitation nurse than Masters and Johnson's because it helps the nurse understand why neurological impairment leads to sexual problems. Most sexual problems can be classified as desire, excitement, or orgasm phase disorders, or combinations of the three. For decades changes in sexual response have been considered normal consequences of aging.

Phase and Physiological Response	Neurological Control	Common Problems in All Adults	Changes with Aging
The desire phase includes the sensations that move one to seek sexual pleasures. Love is a powerful stimulus to sexual desire.	Sexual desire is probably stimulated by endorphins, and the pleasure centers in the brain are stimulated by sex; pain inhibits sexual desire.	Fatigue from work, family, and home responsibilities often interferes with desire.	Desire may or may not change with aging; levels of desire may remain the same throughout life.
The excitement phase consists primarily of myotonia, or increased muscle tone and vasodilation of the genital blood vessels. In men the penis becomes erect. In women the vagina becomes lubricated, the clitoris and vagina become longer and wider, and the labia minora extend outward.	Sexual excitement is controlled by the sympathetic nervous system and fear inhibits sexual excitement.	Occasional difficulty in achieving an erection or vaginal lubrication occurs in most adults throughout the lifespan.	Erections may require more direct stimulation and may be softer. Vaginal lubrication may be decreased and require more direct stimulation.
The orgasm phase is a climatic release of the genital vasodilation and myotonia of the excitement phase.	Orgasm is an automatic spinal reflex response.	Premature ejaculation is common in men. Anorgasmia is common in women.	Ejaculation may not be as forceful. Women's orgasms may feel different.

to be raised and giving permission to talk about the subject

2. *Limited Information:* Providing some specific information related to questions raised or concerns expressed and allowing the person to pursue the issue further if he or she is comfortable

3. *Specific Suggestions:* Assisting people with problem identification, providing specific suggestions to resolve a problem (e.g., suggestions to deal with erectile dysfunction, bowel and bladder concerns, positioning, contraception). Ginsberg (2010) provides additional information on erectile dysfunction.

4. *Intensive Therapy:* Providing expert assistance for intensive discussion and interventions (e.g., psychotherapy for marriage and relationship counseling, medical management of impotence, infertility, childbirth)

F. Common Classes of Medications and Their Effects on Sexual Functioning (**Table 7-9**)

G. Functional Problems and Their Potential Effects on Sexual Relationships (**Table 7-10**)

H. Sex and Intimacy Problems with Chronic Illnesses and Disability (**Table 7-11**)

I. Comfortable Intercourse Positions for Those with Chronic Illness or Disability. Finding a comfortable position for sex can be very difficult for those who have chronic obstructive pulmonary disease or back, hip, or knee pain or who are hemiparetic after a head injury or stroke (**Figure 7-6**).

J. Additional Issues Surrounding Reproduction

1. Contraception: The method should be based on the client's physical ability, cognitive ability to comply, potential medical risks of oral contraceptive use, and personal preferences. An excellent source for information on contraception and chronic illness is Greydanus and Matytsina (2010).

2. Pregnancy, childbirth, and parenting: Options vary according to the disability, available resources, and medical issues.

3. Fertility

   a. Causes of infertility in men: Anejaculation, impaired semen quality, impaired endocrine regulation

   b. For men with spinal cord injury, see the Consortium for Spinal Cord Medicine's "Sexuality and Reproductive Health in Adults with Spinal Cord Injury" (2010b).

K. Safety Issues Related to Sexuality

1. Sexually transmitted diseases

   a. Syphilis, gonorrhea

   b. AIDS

   c. Hepatitis

Table 7-9. Medications and Sexual Functioning

The following groups of medications have been shown to contribute to sexual dysfunction by decreasing sexual desire in men and women, promoting vaginal dryness in women or erectile dysfunction in men, or delaying or preventing orgasm in men or women. These sexual side effects may lessen 6–8 weeks after the medication is started. If the sexual dysfunction persists, a general recommendation for those experiencing sexual dysfunction is to contact the healthcare provider who prescribed the medication and ask whether a different medication from the same class or another class can be prescribed. Sometimes, despite changing medications, the side effects persist and the person taking the medication will need to seek treatment for the sexual dysfunction (Bostwick, 2010; Ginsberg, 2010; Krychman & Kellogg-Spadt, 2009; Mintzer, 2010).

Antidepressants, including tricyclics, monoamine oxidase inhibitors, and selective serotonin reuptake inhibitors, can decrease sexual desire in women and delay or prevent orgasm in both men and women.

Antihypertensives, especially thiazide diuretics and beta blockers. Centrally acting alpha receptor blockers and peripherally acting anti-adrenergics may also cause problems.

Anticholinergics: Probanthine and atropine.

Anticonvulsants: Phenytoin, phenobarbital, carbamazepine.

Histamine 2 blocking agents: Cimetidine, ranitidine

Lipid-lowering agents: Niacin, clofibrate

Digoxin

Opioids

Table 7-10. Functional Problems and Their Potential Effects on Sexual Relationships

Functional Problem	Potential Effect	Suggestion
Sensory/Perception		
Vision	Decreased ability to appreciate visual stimuli, difficulties with depth perception	If unilateral, uninjured partner should lie on unaffected side; use other senses (e.g., verbal, touch)
Sensation	Increased sensitivity or decreased or absent tactile sensation	Define areas of tactile loss, modify stimuli to that part, modify touch to areas of hypersensitivity
Proprioception (position sense)	Injured partner may not know where body parts are without visualizing, making sexual play clumsy or uncomfortable	Allow enough light for visualization; use positioning supports for comfort
Right-left discrimination	Injured partner may not be able to follow through with directions from partner	Direct injured partner by using terms other than right or left; use hand-over-hand guidance
Neglect or denial of deficits	Injured partner may have difficulty recognizing limitation and overstate abilities; may cause embarrassment for both partners if overstated abilities are acted out	Uninjured partner take more active role and gently redirect partner; use positioning with pillows; alternate positions
Communication		
Aphasia or dysarthria	Injured partner may have difficulty correctly interpreting affect of partner or expressing own desires	Use nonverbal communication (touching, gestures).
Concrete thinking	Injured partner may miss subtle cues; sexual play may be concretely focused and one sided	Uninjured partner may need to be very direct with sexual communication and give more specific directions to focus on mutual pleasure
Disinhibition or impulse control	Injured partner may make inappropriate or offending statement to partner; may increase number of sexual partners as a result of impulse control; may show inappropriate public display of sexual impulses or activity	Uninjured partner should give feedback to partner about responses and provide suggestions for better alternatives; enforce privacy and a consistent routine; do not reinforce inappropriate behaviors; may need to implement social skill retraining in matters related to sexual behaviors with the opposite sex

Table 7-10. Functional Problems and Their Potential Effects on Sexual Relationships *continued*

Functional Problem	Potential Effect	Suggestion
Cognition		
Attention or concentration	Injured partner may be restless, unable to focus on sexual play; may affect ability to sustain an erection	Decrease external distractions during sexual play; use relaxation, imagery, or guided fantasy by uninjured partner
Memory or judgment	If short-term memory is impaired, injured partner may persevere on a sexual activity or request or pressure partner for frequent sex; contraceptive use should not rely on memory of injured partner	Log sexual activity; discuss contraceptive options with physician; uninjured partner may need to take responsibility for contraception
Initiative	Injured partner may lack ability to take active role in creating a supportive environment	Uninjured partner may need to initiate, provide romantic environment, encourage
Mobility Impairment		
Paralysis	Inability to move body or a body part to position self or to respond to moves by the uninjured partner	Use pillows, alternate positioning strategies; uninjured partner may need to take more active role
Spasticity	Involuntary muscle contractions of affected parts of body; may interfere with attempts to position or reposition	Use positions that place less stress on muscles that tend to spasm; select positions so that if spasms occur, they will not disrupt activity; use reminders to tend to bowel and bladder needs before initiating foreplay; be aware that pain in another part of the body may set off spasms; pay attention to positioning
Elimination		
Bladder dysfunction	Bladder accidents decrease the appeal of sexual activity; presence of Foley catheter may hinder sexual activity; presence of urostomy may hinder sexual enjoyment	Restrict fluids before sexual activity; complete toileting; keep towel or urinal nearby for potential accidents; if Foley catheter present, can be taped to the side (for women to the thigh, for men to the abdomen or place a condom over the shaft of penis); avoid positions that place pressure on the bladder; cover urostomy or tape to abdomen
Bowel dysfunction	Bowel accidents decrease the appeal of sexual activity; presence of colostomy or ileostomy may hinder sexual activity	Complete bowel regime before sexual activity; avoid positions that place pressure on the bowels; cover ostomy, tape to the side or remove and use an ostomy cap over stoma
Erectile Dysfunction or Anorgasm		
Man is unable to establish or maintain an erection	Decreased ability for penile-vaginal intercourse	Explore alternative forms of sexual satisfaction, stuffing method, exploration of erogenous zones; seek psychological counseling; get referrals for erectile dysfunction assessment; use impotence treatments and medications (e.g., topical, intraurethral, oral, injectable); use external vacuum therapy; use penile implants (e.g., semirigid, inflatable).
Woman is unable to achieve orgasm	Decreased ability to reach climax	Explore alternative forms of sexual satisfaction; seek psychological counseling; educate about potential to have orgasm; encourage use of clitoral stimulation.

Rehabilitation Nursing Foundation. (1995). *Rehabilitation nursing: Directions for practice—a basic rehabilitation nursing course* (3rd ed., pp. 164–170). Glenview, IL: Rehabilitation Nursing Foundation of the Association of Rehabilitation Nurses.

Sipski, M. L., & Alexander, C. J. (1998). Sexuality and disability. In J. A. DeLisa & B. M. Gans (Eds.), *Rehabilitation medicine: Principles and practice* (3rd ed.). Philadelphia: Lippincott-Raven.

Table 7-11. Sex and Intimacy Problems with Chronic Illnesses

Chronic Illness	Common Changes in Sex and Intimacy	Recommendations for Overcoming the Problems
Heart disease Hypertension Peripheral vascular disease	Atherosclerosis and some medications may lead to erectile dysfunction in men and vaginal dryness (dyspareunia) in women. Both men and women may have fear of chest pain during sex. Fatigue may interfere with desire and lead to sexual dysfunction.	Smoking cessation, weight loss, and a consistent exercise program may increase genital circulation and reverse sexual dysfunction. Encourage couples to walk together to increase intimacy and endurance. If medications are leading to vaginal dryness or erectile dysfunction, ask the physician to switch to a different medication in the same drug class.
Diabetes	Peripheral and autonomic neuropathy cause decreased genital sensation, erectile dysfunction, and vaginal dryness. Gastroparesis leads to flatulence. Ketosis leads to bad breath. Fatigue may lead to sexual dysfunction.	Smoking cessation, weight loss, and exercise all may assist in overcoming problems. Keeping the hemoglobin A1c below 7 may reverse clinical manifestations of neuropathy, atherosclerosis, gastroparesis, and ketosis. Explain that clinical manifestations vary over time.
Chronic lung disease	Loss of stamina, fatigue, and chronic cough all may lead to decreased desire and sexual dysfunction. Chronic cough often leads to stress incontinence in older women.	Smoking cessation, weight loss, and exercise all may improve breathing, reduce fatigue, and increase desire and sexual function. Adopt positions that prevent shortness of breath (see Figure 7-3). Wear oxygen cannula during sexual activity.
Arthritis (degenerative joint disease, rheumatoid arthritis, gout)	Impaired mobility and joint pain may limit sexual activity. Chronic pain will decrease sexual desire.	Plan for sex at a time of day when pain is less, often mid morning when pain medications are at peak effect. Adopt sexual positions that don't cause pain (see Figure 7-3). Plan time for intimacy to combat feelings of worthlessness and depression.

Figure 7-6. Comfortable Intercourse Positions for Those with Chronic Illness or Disability

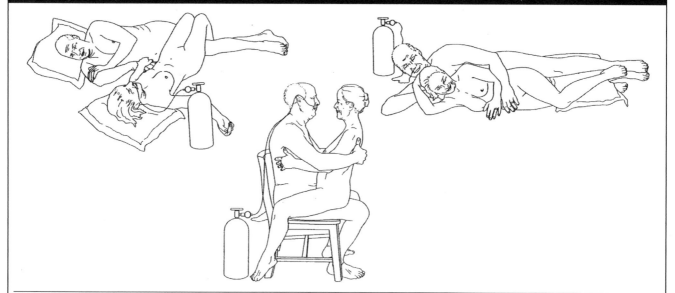

Note. These positions are appropriate when one or both partners cannot breathe well due to lung disease (or is restricted by oxygen tubing), have hip or knee pain due to arthritis, have back pain, or have limitations after a hip or knee replacement. These positions also work well if one or both partners have hemiparesis after a stroke. When side lying, lie on the affected side.

From *Gerontological nursing: Competencies for care* (2nd ed., p. 621), by K. L. Mauk (Ed.), 2010, Sudbury, MA: Jones & Bartlett. Copyright 2010 by Jones & Bartlett. Reprinted with permission.

THE SPECIALTY PRACTICE OF REHABILITATION NURSING

d. Herpes
　　2. Sexual abuse
　L. Age-Specific Issues
　　1. Pediatric: Injury and congenital disorders
　　2. Adolescence: Concerns about acceptance, roles, and relationships. The American Academy of Pediatrics (2001) has published an excellent guideline on sexuality education for children and adolescents.
　　3. Adults: Concerns about fertility, biological parenthood, pregnancy, and parenting
　　4. Older adults: Consideration of the normal effects of aging and their relationship to disability or availability of a partner (see Kautz, 2006, for more information).

References

American Academy of Pediatrics. (2001). Sexuality education for children and adolescents. *Pediatrics, 108*(2), 498–502.

American Diabetes Association, Bantle, J. P., Wylie-Rosett, J., Albright, A. L., Apovian, C. M., Clark, N. G., et al. (2008). Nutrition recommendations and interventions for diabetes: A position statement of the American Diabetes Association. *Diabetes Care, 31*(Suppl. 1), S61–S78.

American Society for Parenteral and Enteral Nutrition. (2009). ASPEN enteral nutrition practice recommendations. *Journal of Parenteral and Enteral Nutrition, 33*(2), 122–167.

American Society for Reproductive Medicine. (2005). *Sperm recovery after spinal cord injury in men.* Birmingham, AL: Author.

Annon, J. S. (1976). The PLISSIT model: A proposed conceptual scheme for behavioral treatment of sexual problems. *Journal of Sex Education Therapy, 2,* 1–15.

Aslan, E., Komurcu, N., Beji, N. K., & Yalcin, O. (2008). Bladder training and Kegel exercises for women with urinary complaints living in a rest home. *Gerontology, 54,* 224–231.

Association of Rehabilitation Nurses. (2008). *Safe patient handling toolkit.* Glenview, IL: Author.

Avidan, A. Y. (2005). Sleep disorders in the older patient. *Primary Care, 32,* 563–583.

Balin, A. K. (1990). Aging of human skin. In W. R. Hazzard, R. Andres, E. L. Bierman, & J. P. Blass (Eds.), *Principles of geriatric medicine and gerontology* (2nd ed., pp. 383–412). New York: McGraw-Hill.

Bostwick, J. M. (2010). A generalist's guide to treating patients with depression with an emphasis on using side effects to tailor antidepressant therapy. *Mayo Clinic Proceedings, 85,* 538–550.

Brain Trauma Foundation. (2007). Management of severe traumatic brain injury. *Journal of Neurotrauma, 24*(1), S1–S95.

Bryant, R. A., & Nix, D. P. (2007). *Acute and chronic wounds: Current management concepts* (3rd ed.). St. Louis: Mosby.

Carlaw, C., & Steele, C. (2009, November). *Implementation of a water protocol in a rehabilitation setting.* Poster presented at the annual convention of the American Speech-Language-Hearing Association, New Orleans, LA.

Chasens, E. R., Williams, L. L., & Umlauf, M. G. (2011). *Excessive sleepiness.* In M. Boltz, E. Capezuti, T. Fulmer, D. Zwicker, & A. O'Meara (Eds.), *Evidence-based geriatric nursing protocols for best practice* (4th ed., pp. 459–476). New York: Spring Publishing Company.

Consortium for Spinal Cord Medicine. (2006). *Bladder management for adults with spinal cord injury: A clinical practice guideline for health care providers.* Washington, DC: Paralyzed Veterans of America.

Consortium for Spinal Cord Medicine. (2010a). *Neurogenic bowel management in adults with spinal cord injury.* Washington, DC: Paralyzed Veterans of America.

Consortium for Spinal Cord Medicine. (2010b). *Sexuality and reproductive health in adults with spinal cord injury.* Washington, DC: Paralyzed Veterans of America.

Department of Health and Human Services, Department of Medicare and Medicaid Services. (2005). *CMS manual system.* Retrieved May 20, 2007, from www.cms.hhs.gov/transmittals/downloads/R8SOM.pdf.

Doughty, D. B. (2006). *Urinary and fecal incontinence: Current management concepts* (3rd ed.). St. Louis: Mosby.

Dowling-Castronovo, A., & Bradway, C. (2008). Urinary incontinence in older adults admitted to acute care. In E. Capezuti, D. Swicker, M. Mezey, & T. Fulmer (Eds.), *Evidence-based geriatric nursing protocols for best practice* (3rd ed., pp. 309–336). New York: Springer.

DuVivier, A. (1993). *Atlas of clinical dermatology* (2nd ed.). London: Times Mirror International Publishers.

Ehrlich-Jones, L., O'Dwyer, L., Stevens, K., & Deutsch, A. (2008). Searching the literature for evidence. *Rehabiliation Nursing, 33*(4), 163–169.

Garcia, J. M., & Chambers, E. IV. (2010). Managing dysphagia through diet modification: Evidence-based help for patients with impaired swallowing. *American Journal of Nursing, 110*(10), 26–33.

Ginsberg, T. B. (2010). Male sexuality. *Clinics in Geriatric Medicine, 26,* 185–195.

Greydanus, D. E., & Matytsina, L. A. (2010). Contraception in adolescent females with chronic illness: A clinical review. *International Journal of Child and Adolescent Health, 3,* 39–52.

Griffith, R., & Tengnah, R. (2007). Consensus guideline on the management of medication related dysphagia. *Nurse Prescribing, 5*(1), 34–36.

Johnson, M., Moorhead, S., Bulechek, G. M., Butcher, H. K., Maas, M. L., & Swanson, E. (2011). *NOC and NIC linkages to NANDA-I and clinical conditions: Supporting critical reasoning and quality care (NANDA, NOC, and NIC linkages)* (3rd ed.). St. Louis: Mosby.

Kaplan, H. S. (1990). Sex, intimacy, and the aging process. *Journal of the American Academy of Psychoanalysis, 18,* 185–205.

Kautz, D. D. (2007). Hope for love: Practical advice for intimacy and sex after stroke. *Rehabilitation Nursing, 32*(3), 95–103.

Kautz, D. D. (2010). Great rehabilitation nurses combine art and science to create magic. *Rehabilitation Nursing, 36*(1), 13–15.

Koenig, S., Teixera, J., & Yetzer, E. (In press). Promoting mobility and function. In K. L. Mauk (Ed.), *Rehabilitation nursing: A contemporary approach to practice* (pp. 136–147). Sudbury, MA: Jones & Bartlett.

Krychman, M. L., & Kellogg-Spadt, S. (2009). Female sexual dysfunction: Working toward new understanding. *Women's Health Care: A Practical Journal for Nurse Practitioners, 8*(5), 37–48.

Langmore, S. E., Terpenning, M. S., Schork, A., Chen, Y., Murray, J. T., Lopatin, D., et al. (1998). Predictors of aspiration pneumonia: How important is dysphagia? *Dysphagia, 13*(2), 68–81.

Mauk, K. L. (Ed.). (2010). *Gerontological nursing: Competencies for care* (2nd ed., p. 621). Sudbury, MA: Jones and Bartlett.

Milne, J. L. (2008). Behavioral therapies for overactive bladder: Making sense of the evidence. *Journal of Wound, Ostomy, and Continence Nursing, 35*(1), 93–101.

Mintzer, S. (2010). Metabolic consequences of antiepileptic drugs. *Current Opinion in Neurology, 23,* 164–169.

Moore, Z. E. H., & Cowman, S. (2005). Wound cleansing for pressure ulcers. *Cochrane Database of Systematic Reviews,* Article CD004983. doi:10.1002/14651858.

Mueller, C., Compher, C., Ellen, D. M., & the American Society of Parenteral and Enteral Nutrition Board of Directors. (2011). ASPEN clinical guidelines: Nutrition screening, assessment, and intervention in adults. *Journal of Parenteral and Enteral Nutrition, 35*(1), 16–24.

National Pressure Ulcer Advisory Panel. (n.d.). *Pressure ulcer category/staging illustrations.* Washington, DC: Author.

National Pressure Ulcer Advisory Panel & European Pressure Ulcer Advisory Panel. (2009). *Prevention and treatment of pressure ulcers: Clinical practice guideline.* Washington, DC: National Pressure Ulcer Advisory Panel.

North American Nursing Diagnosis Association International. (2009–2011). *Nursing diagnoses: Definitions & classification: 2009–20011.* Retrieved January 8, 2011, from www.nanda.org/Marketplace/NANDAIPublications/20092011Taxonomy Print.aspx.

Palmer, P. M. (1999). *Frazier Free Water Protocol.* Retrieved March 27, 2007, from http://dysphagia.com/forum/showthread.html.

Panther, K. (2008). *Frazier Water Protocol: Safety, hydration, and quality of life.* Rockville, MD: ASHA Product Sales.

Pear, S. (2007). Oral care is critical care. *Infection Control Today, 11*(10).

Porth, C. M., & Matfin, G. (2008). *Pathophysiology: Concepts of altered health states* (8th ed.). Philadelphia: Lippincott Wilkins & Williams.

Registered Nurses Association of Ontario. (2005). *Risk assessment and prevention of pressure ulcers.* Toronto, ON, Canada: Author. Retrieved September 12, 2011, from www.rnao.org/Storage/12/638_BPG_Pressure_Ulcers_v2.pdf.

Rehabilitation Nursing Foundation. (1995). *Rehabilitation nursing: Directions for practice—A basic nursing rehabilitation course* (3rd ed., pp. 164–170). Glenview, IL: Author.

Rehabilitation Nursing Foundation. (2002). *Practice guidelines for the management of constipation in adults.* Glenview, IL: Author.

Rye, J., & Mauk, K. L. (in press). Bowel and bladder management. In K. L. Mauk (Ed.), *Rehabilitation nursing: A contemporary approach to practice* (pp. 121–135). Sudbury, MA: Jones & Bartlett.

Schutte-Rodin, S., Broch, L., Buysse, D., Dorsey, C., & Sateia, M. (2008). Clinical guideline for the evaluation and management of chronic insomnia in adults. *Journal of Clinical Sleep Medicine, 4,* 487–504.

Scottish Intercollegiate Guidelines Network. (2010). Management of patients with stroke: Identification and management of dysphagia: A national clinical guideline. Retreived September 12, 2011, from www.sign.ac.uk/pdf/sign119.pdf.

Shimaliyan, T. A., Kane, R. L., Wyman, J., & Wilt, T. J. (2008). Systematic review: Randomized controlled trials of nonsurgical treatments for urinary incontinence in women. *Annals of Internal Medicine, 148*(6), 459–473.

Sievers, A. E. F. (2008). Nursing evaluation and care of the patient with dysphagia. In R. Leonard & K. Kendall (Eds.), *Dysphagia assessment and treatment planning: A team approach* (2nd ed.). San Diego, CA: Plural Publishing.

Sipski, M. L., & Alexander, C. J. (1998). Sexuality and disability. In J. A. DeLisa & B. M. Gans (Eds.), *Rehabilitation medicine: Principles and practice* (3rd ed.). Philadelphia: Lippincott-Raven.

Smith Hammond, C. A., & Goldstein, L. (2006). Cough and aspiration of foods and liquids due to oral-pharyngeal dysphagia: ACCP evidence-based clinical practice guidelines. *Chest, 129,* 154–168.

Stevens, K. A. (2008). Urinary elimination and continence. In S. P. Hoeman (Ed.), *Rehabilitation nursing: Prevention, intervention & outcomes* (4th ed., pp. 334–368). St. Louis: Mosby/Elsevier.

Suiter, D. (Ed.). (2005). *Frazier free water protocol: Evidence and ethics.* Retrieved January 8, 2011, from www.asha.org.

Sussman, C., & Bates-Jensen, B. (Eds.). (2007). Wound healing physiology: Acute and chronic. In *Wound care: A collaborative practice manual for health professionals* (3rd ed., pp. 21–51). Baltimore: Lippincott Williams & Wilkins.

Tosta de Souza, D. M. S., Conceicao de Gouveia Santos, V. L., Iri, H. K., & Oguri, M. Y. S. (2010). Predictive validity of the Braden scale for pressure ulcer risk in elderly residents of long-term care facilities. *Geriatric Nursing, 31*(2), 95–104.

Uniform Data System for Medical Rehabilitation. (1997a). *Functional Independence Measure.* Buffalo, NY: University of Buffalo.

Uniform Data System for Medical Rehabilitation. (1997b). *Functional Independence Measure for Children.* Buffalo, NY: University of Buffalo.

U.S. Department of Health and Human Services and U.S. Department of Agriculture. (2005). *Dietary guidelines for Americans, 2005.* Retrieved June 23, 2010, from www.health.gov/dietaryguidelines/dga2005/document/default.htm.

Wallace, S. A., Row, B., Williams, K., & Palmer, M. (2009). Bladder training for urinary incontinence in adults (review). *Cochrane Database of Systematic Reviews 2004,* Issue 1.

Wound, Ostomy and Continence Nurses Society. (2010). *Guideline for prevention and management of pressure ulcers.* Retrieved September 12, 2011, from www.guideline.gov/content.aspx?id=23868.

Wright, K. J. (2009). Administering medication to adult patients with dysphagia. *Nursing Standard, 23*(29), 61–68.

Young, J. S., Bougeois, J. A., Hilty, D. M., & Hardin, K. A. (2009). Sleep in hospitalized medical patients, part 2: Behavioral and pharmacological management of sleep disturbances. *Journal of Hospital Medicine, 4,* 50–59.

CHAPTER 8
Psychosocial Healthcare Patterns and Nursing Interventions

Cynthia S. Jacelon, PhD RN-BC CRRN FAAN

Rehabilitation nurses must understand the concept of psychosocial health, which involves the influence of psychological processes and social interactions on behavior. Theories of development, self-perception, roles and relationships, coping and stress tolerance, and values and beliefs and concepts such as hope and dignity support psychosocial healthcare patterns. Rehabilitation nurses promote psychosocial health by applying a holistic perspective to the nursing process. The theories and concepts presented in this chapter provide a foundation for rehabilitation nurses to promote psychosocial health during the lifespan.

I. **Developmental Considerations Related to Psychosocial Health**
  A. Cognitive Maturation in Children
    1. Human beings are social creatures. Normal cognitive development involves interacting with other people from the moment of birth. It is a process in which children grow, mature, and interact with their environment. Cognitive deficits can have a profound influence on the life of a developing child; these deficits impair the input, reasoning, and thinking processes needed for normal development.
      a. Children with brain injuries can have impaired cognitive development.
      b. Delays in speech and language development related to deafness, mental deficits, or emotional disturbances can affect the child's psychosocial development.
    2. Piaget's (1952) cognitive development theory and Erikson's (1963) social learning theory provide a theoretical basis for normal cognitive development. (Refer to Chapter 17 for additional information on developmental stages.)
      a. Sensorimotor period (0–2 years)
        1) Description
          a) Learning through feeling, touching, and handling; lack of fully developed object permanence (Piaget, 1952)
          b) The psychosocial development of trust versus mistrust: Disruptions in cognitive achievement during this period impair the psychosocial development of infants and toddlers (Erikson, 1963).
        c) Examples
          (1) An 8-month-old child demonstrates goal-directed activities.
          (2) A 12-month-old child understands means-to-end relationships.
          (3) A 2-year-old child has the beginnings of symbolic thinking.
        2) Nursing interventions: Promote sensory stimulation, security by caregivers, motor coordination, consistent personal attention, and parental education about growth and development.
      b. Preoperational period (2–7 years)
        1) Description: The development of autonomy versus shame, initiative versus guilt, and the beginning of industry versus inferiority; beginning of a sense of self (Erikson, 1963; Piaget, 1952)
          a) Children use representative thought to recall past events, represent the present, and anticipate the future.
          b) Children age 4–7 years use increased symbolic functioning.
        2) Nursing interventions
          a) Conduct initial and ongoing cognitive and physical assessment.
          b) Encourage exploration of the environment.
          c) Encourage participation in age-appropriate activities.
          d) Promote consistent, affectionate caregiving.
          e) Diversify environmental stimuli.
          f) Provide intellectual stimulation.
          g) Promote peer interaction.
          h) Continue parental education about age-appropriate growth and development.
      c. Concrete operational period (7–11 years)
        1) Description
          a) The continued development of industry versus inferiority, characterized by cognitive, concrete operations
          b) Children use logical approaches and rules to solve concrete problems in an effort to feel competent.

2) Nursing interventions
   a) Promote peer interaction and social-ization.
   b) Encourage formal education with peers.
   c) Promote creativity.
   d) Continue parental education about growth and development.
   e) Continue consistent interaction with parents, family, caregivers, and teach-ers.
d. Formal operational period (11–15 years)
   1) Description: The development of identity versus role confusion
      a) Adolescents are capable of logical thought and abstract thinking.
      b) Role expectations include increasing independence, building self-esteem, being socially successful and more mature, increasing autonomy, and in-creasing responsibilities (Satir, 1988).
   2) Research study findings
      a) A study of 14 children between the ages of 5 and 13 years with spinal cord injury (SCI) indicated that the chil-dren's scores for quality of life (QOL) were higher than their parents' scores. One explanation was that the children focused on current life expectations, whereas their parents also considered the long-term picture and future pros-pects (Johnston, Lauer, & Smith, 2006).
      b) A study that surveyed the coping strategies of adolescents with and without disabilities indicated that there was a continuing need to cope with life stressors. There was no dif-ference in the types of coping used be-tween the two groups of adolescents. There was a negative relationship be-tween severity of mobility and both cognitive avoidance and emotional discharge. There was a moderately high correlation between level of in-volvement and both seeking guidance and solving problems. Finally, there was a moderately high correlation be-tween self-esteem levels and methods of coping (Smith, Cook, Frost, Jones, & Wright, 2006).
      c) Adolescents who already have nega-tive life experiences have higher stress levels. Common stressful situations

for adolescents include body changes with puberty, new relationships with peers and family, sexual and moral di-lemmas, and school expectations (Dacey & Margolis, 2006).
   3) Assessment
      a) Conduct initial and ongoing psycho-social and physical assessment.
      b) Assess QOL with the PedsQL instru-ment, which contains the factors of total well-being; physical well-being; psychosocial well-being; and emo-tional, social, and school functioning (Johnston et al., 2006).
   4) Nursing interventions
      a) Treat the adolescent with disability as a normal person.
      b) Allow time for the adolescent to ad-just to changes caused by injury.
      c) Encourage the adolescent to have close bonds with family.
      d) Provide information to reduce fears and misconceptions about the injury.
      e) Provide encouragement, peer support, and motivation.
      f) Foster the adolescent's friendships with peers.
      g) Give the adolescent age- and ability-appropriate responsibilities.
      h) Ensure appropriate parental protec-tiveness.
      i) Ensure that the adolescent is involved with decision making.
      j) Use problem-focused coping ap-proaches (Dacey & Margolis, 2006).
      k) Allow verbalization of frustrations (Dacey & Margolis, 2006).
B. Cognitive Maturation in Young and Middle-Age Adults
   1. Description of social learning theory
      a. This theory explains human behaviors in terms of active, dynamic interactions of be-haviors, personal factors, and environmental influences (Bandura, 1977).
      b. Personal interactions include the person's ability to symbolize behavioral meanings, foresee the outcomes of behaviors, learn through observations and experiences, and self-determine and self-regulate his or her life (Bandura, 1977).
      c. Adults reflect and analyze to give meaning to experiences (Bandura, 1977).

d. Young and middle-age adult development fulfills the psychosocial phases of intimacy versus role confusion and generativity versus stagnation (Erikson, 1963).

e. Cognitive and physical disability can affect the potential and motivation to fulfill developmental phases.

f. The roles of young adults can include positive pairing.
   1) Positive pairing is characterized by willing, knowledgeable, respectful support within the pair and includes relationships based on the equality of value of the couple.
   2) Successful pairing depends on personal autonomy, emotional honesty, expression of needs, responsibility, accountability, freedom of choice, and cooperation (Satir, 1988).

g. The adult faces developmental stresses of career, family, and independence. The adult environment contains stressors that are unavoidable because adults are more aware of the realities of life situations and are more aware of responsibilities (Dacey & Fiori, 2006).

h. Middle-aged adults face unique stressors such as children living at home; children leaving home for marriage, college, or the military; the responsibilities associated with older relatives; and changes in their personal health (Dacey & Fiori, 2006).

2. Nursing interventions
   a. Encourage protective measures of coping such as a supportive family environment, supportive networks, and personal control (Dacey & Fiori, 2006).
   b. Promote trust and balance of decision making.
   c. Promote the ability to adapt and cope with change.
   d. Promote recreational therapy.
   e. Encourage socialization with family and peers.
   f. Ensure access to vocational and academic counseling and education.
   g. Provide family counseling.
   h. Foster autonomy, independence, and personal responsibility.

C. Cognitive Maturation in Older Adults
   1. The last psychosocial developmental phase of ego identity versus despair (Erikson, 1963)
      a. Older adults reflect on their lives and remember worthwhile and unique experiences.

b. Disability and chronic illness can profoundly affect QOL and psychosocial satisfaction.

c. Transition is needed to progress from middle age to older adulthood.
   1) Transitional steps start with acknowledging changes that occur with aging.
   2) Mixed feelings are present with changes in work status and lifestyle.
   3) Life reflection can be positive or negative. Some resent that there may be no opportunity to change poor life decisions (Dacey & Fiori, 2006).
   4) Care of the older adult in poor health is considered one of the most stressful situations in a family, especially for the spouse (Dacey & Fiori, 2006).
   5) Older adults often experience multiple changes in mobility, cognition, social opportunities, financial stability, level of independence, and physical health.
   6) A successful transition is characterized by recognizing the positive aspects of aging and moving toward new challenges.
   7) A successful transition must incorporate positive attitudes, feelings of worth, flexibility, feelings of purpose, positive relationships, and participation in the family and community (Satir, 1988).

2. Assessment
   a. Conduct initial and ongoing assessment of cognitive, social, functional, and physical health.
   b. Assess the relationship and responsibilities of caregivers and the older adult.
   c. Assess the change of role behaviors and responsibilities of spouses (Clark, 2000).
   d. Investigate alternatives in caregiving such as adult care, in-home care providers, and respite care.

3. Nursing interventions
   a. Promote recreational therapy and leisure.
   b. Encourage socialization.
   c. Provide family counseling.
   d. Allow the client to reflect and reminisce.
   e. Foster autonomy, independence, respect, and personal responsibility.
   f. Provide family counseling.

II. **Cognitive Influences on Psychosocial Health**
   A. Cognition
      1. Description
         a. *Cognition* is defined as the concept of thinking and consists of attention, memory,

abstract reasoning, generalization, concept formation, problem solving, and executive function (Grzankowski, 1997); cognitive deficits may involve one or more of these components.

b. Cognitive development allows the processing of information through decoding, encoding, transferring, combining, storage, and retrieval (Travers, 2006).

c. Cognition depends on sensory input, prior experiences, learning, and recall and memory.

d. An injury to the cortex of the brain or the neural pathways interferes with sensory input, cognitive integration, and planning of appropriate responses.

e. The cerebral cortex, internal nuclei, basal ganglia, and the cerebellum process and integrate sensory input and motor planning (**Table 8-1**).

f. Recovery depends on the extent, quality (e.g., edema versus destruction), and area of the injury (Grzankowski, 1997).

2. Assessment

a. Conduct initial and ongoing cognitive assessment.

b. Evaluate the client's ability to determine pertinent and irrelevant stimuli, to learn, to understand situations or conversations, to problem solve, and to follow a plan of action.

c. Obtain a symptom history from the person and family (Shah & Bennett, 2006).

d. Review the medical history and current medications, including alternative medications and treatments.

e. Assess the ability to perform activities of daily living (ADLs; Shah & Bennett, 2006).

f. For clients with brain injury, use the Rancho los Amigos Levels of Cognitive Function Scale as an assessment tool (Flannery, 1998).

g. Assess attention abilities, short- and long-term memory for processing information, recall and retrieval, and problem solving (Travers, 2006).

3. Nursing interventions

a. Use helpful cues (e.g., the client's name, pictures of familiar people or pets) to help the client identify locations.

b. Encourage the client to use daily logs, written schedules, and patterns for ADLs.

c. Use sensory stimulation programs (e.g., visual, auditory, olfactory, cutaneous, taste, motion) that focus on short-term interventions several times a day to increase cognition.

d. Make materials meaningful for each person (Travers, 2006).

e. Use optimal timing when the person is not tired, rushed, hungry, or distracted.

f. Simplify the situation and repeat it for understanding.

g. Ensure a consistent schedule, staff, and environment.

h. Recommend a power of attorney for financial and health decisions (Shah & Bennett, 2006).

Table 8-1. Cognitive Functions Affected by Brain Injury		
Area of Brain	**Function**	**Results of Injury**
Frontal lobe	Controls higher intellectual and social processing	Loss of intellect and inappropriate social behaviors
Temporal lobe	Controls new memory and learning	Impaired learning
Temporal lobe (hippocampus)	—	Temporary memory loss, lack of contralateral orientation, distractibility, hyperactivity, attention deficits, perseveration
Right hemisphere	Controls recognition of geometric patterns, faces, environmental sounds, a second language, music, sense of direction, and memory for pictures	Learning impairments, memory impairments
Left hemisphere	Controls memory for language, letters, works, verbal memory (e.g., reading, writing, speech), arithmetic	Deficits with math and communication
Limbic lobe of the right and left hemispheres	Controls attention that affects socialization	Deficits with socialization

THE SPECIALTY PRACTICE OF REHABILITATION NURSING

4. Research study findings
   a. Children with acquired brain injury often experience cognitive, motor, and *psychosocial* deficits that affect participation in everyday activities. With coaching, the children's behavior improved, although their problem solving did not (Missiuna et al., 2010).
   b. Children with congenital heart disease are at risk for neurological damage related to hypoxia. The impact of neurological damage may include global cognitive deficits, memory deficits, and gross and fine-motor delays and deficits (Townsend, Lohr, & Nelson, 2006).
   c. Clients' cognitive profile affects clients' and therapists' view of their working alliance (WA) in different ways. The weakness of the correlations between cognitive tests and WA ratings may indicate that a good WA is achievable with clients with severe cognitive difficulties (Schönberger, Humle, & Teasdale, 2007).

B. Orientation
   1. Definition: The ability to know about oneself (e.g., name, age, date of birth, home), the time (e.g., current date, month, year), and facts about the environment
   2. Assessment
      a. Conduct an initial and ongoing assessment of orientation.
      b. Distinguish between confusion, disorientation, physical conditions (e.g., electrolyte imbalance, medications, fluid imbalance, fatigue), and sensory deficits (Shah & Bennett, 2006).
      c. Use the Mini-Mental State Examination (MMSE; Folstein, Folstein, & McHugh, 1975).
   3. Nursing interventions
      a. Use cues to orient the client (e.g., familiar photographs of the client, family, or pets; familiar furniture; calendars; holiday decorations; clocks with large, clear numbers; schedules of daily events).
      b. Clearly identify family, relatives, friends, and staff when interacting with the client.
      c. Ensure that the client uses intact, functional sensory aids (e.g., glasses, hearing aids; Remington, Abdallah, Melillo, & Flanagan, 2006).
      d. Provide a consistent environment and staff.
   4. Research study findings: To determine how altered orientation influences rehabilitation outcome in people with stroke and how decreased orientation 6 months after stroke influences ADLs and social activities, Pedersen, Jorgensen, Nakayama, Raaschou, and Olsen (1996) analyzed the independent influence of orientation in acute stroke on rehabilitation. The level of orientation influences basic ADLs and higher-level instrumental ADLs and social activities in acute and chronic stroke. This finding suggests that rehabilitation of memory and attention might be important in people with stroke and impaired orientation.

C. Attention
   1. Definition: The ability to respond to and prioritize relevant information and to ignore or put aside irrelevant information
      a. Older adults are vulnerable for attentional fatigue caused by age-related physiological changes in vision, hearing, touch, and taste.
      b. Attentional capacity is influenced by the capacity to direct attention, attentional demands, attentional fatigue, and restorative activities.
      c. Attention works through global neural inhibitory mechanisms that allow the focusing that is needed for prolonged or intense directed attention (Jansen & Keller, 1998).
   2. Assessment
      a. Assess short-term memory, planning, problem solving, incidence of accidents, irritability, impulsiveness, and frustration (Jansen & Keller, 1998).
      b. Use standard questions to assess attention.
         1) Inquire about home activities that require more or new effort (e.g., physical or environmental factors).
         2) Discern the feelings that the client experiences most often.
         3) Identify times the client would like to but cannot express feelings and share experiences.
      c. Assess changes in the person's feelings, emotions, anger, and frustration, which may accompany loss of motivation (Paterson & Stewart, 2002).
   3. Nursing interventions
      a. Use conservation and restoration measures to reduce neurological fatigue.
         1) Conservation measures: Reduce or limit the extent and number of attentional demands in the internal and external environments; help the client complete necessary and desired activities in a controlled, stable environment.
         2) Restoration measures: Allow rest and recovery by changing activities (e.g., taking a walk in a park, gardening, bird watching).
      b. Prioritize activities for attention.

c. Break the task into parts, focusing on step-by-step instructions.

d. Encourage daily physical activity.

e. Advise the client to avoid alcohol and drugs.

f. Individualize music selections and avoid stressful selections.

g. Modify expectations to fit the reality of the client's status.

h. Provide growth and development opportunities.

i. Allow for variance in the client's attention throughout the day.

j. Identify triggers (e.g., situations, people, places, events) that contribute to intellectual or emotional conflict.

k. Provide client and family education.

l. Avoid denial, devaluation, or demeaning of the client.

m. Participate in group therapy (Paterson & Stewart, 2002).

n. Allow rest to recover from the overwhelming fatigue of dealing with loss of cognitive abilities (Paterson & Stewart, 2002).

4. Research study findings: Findings from a qualitative study of clients' perceptions after closed-head injury found that there were problems in thinking sequentially and conceptually. The participants also had problems dealing with multiple stimuli. These problems affected their ability to concentrate and process thoughts (Paterson & Stewart, 2002).

D. Judgment

1. Description: Remembering, planning, foresight, abstraction, transference of information, and evaluating the appropriateness of an action

2. Assessment

a. Evaluate the client's ability to comprehend physical and cognitive limitations and maintain recommended safety precautions.

b. Observe the client's accuracy with managing money, learning new skills, applying old knowledge in new situations, solving problems, and creating and following through with realistic plans.

c. Periodically reassess the client's judgment deficits to meet his or her increasing or decreasing needs.

3. Nursing interventions: Tailor interventions to match the client's level of cognition.

a. For clients with high cognitive functioning, coordinate counseling, education, crisis management, vocational assessment and planning, and individualized self-care.

b. For clients with moderate cognitive functioning, provide or coordinate scheduled routines, a structured environment, counseling, individualized education, and vocational assessment and planning.

c. For clients with lower cognitive functioning, help coordinate supervised living situations, a protective environment, sheltered vocational opportunities, case management, and legal guardians.

4. Research study findings: An autoethnographic exploration of one woman's illness narrative provides an in-depth understanding of her lived experience of rehabilitation after a traumatic brain injury (TBI) and polytrauma. The narrative confirms the importance of providing people with self-determined choice as a primary component of rehabilitation. The voices and values of clients are integral to professional judgment. This narrative supports clients' personal choice and freedom during the rehabilitation process as a means of increasing their sense of self-determination and empowerment while improving overall health outcomes (Lawson, Delamere, & Hutchinson, 2008).

E. Problem Solving

1. Definition: A high-level cognitive function that involves considering, recalling, and analyzing factors and selecting appropriate choices from various alternatives

2. Assessment

a. Assess the ability to problem solve initially and in an ongoing manner.

b. Assess the ability to plan and organize thoughts and behaviors.

c. Assess the ability to formulate alternative solutions for a problem.

d. Assess the ability to comprehend potential consequences of choices.

3. Nursing interventions

a. Help the client approach problems by taking one step at a time.

b. Encourage the client to differentiate between solutions to a problem and examine the consequences of solutions.

c. Encourage successful problem-solving plans and build on successes.

d. Examine unsuccessful problem-solving plans and discuss ways to select positive action plans.

e. Plan family and caregiver education with a focus on brain function and strategies for dealing with the lack of decision-making skills after stroke or head injury (Williams & Dahl, 2002).

f. Involve the family and caregivers in discharge planning decisions after stroke or head injury.

4. Research study findings

   a. A study of people surviving stroke for 6 months to 8 years indicated that confusion and errors in decision making were noted by both family members and caregivers. Regardless of levels of education, subjects exhibited behaviors of inertia, indifference, cognitive deficits, problems with interpersonal communication, and emotional instability such as panic (Williams & Dahl, 2002).

   b. Spalding (2005) described a mentoring situation for a professional person who had sustained a head injury. The head injury resulted in a high level of cognitive impairment for this person. The problem-solving deficits noted during the mentoring experience included lack of focus and direction, fragmented documentation, impaired memory, anxiety, lack of organization, distraction, impulsivity, lack of flexibility, and lack of appropriate priority judgments. The cognitive impairments severely affected this person's ability to problem solve in the working environment.

   c. As part of a larger study designed to evaluate social communication abilities after TBI, participants completed measures of executive functioning, affect perception, perceived communication ability, and functional outcome (Struchen et al., 2008). Executive functioning performance accounted for 13.3% of the variance in occupational functioning and 16% of explained variance in social integration. These results provide evidence of the value of executive functioning and social communication measures in the prediction of functional outcomes.

F. Motivation

1. Description

   a. Motivation is the external, internal, or combined forces that influence behavior to satisfy needs and achieve goals.

   b. Motivation can be influenced by needs and wants, the cost and rewards of participating in an activity, and personal beliefs about the ability to participate and succeed (Bandura, 1977).

2. Assessment

   a. Assess the amount and persistence of the client's activities toward achieving goals.

   b. Assess the barriers to client motivation (e.g., memory impairment, problem-solving deficits, cultural barriers).

   c. Use the Apathy Evaluation Scale (AES), an 18-item instrument that measures thoughts, actions, and emotions during the previous month. This instrument helps determine motivation that affects discharge function and functional levels after rehabilitation (Resnick, Zimmerman, Magaziner, & Adelman, 1998).

3. Nursing interventions

   a. Help the client establish immediate and long-term goals.

   b. Help the client and family set a realistic plan to achieve goals.

   c. Break long-term goals into small, attainable goals.

   d. Reward successes with family and peer recognition.

   e. Provide resources that lead to the successful achievement of goals.

4. Research study findings: When compared with the dominant English-speaking culture in Australia, people from cultural and linguistic minority groups displayed differences in outcome and levels of distress over role changes after TBI, independent of socioeconomic background and access to rehabilitation (Saltapidas & Ponsford, 2007).

III. **Self-Perception and Self-Concept Issues Related to Psychosocial Health**

A. Self-Concept and Self-Perception

1. Description: The way one thinks about oneself. It is a clear sense of who a person is with respect to others, a sense of being a separate person with strengths and weaknesses. People with strong self-concept acknowledge their emotions and find constructive ways to bring meaning into life. The person with a healthy self-concept views others realistically and is able to relate to them in a satisfying manner, which includes the capacity for intimacy and love. The person with a healthy self-concept handles life's realities and problems with appropriate coping behaviors (Craven & Hirnle, 2009). *Self-concept* is a person's perception of himself or herself as related to others and the environment. Self-concept addresses all aspects of the person.

2. Middle-range theory: People change over time, particularly after incurring a disability. The person's environment also changes over time. These changes affect the person-environment interaction. This framework includes four components of the person's identity (nondisabled, disabled, identity project, and identity imputed by others) and four components of the environment (the given,

the reactive during interaction, modified after interaction, and internalized). The praxis of rehabilitation may be enhanced by taking into account the relationships between these subsets of personal identity and environment in program planning; for instance, in the matching of person and assistive technology or in home support services. This framework may build a theory of person-environment interaction in disability that is compatible with interaction in other forms of difference between individuals (Jahiel & Scherer, 2010).

3. Assessment
   a. Observe for self-concept adjustment (e.g., positive thinking, satisfaction at small successes, interest in appearance).
   b. Observe for self-criticism (e.g., negative thinking, expectations of failure).
   c. Observe for self-diminution (e.g., avoiding, neglecting, or refusing to recognize personal assets; Stuart & Laraia, 1995).
4. Nursing interventions
   a. Encourage activity in community-based social integration programs to develop social skills (Burleigh, Farber, & Gillard, 1998).
   b. Encourage the client to approach life with open, realistic expectations.
   c. Encourage and reinforce the client's evaluations of his or her personal assets.
   d. Encourage the client to interact with family and friends.
   e. Reinforce success, which can academically and vocationally increase self-concept (Brillhart & Johnson, 1997; Hayes, Balfanz-Vertiz, & Ostrander, 2005).
   f. Participation in artistic activities can contribute to positive self-identification (Reynolds, 2003).
5. Research study findings: Soyupek, Aktepe, Savas, and Askin (2010) compared the self-concept of children with cerebral palsy (CP) with that of children without disability to investigate predictive variables that could affect self-concept and QOL. Significant differences in mean scores favoring the control group were found for the Piers-Harris Self-Concept Scale; the Physical Scale of Peds QOL report was a significant predictor of self-concept. Self-concept and QOL of the children with CP were lower than for the children without CP. With the presence of incontinence, the self-concept rating and Gross Motor Function Classification System level were important for predicting domains of QOL.

B. Self-Esteem
   1. Definition: An attitude, feeling of pride in oneself, and self-concept represented by behavior
      a. *Self-esteem* is the person's sense of personal value and ability to consider himself or herself with dignity, love, and reality.
      b. Self-esteem affects the inner person and the person's relationships with others.
      c. Positive self-esteem is fostered by integrity, honesty, responsibility, compassion, and competence.
      d. Self-esteem is based on a personal evaluation of self-worth and competence (Norris & Spelic, 2002).
      e. A person with low self-esteem and self-worth often has a "victim mentality" and expects deprecation.
   2. Middle-range theory: Schreuer and colleagues incorporated variables from the cognitive coping model (self-esteem, appraisal, and social support) and the occupational performance model (engagement in activities, involvement in work or study, time of typing performance, and environmental adaptations) to explore adjustment to disability in 90 adults with severe physical disabilities. Subjects were tested with respect to their adjustment to severe disabilities in their adapted computerized work environment 1 year after occupational therapy consultation. Findings indicated that self-esteem and time of performance were found to be core variables connecting cognitive and functional variables. Age and ADLs were the only background variables that contributed to the model (Schreuer, Rimmerman, & Sachs, 2006).
   3. Assessment
      a. Observe for feelings of defeat, failure, worthlessness (Satir, 1988), weakness, helplessness, hopelessness, fright, vulnerability, fragility, incompleteness, and inadequacy (Antle, 2004; Stuart & Laraia, 1995).
      b. Assess the client to identify a personal situation in which mastery was achieved through positive coping with disability effects (Norris & Spelic, 2002).
   4. Nursing interventions
      a. Allow time for relaxation.
      b. Help the client realize what is occurring and his or her reaction to the situation.
      c. Encourage the client to communicate with family members and share experiences.

d. Encourage the client to listen to others and try to reflect on how both parties perceive the communication.

e. Foster relaxed, flexible family expectations.

f. Encourage the client to declare, "I am unique," "I can love myself," and "I am okay" (Satir, 1988).

g. Encourage family and friends to express that the client is a person of value (Norris & Spelic, 2002).

h. Prepare the client to perform to personally identified standards for life functions and roles (Norris & Spelic, 2002).

i. Encourage spirituality as a basis for self-concept, which has been related to positive rehabilitation outcomes (Faull & Hills, 2006).

5. Research study findings

a. Development of self-esteem and self-efficacy in adolescents with chronic physical illness with and without psychological symptoms was measured for 1 year after a medical inpatient rehabilitation treatment of 4 to 6 weeks. Gender- and diagnosis-related differences were analyzed. A total of 243 chronically ill adolescents were interviewed at the beginning of their rehabilitation treatment and 1 year later. Therapy for chronically ill adolescents in medical rehabilitation affects their self-esteem positively, with differences in self-esteem found between adolescents who show clinically relevant psychological symptoms and those who do not. Only minor changes were noticed in ratings of self-efficacy at school and other social contexts. Gender- and diagnosis-related differences have not been found (Kiera, Stachow, Petermann, & Tiedjen, 2010).

b. To explore the effect of self-esteem level, self-esteem stability, and admission functional status on discharge depressive symptoms in acute stroke rehabilitation, 120 survivors serially completed a measure of state self-esteem during inpatient rehabilitation and completed a measure of depressive symptoms at discharge. Functional status was rated at admission using the Functional Independence Measure (FIM). After potential moderating variables were controlled for, self-esteem level interacted with FIM self-care and cognitive functioning to predict discharge depressive symptoms, such that survivors with lower self-rated self-esteem and poorer functional status indicated higher levels of depressive symptoms. Self-esteem stability interacted with FIM mobility functioning, such that self-esteem instability in the presence of lower mobility functioning at admission was related to higher depressive symptoms at discharge (Vickery, Evans, Sepehri, Jabeen, & Gayden, 2009).

c. Body image

1) Definition of body image: A person's subjective picture of his or her own appearance that is based on observations, comparisons, and reactions by others

2) Middle-range theory: A multidisciplinary, integrated review approach was used to identify the basic elements and the underlying theoretical framework of mirror interventions. Qualitative and quantitative strategies for reviewing evidence were used, and a narrative synthesis approach was used to guide the comprehensive synthesis. Underlying theoretical models were identified, and five elements of mirror interventions (self-knowledge, therapeutic intervention, repetition, homework, and imagery or relaxation) were synthesized from the literature (Freysteinson, 2009).

3) Assessment

a) Observe for grooming and hygiene status.

b) Observe for initiation of self-care activities.

c) Observe the functional abilities for self-care and ADLs.

d) Observe the effect of the client's appearance on family, friends, and the community.

4) Nursing interventions

a) Provide for independent or assisted grooming.

b) Ensure that the client has appropriate street clothing for activities.

c) Coordinate barber and hairdressing services.

d) Encourage the use of prosthetics.

e) Reinforce occupational therapy.

f) Provide recreational therapy and community reentry activities.

g) Encourage the client to recognize successful people with disabilities (e.g., athletes who use wheelchairs).

h) Promote positive public images of people with disabilities in business, politics, and the media.

i) Incorporate people with disabilities into play therapy (e.g., childhood books that include characters with disabilities, dolls in wheelchairs, cartoons with positive images of people with disabilities).

j) Encourage the client to attend support groups for people with disabilities.

5) Research study findings: A qualitative, retrospective, cross-sectional, descriptive study based on interview data from 15 women with SCI was undertaken to explore consumer values important to rehabilitation practice. Four specific values are discussed: genuine interest and respect for the person, fostering autonomy, valuing lay knowledge and expertise, and promoting hopefulness (Yoshida et al., 2009).

C. Grief Associated with Disability

1. Definition: "A state in which an individual or family experiences a natural human response involving psychosocial and physiologic reactions to actual or perceived loss" (Carpenito-Moyet, 2010, p. 198). Worden (1991), who has done substantial work in the area of grief and loss, suggests that grief after a disability consists of four dimensions: feelings, thoughts, behaviors, and physical sensations. In the broader sense, it also includes spiritual or interpersonal dimensions.

2. Middle-range theory

a. Yalom's (1980, 1986) model is used as a foundation to explore the four existential issues of death, freedom and responsibility, loneliness, and meaninglessness. This model is applied to communication disorders based on the work of D. Lutterman (1984, 2001). These four existential issues are juxtaposed with K. Moses's (1989) model of the grief response, which includes denial, anxiety, fear, depression, anger, and guilt. Suggestions for responding within one's scope of practice are provided. Combined, existential and grieving models can offer clinicians new insight into clients' loss resolution work. This inner work constitutes a spiritual journey that may parallel the journey through therapy and rehabilitation. The case has been made that attending to these issues can enhance long-term outcomes of treatment (Spillers, 2007).

b. A systematic review of the literature on predictors of complicated grief (CG) was undertaken. Predictors of CG before the death include previous loss, exposure to trauma, a previous psychiatric history, attachment style, and the relationship to the deceased. Factors associated with the death include violent death, the quality of the caregiving or dying experience, close kinship relationship to the deceased, marital closeness and dependency, and lack of preparation for the death. Perceived social support played a key role after death, along with cognitive appraisals and high distress at the time of the death (Lobb et al., 2010).

3. Assessment

a. Observe for appetite loss, fatigue, apathy, lack of socialization, somatic complaints, and decreased activities.

b. Observe the client's emotions (e.g., feelings of emptiness and numbness, low self-esteem, sadness, guilt; Stuart & Laraia, 1995).

c. Observe the client's level of willingness to participate in rehabilitation.

4. Nursing interventions

a. Encourage family and friends to reassure the client that he or she is loved for himself or herself, not for his or her appearance, physical abilities, or work capacity.

b. Foster peer modeling and mentoring (Davidhizar, 1997).

c. Encourage the client and family to seek psychological counseling.

d. Help the client build a social, cultural, and economic network of support (Davidhizar, 1997).

e. Help the client cultivate a positive and realistic outlook (Davidhizar, 1997).

f. Allow time for adjustment because clients often do not internalize the entire impact of a disability until the rehabilitation phase of treatment (Brillhart & Johnson, 1997).

g. Refer the client for interpersonal psychotherapy, which focuses on grief, interpersonal role disputes, and role transitions (Crowe & Lutz, 2005).

5. Research study findings

a. Focusing beyond survival, the priority of modern burn care is an optimal quality of life. The aim of one study, which was informed by phenomenology, was to describe and identify invariant meanings in the experience of life after major burn injury.

Fourteen adults having sustained a major burn were interviewed, on average, 14 months after injury, and asked about their experience of important aspects of life. The accident meant facing an extreme situation that demanded vigilance, appropriate action, and the need for assistance. The aftermath of the burn injury and treatment included having to put significant effort into creating coherence in their disrupted personal life stories. Continuing life meant accepting the unchangeable, including going through recurrent processes of enduring grief, fatalism, comparisons with others, and new feelings of gratefulness. Furthermore, a continuous struggle to change what was changeable and to achieve personal goals, independence, relationships with others, and a meaningful life were all efforts to regain freedom, aiming for a life as it was before—and sometimes even better (Moi & Gjengedal, 2008).

b. Despite its popularity, few attempts have been made to empirically test the stage theory of grief. This study aimed to replicate and extend the findings of Maciejewski, Zhang, Block, and Prigerson (2007), who found that different states of grieving may peak in a sequence that is consistent with stage theory. The association between time since loss and five grief indicators (focusing on disbelief, anger, yearning, depression, and acceptance) among an ethnically diverse sample of young adults who had been bereaved by natural ($n =$ 441) and violent ($n = 173$) causes was explored. In general, limited support was found for stage theory, alongside some evidence of an "anniversary reaction" marked by heightened distress and reduced acceptance for participants approaching the second anniversary of the death. Overall, sense making emerged as a much stronger predictor of grief indicators than time since the loss, highlighting the relevance of a meaning-oriented perspective (Holland & Neimeyer, 2010).

D. Stigma

1. Definition: The application of set attitudes about and stereotypes of people with disabilities. Stigma begins in the attitudes of others but may be internalized by the person with a disability and eventually influence that person's behaviors (Goffman, 1974).

2. Middle-range theory: The Framework Integrating Normative Influences on Stigma (FINIS) brings together theoretical insights from micro-, meso-, and macro-level research including the understanding that stigma occurs in social relationships. All social interactions take place in a context in which organizations, media, and larger cultures structure normative expectations, which creates the possibility of marking difference. FINIS offers the potential to build a broad-based scientific foundation based on an understanding of the effects of stigma on the lives of people with mental illness and disability, the resources devoted to the organizations and families who care for them, and policies and programs designed to combat stigma (Pescosolido, Martin, Lang, & Olafsdottir, 2008).

3. Assessment

a. Observe for statements of self-deprecation.
b. Observe for self-isolating behaviors.
c. Observe alienation and hostility by others.
d. Note family's and friends' attitudes toward people with disabilities.

4. Nursing interventions

a. Encourage the client to re-evaluate the importance of physique.
b. Encourage a realistic appraisal of the difficulties of dealing with disability.
c. Encourage the evaluation of personal assets and abilities.
d. Encourage the client and family to focus on the total person, not just the disability.
e. Provide counseling on dealing with stigma in the community.
f. Encourage positive images of those with disabilities in the media, business, academia, athletics, and music.
g. Ensure that children and adults with disabilities are mainstreamed into educational and recreational activities.

5. Research study findings: The author used phenomenological (interpretive) ethnography to investigate the experience of physical disability and its attached meanings in relation to self, world, and other for adolescents born with spina bifida. In-depth interviews were conducted with 11 late-stage adolescents (age 18–24 years) and analysis revealed the theme "experiencing self as dissimilar other." Findings imply that adolescents born with spina bifida face biological, psychological, and social challenges that might interfere with normative developmental tasks of adolescence, including identity formation. Greater emphasis must be directed toward humanizing and emancipating the physical and social environment for

young people with physical disabilities to maximize developmental opportunities and potential while fostering positive identity (Kinavey, 2007).

E. Hope and Hopelessness
1. Definition
   a. Hope: An anticipation of a future that is good and is based on relationships with others, purpose, and meaning in life and a sense of the possible (Miller, 2000)
   b. Hopelessness: A sustained subjective emotional state in which a person sees no alternatives or personal choices available to solve problems or to achieve what is desired and cannot mobilize energy on his or her behalf to establish goals (Carpenito-Moyet, 2010)
   c. Associated feelings of hopelessness include powerlessness, despair, helplessness, and apathy.
2. Middle-range theory: The aim of this longitudinal study was to deepen the understanding of the phenomenon of hope and develop a theoretical framework of hope in a context of SCI. Findings revealed nine themes: universal hope, uncertain hope, hope as a turning point, the power of hope, boundless creative and flexible hope, enduring hope, despairing hope, body-related hope, and existential hope. The conceptual model was derived from these themes, illustrated as the battle between hoping and suffering and the road of hope. The interpretations also revealed a distinction between being in hope and having hope, and having a hope of improvements was the main focus at the early stage of rehabilitation, whereas being in hope as being just fine was the main focus after 3–4 years of rehabilitation (Lohne, 2008).
3. Assessment
   a. Observe for the characteristics of powerlessness, despair, and apathy.
   b. Observe for the lack of initiative for self-help.
   c. Observe for depression.
4. Nursing interventions
   a. Enhance the client's sense of power, which precedes hopefulness.
   b. Establish short- and long-term goals with the client and family.
   c. Encourage family and social support.
   d. Encourage spiritual empowerment and strength.
   e. Encourage use of the word *hope,* characterized by active responsibility, rather than *hopeful,* which is more passive (Kautz, 2006).

5. Research study findings: Lohne and Severinsson (2006) conducted a qualitative study to examine the experience of hope for those with SCI. The findings indicated that hope was important because it provided the energy and power to achieve progress and personal development after injury.

F. Powerlessness
1. Definition: The inability to use personal energy to initiate and guide personal behavior
   a. The lack of personal power makes a person powerless, which is destructive to the self (Satir, 1988).
   b. Powerlessness can be learned through negative reinforcement of dependency.
   c. Powerlessness as a reaction to threats can lead to patterns of impotence, withdrawal, and passiveness.
2. Middle-range theory: This review provides the foundations on which to construct a framework of power and powerlessness. Current frameworks, such as antioppressive practice, may be insufficient in being able to identify the range and complexity of power relations that may be enacted within a social situation. A framework for analyzing the operation of different forms of power, one that acknowledges the potential of power to be both damaging and productive, is presented. There is an exploration of how the framework may provide a useful tool for underpinning emancipatory practice (Tew, 2006).
3. Assessment
   a. Note a lack of initiative in goal planning and achievement.
   b. Note passivity.
   c. Note withdrawal from family, social, and vocational decisions and interactions.
   d. Assess apprehension and fear.
4. Nursing interventions
   a. Encourage the client and family to maintain control in decision making and promote environmental predictability and emotional support (Nypaver, Titus, & Brugler, 1996).
   b. Help the client realize that although the injury or illness that led to the disability cannot be changed, his or her response to the disability is a personal choice (Davidhizar, 1997).
   c. Enable the client and family to recognize and mobilize their strengths and resources, feel confident, and use effective coping skills.
   d. Encourage the client to achieve self-direction and self-determination.
   e. Encourage the client and family to seek spiritual support.

f. Encourage and value the client's and family's involvement as participants in the interdisciplinary team.

g. Encourage the client's involvement with group and community support systems.

h. Provide follow-up rehabilitation care in the home setting if applicable.

5. Research study findings

a. Clinical example: Injury or illness leading to disability can destroy a person's normal level of life control and predictability. Relocation stress experienced during the recovery and rehabilitation process and powerlessness are influenced by a decrease in biopsychosocial status, anxiety, depression, apprehension, guilt, denial, and lowered self-esteem (Nypaver et al., 1996).

b. The perspective of clients on their experience of empowerment has been poorly investigated. Aujoulat, Luminet, and Deccache (2007) explored situations and feelings of powerlessness from which a process of empowerment might evolve. They conducted 40 interviews of people with various chronic conditions and looked for the commonalities in their experiences. Powerlessness extends well beyond medical and treatment-related issues and may include distressing feelings of insecurity and a threat to social and personal identities (Aujoulat et al.).

G. Self-Efficacy

1. Definition: A sense of control that consists of coping with, appraising, and managing one's life and leads to the conviction that the person can determine behaviors that lead to desired outcomes (Bandura, 1977)

2. Middle-range theory: Self-efficacy, a core construct of Bandura's social cognitive theory, has wide appeal and usefulness in the health and social sciences. Self-efficacy is frequently used across disciplines to assess a person's beliefs about his or her likelihood to engage in a certain behavior. Several factors contribute to inaccurate or inappropriate assessment, measurement, interpretation, and application of this important construct; numerous scales used to measure efficacy, various contexts, related constructs, and moderating effects of efficacy make best use of efficacy measurement and application difficult. An article outlines the theory of self-efficacy, distinguishes its closely related constructs, summarizes common moderating effects, and provides important considerations for clinical practice and research (O'Sullivan & Strauser, 2009).

3. Assessment

a. Investigate the client's and family's short- and long-term goals.

b. Identify fears of and barriers to self-efficacy.

c. Identify learning needs associated with self-efficacy.

d. Identify resources needed for self-efficacy.

e. Identify the client's ability to provide or direct self-care.

f. Identify the client's ability to manage the vocational and recreational aspects of life.

4. Nursing interventions

a. Individualize self-care education for the client and family.

b. Encourage the client to choose activities.

c. Encourage opportunities for self-responsibility.

d. Encourage behaviors and activities that lead to self-assurance.

e. Encourage alternative solutions for problem solving.

f. Provide opportunities to practice and direct self-care.

g. Provide resources for education and vocational development.

h. Provide opportunities for recreation and socialization.

i. Provide resources for goal achievement.

j. Encourage the client to evaluate the situation completely.

k. Plan with goal setting and identification of resources.

5. Research study findings

a. Exercise adherence after cardiac rehabilitation (CR) is problematic. Effects of an intervention targeting self-efficacy, outcome expectations, and adherence to upper-body resistance exercise after CR were explored. Clients in cardiac rehabilitation ($N = 40$) were randomly allocated to receive either standard exercise recommendations (wait-list control) or an intervention involving a theory-based instructional manual and Thera-Band resistive bands for upper-body resistance exercise. Self-efficacy and outcome expectations were assessed at baseline and 4 weeks later. Participation in resistance exercise was measured 4 weeks after baseline and at 3-month follow-up. The intervention group reported higher levels of self-efficacy, outcome expectations, and resistance exercise volume compared with the control group at the 4-week follow-up. Adherence differences were sustained at

3-month follow-up, with some evidence that self-efficacy for adhering to resistance training mediated the effects of the intervention on follow-up exercise training frequency (Millen & Bray, 2009).

b. Using a pretest-posttest design, Hartley, Vance, Elliott, Cuckler, and Berry (2008) tested the relationships between hope, self-efficacy for rehabilitation, depression, and functional ability reported by people undergoing joint replacement surgery. One hundred community-dwelling older adults were administered measures of hope, self-efficacy for rehabilitation, pain, depression, body mass index, and mental status 1 month before and 6 weeks after joint replacement surgery. Demographic, health information, and functional outcome measures were also obtained. Hope was significantly predictive of presurgery depression, but it was not predictive of depression or functional ability after surgery. Higher levels of self-efficacy were predictive of lower postsurgery depression scores. Results imply that social cognitive constructs may have utility in the prediction of emotional adjustment before and after joint surgery, but they may have limited value in anticipating functional abilities after these surgeries. Theoretical and clinical implications are discussed.

IV. **Roles and Relationships Related to Psychosocial Health**
   A. Types of Families
      1. Description (refer to Chapter 17 for additional information on family roles and theories)
         a. The family unit is an active, operating system.
         b. The person with disability is not in isolation but is considered in the context of family.
         c. Family relationships are the living links that bind the family together.
         d. As a system, the family assigns roles and rules that are established for each member.
         e. Functions of the family include acquiring the means to provide for the necessities of daily life.
         f. The family is essential in dealing with internal change and external disruptions.
      2. Nurturing families
         a. Characteristics include a sense of aliveness, affection, genuineness, honesty, open communication, and love.

b. These families make plans, adjust plans, problem solve without panic, and accept change as part of life.
      3. Troubled families
         a. Characteristics include coldness, rigidity, control, guarded communication, tolerance rather than love, and secrecy.
         b. Adjustment and problem solving are difficult because family members rigidly hold onto assigned roles and responsibilities (Satir, 1988).
      4. The effect of disability on a family
         a. Any family member's disability can cause permanent disruptions in family patterns.
         b. Established roles and responsibilities of the family change.
         c. Life patterns continue to change as children mature, siblings marry, members move away, parents grow older, health status changes within the family, and members die.
         d. Problem solving and adapting to change are necessary skills for positive family life.
      5. Middle-range theory
         a. The concept of family-centered care was introduced to the public more than 4 decades ago, stressing the importance of the family in a child's well-being. Since then, family-centered values and practices have been widely implemented in child and adult health care. Bamm and Rosenbaum (2008) offer an overview of the development and evolution of family-centered theory as an underlying conceptual foundation for contemporary health services. The focus includes key concepts, accepted definitions, barriers, and supports that can influence successful implementation and discussion of the valid quantitative measures of family-centeredness currently available to evaluate service delivery. They also provide the foundation and proposes questions for future research (Bamm & Rosenbaum).
         b. Military personnel returning from war with TBI present with a complex array of stressors encountered during combat and on reentry, often with additional physical and mental health comorbidities. Family-focused therapy is uniquely suited to address the complex issues presented by returning military personnel. The adaptation of an existing family intervention for a chronic condition that focuses on enhancing both individual and family functioning is a useful for working with veterans and others with TBI (Dausch & Saliman, 2009).

6. Assessment
   a. Observe family members' communication patterns.
   b. Observe the family's cohesiveness during change.
   c. Examine the family's planning strategies.
   d. Examine the family's actions, behaviors, and roles.
7. Nursing interventions
   a. Encourage family therapy with a focus on the entire family, which should include information about the injury or illness, strategies for handling emotional distress, assistive services, opportunities to share concerns, and assistance with coping (Butcher, 1994).
   b. Provide training in communication skills (e.g., structured marriage-enrichment programs, effective listening, self-awareness, conflict resolution; Captain, 1995).
   c. Provide the means for lifetime planning for continued care (costs of long-term needs, costs of care and rehabilitation; Deutsch, Allison, & Cimino-Ferguson, 2005).
   d. Help the client and family identify and cope with changes in roles and responsibilities caused by disability (Paterson & Stewart, 2002).
8. Research study findings: The disability of one family member who needs inpatient rehabilitation care can negatively affect all family members and ultimately disrupt family integrity. Current research findings indicate that rehabilitation nurses are in a key position to promote hope and family integrity by facilitating open communication between family members, fostering a tone of togetherness within and between families, and helping families resolve feelings of guilt and move toward forgiveness. These strategies are based on activities form the Nursing Interventions Classification (NIC) intervention "Family Integrity Promotion." Kautz and Van Horn (2009) present a review of research to support these NIC activities and offers practical suggestions so rehabilitation nurses can incorporate these strategies into their daily practice with clients and their family members.

B. Social Support
1. Definition: A multifaceted concept that includes instrumental support (e.g., equipment, services), affective support (e.g., concern, being loved, feeling important, support presence), and cognitive support (e.g., education, advice, information, role modeling, counseling; Rintala, Young, Spencer, & Bates, 1996)

2. Middle-range theory: Through in-depth interviews, the process of recovery following total hip replacement (THR) surgery from the perspective of the older adult was explored. In-depth interviews were conducted with 10 people older than 65 years old who had been discharged from the hospital for a period of 4–6 months after THR surgery. Findings showed that three distinct but interrelated processes constitute the physical, psychological, and social recovery process: reclaiming physical ability, re-establishing roles and relationships, and refocusing self. Intervening conditions affecting the recovery process include comorbid conditions, the personal outlook of the client, clients' relationships, and social support. The recovery process can lead to changes in personal and social functioning that clients might not anticipate (Grant, St. John, & Patterson, 2009).
3. Assessment
   a. Observe for barriers in socialization (e.g., fatigue, multiple problems, isolation, lack of self-confidence, apathy; Abjornsson, Orbaek, & Hagstadius, 1998).
   b. Observe the frequency of contact with family and friends and leisure and physical activities.
   c. Use the Life Satisfaction Index (Diener, 1984).
   d. Use the Sickness Impact Profile (De Bruin, Diederiks, De White, Stevens, & Philipsen, 1994).
   e. Use the Community Integration Questionnaire (Willer, Ottenbacher, & Coad, 1994).
   f. Use the Quality of Social Support instrument (Bethoux, Calmels, Gautheron, & Minaire, 1996).
   g. Observe the client's patterns of behaviors such as alcohol use after injury. Increased consumption of alcohol is associated with lower levels of social support (Boraz & Heinemann, 1996).
4. Nursing interventions
   a. Encourage the client to use problem- and emotion-focused coping skills.
   b. Encourage social networking (Cormier-Daigle & Stewart, 1997).
   c. Involve the spouse with instrumental (task-oriented) and emotional support.
   d. Encourage the client to engage in meaningful, rewarding activities.
   e. Encourage social roles for identity, power, and family position (Nir, Wallhagen, Doolittle, & Galinsky, 1997).

f. Encourage the client to attend support groups.

g. Provide crisis therapy and stress management.

h. Encourage cognitive activation and memory training (Abjornsson et al., 1998).

i. Encourage the use of support groups using computer-based systems. This is especially helpful for those in rural areas or those with fewer transportation resources (Hill, Schillo, & Weinert, 2004).

j. Provide access for social support to promote participation in life situations (Lund, Nordlund, Nygard, Lexell, & Bernspang, 2005).

k. Encourage the peer mentoring experience as a complement to social support (Sherman, Sperling, & DeVinney, 2004).

l. Encourage emotion-focused coping to promote social reintegration. Other pertinent factors for social reintegration include family support, information, and removal of social barriers (Song, 2005).

5. Research study findings

a. Isaksson, Skar, and Lexell (2005) conducted a qualitative study among women with SCI to investigate perceptions of social networking. Data analysis indicated that the subjects needed the social support to function in their occupations. The subjects also reported that they established new relationships with other people who had disabilities.

b. Fairfax (2002) investigated QOL among stroke survivors. Analysis of data from 102 adults indicated a positive but nonsignificant relationship of QOL and social support. Level of disability contributed to 27% of prediction of QOL.

c. Ferguson, Richie, and Gomez (2004) conducted a qualitative study to investigate the psychological factors contributing to recovery for those with traumatic amputations. Results of the study indicated that acceptance of the loss and level of psychological recovery were greatly influenced by social support and societal attitudes toward the disabled.

C. Independence and Dependence

1. Independence can be fostered when people with disabilities have responsibility for self-care and are expected to participate in family roles.

2. Dependence can result when clients are not encouraged to take control of their situations.

3. Middle-range theory: Self-responsibility and self-control are meaningful values in the activities and decisions of everyday life. Dignity and being respected as an individual are closely connected to being able to manage on one's own and being independent of others' help. Including other people into one's life situation can be an important sign of self-management. However, the critical interpretation shows that it is the view of the human being that determines whether help from others and self-managing on one's own can be combined. With a relational view of the human being (i.e., the basic condition that people always enter into relationships of dependence), there is no contradiction between independence and dependence. The objective of the interview study was to highlight themes in the clients' views of health and illness related to their chronic condition and the significance of these views for their mastery of everyday life (Delmar et al., 2006).

4. Assessment

a. Observe for initiation of ADLs.

b. Assess the client's level of functional abilities.

c. Assess the client's cognitive abilities.

d. Use the FIM instrument to assess cognitive and functional abilities and the need for supervision, especially for clients with TBI (Smith & Schwirian, 1998).

e. Observe participation in academic and vocational activities.

f. Assess for initiation of recreational activities.

g. Assess for perceptions of poor health and emotional distress, which are often associated with increased dependency (Riegel, Dracup, & Glaser, 1998).

h. Use the FAMTOOL (a family health assessment tool) to evaluate communication; shared beliefs; shared work and play; value connectedness; and effort toward physical, emotional, social, and spiritual health (Weeks & O'Connor, 1997).

i. Assess role expectations from the different viewpoints of family members, especially those focusing on pressures, demands, personal resources, and family structure (Satir, 1988).

j. Use the QOL Scale (Ferrans, 1996).

5. Nursing interventions

a. Encourage independence within the family unit.

b. Provide more intensive family support during transitional periods (e.g., moving from acute care to rehabilitation, rehabilitation to home, home to independence).

c. Eliminate environmental barriers.

d. Provide resources for adaptive housing, equipment, and attendant care (Brillhart & Johnson, 1997).

e. Encourage thoughts such as "I have control of my life," "I can do things," "I feel close to others," and "Others understand me" to promote independence (Secrest, 2006).

f. Encourage family counseling
   1) Appropriate support for the client
   2) Education about the client's discomfort with being a unilateral receiver and burden rather than a bidirectional receiver and giver
   3) The appropriate help needed by the client (Rintala et al., 1996)

g. Encourage the family to reestablish life trajectories, meet development needs, and reintegrate the survivor into the family (Brzuzy & Speziale, 1997).

6. Research study findings
   a. Elfstrom, Ryden, Kreuter, Taft, and Sullivan (2005) investigated the relationship between coping strategies and QOL among 256 people with SCI. The findings of this study indicated that revaluation of life values (acceptance) and fewer dependency behaviors (social reliance) were positively related to QOL.

   b. In their article, Stephens and Yoshida (1999) examine issues of autonomy and independence in the lives of people with rheumatoid arthritis. The subjective experiences of the informants were examined using qualitative interviews. The data show that the personal meanings people give to being independent or dependent involve issues of autonomy. Autonomy issues are manifested in restricted choice and control regarding one's body and disease, everyday tasks and routines (and related use of assistance and aids), lifestyle patterns, and major life decisions. Although independence and autonomy are interrelated concepts, the connection has not received much attention in the rehabilitation literature because of the dominance of the ADL perspective. This article argues that attention to everyday autonomy furthers our understanding of the personal and social impact of a disabling condition (Stephens & Yoshida).

D. Helplessness
   1. Definition: The belief that a person is dependent on others for support for a situation that seems to be impossible to change. The person may perceive that events are beyond his or her control.

2. Middle-range theory: Faulkner (2001) investigated the relevance of learned helplessness (LH) and learned mastery (LM) theories in the respective development of dependence and independence in older hospitalized people. Participants exposed to the LH-inducing strategy demonstrated LH effects within both the meal and psychomotor tasks. These effects were alleviated through exposing participants to the LM-inducing intervention. Exposing older hospitalized people to uncontrollable or disempowering circumstances may potentially lead them to develop an LH-induced dependence. This may be alleviated by increasing the client's expectation of control, leading to the development of LM.

3. Assessment
   a. Observe for inactivity and nonparticipation in rehabilitation.
   b. Observe for self-isolation and withdrawal.
   c. Observe for general behaviors (e.g., slow movements, low voice tones, sitting alone quietly).
   d. Observe for disturbances in motivation, cognition, and emotion.
   e. Observe for the absence of voluntary response to a situation.
   f. Observe for learned dependence (i.e., the inability to act and make decisions).
   g. Observe for fear and depression.
   h. Observe for suicidal ideation and behaviors.

4. Nursing interventions
   a. Foster voluntary responses and independence.
   b. Encourage learning and reinforce successes.
   c. Form the expectation of independence for the client and family.
   d. Encourage the client to evaluate his or her personal assets and affirm his or her feelings or expressions of hope.
   e. Encourage memory and increased coping abilities (Davidhizar, 1997).
   f. Refer the client for psychotherapy as necessary.

5. Research study findings: The outcome expectation for exercise (OEE), helplessness, and literacy on arthritis outcomes in two community-based randomized controlled trials were examined. Findings indicated that disability after intervention was not predicted by helplessness, literacy, or OEE. Helplessness predicted pain, fatigue, and stiffness (Bhat, DeWalt, Zimmer, Fried, & Callahan, 2010).

V. Coping and Stress Tolerance
A. Coping
1. Description
   a. *Coping* is defined as cognitive and behavioral efforts directed at managing demanding and stressful situations.
      1) Problem-focused coping efforts are directed at lowering or eliminating threats.
      2) Emotion-focused coping efforts are directed at decreasing negative emotions.
   b. Personal competence with coping includes many factors (Satir, 1988) such as
      1) The components of relationships (being content with self and others)
      2) Differentiation (distinguishing between self and others)
      3) Autonomy (relying on self, separate and distinct from others)
      4) Self-esteem (feeling worthy about self)
      5) Power (using energy to initiate and guide behaviors)
      6) Productivity (manifesting competence)
      7) Love (being compassionate, accepting, and giving as well as receiving affection)
   c. The antecedents of stress require coping skills, including
      1) Personal and environmental demands that exceed resources
      2) Ambiguity and uncertainty
      3) Loss of control
      4) Loss of social support
   d. Many variables influence coping efforts, such as
      1) Developmental age
      2) Severity of disability
      3) Visibility of disability
      4) Threat of chronicity
      5) Sense of control
      6) Prior coping abilities
      7) Self-esteem
      8) Values
      9) Perceived social support
2. Middle-range theory: Factors associated with the development and persistence of work disability can be related to the worker, work environment, compensation policies, healthcare system, and insurance system. Workers' understanding and representations of their disability are associated with coping behaviors aimed at helping them adapt to or solve their health problem. Theories from anthropology, sociology, and psychology are analyzed to gain a better understanding of their application to people with work-related injuries. The identified models are mainly descriptive. Integrating unique perspectives and taking social interactions into account will enhance understanding of workers' representations and the behaviors they adopt to manage their musculoskeletal disorder-related disability (Coutu, Baril, Durand, Côté, & Rouleau, 2007).
3. Assessment
   a. Assess the level and sources of stress expressed by the client and family.
   b. Assess the client's ability to solve problems.
   c. Note changes in the client's and family's abilities to meet their needs.
   d. Note changes in communication patterns that reflect frustration (e.g., verbal manipulation, hostility).
   e. Note inappropriate behavior, activity, and responses that reflect frustration.
   f. Use the Assessment Instrument of Problem-Focused Coping, a self-report instrument that focuses on a person's own assessment of competence in coping with ADLs, personal problems, and level of satisfaction with ADLs (Tollen & Ahlstrom, 1998).
   g. Use the Multidimensional Acceptance of Loss Scale, developed by Ferrin (2002), which evaluates the ability to enlarge the scope of values, contain the disability, subordinate the physique, and change comparative status values to asset values.
   h. Assess the continuing impact of chronic illness and exacerbation of symptoms (Stuifbergen, 2005).
   i. Assess spirituality as a factor in QOL (Brillhart, 2005).
4. Nursing interventions
   a. Provide rehabilitation and education and locate resources beyond personal care and independence, which can allow people with disability to expand their leisure and productive roles and promote socioeconomic integration (Pentland, Harvey, & Walker, 1998).
   b. Explore the meaning of illness for the client and family, which can lead to understanding of their behaviors and responses.
      1) The meaning the client or family associates with illness can have a profound effect on coping and adjustment and can influence relationships with the healthcare team.
      2) The meaning of illness is influenced by cultural beliefs, religion, values, life philosophy, and past experiences (Howell, 1998).

c. Encourage purposeful and meaningful time expenditure, which contributes to an improved QOL even more than the ability to be independent with ADLs (Cardol, Elvers, Oostendorp, Brandsma, & deGroot, 1996).

d. Understand the unique experience of the person with disability as influenced by his or her psychological, emotional, and spiritual needs and develop appropriate interventions to promote coping (Berman & Rose, 1998).

e. Encourage personal spirituality with the nurturing of friends, community, and family (Walton, Craig, Derwinski-Robinson, & Weinert, 2004).

f. Educate the family about the impact of chronic illness on the roles and responsibilities of those with chronic illness (Walton et al., 2004).

5. Research study findings

a. Polio survivors have been known for positive coping, resulting in achievements in family, social, and professional lives. Postpolio syndrome presents new challenges to independence and functional abilities. Life satisfaction scores of polio survivors are high, but postpolio syndrome is associated with declining scores. People with postpolio syndrome have new challenges such as muscle weakness, scoliosis, elimination problems, fatigue, and pain (Stuifbergen, 2005).

b. A survey of 230 people with SCI indicated that there was a significantly positive correlation between life satisfaction and spirituality. This study supported prior research demonstrating that levels of life satisfaction correlated with levels of spirituality. Spirituality included the concepts of faith, submission, and peace of mind (Brillhart, 2005).

c. In a descriptive study examining the role of coping strategies as predictors of physical function and social adjustment in people with SCI, a sample of 128 community-residing people with SCI completed a structured questionnaire that included demographic characteristics and the Ways of Coping Questionnaire, Modified Barthel Index, and Social Adjustment Scale to measure coping, physical function, and social adjustment, respectively. Among the eight factors of the Ways of Coping Questionnaire, planful problem solving was used most often by the participants (Song & Nam, 2010).

d. Parents of school-aged children with disabilities indicated by survey that parental coping

was enhanced most often by spiritual support, passive appraisal, reframing, and mobilizing the family to accept help. The least common mechanisms for coping included maintaining family integration and understanding the child's health condition (Smith, Jackson, & Sharpe, 2006).

B. Stress

1. Definition: The cognitive awareness of any external or internal unmet demands on a person that unbalance the equilibrium. Effects of stress are expressed physically, emotionally, intellectually, spiritually, and socially (Barry, 1996).

2. Middle-range theory: Testing a portion of the stress, appraisal, and coping model, Strom and Kosciulek (2007) developed a theoretical model that indicated that higher levels of perceived stress predicted higher levels of self-reported depression, higher levels of depression predicted lower levels of dispositional hope, and dispositional hope predicted increased life satisfaction and work productivity.

3. Assessment

a. Observe for physiological manifestations of stress (e.g., gastrointestinal distress, cardiac palpitations, anxious facial expressions, tremors).

b. Observe for emotional manifestations of stress (e.g., anxiety, emotional lability, restlessness, fright).

c. Observe for intellectual manifestations of stress (e.g., difficulty in concentration and memory, poor coping strategies).

d. Observe for spiritual manifestations of stress (e.g., value conflicts).

e. Observe for social manifestations of stress (e.g., role conflict, status incongruity, withdrawal, antagonism, role rigidity).

4. Nursing interventions

a. Examine the source of stress (e.g., fears of failure, lack of resources, lack of support system, role loss, ambiguity).

b. Examine and reinforce prior successful coping measures.

c. Provide crisis management.

d. Consult with the client's case managers and social workers.

e. Encourage the client to appraise stressors and his or her responses to stress and approaches to problem solving.

f. Encourage the client and family to be flexible with roles and problem solving.

g. Promote psychological hardiness by fostering control, commitment, and challenge for growth and development.

h. Encourage the client to seek spiritual counseling and support (Barry, 1996; Lazarus & Folkman, 1984).

i. Encourage prayer in times of stress, set limits on activities, and give rationale to others for relief of activities leading to stress (Walton et al., 2004).

j. Encourage guided imagery as a relaxation technique to decrease stress (Nathenson, 2006).

5. Research study findings

a. Rintala, Robinson-Whelen, and Matamoros (2005) reported that stressors among men with SCI were focused on problems with physical abilities, health, and finances. Stress was positively related to depression and anxiety and negatively related to life satisfaction. Finally, those with low levels of social support were more vulnerable to negative effects of stress.

b. Ostwald, Swank, and Khan (2008) identified predictors of functional independence and perceived stress for stroke survivors discharged home from inpatient rehabilitation with a spousal caregiver. Stroke survivors perceived a 50% recovery in their function upon discharge from inpatient rehabilitation. Variables that predict the stroke survivors' recovery are complex because the severity of the stroke combines with demographic and economic variables and depression to predict functional independence and perceived stress.

C. Posttrauma Syndrome or Posttraumatic Stress Disorder (PTSD)

1. Definition: "The state in which an individual experiences a sustained painful response for more than one month to one or more overwhelming traumatic events that have not been assimilated" (Carpenito-Moyet, 2010, p. 327).

2. Middle-range theories: Exposure to reminders of trauma underlies the theory and practice of most treatments for PTSD, yet exposure may not be the most important treatment mechanism. Interpersonal features of PTSD influence its onset, chronicity, and possibly its treatment. Markowitz, Milrod, Bleiberg, & Marshall (2009) reviewed interpersonal factors in PTSD, including the critical but underrecognized role of social support as protective after trauma and as a mechanism of recovery. They discussed interpersonal psychotherapy as an alternative treatment for PTSD and presented encouraging findings from two initial studies. Highlighting the potential importance of attachment and interpersonal relationships, the authors proposed a mechanism to explain why improving relationships may ameliorate PTSD symptoms (Markowitz et al.).

3. Assessment (Carpenito-Moyet, 2010, p. 329)

a. Reexperiencing the traumatic event in one or more of the following ways:
1) Flashbacks
2) Repetitive dreams or nightmares
3) Excessive verbalization of the event
4) Survival guilt
5) Painful emotions, self-blame, shame
6) Fear of repetition
7) Anger outbursts
8) Reduced interest in significant activities

b. Psychic or emotional numbness

c. Altered lifestyle

4. Interventions (NIC; Carpenito-Moyet, 2010, p. 329)

a. Counseling
b. Anxiety reduction
c. Emotional support
d. Support system enhancement
e. Coping enhancement
f. Active listening
g. Presence
h. Grief work facilitation
i. Referral

5. Research study findings: Treatment of complex PTSD, often associated with comorbid conditions, has been insufficiently studied and somewhat resistant to traditional treatment interventions. More recent research in the neurobiology of PTSD offers information about the reasons for such intractability. Neuroscience studies suggest possible reasons for the inabilities of people with complex PTSD to verbalize their experiences. As a result, healthcare practitioners are challenged to find more effective interventions in these situations and to stay abreast of the newest research. Kempson (2007) reviewed empirical findings of alternative or complementary interventions with a specific focus on body-oriented therapies in facilitating return to normal neurobiological functioning, thereby enhancing efficacy of talk therapies in resolution of PTSD.

References

Abjornsson, G., Orbaek, P., & Hagstadius, S. (1998). Chronic toxic encephalopathy: Social consequences and experiences from a rehabilitation program. *Rehabilitation Nursing, 23*(1), 38–43.

Antle, B. J. (2004). Factors associated with self-worth in young people with disabilities. *Health and Social Work, 29*(3), 167–175.

Aujoulat, I., Luminet, O., & Deccache, A. (2007). The perspective of patients on their experience of powerlessness. *Qualitative Health Research, 17*(6), 772–785.

Bamm, E. L., & Rosenbaum, P. (2008). Family-centered theory: Origins, development, barriers, and supports to implementation in rehabilitation medicine. *Archives of Physical Medicine & Rehabilitation, 89*(8), 1618–1624.

Bandura, A. (1977). Self-efficacy: Toward a unifying theory of behavioral change. *Psychological Review, 84,* 191–215.

Barry, P. D. (1996). *Psychosocial nursing care of physically ill patients and their families* (3rd ed.). New York: Lippincott.

Berman, C., & Rose, L. (1998). Examination of a patient's adaptation to quadriplegia. *Physical Therapy Case Reports, 1*(3), 148–156.

Bethoux, F., Calmels, P., Gautheron, V., & Minaire, P. (1996). Quality of life of spouses of stroke patients: A preliminary study. *International Journal of Rehabilitation and Health, 2*(3), 189–198.

Bhat, A. A., DeWalt, D. A., Zimmer, C. R., Fried, B. J., & Callahan, L. F. (2010). The role of helplessness, outcome expectation for exercise and literacy in predicting disability and symptoms in older adults with arthritis. *Patient Education, 81*(1), 73–78.

Boraz, M., & Heinemann, A. (1996). The relationship between social support and alcohol abuse in people with spinal cord injuries. *International Journal of Rehabilitation and Health, 2*(3), 189–199.

Brillhart, B. (2005). A study of spirituality and life satisfaction among persons with spinal cord injury. *Rehabilitation Nursing, 30*(1), 31–34.

Brillhart, B., & Johnson, K. (1997). Motivation and the coping process of adults with disabilities: A qualitative study. *Rehabilitation Nursing, 22*(5), 249–256.

Brzuzy, S., & Speziale, B. (1997). Persons with traumatic brain injuries and their families: Living arrangements and well-being post injury. *Social Work in Health Care, 26*(1), 77–88.

Burleigh, S. A., Farber, R. S., & Gillard, M. (1998). Community integration and life satisfaction after traumatic brain injury: Long-term findings. *American Journal of Occupational Therapy, 52*(1), 45–52.

Butcher, L. A. (1994). A family-focused perspective on chronic illness. *Rehabilitation Nursing, 19*(2), 70–74.

Captain, C. (1995). The effects of communication skills training on interaction and psychosocial adjustment among couples living with spinal cord injury. *Rehabilitation Nursing Research, 4*(4), 111–118.

Cardol, M., Elvers, J., Oostendorp, R., Brandsma, J., & deGroot, I. (1996). Quality of life in patients with amyotrophic lateral sclerosis. *Journal of Rehabilitation Sciences, 9*(4), 99–103.

Carpenito-Moyet, L. J. (2010). *Handbook of nursing diagnosis.* Philadelphia: Lippincott Williams, & Wilkins.

Clark, M. S. (2000). Patient and spouse perceptions of stroke and its rehabilitation. *International Journal of Rehabilitation Research, 23*(1), 19–29.

Cormier-Daigle, M., & Stewart, M. (1997). Support and coping of male hemodialysis-dependent patients. *International Journal of Nursing Studies, 34*(6), 420–430.

Coutu, M. F., Baril, R., Durand, M. J., Côté, D., & Rouleau, A. (2007). Representations: An important key to understanding workers' coping behaviors during rehabilitation and the return-to-work process. *Journal of Occupational Rehabilitation, 17*(3), 522–544.

Craven, R., & Hirnle, C. (2009). *Fundamentals of nursing: Human health and function* (6th ed.). Philadelphia: Lippincott, Williams & Wilkins.

Crowe, M., & Lutz, S. (2005). Nonpharmacological treatments for older adults with depression. *Geriatrics & Aging, 8*(8), 30–33.

Dacey, J., & Fiori, L. (2006). Psychological development: Challenges of adulthood. In K. Theis & J. Travers (Eds.), *Handbook of human development for health care professionals* (pp. 219–242). Boston: Jones & Bartlett.

Dacey, J., & Margolis, D. (2006). Psychological development: Adolescence and sexuality. In K. Thies & J. Travers (Eds.), *Handbook of human development for health care professionals* (pp. 191–218). Boston: Jones & Bartlett.

Dausch, B. M., & Saliman, S. (2009). Use of family focused therapy in rehabilitation for veterans with traumatic brain injury. *Rehabilitation Psychology, 54*(3), 279–287.

Davidhizar, R. (1997). Disability does not have to be the grief that never ends: Helping patients adjust. *Rehabilitation Nursing, 22*(1), 32–35.

De Bruin, A. F., Diederiks, J. P. M., De Witte, L. P., Stevens, F. C. J., & Philipsen, H. (1994). The development of a short generic version of the Sickness Impact Profile. *Journal of Clinical Epidemiology, 47,* 407–418.

Delmar, C., Bøje, T., Dylmer, D., Forup, L., Jakobsen, C., Møller, M., et al. (2006). Independence/dependence: A contradictory relationship? Life with a chronic illness. *Scandinavian Journal of Caring Sciences, 20*(3), 261–268.

Deutsch, P. M., Allison, L., & Cimino-Ferguson, S. (2005). Life care planning assessments and their impact on life in spinal cord injury. *Topics in Spinal Cord Rehabilitation, 10*(4), 135–145.

Diener, E. (1984). Subjective well-being. *Psychological Bulletin, 95*(3), 542–575.

Elfstrom, M. L., Ryden, A., Kreuter, M., Taft, C., & Sullivan, M. (2005). Relations between coping strategies and health-related quality of life in patients with spinal cord lesion. *Journal of Rehabilitation Medicine, 31*(1), 9–16.

Erikson, E. (1963). *Childhood and society.* New York: W. W. Norton.

Fairfax, J. (2002). *Theory of quality of life of stroke survivors.* Doctoral dissertation, Wayne State University, Detroit, MI.

Faulkner, M. (2001). The onset and alleviation of learned helplessness in older hospitalized people. *Aging & Mental Health, 5*(4), 379–386.

Faull, K., & Hills, M. (2006). The role of the spiritual dimension of the self as the prime determinant of health. *Disability and Rehabilitation, 28*(11), 729–740.

Ferguson, A. D., Richie, B. S., & Gomez, M. J. (2004). Psychological factors after traumatic amputation in landmine survivors: The bridge between physical healing and full recovery. *Disability and Rehabilitation, 26*(14/15), 931–938.

Ferrans, C. E. (1996). Development of a conceptual model of quality of life. *Scholarly Inquiry for Nursing Practice: An International Journal, 10*(3), 293–304.

Ferrin, J. M. (2002). *Acceptance of loss after an adult-onset disability: Development and psychometric validation of the Multidimensional Acceptance of Loss Scale.* Doctoral dissertation, University of Wisconsin–Madison.

Flannery, J. (1998). Using the Levels of Cognitive Functioning Assessment Scale with patients with traumatic brain injury in an acute care setting. *Rehabilitation Nursing, 23*(3), 88–94.

Folstein, M. F., Folstein, S. E., & McHugh, P. R. (1975). "Mini-mental state." A practical method for grading the cognitive state of patients for the clinician. *Journal of Psychiatric Research, 12*(3), 189–198.

Freysteinson, W. M. (2009). Therapeutic mirror interventions: An integrated review of the literature. *Journal of Holistic Nursing, 27*(4), 241–255.

Goffman, E. (1974). *Stigma.* New York: Jason Aronson.

Grant, S., St. John, W., & Patterson, E. (2009). Recovery from total hip replacement surgery: "It's not just physical." *Qualitative Health Research, 19*(11), 1612–1620.

Grzankowski, J. A. (1997). Altered thought processes related to traumatic brain injury and their nursing implications. *Rehabilitation Nursing, 22*(1), 24–28.

Hartley, S. M., Vance, D. E., Elliott, T. R., Cuckler, J. M., & Berry, J. W. (2008). Hope, self-efficacy, and functional recovery after knee and hip replacement surgery. *Rehabilitation Psychology, 53*(4), 521–529.

Hayes, E., Balfanz-Vertiz, K., & Ostrander, R. N. (2005). Building pathways to education and employment among individuals with spinal cord injury. *SCI Psychosocial Process, 18*(1), 17–26.

Hill, W., Schillo, L., & Weinert, C. (2004). Effect of a computer-based intervention on social support for chronically ill rural women. *Rehabilitation Nursing, 29*(5), 169–173.

Holland, J. M., & Neimeyer, R. A. (2010). An examination of stage theory of grief among individuals bereaved by natural and violent causes: A meaning-oriented contribution. *Omega: Journal of Death & Dying, 61*(2), 103–120.

Howell, D. (1998). Reaching to the depths of the soul: Understanding and exploring meaning in illness. *Canadian Oncology Nursing Journal, 8*(1), 22–23.

Isaksson, G., Skar, L., & Lexell, J. (2005). Women's perceptions of changes in the social network after a spinal cord injury. *Disability and Rehabilitation, 27*(17), 1013–1021.

Jahiel, R. I., & Scherer, M. J. (2010). Initial steps towards a theory and praxis of person-environment interaction in disability. *Disability & Rehabilitation, 32*(17), 1467–1474.

Jansen, D., & Keller, M. (1998). Identifying the attention demands perceived by elderly people. *Rehabilitation Nursing, 23*(1), 12–19.

Johnston, T., Lauer, R. T., & Smith, B. T. (2006). Differences in scores between children with spinal cord injury and their parents using the Pediatric Quality of Life Inventory. *Pediatric Physical Therapy, 18*(1), 94–96.

Kautz, D. D. (2006, October). *Inspiring hope in our patients, their families, and ourselves.* Paper presented at the conference of the Association of Rehabilitation Nurses, Chicago, IL.

Kautz, D. D., & Van Horn, E. (2009). Promoting family integrity to inspire hope in rehabilitation patients: Strategies to provide evidence-based care. *Rehabilitation Nursing, 34*(4), 168–173.

Kempson, D. A. (2007). Overwhelming grief in a traumatized world: Evolving perspectives in treatment. *Illness, Crisis & Loss, 15*(4), 297–314.

Kiera, S., Stachow, R., Petermann, F., & Tiedjen, U. (2010). Medical inpatient rehabilitation influences on self-esteem and self-efficacy of chronically ill adolescents. *Rehabilitation, 49*(4), 248–255.

Kinavey, C. (2007). Adolescents born with spina bifida: Experiential worlds and biopsychosocial developmental challenges. *Issues in Comprehensive Pediatric Nursing, 30*(4), 147–164.

Lawson, S., Delamere, F. M., & Hutchinson, S. L. (2008). A personal narrative of involvement in post-traumatic brain injury rehabilitation: What can we learn for therapeutic recreation practice? *Therapeutic Recreation Journal, 42*(4), 236–250.

Lazarus, R. S., & Folkman, S. (1984). *Stress, appraisal, and coping.* New York: Springer.

Lobb, E. A., Kristjanson, L. J., Aoun, S. M., Monterosso, L., Halkett, G. K. B., & Davies, A. (2010). Predictors of complicated grief: A systematic review of empirical studies. *Death Studies, 34*(8), 673–698.

Lohne, V. (2008). The battle between hoping and suffering: A conceptual model of hope within a context of spinal cord injury. *Advances in Nursing Science, 31*(3), 237–248.

Lohne, V., & Severinsson, E. (2006). The power of hope: Patients' experiences of hope a year after acute spinal cord injury. *Journal of Clinical Nursing, 15*(3), 315–523.

Lund, M. L., Nordlund, A., Nygard, L., Lexell, J., & Bernspang, B. (2005). Perceptions of participation and predictors of perceived problems with participation in persons with spinal cord injury. *Journal of Rehabilitation Medicine, 37*(1), 3–8.

Lutterman, D. (1984). *Counseling with the communicatively disordered and their families.* Boston: Little, Brown.

Lutterman, D. (2001). *Counseling persons with communication disorders and their families* (4th ed.). Austin, TX: Pro-Ed.

Maciejewski, P. K., Zhang, B., Block, S. D., & Prigerson, H. G. (2007). An empirical examination of the stage theory of grief. *Journal of the American Medical Association, 297*(7), 716–723.

Markowitz, J. C., Milrod, B., Bleiberg, K., & Marshall, R. D. (2009). Interpersonal factors in understanding and treating posttraumatic stress disorder. *Journal of Psychiatric Practice, 15*(2), 133–140.

Millen, J. A., & Bray, S. R. (2009). Promoting self-efficacy and outcome expectations to enable adherence to resistance training after cardiac rehabilitation. *Journal of Cardiovascular Nursing, 24*(4), 316–327.

Miller, J. F. (2000). *Coping with chronic illness: Overcoming powerlessness* (3rd ed.). Philadelphia: F. A. Davis.

Missiuna, C., DeMatteo, C., Hanna, S., Mandich, A., Law, M., Mahoney, W., et al. (2010). Exploring the use of cognitive intervention for children with acquired brain injury. *Physical & Occupational Therapy in Pediatrics, 30*(3), 205–219.

Moi, A. L., & Gjengedal, E. (2008). Life after burn injury: Striving for regained freedom. *Qualitative Health Research, 18*(12), 1621–1630.

Moses, K. (1989). *Fundamentals of grieving: Relating to parents of the disabled.* Evanston, IL: Resource Networks.

Nathenson, N. (2006, October). *A new model in outpatient cardiac rehabilitation.* Paper presented at the conference of the Association of Rehabilitation Nurses, Chicago, IL.

Nir, Z., Wallhagen, M., Doolittle, N., & Galinsky, D. (1997). A study of the psychosocial characteristics of patients in a geriatric rehabilitation unit in Israel. *Rehabilitation Nursing, 22*(3), 143–151.

Norris, J., & Spelic, S. S. (2002). Supporting adaptation to body image disruption. *Rehabilitation Nursing, 27*(1), 8–10.

Nypaver, J., Titus, M., & Brugler, C. (1996). Patient transfer to rehabilitation: Just another move? *Rehabilitation Nursing, 21*(2), 94–97.

Ostwald, S. K., Swank, P. R., & Khan, M. M. (2008). Predictors of functional independence and stress level of stroke survivors at discharge from inpatient rehabilitation. *Journal of Cardiovascular Nursing, 23*(4), 371–377.

O'Sullivan, D., & Strauser, D. R. (2009). Operationalizing self-efficacy, related social cognitive variables, and moderating effects: Implications for rehabilitation research and practice. *Rehabilitation Counseling Bulletin, 52*(4), 251–258.

Paterson, J., & Stewart, J. (2002). Adults with acquired brain injury: Perceptions of their social world. *Rehabilitation Nursing, 27*(1), 13–18.

Pedersen, P. M., Jorgensen, H. S., Nakayama, H., Raaschou, H. O., & Olsen, T. S. (1996). Orientation in the acute and chronic stroke patient: Impact on ADL and social activities. The Copenhagen Stroke Study. *Archives of Physical Medicine & Rehabilitation, 77*(4), 336–339.

Pentland, W., Harvey, A., & Walker, J. (1998). The relationships between time use and health and well-being in men with spinal cord injury. *Journal of Occupational Science, 5*(1), 14–25.

Pescosolido, B. A., Martin, J. K., Lang, A., & Olafsdottir, S. (2008). Rethinking theoretical approaches to stigma: A Framework Integrating Normative Influences on Stigma (FINIS). *Social Science & Medicine, 67*(3), 431–440.

Piaget, J. (1952). *The origins of intelligence in children.* New York: Norton.

Remington, R., Abdallah, L., Melillo, K., & Flanagan, K. (2006). Managing problem behaviors associated with dementia. *Rehabilitation Nursing, 31*(5), 186–191.

Resnick, B., Zimmerman, S., Magaziner, J., & Adelman, A. (1998). Use of the Apathy Evaluation Scale as a measure of motivation in elderly people. *Rehabilitation Nursing, 23*(3), 141–147.

Reynolds, F. (2003). Reclaiming a positive identity in chronic illness through artistic occupation. *Occupation, Participation and Health, 23*(3), 118–127.

Riegel, B., Dracup, K., & Glaser, D. (1998). A longitudinal model of cardiac invalidism following myocardial infarction. *Nursing Research, 47*(5), 285–292.

Rintala, D. H., Robinson-Whelen, S., & Matamoros, R. (2005). Subjective stress in male veterans with spinal cord injury. *Journal of Rehabilitation Research and Development, 42*(3), 291–304.

Rintala, D., Young, M., Spencer, J., & Bates, P. (1996). Family relationships and adaptation to spinal cord injury: A qualitative study. *Rehabilitation Nursing, 21*(2), 67–74.

Saltapidas, H., & Ponsford, J. (2007). The influence of cultural background on motivation for and participation in rehabilitation and outcome following traumatic brain injury. *Journal of Head Trauma Rehabilitation, 22*(2), 132–139.

Satir, V. (1988). *The new peoplemaker.* Mountain View, CA: Science and Behavior Books.

Schönberger, M., Humle, F., & Teasdale, T. W. (2007). The relationship between clients' cognitive functioning and the therapeutic working alliance in post-acute brain injury rehabilitation. *Brain Injury, 21*(8), 825–836.

Schreuer, N., Rimmerman, A., & Sachs, D. (2006). Adjustment to severe disability: Constructing and examining a cognitive and occupational performance model. *International Journal of Rehabilitation Research 29*(3), 201–207.

Secrest, J. A. (2006, October). *The relationship of continuity, functional ability, depression, quality of life over time in stroke survivors.* Paper presented at the conference of the Association of Rehabilitation Nurses, Chicago, IL.

Shah, R. C., & Bennett, D. A. (2006). Diagnosis and management of mild cognitive impairment. *Geriatrics & Aging, 8*(8), 53–56.

Sherman, J. E., Sperling, K. B., & DeVinney, D. J. (2004). Social support and adjustment after spinal cord injury: Influence of past peer-mentoring experiences and current live-in partner. *Rehabilitation Psychology, 49*(2), 140–149.

Smith, A., & Schwirian, P. (1998). The relationship between caregiver burden and the TBI survivor's cognition and functional ability after discharge. *Rehabilitation Nursing, 23*(5), 252–257.

Smith, C. R., Cook, S., Frost, K., Jones, M., & Wright, P. (2006). A comparison of coping strategies of adolescents with and without physical disabilities. *Pediatric Physical Therapy, 18*(1), 105–106.

Smith, C. R., Jackson, L., & Sharpe, L. (2006). Coping behaviors of parents with school age/latency age children with disabilities. *Pediatric Physical Therapy, 18*(1), 106.

Song, H. (2005). Modeling social reintegration in persons with spinal cord injury. *Disability and Rehabilitation, 27*(3), 131–141.

Song, H., & Nam, K. A. (2010). Coping strategies, physical function, and social adjustment in people with spinal cord injury. *Rehabilitation Nursing, 35*(1), 8–15.

Soyupek, F., Aktepe, E., Savas, S., & Askin, A. (2010). Do the self-concept and quality of life decrease in CP patients? Focussing on the predictors of self-concept and quality of life. *Disability & Rehabilitation, 32*(13), 1109–1115.

Spalding, J. A. (2005). Challenges of mentoring a brain-injured peer. *Rehabilitation Nursing, 30*(1), 3, 6.

Spillers, C. S. (2007). An existential framework for understanding the counseling needs of clients. *American Journal of Speech–Language Pathology, 16*(3), 191–197.

Stephens, M., & Yoshida, K. K. (1999). Independence and autonomy among people with rheumatoid arthritis. *Canadian Journal of Rehabilitation, 12*(4), 229–243.

Strom, T. Q., & Kosciulek, J. (2007). Stress, appraisal and coping following mild traumatic brain injury. *Journal of Brain Injury, 21*(11), 1137–1145.

Struchen, M. A., Clark, A. N., Sander, A. M., Mills, M. R., Evans, G., & Kurtz, D. (2008). Relation of executive functioning and social communication measures to functional outcomes following traumatic brain injury. *NeuroRehabilitation, 2008, 23*(2), 185–198.

Stuart, G. W., & Laraia, M. T. (1995). *Principles and practice of psychiatric nursing.* St. Louis: Mosby.

Stuifbergen, A. (2005). Secondary conditions and life satisfaction among polio survivors. *Rehabilitation Nursing, 30*(5), 173–178.

Tew, J. (2006). Understanding power and powerlessness: Towards a framework for emancipatory practice in social work. *Journal of Social Work, 6*(1), 33–51.

Tollen, A., & Ahlstrom, G. (1998). Assessment instrument for problem-focused coping: Reliability of APC, Part I. *Scandinavian Journal of Caring Sciences, 12*(1), 18–24.

Townsend, E., Lohr, J. L., & Nelson, C. A. (2006). Neurocognitive sequelae of repaired congenital heart disease. *Pediatric Physical Therapy, 18*(1), 107.

Travers, J. (2006). Cognitive development. In K. Theis & J. Travers (Eds.), *Handbook of human development for health care professionals* (pp. 113–138). Boston: Jones & Bartlett.

Vickery, C. D., Evans, C. C., Sepehri, A., Jabeen, L. N., & Gayden, M. (2009). Self-esteem stability and depressive symptoms in acute stroke rehabilitation: Methodological and conceptual expansion. *Rehabilitation Psychology, 54*(3), 332–342.

Walton, J., Craig, C., Derwinski-Robinson, B., & Weinert, C. (2004). I am not alone: Spirituality of chronically ill rural dwellers. *Rehabilitation Nursing, 29*(5), 164–168.

Weeks, S., & O'Connor, P. (1997). The FAMTOOL family assessment tool. *Rehabilitation Nursing, 22*(4), 188–191.

Willer, B., Ottenbacher, K. J., & Coad, M. L. (1994). The community integration questionnaire: A comparative examination. *American Journal of Physical Medicine & Rehabilitation, 73*(2), 103–111.

Williams, A. M., & Dahl, C. W. (2002). Patient and caregiver perceptions of stroke survivor behavior: A comparison. *Rehabilitation Nursing, 27*(1), 19–24.

Worden, J. W. (1991). Grieving a loss from AIDS. *Hospice Journal, 7*(1/2), 143–150.

Yalom, I. (1980). *Existensial psychotherapy.* New York: Basic Books.

Yalom, I. (1986). *Love's executioner.* New York: Basic Books.

Yoshida, K. K., Self, H., Renwick, R. M., Forma, L. L., King, A. J., & Fell, L. A. (2009). Consumer values as a basis for future SCI practice models: Application to women with SCI and body issues. *Topics in Spinal Cord Injury Rehabilitation, 15*(1), 1–14.

Nursing Management of Clients with Common Rehabilitation Disorders

CHAPTER 9
Neuroanatomy

Cynthia K. Fine, MSN CRRN

Neurological injuries and illnesses are catastrophic events for clients and families. Many people have never known anyone who has survived such an event, much less had to care for someone with neurological deficits. Therefore, clients and their families need nurses experienced in rehabilitation and knowledgeable about neuroanatomy and pathophysiology to manage an array of complex needs. A solid understanding of neuroanatomy provides rehabilitation nurses with the foundation for providing optimal rehabilitation nursing interventions. It also can assist nurses in explaining what the client is going through. Rehabilitation nurses can use their knowledge of neuroanatomy to help clients and their families set realistic, outcome-oriented goals based on expected functional and cognitive levels.

It is important for nurses who work with people with neurological illnesses and injuries to understand key anatomical and functional aspects of the central nervous system (CNS), peripheral nervous system (PNS), autonomic nervous system (ANS), and the associated musculoskeletal system. The importance of this level of knowledge lies in the fact that the nature and location of injury in the nervous system affect the presentation of the client in both the short term and the long term. This allows the nurse, client, and family to comprehend the basics of the deficits that have occurred and ways to best compensate for the temporary or permanent changes. It is also important to keep in mind that neurologic trauma rarely affects only one portion of the nervous system; rather it impacts many different portions of the neurologic system.

I. **Anatomy of the Brain**
   A. Meninges (Lewis, Heitkemper, & Dirksen, 2004)
      1. Three layers of protective membranes that surround the brain and spinal cord and help to protect the nervous tissue (**Figure 9-1**).
      2. Composed of pia mater, arachnoid mater, and dura mater (PAD)
         a. Pia mater (P)
            1) The innermost layer, which adheres to the brain and spinal cord
            2) A highly vascularized layer that provides nourishment to the CNS
         b. Arachnoid mater (A): A thin, delicate, cobweb-like layer
         c. Dura mater (D)
            1) The outermost layer that lies against the skull and vertebrae

2) Composed of tough, white, fibrous tissue
3) Includes the tentorium cerebelli, which is a fold of dura that separates the cerebellum from the cerebrum in the occipital lobe, and the falx cerebri, which is a fold of the dura that separates the two hemispheres and prevents expansion of brain tissue in situations such as the presence of a rapidly growing tumor or acute hemorrhage (Lewis et al., 2004)
4) Is the location of a condition called tentorial herniation, which occurs when intracranial pressure (ICP) causes the brain to push down through the tentorial notch, compressing the brainstem
5) Creates spaces known as sinuses, through which cerebrospinal fluid (CSF) is reabsorbed into the bloodstream
   B. Spaces (Mosby, 2006)
      1. Subarachnoid space
         a. Space between the pia mater and arachnoid mater that is filled with CSF.
         b. CSF flows from the ventricles to sinuses via the subarachnoid space.
         c. Subarachnoid hemorrhage occurs when bleeding occurs in this space. It is caused by trauma, rupture of an aneurysm, or an arteriovenous anomaly.

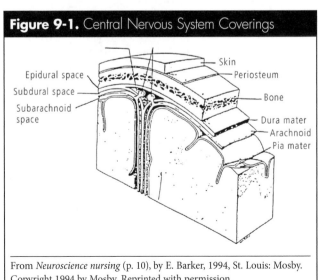

Figure 9-1. Central Nervous System Coverings

From *Neuroscience nursing* (p. 10), by E. Barker, 1994, St. Louis: Mosby. Copyright 1994 by Mosby. Reprinted with permission.

2. Subdural space
   a. Space between the arachnoid and dura mater that is a potential (empty) space
   b. Subdural hematoma occurs when venous blood leaks into this space, most commonly caused by injury. The bleed can be rapid or slow (Mosby, 2006).
   c. Subdural hygroma occurs when CSF leaks into the subdural space. This is believed to be caused by a tear in the arachnoid mater.
3. Epidural space
   a. Space between the dura mater and the bone that is a potential (empty) space
   b. Epidural hematoma results from bleeding between the dura and the inner surface of the skull, typically when the middle meningeal artery bleeds rapidly into the epidural space.

C. Ventricles (Barker, 2010; **Figure 9-2**)
   1. Spaces in the brain where CSF is found and produced
   2. Two lateral ventricles (one in each hemisphere); CSF is formed here
   3. The third and fourth ventricles are more centrally located and allow CSF to continually flow from the brain to the spinal cord.

D. CSF (Lewis et al., 2004)
   1. Cushions and protects the brain and spinal cord; circulates within the subarachnoid space
   2. Functions similarly to blood, carrying nutrients to the CNS and removing wastes
   3. ICP is the hydrostatic force measured in the brain CSF compartment of the brain. Normal ICP is the pressure exerted by the total volume from the brain tissue, blood, and CSF (Lewis et al., 2004).
   4. Hydrocephalus is an abnormal accumulation of CSF in the cranial vault caused by an overproduction of CSF, obstruction of CSF flow, or defective reabsorption of CSF (Mosby, 2006). Pressure may remain within normal limits, causing normal-pressure hydrocephalus (Figure 9-2).

E. Cerebrum (Cerebral Cortex; Barker, 2010)
   1. Believed to contain approximately 14 billion neurons, which are the building blocks of the CNS; pressure or damage to the cerebrum results in damage that is specific to the area injured
      a. Composition of neurons: Three components
         1) A cell body (perikaryon) and elongated processes that come from the body
         2) Dendrites, which conduct impulses toward the perikaryon
         3) Axons, which conduct impulses away from the perikaryon (**a**xon = **a**way)
      b. Types of neurons

         1) Pseudounipolar
            a) Appear to have only one process originating from the perikaryon, which then divides into two processes; one branch goes to the skin, and the other enters the CNS
            b) Typically found in the sensory ganglia of peripheral nerves
         2) Bipolar
            a) Have two processes originating from the perikaryon; one functions as the dendrite, the other as an axon
            b) Have limited distribution in the CNS
            c) Found primarily in the visual, auditory, and olfactory systems
         3) Multipolar
            a) Possess one axon and many dendrites
            b) Are the most plentiful type of neuron
            c) Can be found throughout the CNS and PNS
   2. Gyri (bumps), sulci (small grooves), and fissures (deeper grooves) form the geography of the cerebral cortex.
   3. Composed of myelinated white matter, which is located deep inside the brain, and gray matter, which is made up of cell bodies located on the outer portion of the brain
   4. Divided into two halves (hemispheres)
      a. Hemispheres are connected by nerve fibers called corpus callosum that allow communication between the two sides. Destruction of the corpus callosum leads to inability of the hemispheres to communicate (hemispheric independence), or "split brain" (Wong, 1999).
      b. One hemisphere usually is dominant.
         1) The dominant hemisphere is responsible for speech and is most often located in the left hemisphere.
         2) Dominance is also related to a dominant hand and foot.
            a) 90% of the population is right handed. 99% of these people have a dominant left hemisphere.
            b) 10% of the population is left handed. 60% of these people have a dominant left hemisphere; however, 80% of all left-handed people have some mixed dominance.
   5. Contains the lobes of the brain (Hickey, 2008; **Figure 9-3**)
      a. Frontal lobes
         1) The anterior portion controls emotions, personality, complex intelligence

Figure 9-2. Circulation of the CSF

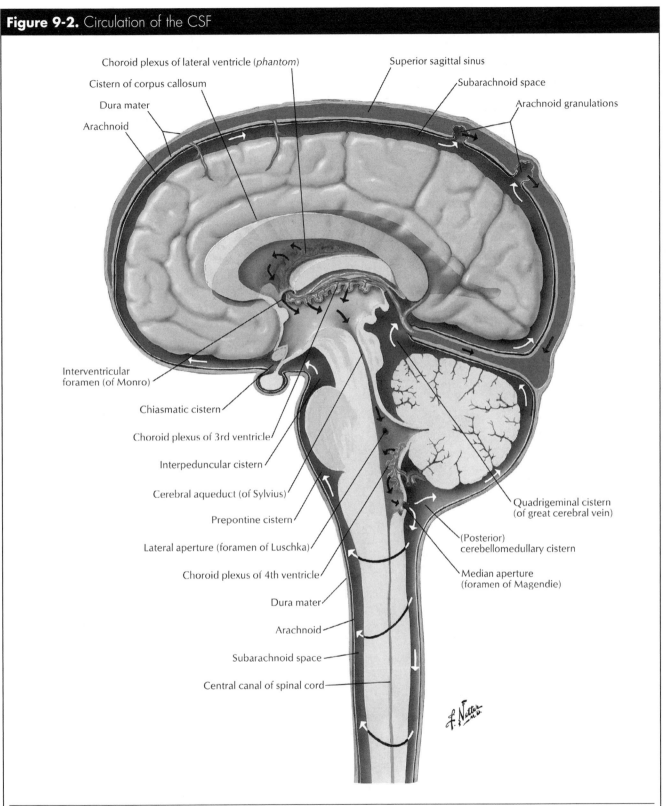

Choroid plexus of lateral ventricle (*phantom*)

Cistern of corpus callosum

Dura mater

Arachnoid

Superior sagittal sinus

Subarachnoid space

Arachnoid granulations

Interventricular foramen (of Monro)

Chiasmatic cistern

Choroid plexus of 3rd ventricle

Interpeduncular cistern

Cerebral aqueduct (of Sylvius)

Prepontine cistern

Lateral aperture (foramen of Luschka)

Choroid plexus of 4th ventricle

Dura mater

Arachnoid

Subarachnoid space

Central canal of spinal cord

Quadrigeminal cistern (of great cerebral vein)

(Posterior) cerebellomedullary cistern

Median aperture (foramen of Magendie)

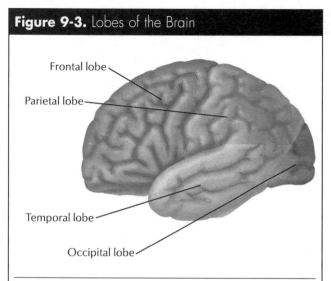

Figure 9-3. Lobes of the Brain

From *Atlas of human anatomy* (5th ed., p. 104), by F. H. Netter, 2010, Philadelphia: Saunders. Retrieved August 23, 2011, from www.netterimages.com (Image #5274). Copyright 2010 by Saunders. Reprinted with permission.

(i.e., executive functions such as problem solving and organizational skills), and cognition.

2) The posterior portion controls voluntary motor movements.

3) Broca's area, which is responsible for the motor component of speech, is located in the left hemisphere.

4) Injury to this area may be indicated by emotional lability, difficulty with executive functions, personality changes, difficulty initiating voluntary movements, and Broca's aphasia.

5) Broca's aphasia, also called nonfluent aphasia, is an expressive aphasia that is characterized by impairment in forming language or expressing thoughts. The client's comprehension and ability to conceptualize thoughts usually are not impaired. Frustration and anger can result from the patient's awareness of the deficit (Barker, 1994).

b. Parietal lobes

1) Receive and interpret sensory input (e.g., pain, temperature, pressure, size, shape, texture, body image, left-right discrimination, and spatial orientation)

2) Injury to this area usually is indicated by difficulty with left-right discrimination, spatial orientation, body image perception, and atopognosia, or loss of the power of topognosia (ability to correctly locate a sensation).

c. Occipital lobes

1) Receive and interpret visual stimuli

2) Responsible for depth perception

3) Injury to this area is indicated by difficulty interpreting visual clues or stimuli (results in functional blindness).

d. Temporal lobes

1) Control hearing, taste, and smell

2) Include Wernicke's area, which enables speech reception (usually in left hemisphere) and interpretation of sounds as words

3) Control memory functions

4) Injury to this area involves loss of smell, hearing deficits, loss of taste, memory deficits, and Wernicke's aphasia.

5) Wernicke's aphasia is characterized by fluent speech that does not make sense.

6. Cerebral hemorrhages are classified by

a. Location: Subarachnoid, extradural, subdural

b. Vessel type: Arterial, venous, capillary

c. Origin: Traumatic, degenerative

d. Bleeds can be slow and occur over a long period of time or can be rapid in onset.

F. Other Structures in the Brain (**Figure 9-4**)

1. The limbic system includes structures in the brain involved in emotion, motivation, and emotional association with memory.

a. Composed of a group of structures deep inside the brain associated with the hypothalamus

b. Involved in primitive emotions (e.g., anger, rage, sexual arousal and behavior, pleasure, sadness) and the fight-or-flight response

c. Affects motivation, attention, and biological rhythm

d. Injury to this system usually results in a hyperaroused state, which is indicated by a person's disinhibited behaviors.

2. Basal ganglia

a. A mass of gray matter deep within the cerebrum

b. A group of nuclei associated with motor and learning functions

c. The cerebellum is excitatory and the basal ganglia are inhibitory, which allows steady voluntary movements and suppression of meaningless and unintentional movements.

d. Injury to this system usually results in dyskinesias (i.e., abnormal involuntary movements) and muscle tone alteration (i.e., rigidity and bradykinesia).

1) Tremors: Rhythmic and purposeless movements that occur at rest and disappear during intentional movements

2) Athetosis: Slow, snakelike, writhing movements of the extremities, face, and neck

3) Chorea: Rapid, purposeless, jerky movements that often are associated with facial grimacing

3. Diencephalon: Located between the cerebrum and the mesencephalon. It consists of the hypothalamus, thalamus, metathalamus, epithalamus, and most of the third ventricle (Lewis et al., 2004). It contains diffuse fibers that compose the reticular activating system (Wong, 1999).

   a. Thalamus

1) Rounded mass that forms most of the lateral wall of the third ventricle and part of the fourth ventricle (Wong, 1999)

2) Functions as a relay station for some sensory messages, particularly pain, touch, and pressure

3) Helps to distinguish pleasant feelings from unpleasant feelings

4) Lesions tend to be associated primarily with sensory loss.

5) Activates the cerebral cortex

6) Thalamic syndrome is a vascular disorder

Figure 9-4. Other Structures in the Brain

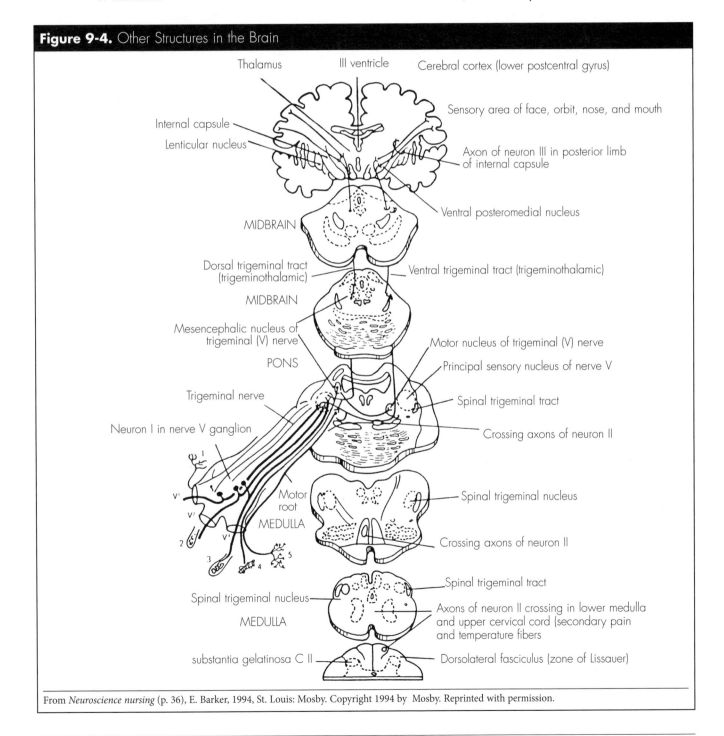

From *Neuroscience nursing* (p. 36), E. Barker, 1994, St. Louis: Mosby. Copyright 1994 by Mosby. Reprinted with permission.

that causes disturbances of sensation and partial or complete paralysis of one side of the body (Mosby, 2006). It is also characterized as a nonspecific, spontaneous, intolerable pain that cannot be relieved pharmaceutically.

   b. Hypothalamus
     1) Located below the thalamus and forms the floor of the fourth ventricle
     2) Is the master controller of both divisions (parasympathetic and sympathetic) of the ANS
     3) Plays a role in producing two hormones that are stored and released from the pituitary gland
       a) Antidiuretic hormone (ADH) increases reabsorption of water in the kidneys
         (1) Too much ADH leads to a syndrome of inappropriate ADH secretion, which leads to water retention. It is common to see this syndrome in clients with trauma.
         (2) Too little ADH leads to diabetes insipidus and excessive water loss.
       b) Oxytocin stimulates uterine contractions. Recent studies have begun to investigate oxytocin's role in various behaviors, including orgasm, social recognition, pair bonding, anxiety, and maternal behaviors (Lee, Macbeth, Pagani, & Young, 2009).
     4) The impairment of the hypothalamus results in somnolence, coma, anorexia, loss of libido, and endocrine disorders.

4. Brainstem: Includes the midbrain, pons, medulla oblongata, and reticular formation. It extends from the cerebral hemisphere to the spinal cord. The cell bodies of cranial nerves (CNs) III through XII are in the brainstem (Lewis et al., 2004).
   a. Midbrain
     1) Approximately 2 cm long
     2) Composed of two structures
       a) Substantia nigra: Motor nuclei that are concerned with muscle tone. This area is impaired in people with Parkinson's disease.
       b) Red nucleus: Large motor nuclei associated with flexor rigidity
     3) Injury to the midbrain is associated with decorticate posturing (i.e., abnormal flexion).
   b. Pons
     1) A bridge between the cerebellar hemispheres

     2) Contains two areas that help control breathing
       a) The apneustic center initiates inspiration.
       b) The pneumotaxic center inhibits inspiration.
     3) Injury to the pons usually involves abnormal breathing patterns.
       a) Central neurogenic hyperventilation: Sustained regular, rapid, deep breaths
       b) Apneustic breathing: Sustained, cramplike inspiratory efforts that pause when inspiration is complete; there also may be an expiratory pause
     4) Two reflexes that are tested in comatose people to determine pontine and brainstem involvement
       a) Oculocephalic reflex (doll's eyes): In this reflex, the eyes move in sync with head movement. In normal pontine activity, movement of the eyes lags behind.
       b) Oculovestibular reflex (caloric test): To test for this reflex, water is placed in the ear canal. In pontine lesions, the eyes do not deviate toward the stimulated ear. In normal pontine function, the eyes deviate toward the stimulated ear.
     5) Pontine lesions produce a "locked-in" syndrome in which the person has no movement except for the eyelids, but the person is conscious, has sensation, and cognition typically is intact.
   c. Medulla oblongata
     1) Houses the respiratory center
       a) Inspiratory dominant: The medulla senses the need to inspire; exhalation is a passive process.
       b) Produces rhythmic breathing
       c) Involves chemoreceptors that are sensitive to CO_2 levels in the blood and cause an increase in ventilation when CO_2 is elevated
       d) Injuries to this area result in ataxic breathing in which breathing is irregular with both shallow and deep inspiratory efforts.
     2) Controls temperature; Regulates hunger, thirst, and sleep-wake patterns
     3) Houses the vasodilation and vasopressor centers
     4) The swallowing and vomiting centers originate here.

5) Injuries to this area also result in flaccid muscle tone.

d. Reticular formation
1) Located in the brainstem
2) Receives sensory input from all sensory organs and acts as a relay station to determine which area of the brain receives the input; influences excitatory and inhibitory control of spinal motor neurons
3) The reticular activating system is part of the reticular formation and usually is associated with controlling states of consciousness.
4) Particularly susceptible to trauma
5) Involves the following functions:
   a) Motor control modulation: Coordinates (but does not inhibit) movement and plays a role in the extrapyramidal system
   b) Visceral functioning: Controls the state of consciousness
   c) Sensory filtering: Plays an inhibitory role to prevent the brain from becoming overstimulated
   d) Inhibition of stimuli: Helps to narrow down stimuli to allow selective attention and plays a major role in attention and concentration
   e) Arousal and alertness
6) Injury to this area may cause coma.

5. Cerebellum
a. Located below the cerebrum
b. Involves two hemispheres and a medial portion called the vermis
c. Contains gray matter on the outside of the cerebellar cortex and white matter on the inside of the cortex
d. Receives sensory and motor impulses
e. Responsible for the following functions:
1) Coordination of all reflex activity and voluntary motor activity
2) Regulation of muscle tone and trunk stability
3) Influence and maintenance of equilibrium
f. Injury to this area can produce a variety of signs of dysfunction related to muscular control.
1) Deficits on the same (ipsilateral) side of the body as the injury
2) Hypotonia: Decreased resistance to passive movement
3) Postural changes and wide-based gait to compensate for loss of muscle tone
4) Ataxia: Impaired ability to coordinate movement
   a) Intentional tremors

b) Jerky movements
c) Dysmetria: Inability to judge movement within space, causing loss of control of motor activity
d) Dysdiadochokinesis: Inability to perform alternating movements rapidly or regularly
e) Nystagmus: Disorders or ataxia of ocular movement
f) Ataxia of speech muscles (slurred speech)

G. Cranial Nerves (Barker, 2010)
1. Twelve CNs (**Table 9-1**)
a. CN I: Olfactory (smell)
b. CN II: Optic (vision)
c. CN III: Oculomotor (eye movement [e.g., elevating eyelids, moving eyes in and out, constricting pupil, accommodating for light])
d. CN IV: Trochlear (eye movement down and outward)
e. CN V: Trigeminal (chewing; sensations of face, scalp, and teeth)
f. CN VI: Abducens (outward eye movement)
g. CN VII: Facial (facial expression, taste [anterior two-thirds of tongue], salivation, crying)
h. CN VIII: Acoustic (also called vestibulocochlear; hearing and sense of balance)
i. CN IX: Glossopharyngeal (secretes saliva, swallowing, controls gag reflex, sensation in the throat, and taste)
j. CN X: Vagus (swallowing, voice production, heart rate, rate of peristalsis, sensation of throat, thoracic and abdominal viscera)
k. CN XI: Spinal accessory (shoulder and head movement)
l. CN XII: Hypoglossal (tongue movement)
2. Mnemonic tip for remembering the cranial nerves (see below)

H. Components That Provide Vascular Supply to the Brain (Barker, 2010; **Figure 9-5**)
1. Internal carotid arteries (right and left)
a. Supply 80% of the blood supply to the brain
b. Divide to form the anterior cerebral artery and the middle cerebral artery

Mnemonic for Names

On Old Olympus's Towering Tops, A Finn And German Viewed Some Hops.

Mnemonic for Function

S = Sensory, M = Motor, B = Both
Some Say Marry Money But My Brother Says Bad Business Marry Money.

Table 9-1. Cranial Nerves

Cranial Nerve (CN)	Origin and Course	Function
CN I: Olfactory		
Sensory	Mucosa of nasal cavity; only CN with cell body located in peripheral structure (nasal mucosa). Pass through cribriform plate of ethmoid bone and go on to olfactory bulbs at floor of frontal lobe. Final interpretation is in temporal lobe.	Smell; however, system is more than receptor and interpreter for odors; perception of smell also sensitizes other body systems and responses such as salivation, peristalsis, and even sexual stimulus. Loss of sense of smell is called anosmia.
CN II: Optic		
Sensory	Ganglion cells of retina converge on the optic disc and form optic nerve. Nerve fibers pass to optic chiasm, which is above pituitary gland. Some fibers decussate, others do not. The two tracts then go to the lateral geniculate body near the thalamus and then on to the end station for interpretation in the occipital lobe.	Vision
CN III: Oculomotor		
Motor	Originates in midbrain and emerges from brainstem at upper pons	Extraocular movement of eyes
	Motor fibers to superior, medial, inferior recti, and inferior oblique for eye movement; levator muscle of the eyelid	Raise eyelid
Parasympathetic	Parasympathetic fibers to ciliary muscles and iris of eye	Constrict pupil; change shape of lens
CN IV: Trochlear		
Motor	Comes from lower midbrain area to innervate superior oblique eye muscle	Allows eye to move down and inward
CN V: Trigeminal		
Sensory	Originates in fourth ventricle and emerges at lateral parts of pons. Has three branches to face: ophthalmic, maxillary, and mandibular	Ophthalmic branch: Sensation to cornea, ciliary body, iris, lacrimal gland, conjunctiva, nasal mucosal membranes, eyelids, eyebrows, forehead, and nose
		Maxillary branch: Sensation to skin of cheek, lower lid, side of nose and upper jaw, teeth, mucosa of mouth, spheno-polative-pterygoid region, and maxillary sinus
		Mandibular branch: Sensation to skin of lower lip, chin, ear, mucous membrane, teeth of lower jaw and tongue
Motor	Goes to temporalis, masseter, pterygoid gland, anterior part of digastric muscles (all for mastication), and the tensor tympani and tensor veli palatin muscles (clench jaws)	Muscles of chewing and mastication and opening jaw
CN VI: Abducens		
Motor	Arises from a nucleus in pons to innervate lateral rectus eye muscle	Allows eye to move outward
CN VII: Facial		
Sensory	Lower portion of pons goes to anterior two-thirds of tongue and soft palate	Taste anterior two-thirds of tongue; sensation to soft palate
Motor	Pons to muscles of forehead, eyelids, cheeks, lips, ear, nose, and neck	Movement of facial muscles to produce facial expressions, close eyes
Parasympathetic	Pons to salivary gland and lacrimal glands	Secretory for salivation and tears

continued

THE SPECIALTY PRACTICE OF REHABILITATION NURSING

Table 9-1. Cranial Nerves *continued*

Cranial Nerve (CN)	Origin and Course	Function
CN VIII: Acoustic		
Sensory	Cochlear division: Originates in spinal ganglia of the cochlea, with peripheral fibers to the organ of Corti in the internal ear. Goes to pons, and impulses are transmitted to the temporal lobe.	Hearing
	Vestibular division: Originates in otolith organs of the semicircular canals in the inner ear and in the vestibular ganglion. Terminates in pons, with some fibers continuing to cerebellum. Only cranial nerve originating wholly within a bone, petrous portion of temporal bone.	Equilibrium
CN IX: Glossopharyngeal		
Sensory	Posterior one-third of tongue for taste sensation and sensations from soft palate, tonsils, and opening to mouth in back of oral pharynx (fauces). Fibers go to medulla and then to the temporal lobe for taste and sensory cortex for other sensations.	Taste in posterior one-third of tongue. Sensation in back of throat; stimulation elicits a gag reflex.
Motor	Medulla to constrictor muscles of pharynx and stylopharyngeal muscles	Voluntary muscles for swallowing and phonation
Parasympathetic	Medulla to parotid salivary gland via otic ganglia	Secretory, salivary glands; carotid reflex
CN X: Vagus		
Sensory	Sensory fibers in back of ear and posterior wall of external ear go to medulla oblongata and on to sensory cortex.	Sensation behind ear and part of external ear meatus
Motor	Fibers go from medulla oblongata through jugular foramen with glossopharyngeal nerve and on to pharynx, larynx, esophagus, bronchi, lungs, heart, stomach, small intestines, liver, pancreas, kidneys.	Voluntary muscles for phonation and swallowing. Involuntary activity of visceral muscles of heart, lungs, and digestive tract.
Parasympathetic	Medulla oblongata to larynx, trachea, lungs, aorta, esophagus, stomach, small intestines, and gall bladder	Carotid reflex; autonomic activity of respiratory tract, digestive tract including peristalsis and secretion from organs
CN XI: Spinal Accessory		
Motor	This nerve has two roots, cranial and spinal. Cranial portion arises at several rootlets at side of medulla, runs below vagus, and is joined by spinal portion from motor cells in cervical cord. Some fibers go along with the vagus nerve to supply motor impulse to the pharynx, larynx, uvula, and palate. Major portion to sternomastoid and trapezius muscles, branches to cervical spinal nerves C2–C4.	Some fibers for swallowing and phonation. Turn head and shrug shoulders.
CN XII: Hypoglossal		
Motor	Arises in medulla oblongata and goes to muscles of tongue	Movement of tongue necessary for swallowing and phonation.

From *Neuroscience nursing* (pp. 78–79), by E. Barker, 1994, St. Louis: Mosby. Copyright 1994 by Mosby. Reprinted with permission.

2. Vertebral arteries (right and left)
   a. Supply 20% of the blood supply to the brain
   b. Join to form the basilar artery as it passes over the pons and then splits and becomes the posterior cerebral arteries at the level of the cerebrum
3. Communicating arteries
   a. Posterior: Connects the posterior cerebral

and middle cerebral arteries
  b. Anterior: Connects the two anterior cerebral arteries
4. Circle of Willis
  a. Formed by the anastomosis of the two internal carotid arteries and the two vertebral arteries
  b. Composed of the following arteries:
    1) Anterior cerebral
    2) Posterior cerebral
    3) Anterior communicating (supplies the medial portion of the frontal lobes)
    4) Posterior communicating
    5) Internal carotid
  c. Allows blood that enters the internal carotid arteries or the vertebral arteries to be distributed to the brain and acts as a safety valve when differential pressures are present in these arteries. It may also function as an anastomotic pathway when occlusion of a major artery on one side of the brain occurs (Lewis et al., 2004).
  d. Located at the base of the skull in the subarachnoid space
    1) The site of many congenital aneurysms
    2) If an aneurysm bursts or vessels are sheared or torn, a subarachnoid hemorrhage occurs.
I. Skull (Lewis et al., 2004; **Figure 9-6**)
  1. Composed of eight cranial bones and 14 facial bones. The structure of the skull cavity often explains the physiology of head injuries because of the many ridges, prominences, and foramina.
  2. Outermost protection of the brain
  3. During the first year of life, the skull is larger than the facial components of the cranial vault. The brain is 25% of its adult size at birth and by age 15 has reached 98% of its adult size. The cranium accommodates for this (Wong, 1999).
  4. Skull fractures often occur with head trauma.
    a. Linear: Break in continuity of bone caused by low-velocity injuries
    b. Depressed: Inward indentation of skull caused by powerful blow
    c. Simple: Linear or depressed skull fracture without fragmentation or communicating lacerations, caused by low to moderate impact
    d. Comminuted: Multiple linear fractures with fragmentation of bone into many pieces, caused by direct, high-momentum impact

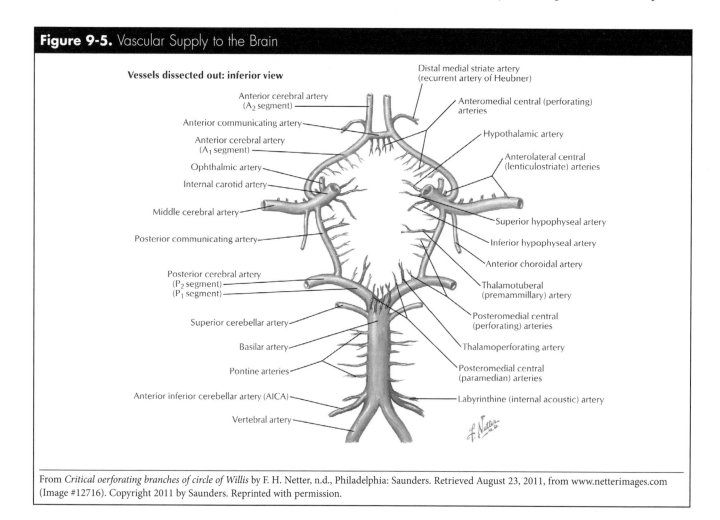

Figure 9-5. Vascular Supply to the Brain

From *Critical oerforating branches of circle of Willis* by F. H. Netter, n.d., Philadelphia: Saunders. Retrieved August 23, 2011, from www.netterimages.com (Image #12716). Copyright 2011 by Saunders. Reprinted with permission.

THE SPECIALTY PRACTICE OF REHABILITATION NURSING

Figure 9-6. The Skull

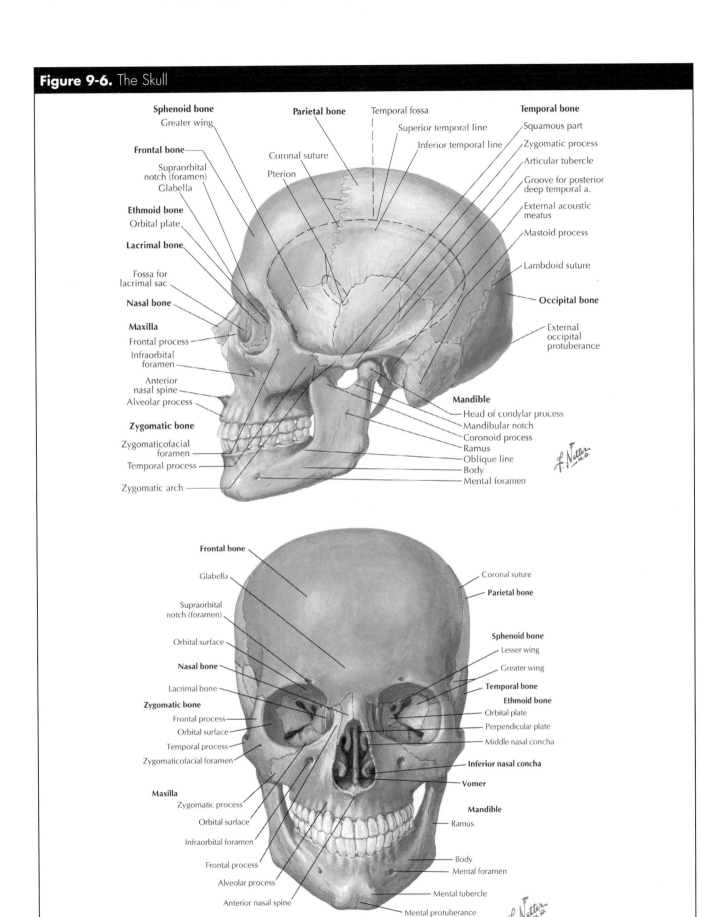

From *Netter's head and neck anatomy for dentistry* (p.27), by N. S. Norton, 2006, Philadelphia: Saunders. Retrieved August 23, 2011, from www. netterimages.com (Image #11485 and #10775). Copyright 2006 by Saunders. Reprinted with permission.

e. Compound: Depressed skull fracture and scalp laceration with communicating pathway to intracranial activity, caused by severe head trauma

II. Anatomy of the Spinal Cord

A. Spinal Column: The bony structure that surrounds and protects the delicate nervous tissue of the spinal cord (**Figure 9-7**).
   1. Vertebrae
      a. Seven cervical vertebrae
         1) The C1 vertebra is called the atlas.
         2) The C2 vertebra, also called the axis, has a finger-like projection called the odontoid process (dens) that articulates with the anterior arch of the atlas.
      b. Twelve thoracic vertebrae
      c. Five lumbar vertebrae
      d. Five fused sacral vertebrae
      e. Five fused coccygeal vertebrae
      f. The anterior portion of the vertebra is the body.

Figure 9-7. The Spinal Column

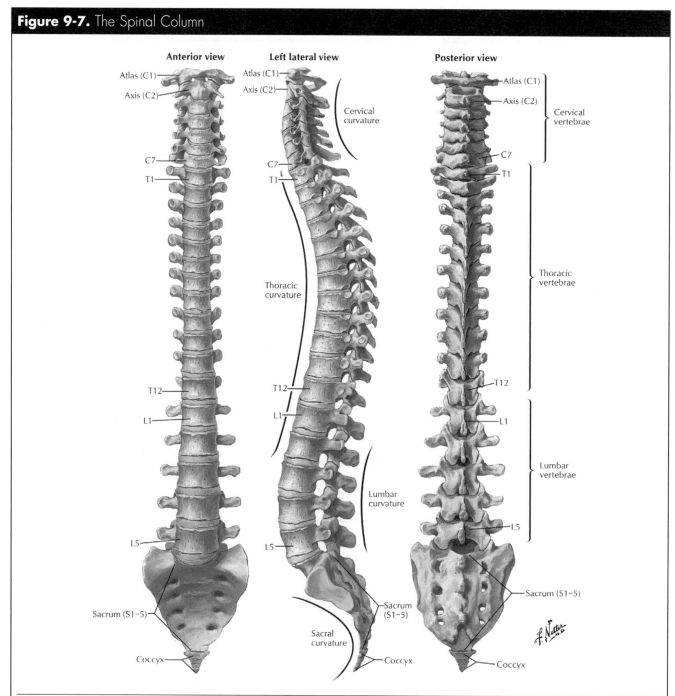

From *Atlas of human anatomy* (5th ed., p. 150), by F. H. Netter, 2010, Philadelphia: Saunders. Retrieved August 23, 2011, from www.netterimages.com (Image #4804). Copyright 2010 by Saunders. Reprinted with permission.

g. The posterior portion of the vertebra is the arch. The arch is formed from two transverse processes, one spinous process, and two superior and inferior facets. Two laminae form the roof of the arch, and two pedicles attach the arch to the body of the vertebra.

2. Intervertebral discs
    a. Situated between vertebral bodies and act as shock absorbers
    b. The disc is formed from an outer fibrous cartilage ring (annulus fibrosis) containing a spongy inner material (nucleus pulposus).

3. Ligaments
    a. Anterior and posterior longitudinal ligaments are the two main supporting ligaments that run from the atlas to the sacrum.
    b. Short, dense ligaments are located between the vertebral arches.
    c. Ligamenta flava run between the laminae.
    d. Supraspinal and interspinal ligaments run between the spinous processes.
    e. Transverse ligaments run between the transverse processes.

B. Spinal Cord (**Figure 9-8**)
    1. The spinal cord begins at the caudal end of the medulla oblongata and leaves the cranial vault by extending through the foramen magnum into the vertebral canal and in the adult usually terminates at the intervertebral disc between L1 and L2 (Goshgarian, 2003).
        a. Conus medullaris: The cone-shaped area from T10 to T12
        b. Cauda equina (horse's tail): The area at the end of the conus medullaris that is not

actually a part of the spinal cord but is composed of peripheral spinal nerves

2. Neuroanatomic organization of the spinal gray and white matter: Major afferent or ascending, sensory tracts (**Figure 9-9**); the names indicate the direction in which the impulses travel
    a. In a transverse section of the spinal cord, the white matter is located peripherally, whereas gray matter (shaped like a butterfly) is centrally located. This is the opposite of the brain's makeup of white and gray matter.
    b. White matter contains ascending and descending bundles of fibers contained in fiber tracts and glial cells and appears white because it contains myelin (Goshgarian, 2003; Zejdlik, 1992).
        1) Major afferent, ascending tracts
            a) Posterior spinocerebellar tract and posterior columns: Proprioception from muscles, tendons, and joints; sensations of deep touch, proprioception, and vibration and most bowel and bladder sensations
            b) Lateral spinothalamic tract: Transmission of pain and temperature sensations; the fibers cross at the level of the cord after ascending one or two segments and ascend on the contralateral side of the cord
            c) Anterior spinothalamic tract: Light touch and sensation and some pain transmission
        2) Major efferent, descending tracts
            a) Lateral corticospinal tracts: Neurons found in the cerebral cortex; most of these fibers cross at the medulla before traveling to their target muscles
            b) Anterior (ventral) corticospinal: Fine tuning of muscle tone
    c. Gray matter consists predominantly of neurons, their processes, and glial cells and has an enriched blood supply (Goshgarian, 2003).

3. Spinal nerves (American Spinal Injury Association [ASIA], 2002)
    a. The nerve roots that come from the spinal cord contain both a motor and sensory component. Each root has a dorsal (posterior) sensory root that transmits afferent impulses to the cord and a ventral (anterior) motor root that transmits efferent impulses from the cord to target muscles and organs.
    b. There are 31 pairs of spinal nerves: 8 cervical (C), 12 thoracic (T), 5 lumbar (L), 5 sacral (S), and 1 coccygeal (C; **Figure 9-10**).

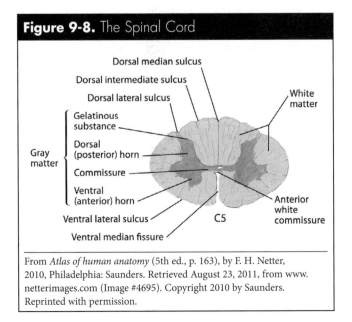

Figure 9-8. The Spinal Cord

Dorsal median sulcus
Dorsal intermediate sulcus
Dorsal lateral sulcus
White matter
Gelatinous substance
Gray matter
Dorsal (posterior) horn
Commissure
Ventral (anterior) horn
Anterior white commissure
Ventral lateral sulcus
C5
Ventral median fissure

From *Atlas of human anatomy* (5th ed., p. 163), by F. H. Netter, 2010, Philadelphia: Saunders. Retrieved August 23, 2011, from www.netterimages.com (Image #4695). Copyright 2010 by Saunders. Reprinted with permission.

Figure 9-9. Major Sensory Tracts

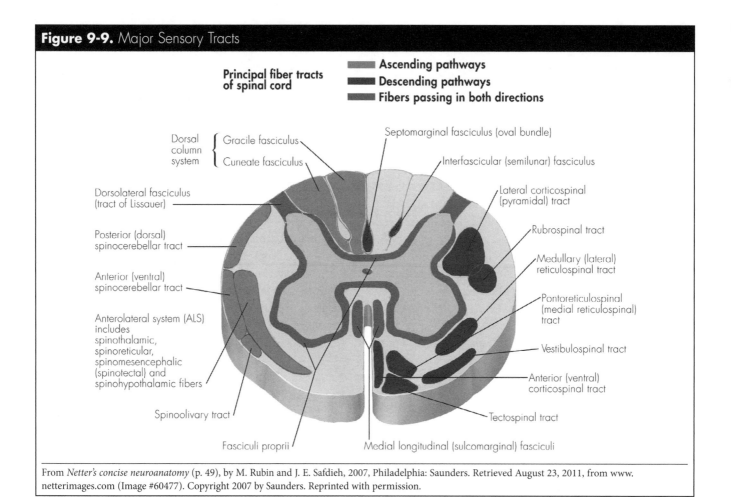

Principal fiber tracts of spinal cord

Ascending pathways
Descending pathways
Fibers passing in both directions

Dorsal column system { Gracile fasciculus / Cuneate fasciculus

Septomarginal fasciculus (oval bundle)

Interfascicular (semilunar) fasciculus

Dorsolateral fasciculus (tract of Lissauer)

Lateral corticospinal (pyramidal) tract

Rubrospinal tract

Posterior (dorsal) spinocerebellar tract

Medullary (lateral) reticulospinal tract

Anterior (ventral) spinocerebellar tract

Pontoreticulospinal (medial reticulospinal) tract

Anterolateral system (ALS) includes spinothalamic, spinoreticular, spinomesencephalic (spinotectal) and spinohypothalamic fibers

Vestibulospinal tract

Anterior (ventral) corticospinal tract

Spinoolivary tract

Tectospinal tract

Fasciculi proprii

Medial longitudinal (sulcomarginal) fasciculi

c. Cervical: The C1 nerve roots exit over the top of the body of C1. The C2 nerve roots exit between C1 and C2. All other cervical nerve roots exit over the top of the caudal vertebrae until C8, which exits between C7 and T1. The thoracic nerve roots pass below the vertebrae.

1) C1: Innervates the chin for sensation
2) C2: Innervates the lateral neck muscles that provide head support
3) C3: Innervates the anterior and posterior neck muscles that provide head support
4) C4: Innervates the deltoids and diaphragm (C3–C5 forms the phrenic nerve and innervates the diaphragm)
5) C5: Elbow flexors (biceps, brachialis)
6) C6: Wrist extensors (extensor carpi radialis longus and brevis)
7) C7: Elbow extensors (triceps)
8) C8: Finger flexors (flexor digitorum profundus) to the middle finger

d. Thoracic

1) T1: Small finger abductors (abductor digiti minimi)
2) T1–T6: Intercostal muscles

3) T7–T12: Upper and lower abdominal muscles, thoracic muscles, quadratus lumborum flexors

e. Lumbar

1) L1–L2: Hip flexors (iliopsoas)
2) L3: Knee extensors (quadriceps)
3) L4: Ankle dorsiflexors (tibialis anterior)
4) L5: Long toe extensors (extensor hallucis longus)

f. Sacral

1) S1: Ankle plantar flexors (gastrocnemius, soleus)
2) S2–S4: Innervates specific motor and sensory functions, including anorectal muscles, perineal sensation, sphincter control, genitalia, and sexual function

4. Spinal reflexes, which are necessary for normal neurological function (Barker, 1994; **Figure 9-11**)

a. The brain is able to inhibit approximately 80% of spinal reflexes to maintain voluntary control over posture and movement.

b. A normal spinal cord reflex involves the following:

1) Sensory input, which ascends to the cell body, where it synapses with a motor neuron

2) The motor cell body, which sends an impulse down to initiate motor activity

c. The brain is able to prevent or speed up a synapse if the stimulus is anticipated (i.e., the brain maintains ultimate control over the spinal cord).

d. When a person sustains a spinal cord injury (SCI), reflex activity resumes after spinal shock; however, the connection between the brain and spinal cord is missing and therefore the brain can no longer inhibit or facilitate spinal reflexes, which causes spasticity.

e. If damage occurs to the peripheral nerves or the cauda equina, reflex activity does not occur.

f. Reflex activity may not return at the level of injury because of damaged or destroyed neurons at the level of injury.

5. Blood supply to the spinal cord (Goshgarian, 2003; **Figure 9-12**)

a. The spinal cord is a highly vascularized organ that receives its blood supply from the vertebral arteries.

1) Damage to the arteries can be a result of damage to the vertebrae or vertebral alignment.

2) Damage can be caused by trauma, vascular anomalies, infarcts, or vascular surgery.

b. The anterior spinal artery (one artery) provides the blood supply to the anterior two-thirds of the spinal cord. Occlusion can cause anterior artery syndrome.

c. The posterior spinal arteries (two arteries) provide the blood supply to the posterior one-third of the spinal cord. These arteries provide the needed blood supply to the posterior one-third of the white matter and some of the posterior portions of the meninges.

d. Radicular arteries contribute to the anterior and posterior blood supply of the spinal cord.

C. Classifications of Incomplete SCI or Clinical Syndromes (ASIA, 2002)

1. Central cord syndrome

a. A lesion that occurs almost exclusively in the cervical region

b. Central damage to the cord

c. Produces sacral sensory sparing and greater weakness in the upper limbs than the lower limbs

2. Brown-Sequard syndrome

a. Damage to one side of the spinal cord

b. Produces greater ipsilateral proprioceptive and

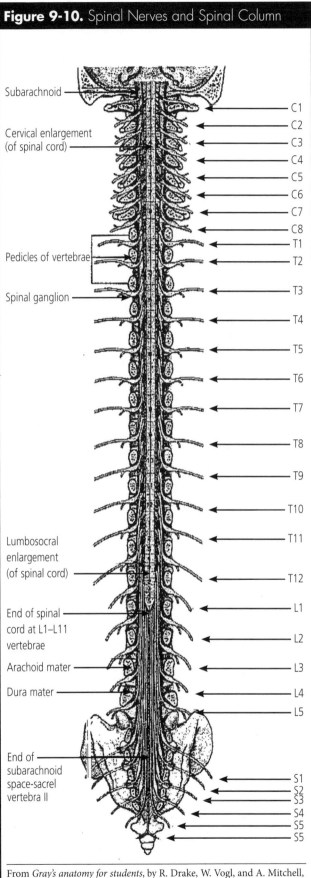

Figure 9-10. Spinal Nerves and Spinal Column

Subarachnoid

Cervical enlargement (of spinal cord)

Pedicles of vertebrae

Spinal ganglion

Lumbosocral enlargement (of spinal cord)

End of spinal cord at L1–L11 vertebrae

Arachoid mater

Dura mater

End of subarachnoid space-sacral vertebra II

C1
C2
C3
C4
C5
C6
C7
C8
T1
T2
T3
T4
T5
T6
T7
T8
T9
T10
T11
T12
L1
L2
L3
L4
L5
S1
S2
S3
S4
S5
S5

From *Gray's anatomy for students*, by R. Drake, W. Vogl, and A. Mitchell, 2005, Philadephia: Elsevier. Copyright 2005 by Elsevier. Reprinted with permission.

Figure 9-11. Spinal Reflexes

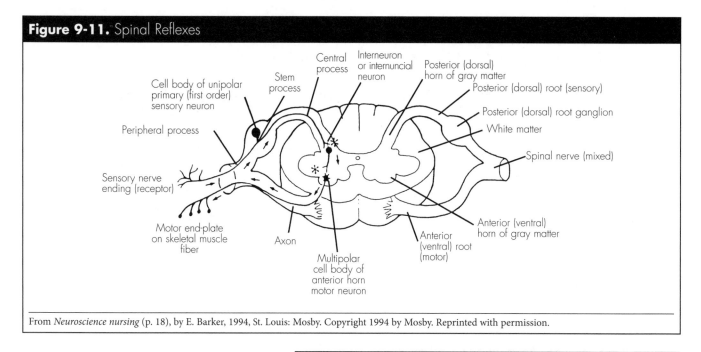

From *Neuroscience nursing* (p. 18), by E. Barker, 1994, St. Louis: Mosby. Copyright 1994 by Mosby. Reprinted with permission.

motor loss and contralateral loss of sensitivity to pain and temperature

3. Anterior cord syndrome
   a. Damage to or disruption of blood supply to the anterior two-thirds of the spinal cord
   b. Produces variable loss of motor function and of sensitivity to pain and temperature while preserving proprioception
4. Conus medullaris syndrome
   a. Injury of the sacral cord (conus) and lumbar nerve roots within the spinal canal
   b. Usually results in areflexic bladder, bowel, and lower limbs
5. Cauda equina syndrome
   a. Injury to lumbosacral nerve roots within the neural canal
   b. Results in areflexic bladder, bowel, and lower limbs

III. **Autonomic Nervous System (Figure 9-13)**
   A. Overview (Barker, 2010)
      1. The part of the peripheral nervous system that controls the viscera at an unconscious level
      2. Involves major effector organs
         a. Smooth muscle
         b. Cardiac muscle
         c. Glands
      3. Carries messages from the CNS to the peripheral effector organs
      4. Includes two divisions, sympathetic and

Figure 9-12. Blood Supply to the Spinal Cord

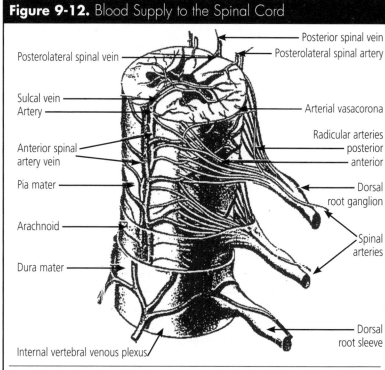

From *Spinal cord medicine: Principles and practice* (p. 31), by V. W. Lin (Ed.), 2003. New York: Demos. Copyright 2003 by Demos. Reprinted with permission.

parasympathetic, that are parallel but act in an opposing manner (Barker, 2010)
   a. Sympathetic division
      1) Prepares the body to meet crises
      2) Produces a fight-or-flight pattern, which is characterized by elevated heart rate and blood pressure and dilation of the pupil of the eye
      3) Slows peristalsis and closes the bladder neck

b. Parasympathetic division
   1) Is more vegetative in action
   2) Operates in calm moments
      and allows the body to restore
      itself
   3) Slows the heart rate, lowers
      blood pressure, increases gas-
      trointestinal activity, and
      shunts blood from the periph-
      ery to the internal organs
5. Functions independently of the hypothalamus and vasomotor centers in
   the brainstem
6. Responds to local stimulation; both
   inhibitory and facilitative influences
   from higher centers are blocked
7. Autonomic dysfunction can result in
   the following conditions:
   a. Autonomic dysreflexia
   b. Orthostatic hypotension
   c. Poikilothermia (inconsistent body
      temperature regulation)

IV. **Neurological Assessment**
   A. Neurological Assessment: For the reha-
      bilitation nurse, monitoring neurological
      status for changes is very important and
      is a fundamental component of a com-
      prehensive functional assessment.
   B. Team Approach: A team approach pro-
      vides the client and the team with data
      that will help them determine an appro-
      priate plan of care. The treatment team
      varies by client diagnosis but may include
      a physician, nurse, physical therapist, oc-
      cupational therapist, speech therapist,
      recreational therapist, neuropsychologist,
      dietitian, respiratory therapist, chaplain,
      alternative medicine practitioner, or others.
   C. Comprehensive Assessment: A comprehensive as-
      sessment of a client with neurological needs includes
      multiple domains (Chin, 1998)
      1. Cognitive, motor, and sensory function
      2. Disability
      3. Activities of daily living
      4. Affective assessment
      5. Learning needs
      6. Quality of life
   D. Spinal Shock: This is a result of the concussive effect
      of the primary SCI on the nervous system (Bader &
      Littlejohns, 2004). This concussive effect results in
      transient depression of all reflexes, including loss of
      deep tendon reflexes, paralysis, loss of sensation, loss

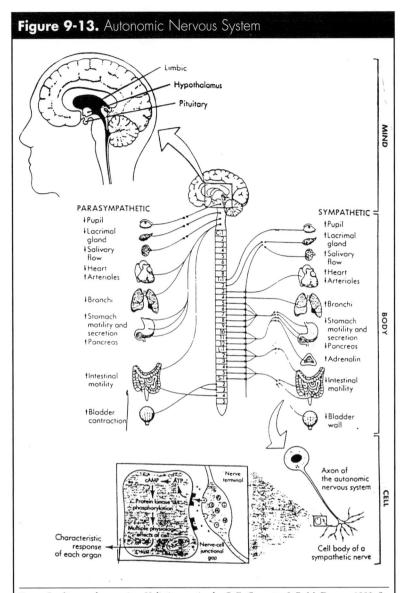

Figure 9-13. Autonomic Nervous System

From *Cardiovascular nursing: Holistic practice,* by C. E. Guzzetta & B. M. Dassey, 1992, St. Louis: Mosby. Copyright 1992 by Mosby. Reprinted with permission.

of autonomic function, and loss of bowel and bladder control. The duration of spinal shock may range
from days to months (Tator, 2000). It is not possible
to determine completeness of SCI until spinal shock
resolves (Bader & Littlejohns). Resolution of spinal
shock is indicated by return of a functioning bulbo-
cavernosus reflex.
   E. Classification of SCI (ASIA, 2002)
      1. Tetraplegia
         a. Impairment or loss of motor and sensory
            function in the cervical segments of the cord
         b. Results in loss of function in the upper and
            lower extremities and the trunk, including
            the pelvic organs
      2. Paraplegia
         a. Impairment or loss of motor and sensory

function in the thoracic, lumbar, or sacral segments of the cord

b. Results in loss of function in the lower extremities and the trunk, including the pelvic organs

F. ASIA Impairment Scale (ASIA, 2002; **Figure 9-14**)

1. A = Complete. No sensory or motor function is preserved in the sacral segments S4–S5.

2. B = Incomplete. Sensory but not motor function is preserved below the neurological level and includes the sacral segments S4–S5.

3. C = Incomplete. Motor function is preserved below the neurological level and more than half of key muscles below the neurological level have a muscle grade lower than 3.

4. D = Incomplete. Motor function is preserved below the neurological level and at least half of key muscles below the neurological level have a muscle grade higher than or equal to 3.

5. E = Normal. Sensory and motor functions are normal.

6. Motor examination: Used to quantify degree of muscle using standard measurements of strength in key muscles (ASIA, 2002)

a. Grade 0 = total paralysis

b. Grade 1 = palpable or visible contraction

c. Grade 2 = active movement, full range of motion (ROM) with gravity eliminated

d. Grade 3 = active movement, full ROM against gravity

e. Grade 4 = active movement, full ROM against moderate resistance

f. Grade 5 (normal) = active movement, full ROM against full resistance

G. Classification of Neurogenic Function

1. Upper motor neurons: Long neurons that originate in the brain and travel in bundles or tracts within the spinal cord. The cell bodies are located in the brain, with the axons extending down the spinal cord. They terminate at each segmental level throughout the cord to synapse with the lower motor neurons. These neurons of the motor cortex contribute to formation of the corticospinal and corticonuclear tracts. Although not motor neurons in the strict sense, they are classified as motor neurons because their stimulation produces movement and their destruction causes moderate to severe disorders of movement.

a. Impairment occurs in SCI when the damage to the cord is above the conus medullaris and the reflex center remains intact (S2–S4).

b. Often used to classify bladder, bowel, and sexual function

c. SCI above T12 generally results in impaired bladder, bowel, and sexual organ function.

d. Impairment is characterized by presence of muscle tone, spastic paralysis, positive reflexes, and sphincter tone.

2. Lower motor neurons: Lower motor neurons originate in the spinal cord and travel outside the CNS. They form the spinal nerve and subsequent branches of the PNS. These are the final motor neurons that innervate the skeletal muscles.

a. Impairment occurs in SCI of the sacral cord segments in the conus medullaris or the sacral nerve roots in the cauda equina.

b. Impairment is characterized by flaccid paralysis, loss of muscle, absent reflexes, and loss of sphincter tone.

V. **Neural Recovery**

A. Past Thinking: Historically, it was believed that the CNS was unable to replace or repair neurons. It was thought that you were born with a certain number of neurons and that was all you had.

B. Current Treatment: The care and treatment of a person with an SCI begins with the emergency medical care that is first given at the scene of the injury. Movement of the spinal column or other resuscitation efforts can cause further injury.

1. Prevention of secondary damage: In 1990 a study was published that cited the use of methylprednisolone (steroid) as a first-line treatment in helping to protect the spinal cord shortly after injury.

a. The first step in acknowledging that secondary injury to nervous tissue was preventable

b. Current research is focusing on two areas: cell death and immune system reactions. Initial work was done with people who had cerebral vascular trauma. The information in this section applies to both brain injuries (traumatic and vascular) and SCI.

1) Cells die in one of two ways: necrosis or apoptosis. Necrosis is an uncontrolled process in which cells swell, break open, and then leak neurotoxins that are toxic to neighboring cells. Apoptosis is programmed cell death in which an ordered sequence of events leads to the cell dying. There is little damage to surrounding cells. Apoptosis is generally limited to the area right around the initial damage and occurs within 8 hours after the insult. This also occurs again at Day 7 after injury and causes the zone of neurological damage to increase. These processes are

Figure 9-14. ASIA Impairment Scale

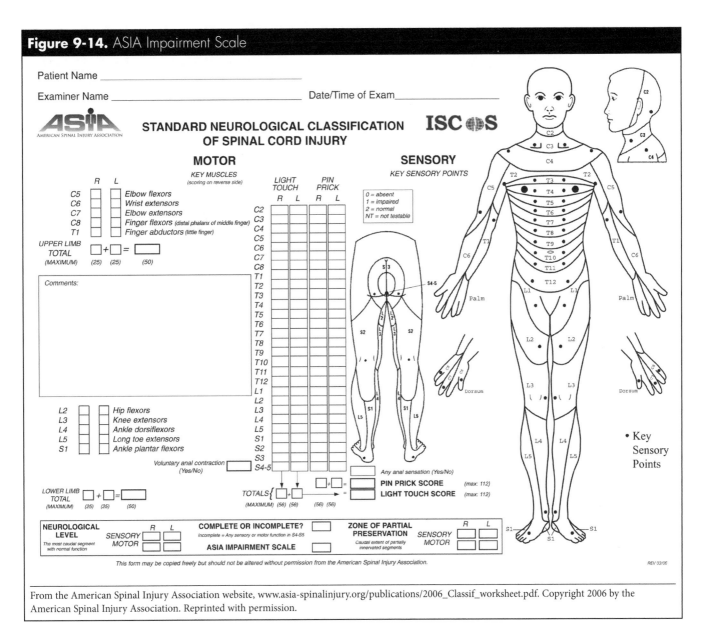

From the American Spinal Injury Association website, www.asia-spinalinjury.org/publications/2006_Classif_worksheet.pdf. Copyright 2006 by the American Spinal Injury Association. Reprinted with permission.

just beginning to be understood (National Institute of Neurologic Disorders and Stroke [NINDS], 1996).

2) Immune system: Its role in neurological damage and recovery is poorly understood. After damage occurs, the immune system does respond. Some cells remove cellular debris, and others release substances that are beneficial to neuron recovery. These are the cells that we need to learn how to trigger. Other immune system cells are detrimental to neural repair and learning how to turn them off is a key to promoting neural recovery (NINDS, 1996).

3) Cooling of neurological tissue: Mild hypothermia (therapeutic hypothermia)

appears to protect neurological tissue by blocking the cascade of events that occur shortly after the insult has occurred.

a) Risks appear to be low.

b) Can be done externally or internally

c) Still need to do controlled studies with multiple sites using the same protocol (www.neurologyreviews.com)

2. Regeneration: For successful regeneration to occur, damaged nerve cells and surrounding cells must survive or be replaced. Axons must be able to be targeted to appropriate connections. It is now thought that even if a small amount of neurons regenerate, a significant amount of neural recovery will occur (NINDS, 1996).

a. Nerve cell differentiation occurs during embryonic development.

b. Nervous tissue gives off signals that help to differentiate one section from another and different neurochemical transmitters (NINDS, 1996).

c. For regeneration to be successful, the neurons must not only grow but also be able to locate and connect to appropriate targets.

d. Regeneration also requires that the appropriate environment be available for the nervous tissue to grow. Different areas need different trophic factors to be present.

e. Scientists are now beginning to apply this knowledge to animal models of spinal cord and brain injury.

3. Transplantation: By transplanting peripheral nerves into the area of neural damage, you can form a bridge over the damaged area. This appears to work better in newborn animal models than in adult ones (NINDS, 1996).

4. Locomotor pathways: Using "patterning" via a treadmill and harness system, it has been shown that when appropriately stimulated with neurotransmitters from sensory nerves, the spinal cord has a "central pattern generator" that allows the motor nerves to fire. Stimulation of these pathways has helped to speed recovery in some people. This appears to assist people with all types of neurological disorders.

C. Current Thought: It will probably take more than one modality to cure neurological injuries. The devastation that occurs with each injury will have to be looked at individually to determine which modality may be the most appropriate to use on that person. However, today the research community is hopeful that soon an algorithm for curing neurological devastation will be developed.

References

American Spinal Injury Association. (2002). *Standards for neurological classification of spinal injury patients* (6th ed.). Chicago: American Spinal Injury Association.

Bader, M. K., & Littlejohns, L. R. (2004). *AANN core curriculum for neuroscience nursing* (4th ed.). Philadelphia: Saunders.

Barker, E. (1994). *Neuroscience nursing: A spectrum of care.* St. Lous: Mosby.

Barker, E. (2004). *Neuroscience nursing* (1st ed.). St. Louis, Mosby.

Barker, E. (2010). *Neuroscience nursing* (3rd ed.). St. Louis: Mosby.

Chin, P. A. (1998). Nursing process and nurse client relationship. In P. A. Chin, D. Finocchiaro, & A. Rosebrough (Eds.), *Rehabilitation nursing practice* (pp. 61–76). New York: McGraw-Hill.

Goshgarian, H. G. (2003). Anatomy and function of the spinal cord. In V. W. Lin (Ed.), *Spinal cord medicine: Principles and practice.* New York: Demos.

Hickey, J. V. (2008). *The clinical practice of neurological and neuroscience nursing* (6th ed.). Houston, TX: J. B. Lippincott.

Lee, H. J., Macbeth, A. H., Pagani, J. H., & Young, W. S. (2009, June). Oxytocin: The great facilitator of life. *Progress in Neurobiology, 88*(2), 127–151.

Lewis, S. M., Heitkemper, M. M., & Dirksen, S. R. (2004). *Medical-surgical nursing: Assessment and management of clinical problems* (6th ed.). St. Louis: Mosby.

Mosby. (2006). *Mosby's dictionary of medical, nursing & health professions* (7th ed.). St. Louis: Mosby Elsevier.

National Institute of Neurologic Disorders and Stroke. (1996). *Spinal cord injury: Emerging concepts.* Retrieved September 6, 2011, from www.ninds.nih.gov/news_and_events/proceedings/sci_report.htm.

Tator, C. H. (2000). Clinical manifestations of acute spinal cord injury. In C. H. Tator & E. C. Benzel (Eds.), *Contemporary management of spinal cord injury: From impact to rehabilitation* (pp. 21–32). Park Ridge, IL: American Association of Neurological Surgeons.

Wong, D. (1999). *Whaley & Wong's nursing care of infants and children* (6th ed.). St. Louis: Mosby.

Zejdlik, C. M. (1992). *Management of spinal cord injury.* Boston: Jones & Bartlett.

Suggested Resources

American Association of Neuroscience Nurses. (2004). *AANN core curriculum for neuroscience nursing* (4th ed.). Glenview, IL: Author.

Barker, E. (2010). *Neuroscience nursing.* St. Louis: Mosby.

Brain Injury Association of America: www.biausa.org

Clayman, C. (1995). *The human body: An illustrated guide to its structure, function, and disorders.* New York: DK Publishing.

Netter, F. (2006). *Atlas of human anatomy* (4th ed.). Philadelphia: Saunders Elsevier.

CHAPTER 10
Clients with Acute and Chronic Neurological Diseases

Joan P. Alverzo, PhD CRRN • Michele Russell Ward, BS CRRN

Life with a chronic illness is still life.

Rehabilitation nurses play an important role in caring for people with a wide variety of chronic illnesses and disabilities. This chapter covers the following specific disease processes that warrant rehabilitation interventions:

- Multiple sclerosis (MS)
- Parkinson's disease (PD)
- Amyotrophic lateral sclerosis (ALS)
- Guillain-Barré syndrome (GBS)
- Myasthenia gravis (MG)
- Postpolio syndrome (PPS)

Coping with a chronic condition is very stressful. Rehabilitation nurses are the ideal practitioners to provide and coordinate client and family education and interventions to help clients integrate the effects of their illness into daily life and become as independent as possible. It is important for rehabilitation nurses to have current knowledge and the requisite skills to prevent complications and modify the effects of chronic conditions regardless of the practice setting.

I. Multiple Sclerosis (MS)

A. Overview
1. A chronic neuroimmunologic condition that affects the white matter of the central nervous system (CNS)
2. Affects primarily adults in the prime years of life, with an increasing incidence in children and adolescents
3. Characterized by numerous etiologic possibilities, an uncertain prognosis, and a course that consists of episodes of remission and relapse
4. An unpredictable disease that can result in diverse neurologic impairments and necessitates a collaborative approach to care
5. A degenerative progressive disease characterized by inflammation, demyelination (loss of the myelin sheath that surrounds the nerve fiber tracts), plaques in the white matter of the CNS, and scarring of the myelin sheath in the CNS
6. Involves partial or complete destruction of the myelin sheath followed by sclerotic plaques or scar tissue formation
7. Associated with various signs and symptoms caused by the loss of myelin sheath integrity that interferes with the efficiency of nerve impulse conduction in the CNS

8. The name *multiple sclerosis* signifies that myelin is lost in multiple areas, leaving scar tissue.

B. Epidemiology
1. Incidence
   a. Currently there are approximately 350,000–500,000 people affected with MS in the United States and 2.5 million people worldwide (Multiple Sclerosis Foundation, 2009; National Multiple Sclerosis Society, 2010).
   b. Approximately 200 MS cases are diagnosed every week (National Multiple Sclerosis Society, 2010).
   c. A major cause of disability and economic hardship in young adults between the ages of 20 and 40
   d. Occurs more often in women than men, in people who live in colder northern latitudes, in Caucasians, and in people who have first-degree relatives with MS (Monahan, Sands, Neighbors, Marek, & Green, 2007)
   e. Strong association between ultraviolet radiation and MS distribution, with a higher rate in areas with a low ultraviolet index (Beretich & Beretich, 2009)
   f. The number of children with MS is climbing, and statistics suggest there may be 20,000 undiagnosed pediatric MS cases in the United States. Healthcare providers do not typically associate MS with children (Steefel, 2006).
   g. MS onset during childhood and adolescence presents unique diagnostic challenges and requires specialized multidisciplinary care for optimal management (Venkateswaran & Banwell, 2010).
   h. There is recent early evidence of an increased risk of MS with vitamin D deficiency, but further research is needed. This may have implications for sunscreen use for those who live in northern climates (Smolders, 2010).
   i. The overall pattern of lower paid employment among people with MS compared with other chronic diseases is related to delayed symptom management, with men likely to leave the workplace earlier than women (Simmons, Tribe, & McDonald, 2010).
2. Disease patterns

a. Relapsing-remitting MS: The most typical pattern of the disease
    1) Defined by episodes with clear relapses (also known as exacerbations or acute attacks) followed by complete or partial recovery periods (remission) free of disease progression
    2) Involves no disease progression between relapses
b. Secondary progressive MS
    1) Can begin as a relapsing-remitting course followed by progression that is unpredictable
    2) Involves acute attacks that can result in a progressive worsening level of disability
c. Primary progressive MS: Identified by a slow but continuous worsening of the client's disability but with no actual relapses or remissions
d. Progressive relapsing MS
    1) Marked by disease progression from the onset with definite acute relapses
    2) Involves disease progression that continues to escalate between relapses

C. Etiology
1. The specific cause remains unknown.
2. Factors that may be involved in causing MS are viral, immunologic, and genetic susceptibility.
    a. A latent viral infection may cause inflammation of white matter or trigger an autoimmune reaction that precipitates demyelination.
    b. Although there is no specific genetic pattern of transmission for MS, researchers support a multigenic predisposition that makes certain people susceptible to the disease (National Multiple Sclerosis Society, 2010).
    c. Various stressors including emotional stress, fatigue, pregnancy, viral infection, extreme physical exertion, trauma, and secondary illness have been suggested as triggers for MS.

D. Pathophysiology
1. Overview
    a. Normally, an intact blood-brain barrier protects the brain from immune-cell activity. In MS, the protective barrier is breached as activated T cells migrate into the CNS, triggering antibody-antigen reaction and resulting in inflammation, leading to loss of myelin, disappearance of oligodendrocytes, and proliferation of astrocytes or scavenger cells that remove the damaged myelin, forming scar tissue over the affected area (Lewis et al., 2004; Monahan et al., 2007).
    b. Inflammation and oligodendrocyte loss are found in MS, but determining which comes first has been a focus of recent research (Lewis et al., 2004).
    c. Demyelination appears as diffuse, discrete lesions (plaques) throughout the brain and spinal cord.
        1) Although natural healing (remyelination) by oligodendrocytes may restore some myelin function, the characteristic plaque formation or sclerosis interferes with normal nerve conduction.
        2) Nerve impulses slow down initially; eventually, with permanently damaged nerve fibers the impulses are completely blocked.
        3) Plaques or lesions vary in diameter from 1–2 mm to several centimeters and have an affinity for the optic nerves, periventricular white matter, brainstem, cerebellum, and spinal cord white matter.
        4) Sites of demyelination can occur anywhere in the CNS, producing a wide range of signs and symptoms; however, progressive scarring leads to progressive deterioration in neurological function (Lewis et al., 2004).

2. Clinical manifestations (**Table 10-1**)
    a. Primary symptoms
        1) Occur as the result of the nerve conduction deficits caused by demyelination and plaque formation
        2) Reflect a specific area of dysfunction in the CNS
        3) Symptoms may range from mild to severe; symptoms are unpredictable and vary from person to person and from time to time in the same person.
    b. Secondary symptoms
        1) Occur as a consequence of primary symptoms
        2) Include problematic complications resulting from decreased neurologic function
    c. Tertiary symptoms
        1) Evolve as the cumulative and detrimental effects of the disease affect all aspects of the person's life
        2) Include psychosocial, vocational, financial, and emotional problems

3. Diagnosis
    a. There is no specific laboratory or radiologic test to definitively diagnose MS.
    b. Because MS can mimic other diseases and the initial symptomatic presentation varies and fluctuates so greatly in severity, the diagnosis

Table 10-1. Symptomatic Manifestations of Multiple Sclerosis

Primary Symptoms	Secondary Symptoms	Tertiary Symptoms
Muscle weakness, paralysis, spasticity, and hyperreflexia	Falls, fractures, skin breakdown, contractures, and other injuries	Loss of job
Mild to disabling fatigue	Marked reduction in carrying out all aspects of self-care	Complete change in roles
Visual impairments (e.g., diplopia, scotoma, decreased acuity)	Decreased safety caused by decreased visual input	Social isolation
Numbness, tingling, pain, and tremors	Interruption in rest and disrupted sleep	Divorce
Bowel, bladder, and sexual dysfunction	Urinary tract infections, bowel and bladder incontinence or retention, and marked decline in libido and orgasmic ability	Ineffective coping with anxiety, denial, anger, reactive depression, and suicide
Ataxia, nystagmus, dysarthria (scanning speech), and dysphagia	Problems affecting a safe gait pattern, communication ability, and swallowing function	Loss of financial stability, self-esteem, and self-worth
Cognitive changes (e.g., memory loss, impaired judgment), emotional lability, and depression	Marked decline in healthy and effective coping strategies	

of MS is a challenge and a process of eliminating all other possibilities.

c. Diagnostic tests that can support a suspected MS diagnosis include the following:

1) Magnetic resonance imaging (MRI)

   a) Extremely sensitive to white matter lesions and useful in identifying demyelinated plaque in the CNS

   b) Is used to distinguish between old and new lesions and to monitor disease progression

2) Cerebrospinal fluid analysis reveals elevated immunoglobulin G and the presence of oligoclonal (immunoglobulin G) bands and increased protein.

3) Evoked potential studies (somatosensory, auditory, visual) demonstrate a slow, absent, or abnormal response in electrical impulse conduction.

4) The Schumacher criteria and the revised McDonald criteria are commonly used criteria for diagnosis of MS.

   a) Schumacher criteria include an abnormal neurologic exam; white matter involvement; two or more sites of the CNS; pattern of relapsing, remitting, and progressing; age 10 to 50; and no other explanation of symptoms (Mattson, 2002).

   b) McDonald criteria include number of clinical attacks, number of objective lesions on MRI, in some categories other required evidence, in some categories cerebrospinal fluid (CSF) findings (Mattson, 2002).

E. Management Options

1. Goal: To decrease the number and frequency of relapses, enhance recovery from exacerbations, alleviate symptoms, maintain independence, and ensure the highest quality of life (Lewis et al., 2004; Monahan et al., 2007)

2. Pharmacotherapy (**Figure 10-1**)

   a. The necessity of early treatment for MS has been established to provide an opportunity to intervene early and potentially mitigate the progression of the disease.

   b. Treatments to change the course of the disease (Multiple Sclerosis Foundation, 2009)

   1) Interferon-beta products shut down the inflammation of lesions and are given by subcutaneous injection. These drugs include Betaseron, Avonex, and Rebif.

   2) Glatiramer acetate (Copaxone) suppresses the immune system's attack on myelin and is administered by subcutaneous injection.

   3) Monoclonal antibody (Tysabri) is a humanized monoclonal antibody and works by blocking the white blood cell receptors that allow them to enter the brain and spinal cord, leading to decreased inflammation.

   4) Mitoxantrone (Novantrone) slows the progression of the disease by suppressing the activity of T cells and B cells.

   5) Steroid treatment is used to shorten the duration of acute attacks but does not reduce the frequency of exacerbations.

   c. Treatment to manage symptoms may be extensive (**Table 10-2**).

   d. Baclofen is most often used to treat spasticity and tremor.

Figure 10-1. Pharmacotherapeutic Agents Used to Treat MS

Treatment of Acute Relapses
Short course of anti-inflammatory corticosteroids
- Methylprednisolone (Solu-Medrol)
- Adrenocorticotropic hormone
- Prednisone

Treatment to Reduce the Frequency of Relapses
Parenteral injections of immunomodulators (effective for only one or two MS disease patterns)
- Interferon beta-1b (Betaseron)
- Interferon beta-1a (Avonex, Rebif)
- Glatiramer acetate (Copaxone)

Treatment of Disease Progression
Immunosuppressants that halt disease progression
- Azathioprine (Imuran)
- Methotrexate (Rheumatrex)

Treatment of Spasticity and Tremor
- Baclofen (Lioresal)
- Dantrolene (Dantrium)
- Tizanidine (Zanaflex)
- Diazepam (Valium)
- Clonazepam (Klonopin)
- Botulinum toxin (Botox)

Treatment of Urinary Retention
- Bethanechol chloride (Urecholine)

Treatment of Urinary Frequency and Urgency
- Propantheline (Pro-Banthine)
- Oxybutynin (Ditropan)

Treatment of Chronic Pain, Fatigue, and Depression
- Carbamazepine (Tegretol)
- Pemoline (Cylert)
- Amitriptyline (Elavil)
- Imipramine (Tofranil)
- Fluoxetine (Prozac)

e. Injections of glatiramer acetate or interferon may produce local reactions, including itching, pain, swelling, or redness and reduce adherence to the regimen (Pardo, Boutwell, Conner, Denney, & Loeen-Burkey, 2010).

3. MS has become increasingly expensive to manage because of medication prices, but this has been counterbalanced by a decrease in exacerbation and hospitalizations, influencing many national insurance companies to cover these medications (Lad et al., 2010).

4. Alternative approaches (e.g., bee venom therapy, massage, herbal treatment, dietary modifications; National Multiple Sclerosis Society, 2010)

   a. Approximately 75% of people with MS use some form of complementary and alternative medicine.

   b. Clients using alternative therapies should inform their physicians because of potential interactions with other medications.

   c. Alternatives should not be substituted for conventional therapies.

   d. Research on the impact of these alternative approaches is difficult because the course of the disease is so variable.

5. Use of a collaborative team of professionals, including physicians, physical and occupational therapists, spiritual advisers, social workers, psychologists, vocational rehabilitation specialists, legal advisors, and nurses

6. Exercise

   a. Aquatic or water therapy gives buoyancy to the body, allowing performance of activities that otherwise would not be possible.

   b. Yoga and tai chi can be beneficial.

   c. Exercises that are fatiguing should be avoided.

7. Nutritional therapy

   a. A high-protein, low-fat, and low-cholesterol diet with supplemental vitamins is recommended (Lewis et al., 2004; Multiple Sclerosis Foundation, 2009).

   b. Natural fiber is encouraged to promote bowel regularity.

8. Cognitive-behavioral programs have improved outcomes for many clients, particularly women (Sinclair & Scroggie, 2005).

9. Neuropathic pain, including central neuropathic pain, occurs in more than 40% of people with MS and is described as constant, often spontaneous burning, most often in the lower limbs (Solaro & Messmer Uccelli, 2010).

   a. Treatment includes tricyclic antidepressants and antiepileptic medication. Cannabinoids can be useful for some people.

   b. Antispasticity medications such as baclofen and benzodiazepines are often used to manage spasticity-related pain.

10. Spasticity and incontinence symptoms may be treated with botulinum toxin injections, but the studies to confirm its efficacy are still pending (Habek, Kami, Balash, & Gurevich, 2010).

F. Nursing Process

1. Assessment

   a. Obtain a complete health history and information about current symptoms, time of onset, and past history of relapses, including recent or past viral infections or vaccinations, physical or emotional stress, pregnancy, or exposure to extremes of heat and cold based

Table 10-2. Pharmacologic Treatment Options for Primary Multiple Sclerosis Symptoms

Symptom	Drug and Dose	Adverse Effects
Spasticity	Baclofen (Lioresal) 5–20 mg tid up to 80 mg/d; continuous intrathecal pump if cannot tolerate or unresponsive to oral therapy	Drowsiness, vertigo, ataxia, weakness
	Tizanidine 4 mg qhs increased to bid or tid frequency up to 36 mg/d	Dry mouth, elevation of liver enzymes, daytime drowsiness
	Diazepam (Valium) 0.5–10 mg 2–4 times/d	Drowsiness, fatigue
	Dantrolene (Dantrium) 25 mg daily up to 100 mg bid-qid	Increased muscle weakness, drowsiness, diarrhea
Urinary (urgency, incontinence, frequency, nocturia)	Oxybutynin (Ditropan) 2.5–5 mg bid or tid up to 5 mg qid; extended-release product 5 mg daily up to 30 mg daily	Dry mouth, constipation, drowsiness
	Tolterodine (Detrol) 1–2 mg bid; extended-release product 2–4 mg daily	Dry mouth
	Tarrisulosin (Flomax) 0.4–0.8 mg daily	Headache, dizziness
Fatigue	Amantadine (Symmetrel) 100–200 mg bid	Hypotension, depression, irritability
	Modafinil (Provigil) 100–200 mg daily up to 400 mg/d	Headache, nausea
Sensory (burning, itching, neuralgia)	Carbamazepine (Tegretol) 100 mg bid-tid up to 1,200 mg/d	Dizziness, hyponatremia, nausea, ataxia
	Gabapentin (Neurontin) 100 mg tid up to 4,800 mg/d	Somnolence, dizziness, ataxia, fatigue
	Amitriptyline (Elavil) 25 mg qhs up to 100 mg/d	Dry mouth, sedation, hypotension
Tremors	Propranolol (Inderal) 20 mg bid up to 320 mg/d	Bradycardia, bronchospasm
	Primidone (Mysoline) 125 mg qhs up to 2,000 mg/d in divided doses 3–4 times/d	Drowsiness, ataxia, nausea
	Clonazepam (Klonopin) 0.25 mg bid up to 2 mg/d	Drowsiness, ataxia
Depression	Sertraline (Zoloft) 25 mg daily up to 200 mg/d	Insomnia, dizziness, headache
	Citalopram (Celexa) 20 mg daily up to 60 mg/d	Somnolence, insomnia, nausea
Sexual	Sildenafil (Viagra) 50 mg given 30 min–4 hr before sexual activity; avoid with concurrent use of nitroglycerin	Headache, flushing

From "Pharmacologic management of neuroscience patients" (p. 260), by T. F. Lassiter & A. L. Henkel, 2008. In J. V. Hickey (Ed.), *The clinical practice of neurological and neurosurgical nursing* (6th ed.), Philadelphia: Lippincott Williams & Wilkins. Copyright 2008 by Lippincott Williams and Wilkins. Reprinted with permission.

on their potential to trigger an exacerbation (Hickey, 2009).

b. Pay particular attention to mental state and overt coping abilities.

c. Determine how the disease has affected the client's lifestyle and family.

d. Observe the client's overall appearance.

e. Investigate physical mobility, urinary elimination, self-care activities, and safety concerns.

f. Assess for spasticity, weakness, incontinence, and visual impairments.

g. Investigate use of and compliance in taking prescription medications and alternative approaches.

2. Plan of care

a. Nursing diagnoses

1) Impaired physical mobility related to neuromuscular impairment (weakness, spasticity, and tremor)

2) Fatigue related to the MS disease process

3) Self-care deficits (e.g., bathing, dressing, feeding, toileting) related to weakness, spasticity, and tremor

4) Altered urinary elimination (e.g., retention, frequency, urgency) related to spinal cord involvement and decreased functional ability

5) Knowledge deficit related to the variable nature of symptoms and multifaceted treatment options

6) Ineffective individual coping related to the variability of the disease course, cognitive impairments, decreased independence, and changes in family and vocational roles
7) Sensory perception alterations: Visual, related to optic nerve involvement (diplopia, nystagmus, blurred vision)
8) Chronic pain related to neuropathy
9) Impaired communication related to impaired muscles of speech
10) High risk for aspiration related to impaired muscles for swallowing
11) Ineffective breathing patterns related to impaired respiratory muscles
12) Altered nutrition, less than required, related to inability to swallow (Hickey, 2009)

b. Goals
1) Maintain maximal level of mobility.
2) Demonstrate safety in mobility and recognize the need for appropriate assistive devices.
3) Conserve energy and verbalize understanding of ways to integrate energy conservation principles into daily activities.
4) Attain maximal level of function in activities of daily living (ADLs).
5) Maintain continence and identify symptoms of urinary tract infection.
6) Verbalize understanding of the disease process, significant implications, and prescribed regimens.
7) Verbalize appropriate plans for coping with stress.
8) Attain maximal visual functioning and demonstrate satisfactory use of compensatory measures when needed.
9) Verbalize satisfactory pain relief.

3. Nursing interventions
a. Improve mobility and neuromuscular function.
1) Encourage progressive, resistive exercises according to the prescribed physical therapy program to maintain function of the uninvolved nerves.
2) Gradually build up tolerance through a daily exercise program.
3) Use assistive devices (e.g., walker, cane, wheelchair, motorized scooter).
4) Avoid physical and emotional stressors.
5) Avoid exposure to extreme heat and schedule activities to occur during the cooler part of the day; ensure that air conditioning is available in warm weather.
b. Conserve energy.

1) Avoid vigorous exercise.
2) Ensure adequate sleep and frequent rest periods.
3) Space out activities and allow rest periods.
c. Maintain independence in ADLs.
1) Encourage a balance between assisted and independent activities.
2) Encourage the use of assistive devices to promote independence.
3) Avoid extremes in body temperature and use air conditioning when needed.
d. Improve bladder function and prevent complications.
1) Avoid caffeinated beverages and encourage high daily fluid intake (approximately 3,000 mL per day).
2) Administer medications to improve muscle tone of bladder and facilitate emptying and instruct client on effective use of medication.
3) Teach intermittent self-catheterization or external catheter procedures.
4) Use Credé's maneuver or manual reflex stimulation for emptying reflexic bladder (unless contraindicated by complications such as detrusor sphincter dyssynergia).
5) Instruct the client to identify and prevent urinary tract infections.
e. Improve knowledge.
1) Provide information to help manage the disease on a continuous basis.
2) Encourage the client to ask questions.
3) Review educational information with the client and family.
f. Develop effective coping strategies to adjust to the illness.
1) Encourage the client and family to verbalize feelings and concerns.
2) Refer the client and family to support groups (e.g., Multiple Sclerosis Association of America, National Multiple Sclerosis Society).
3) Make referrals for psychological counseling as necessary.
g. Maintain visual functioning.
1) Administer treatment as needed (eye patch or occluder, medications).
2) Instruct clients to rest their eyes when fatigue is noticed.
3) Advise clients of availability of large-type material and talking books.
h. Promote comfort.

      1) Provide medication as ordered for pain control and instruct on effective use of medications and precautions.

      2) Manage spasticity, including a medication regimen and positioning or movement to reduce the incidence of spasticity.

      3) Encourage use of alternative pain relief measures (distraction, relaxation, imagery, music, massage).

      4) Assess effectiveness of pain relief measures.

II. Parkinson's Disease (PD)

A. Overview

1. PD is a slowly progressive neurodegenerative disease of the brain.

2. PD involves manifestations that occur when there is significant damage to or destruction of dopamine-producing neurons in the substantia nigra within the basal ganglia of the brain.

3. PD begins insidiously and is characterized by a prolonged course of illness.

4. Loss of dopamine causes neurons to fire out of control, leading to marked disability with the initiation and execution of smooth, coordinated voluntary movements and balance.

5. There is no known way to stop or cure the disease.

6. PD is one of the more common chronic diseases of the nervous system.

7. Types

    a. Primary PD

      1) A chronic debilitating disease caused by an idiopathic dopamine deficiency in the basal ganglia of the brain

      2) Characterized by tremor, rigidity, bradykinesia, and postural instability

    b. Secondary parkinsonism or parkinsonism syndrome: A group of symptoms (e.g., tremors, stiffness, slow movements) in which there is a known cause of injury to the dopamine-producing cells

B. Epidemiology and Incidence

1. Approximately 1 million Americans have PD. The disease shows no socioeconomic or cultural preferences. Approximately 4 million people worldwide are living with PD (Parkinson's Disease Foundation, 2010).

2. Approximately 60,000 new cases are diagnosed annually in the United States (Parkinson's Disease Foundation, 2010).

3. PD occurs in men slightly more often than women.

4. PD most commonly occurs after age 55. With an aging population, the prevalence of PD is likely to increase. The mean age of onset for PD is 60 (Hayes, Fung, Kimber, & O'Sullivan, 2010).

5. Approximately 10% of people with PD are younger than age 40; however, the incidence in younger people has been growing (Monahan et al., 2007).

C. Etiology

1. Primary PD is idiopathic.

2. A number of theories of causation for PD are being tested, including viral, vascular, metabolic, environmental, event, and genetic, although PD is currently believed to be associated with a combination of genetic and environmental factors (e.g., viruses, toxins, free radical exposure; Monahan et al., 2007).

3. There is some suggestion that the use of nonsteroidal anti-inflammatory drugs may provide some protection from developing the disease (Gagne & Power, 2010).

4. Secondary parkinsonism may be linked to a variety of causes: Response to antipsychotic, antihypertensive, or neuroleptic agents or illicit drug use; response to brain trauma, tumors, ischemia, encephalitis infections, and arteriosclerosis; response to neurotoxins such as cyanide, manganese, carbon monoxide, and pesticides (Monahan et al., 2007)

D. Pathophysiology

1. Overview

    a. The Braak hypothesis proposes that the earliest evidence of PD is found in the medulla and olfactory bulb and that the disease progresses to the substantia nigra and cortex (Hayes et al., 2010).

    b. Degenerative changes in several areas in the basal ganglia deplete the inhibitory neurotransmitter dopamine, normally provided to the basal ganglia by the neurons in the substantia nigra.

      1) Dopamine is a neurotransmitter essential for the functioning of the extrapyramidal system, which includes control of upright posture, support, and voluntary motion.

      2) Normally, there is a balance between the neurotransmitters dopamine and acetylcholine (ACh), which are responsible for controlling and refining motor movements and have opposing effects.

    c. An increase in the excitatory effects of ACh caused by depletion of dopamine causes the manifestations of PD and prevents affected brain cells from performing their normal inhibitory function in the CNS.

    d. A shift in the balance of neurotransmitter

activity is responsible for the client's difficulty in controlling and initiating voluntary movements (Lewis et al., 2004).

    e. As the disease progresses, dopamine receptors in the basal ganglia are reduced.

2. Clinical features: Classic manifestations (Monahan et al., 2007)

    a. Tremor

        1) Occurs in the tongue, lips, jaw, chin, head, and limbs

        2) May involve a pill-rolling movement of the thumb and finger

        3) Is present at rest and diminishes with active movement

    b. Rigidity or cogwheeling: Resistance to movement caused by constant contraction of opposing muscle groups, caused by abnormal muscle stiffness and jerky movements with passive motion

    c. Bradykinesia or akinesia: Inability to initiate movement or change movement, which results in abnormal slowness.

    d. Postural instability, which causes a stooped-over, flexed posture and a shuffling propulsive gait with no arm swing. Diminished postural reflexes lead to frequent falls that are associated with balance and coordination problems.

    e. Other symptoms: Mask-like facial appearance; difficulty with chewing, swallowing, and voice changes; autonomic disturbances (e.g., orthostatic hypotension, constipation, excessive perspiration, oily skin); and numerous cognitive losses (e.g., memory, problem solving, depression)

3. Diagnosis (Monahan et al., 2007)

    a. Diagnosis is made clinically from the client's history and presenting symptoms.

    b. No specific laboratory or radiologic studies are available to support a positive diagnosis.

    c. Positron emission tomography (PET) scan may detect low levels of dopamine (not typically done because of high cost and unavailability).

    d. Definitive diagnosis may be confirmed after assessment of the client's response to antiparkinson medications.

E. Management Options

1. General notes

    a. Currently, there is no known treatment that halts or reverses neuronal degeneration (Hayes et al., 2010).

    b. Current options provide symptom relief and improve quality of life.

    c. Nonmotor symptoms (sleep dysfunction, sensory symptoms, autonomic dysfunction, mood disorders, and cognitive abnormalities) add to the morbidity and are often underrecognized (Zesewicz et al., 2010).

2. Types of treatment

    a. Pharmacotherapy involves the use of drugs from various classes (e.g., monoamine oxidase B inhibitor, levodopa, dopamine agonist, antiviral, anticholinergic, and catechol-O-methyltransferase inhibitor; Monahan et al., 2007; **Table 10-3**).

        1) Levodopa is the gold standard for efficacy, but its chronic use is associated with potentially disabling motor complications (Poewe, 2009).

        2) The mode of administrating levodopa is key, and best results are achieved by subcutaneous or intraduodenal delivery of levodopa (Poewe, 2009).

Table 10-3. Drugs Prescribed for Symptomatic Control of Parkinson's Disease

Drug Category and Name	Action
Monoamine oxidase B inhibitor: selegiline (Eldepryl)	Used in the early stages of PD to delay the breakdown of naturally occurring dopamine
Carbidopa–levodopa (Sinemet)	Is the first-line, gold-standard therapy that restores deficient dopamine to the brain without causing extreme, uncomfortable peripheral side effects
Dopamine agonists: bromocriptine (Parlodel), pergolide (Permax), pramipexole (Mirapex), ropinirole (ReQuip)	Directly stimulates the dopamine receptors in the brain to produce more dopamine
Antiviral: amantadine (Symmetrel)	Acts by releasing dopamine from neuronal storage sites
Anticholinergic: benztropine (Cogentin), trihexyphenidyl (Artane)	Counteracts the action of acetylcholine in the central nervous system
Catechol-O-methyltransferase inhibitor: tolcapone (Tasmar)	Used in combination with Sinemet to block the enzyme that metabolizes levodopa, allowing more levodopa to be available for conversion to dopamine

b. Surgical interventions offer some people relief from some symptoms; however, they cannot improve the disease course or guarantee long-lasting disease improvement (Monahan et al., 2007).
   1) Pallidotomy and thalamotomy destroy groups of brain cells of the thalamus or basal ganglia to prevent involuntary movements, some of the most distressing symptoms.
   2) Thalamic or deep-brain stimulators have been approved by the Food and Drug Administration to treat tremor.
      a) Electrodes are surgically implanted into the thalamus, globus pallidus, or subthalamic nuclei and connected to a neurostimulator (pulse generator) implanted under the skin of the chest (like a pacemaker).
      b) After the system is in place, the device is programmed to deliver electrical stimulation sent from the neurostimulator up along the extension wire and the lead and into the brain to targeted areas that control movement, blocking the abnormal nerve signals that cause tremor and PD symptoms.
      c) The client can self-activate the device.
      d) Currently, the procedure is used only for people whose symptoms cannot be adequately controlled with medications.
      e) Many people experience reduction of their PD symptoms after undergoing deep-brain stimulation and are able to greatly reduce their medications (Deuschl et al., 2006).
c. Transplantation: Still in experimental stages, transplantation of fetal neural tissue into the brain is designed to provide dopamine-producing cells in the brain, allowing these cells to grow and process dopamine with a goal of either halting or reversing disease process (Brundin, Barker, & Parmar, 2010).
d. Nutritional intervention
   1) Diet should contain adequate roughage and fruit to prevent constipation
   2) Low-protein diet with less fat and more carbohydrates; foods high in protein can decrease absorption of levodopa (Lewis et al., 2004)
   3) Food should be cut into bite-size pieces, and ample time should be planned for eating.

e. Gastrointestinal, urological, and sexual dysfunction are common complications of PD and affect quality of life. Recognition and management of these conditions are critical to optimal clinical management (Pfeiffer, 2010).
f. Mood disorders, cognitive impairment, autonomic dysfunction, and sleep disorders are responsible for significant morbidity (Hayes et al., 2010).
   1) Psychosis is treated with the reduction of antiparkinson drugs and the use of atypical antipsychotics such as mianserin hydrochloride that do not exacerbate motor symptoms (Fujimoto, 2009).
   2) Orthostatic hypotension can be treated with isometric leg-holding exercises (Fujimoto, 2009).
   3) Mood disorders are difficult to treat because of the potential secondary effect on dopamine receptors (Fujimoto, 2009).
F. Nursing Process
   1. Assessment
      a. Obtain a complete health history and information about current symptoms, time of onset, and progression, including CNS trauma, exposure to metals and carbon dioxide, encephalitis, and use of tranquilizers or antipsychotic medications.
      b. Pay particular attention to mental status, ability to answer questions, and overt coping abilities.
      c. Determine how the disease has affected the client and family and ask about what aspects of the disease are most troublesome.
      d. Observe overall appearance, posture, and gait pattern.
      e. Determine level of extremity stiffness, tremors, and ability to move.
      f. Investigate safe mobility, self-care activities, nutritional intake, and verbal communication.
   2. Plan of care
      a. Nursing diagnoses (Monahan et al., 2007)
         1) Ineffective individual coping related to depression and increasingly severe physical limitations
         2) Knowledge deficit related to disease progression, treatment, ongoing adaptations, and availability of support systems
         3) Impaired physical mobility related to tremor, rigidity, bradykinesia, and postural instability
         4) Self-care deficits (e.g., bathing, dressing, feeding, toileting) related to tremor, rigidity, bradykinesia, and postural inability

5) Inadequate nutrition related to difficulty with chewing, swallowing, and drooling
6) Impaired verbal communication related to low voice, slow speech, and difficulty moving facial muscles
7) Risk of injury (falling) related to tremors, bradykinesia, and altered gait (Kerr et al., 2010)

b. Goals
1) Verbalize appropriate plans for coping with stress.
2) Verbalize understanding of the disease process, significant implications, and prescribed regimen.
3) Maintain maximal level of mobility.
4) Attain maximal level of function in ADLs.
5) Verbalize understanding of diet management and achieve adequate hydration and nutritional balance.
6) Communicate effectively.
7) Demonstrate safety in mobility and recognize the need for appropriate assistive devices.

3. Interventions
a. Develop positive coping mechanisms.
1) Allow the client to freely verbalize feelings and concerns.
2) Encourage participation in support groups (e.g., Parkinson's Disease Foundation, Parkinson's Support Groups of America, National Parkinson Foundation).
3) Encourage the client to establish realistic, attainable goals.
4) Support the use of prescribed psychotherapy and medication to combat depression.
b. Develop a sound knowledge base about the disease and treatments.
1) Teach the client about the common signs, symptoms, and progression of PD.
2) Discuss aspects of the disease that are unique to PD and the use of antiparkinson drugs (e.g., "on-off," "wearing off," and "freezing" phenomena).
3) Educate the client and family about the desired effects and side effects of prescribed medications and surgical treatments.
4) Offer suggestions to make living with PD easier, including energy conservation, home modifications, and assistive devices for walking or transfers from one surface to another.
5) Inform the client and family of local and national support groups for assistance and education.
c. Improve mobility and maximize neuromuscular function.
1) Encourage active and passive range of motion (ROM) exercises according to the prescribed physical therapy program.
2) Allow time for rest after activity and avoid rushing.
3) Administer medications as prescribed to avoid exacerbation of symptoms.
4) Use warm baths and massage to help relax muscles.
5) Teach to concentrate on walking erect by consciously using a wide-based gait and deliberately swinging the arms; teach the client to pretend to cross over an imaginary line or rock side to side to initiate leg movement to help deal with "freezing" while walking.
6) Provide muscle stretching and massage to reduce rigidity.
d. Maintain independence in ADLs.
1) Encourage the use of devices to make self-care easier (e.g., raised toilet seats, trapeze bar, grab bars, long-handled shoehorns, elastic shoelaces).
2) Allow adequate time to accomplish self-care.
3) Make environmental modifications to increase safety and independence.
e. Achieve satisfactory hydration and nutritional status.
1) Encourage clients to sit upright for all meals.
2) Offer semisolid foods and thickened liquids if choking occurs.
3) Use stabilized plates, plate guards, non-spill cups, and large-handled utensils.
4) Augment caloric intake with supplementary feedings.
5) Monitor weight weekly.
f. Improve verbal communication.
1) Reinforce exercises prescribed by the speech and language therapist.
2) Inform family and friends to wait for the client to answer questions.
3) Encourage the client to engage in conversation and read aloud.
g. Maintain safety.
1) Modify the environment to remove hazards and improve lighting.
2) Install devices for safety (e.g., grab bars, raised toilet seat).

THE SPECIALTY PRACTICE OF REHABILITATION NURSING

3) Change position slowly with orthostatic hypotension.

III. Amyotrophic Lateral Sclerosis (ALS)

A. Overview
1. A rapidly progressive neurodegenerative disease involving the destruction of motor neurons in the brainstem and the anterior gray horns of the spinal cord and degeneration of pyramidal tracts
2. Variations in disease progression exist. Functional loss may begin with upper-motor neurons, lower-motor neurons, bulbar symptoms only, or a combination.
3. Characterized by muscle weakness, wasting, and atrophy, followed by spasticity and hyperreflexia
4. Onset is often subtle, and first symptoms may be disregarded. Diagnosis consists of a combination of tests. No single test exists to diagnose ALS.
5. There is no known prevention and no known cure for ALS, but treatments exist to assist in slowing deterioration.
6. Rehabilitation focuses on adaptation to increasing losses of function. Caregiver training will be necessary as the disease progresses and the client loses self-care abilities.
7. This disease was historically called Lou Gehrig's disease because of the national and international attention the baseball star brought to ALS after his 1939 diagnosis, but a new study has cast doubt on whether he had ALS or another neurological condition (Schwarz, 2010).

B. Epidemiology
1. Approximately 30,000 people in the United States have ALS at any given time. The incidence ranges from 1.5–2.5 per 100,000 people (Logroscino et al., 2008).
2. Approximately 15 new cases are diagnosed per day in the United States (Cronin, Hardiman, & Trayor, 2007).
3. Prevalence in men is higher. According to the ALS database in 2008, 60% were male.
4. ALS occurs typically during midlife, between 40 and 70 years of age. The most common age group is 40–60, and the most common ethnic group is Caucasian (Cronin et al., 2007).
5. Life expectancy is 2–5 years from the time of diagnosis. More than half of those with ALS live longer than 3 years (ALS Association, 2010).

C. Etiology
1. Sporadic, unknown cause (90%–95% of cases)
2. Genetic (5%–10% of cases), an inherited autosomal dominant trait (Hickey, 2009)

D. Pathophysiology

1. Overview
a. ALS is characterized by destruction of motor neurons primarily in the motor nuclei of the brainstem, anterior horn cells of the spinal cord, corticospinal tracts, and Betz's and pre-central cells of the frontal cortex.
b. Asymmetric muscle weakness and wasting occurs most often, leading to paresis, and progression of functional loss varies.
1) Upper-motor neuron involvement will cause reduced strength and spasticity, often beginning with the intrinsic muscles of the hands.
2) Lower motor neuron involvement will cause weakening, muscular atrophy, and paralysis.
c. Although intellectual ability, vision, hearing, and sensation are generally not affected throughout the disease process, some people do experience cognitive deficits.
2. Differentiation of ALS from motor neuron disease with variants (Polak, Richman, Lorimer, Bonton Despulveda, & Del Bene, 2004)
a. Motor neuron disease with variants
1) Primary lateral sclerosis, with limited upper motor neuron component, with the longest survival (in the decades) and progressive decline
2) Progressive bulbar palsy, with bulbar symptoms and upper or lower motor neuron involvement, with a poor prognosis
3) Progressive muscular atrophy, with lower motor neuron changes and a prognosis similar to that of ALS
b. ALS
1) Asymmetric distal weakness greater than proximal weakness
2) Upper and lower motor neuron symptoms as well as bulbar and thoracic symptoms
3. Theoretical models (Polak et al., 2004)
a. Excitotoxicity: Glutamate defect in possibly metabolism, transport, or storage
b. Oxidative stress caused by excessive free radicals
c. Autoimmune
1) Antibodies to calcium channels
2) Activated T lymphocytes
3) Monoclonal paraproteinemia
d. Cytoskeletal
e. Neurofilament abnormalities: Abnormal accumulation and damage to structure
4. Clinical manifestations

a. Asymmetric weakness in all extremities occurs progressively with no remission. Ability to perform ADLs and instrumental ADLs is lost as function decreases.

b. Intrinsic muscles of hands lose function, resulting in inability to perform fine motor movement (e.g., buttoning pants, tying shoes, writing).

c. Weakening and loss of gross motor muscles result in inability to walk or stand.

d. Bulbar symptoms affect swallowing ability. Not every person experiences this symptom.

e. Brainstem involvement can account for cranial nerve function loss. Fasciculation, flaccidity, or spasticity can occur in the tongue, hands, and upper extremities.

f. Frontal lobe involvement can result in emotional lability regardless of intact intellect.

g. Loss of bowel and bladder function and eye movement often occur late in disease progression.

h. Complete paresis often occurs as the disease progresses.

i. Respiratory muscle involvement inhibits proper breathing, necessitating mechanical support at the client's discretion.

j. Dysarthria in ALS is related to quality of life, and maintaining effective communication is a priority of treatment (Tomik & Gulloff, 2010).

k. Pain is a common symptom in the later stages. There is little research about how to manage pain in ALS, so conventional pain management strategies should be used (Brettschneider, Kurent, Ludolph, & Mitchell, 2008).

l. Cognitive impairments can be grouped into two types: those with clear frontotemporal dementia with cognitive decline and increased apathy and those with mild cognitive impairments with no detectable progression (Woolley & Katz, 2008).

5. Diagnosis

a. A combination of laboratory testing, electrophysiology studies, neuroimaging studies, and muscle biopsy will be combined with history and physical to determine a diagnosis of ALS. There is no single test to diagnose ALS (**Table 10-4**).

b. Diagnosis is typically made late in the disease. Individual muscle group involvement early on may be mistaken for other health problems.

E. Management Options

1. A multidisciplinary approach is needed to meet the host of client problems that occur as the disease progresses (Miller et al., 2009). High-risk issues include the following:

   a. Aspiration pneumonia
   b. Malnutrition
   c. Loss of ability to speak
   d. Muscle spasticity and wasting
   e. Respiratory insufficiency
   f. Depression
   g. Preparation for disease progression
   h. Preparation for death

2. The focus should be on palliative care and comfort.

3. Key decisions related to management must be discussed in advance of a crisis (Rowland & Shineider, 2001).

4. A teaching plan is developed and individualized to the client and family.

5. The client is assisted to be as independent as possible for as long as possible with the use of assistive techniques and devices.

6. Education about symptom management is prepared and implemented.

7. The client and family are assisted to reduce the development of complications.

8. Referrals are provided to support groups, medical professionals, and community resources.

9. The client and family are assisted to prepare for decisions including gastrostomy tube placement and the use of mechanical ventilation.

10. The client and family are assisted to prepare for end-of-life decisions such as advance directives and hospice care and to resolve personal affairs.

Table 10-4. Diagnostics for Amyotrophic Lateral Sclerosis

- History
- Physical, including thorough neurological exam
- Electromyography to measure fasciculation potentials
- Nerve conduction velocity study
- Blood and urine studies
  - High resolution serum protein electrophoresis
  - Thyroid and parathyroid hormone levels
  - 24-hour urine collection for heavy metals
- Spinal tap
- X rays and magnetic resonance imaging
- Myelogram of cervical spine
- Muscle and/or nerve biopsy
- Ttranscranial magnetic stimulation can be used to measure the connection between the primary motor cortex and the muscle

From "Neuromuscular disorders" (p. 435), by L. Neal Boylan, 2008. In S. P. Hoeman (Ed.), *Rehabilitation nursing: Prevention, intervention, & outcomes* (4th ed.), St. Louis, Mosby. Copyright 2008 by Mosby. Reprinted with permission.

F. Nursing Process
  1. Assessment
    a. Obtain a complete health history, including family incidence of ALS and onset of symptoms.
    b. Assess current level of function and ability to perform ADLs and instrumental ADLs.
    c. Ask for a timeline of changes in function to understand progression of the client's disease.
    d. Evaluate functional status.
    e. Observe gait and evaluate strength and stability.
    f. Assess flaccidity, spasticity, and reported fasciculation in each muscle group.
    g. Evaluate swallowing and chewing ability.
    h. Evaluate respiratory status.
    i. Evaluate bowel and bladder function and the client's ability to use the bathroom, commode, or bedpan.
    j. Perform a skin assessment for wounds caused by decreased mobility.
    k. Observe client and family interactions. Consider how they discuss the disease process, their coping strategies, and their preparedness.
  2. Plan of care: Nursing diagnoses
    a. Impaired physical mobility related to muscle wasting, weakness, and spasticity
    b. Self-care deficit related to weakness, loss of function
    c. Impaired communication related to impairment of muscles for speech
    d. Ineffective breathing pattern related to impairment of diaphragm and accessory muscles
    e. Altered nutrition: Less than body requirements related to impaired bulbar muscles
    f. High risk for aspiration related to impaired bulbar muscles
    g. Potential for anxiety related to prognosis
    h. Risk for ineffective coping related to situation and prognosis
    i. Interrupted family processes related to change in health status in family member, modification of family roles, and foreseen loss of family member
    j. Risk for caregiver role strain related to severity of impairment from disease process
  3. Goals
    a. Maintain a maximum level of independence with ADLs.
    b. Demonstrate safety in activity and use of appropriate assistive devices.
    c. Limit complications from loss of function.
    d. Maintain nutrition intake.
    e. Maintain skin integrity.
    f. Verbalize an understanding of the disease process.
    g. Ensure comfort.
  4. Interventions
    a. Maintain independence with ADLs.
      1) Seek consultation with occupational therapist.
      2) Educate the client and family on available adaptive devices.
      3) Assess safety with use of mobility aids (cane, walker).
      4) Encourage expression of feelings about loss of independence to understand what is most important to the client.
    b. Limit complications from progressive loss of function.
      1) Ineffective breathing
        a) Consult with a respiratory therapist.
        b) Review energy-conservation techniques.
        c) Assess breathing pattern and presence of cyanosis or other signs of hypoxia.
        d) Provide suction as needed for stasis of secretions due to immobility.
        e) Teach use of equipment (e.g., oxygen, bilevel positive airway pressure, continuous positive airway pressure) as it is prescribed for the client.
      2) Impaired swallowing and decrease in nutritional intake
        a) Consult with a speech pathologist.
        b) Consult with a dietitian.
        c) Auscultate lungs for abnormal sounds.
        d) Evaluate weakness of facial and oral muscles.
        e) Implement dietary modifications as necessary based on the ability to swallow different consistencies of food.
        f) Teach the client to eat only one consistency at a time.
        g) Avoid milk products and sticky foods (peanut butter, white bread).
        h) Ingest smaller, more frequent meals.
        i) Provide information to assist the client in decision making about placement of gastrostomy tube as the disease progresses.
      3) Impaired communication
        a) Provide communication tools such as language boards, paper and pen if the client can still write, or a computer if the client can type.

b) Designate a system of blinking to spell out words when the client can no longer point at a language board.

c) Encourage patience from family members to ensure that the client is allowed to fully communicate needs.

c. Maintain skin integrity.

1) Assess skin for signs of pressure and breakdown.

2) Assess nutritional and fluid intake.

3) Educate the client and family about identifying the beginning of skin breakdown.

4) Educate the client and family about weight shifting and turning in bed to avoid pressure ulcers as mobility decreases.

5) When the client is no longer independent with bed mobility, turn him or her every 2 hours and weight shift every 20 minutes if the client is in a wheelchair.

6) Educate on keeping skin clean and dry and suggest use of proper lotions.

d. Discuss the disease process with the client and family.

1) Provide an open and trusting relationship with the client and family.

2) Encourage expression of feelings.

3) Educate the client and family about changes in function that will occur with disease progression and discuss their plan for adjustment at each stage.

4) Provide information to assist the family and client in decision making about advance directives, gastrostomy tube placement, and mechanical ventilation.

5) Provide referrals to support groups and medical professionals as needed.

6) Assess coping skills and seek consultation as appropriate.

7) Refer to hospice, palliative, or end-of-life care resources as appropriate.

8) Ensure that the client is comfortable.

9) Assess for pain due to immobility or contractures.

10) Provide medication as ordered for pain control and instruct the client on effective use of medications and precautions.

11) Encourage the use of alternative pain-relief measures (distraction, relaxation, imagery, music, massage).

12) Assess effectiveness of pain-relief measures.

IV. **Guillain-Barré Syndrome (GBS)**
    A. Overview

1. Classified as acute inflammatory polyneuropathy

2. An acute, inflammatory disease affecting the myelin of the nerves in the peripheral nervous system primarily. In some cases axonal degeneration can occur (Polak et al., 2004).

3. Autoimmune response that is triggered by a viral or bacterial infection

4. Onset can be a course of hours to about 3 weeks, and this phase ends when no addition deterioration is occurring.

5. The duration can span 3 years.

6. GBS can cause near complete paralysis, and rehabilitation will need to be a comprehensive program to assist and support the regaining of function in all body systems.

7. Residual weakness including pain and fatigue that may persist for months or years occurs in approximately 15%–25% of clients (Polak et al., 2004; van Doorn, Ruts, & Jacobs, 2008).

8. Very few clients remain totally paralyzed.

9. The disease can be life threatening and is considered a medical emergency, with mortality of 3%–10% due to complications of disease, not from the disease itself (van Doorn et al., 2008).

10. Twenty percent of clients are unable to walk 6 months after GBS (van Doorn, 2009).

11. Cognitive function and level of consciousness are not affected by GBS.

B. Epidemiology

1. Incidence

a. The annual incidence of GBS is between 1.1 and 1.8 per 100,000 people (McGrogan, Madle, Seaman, & de Vries, 2009), with GBS in children (15 years and younger) between 0.34 and 1.34 per 100,000.

b. Both genders, all ages, and all ethnicities are equally affected.

c. The incidence increases in those 50 years and older (McGrogan et al., 2009).

d. Hospitalization for GB has decreased in the past several years, probably because of the widespread availability of intravenous immunoglobulin (van Doorn, 2009).

2. Subtypes exist that vary in symptoms and pattern and in geographic distribution.

a. Acute inflammatory demyelination polyneuropathy (AIDP): Classic GBS, accounting for 90% of all cases in Western world (Vucic, Kiernan, & Cornblath, 2009)

b. Acute motor axonal neuropathy (AMAN): More prevalent in Asia and South and Central America (Vucic et al., 2009)

c. Acute motor sensory axonal neuropathy

(AMSAN): More prevalent in Asia and South and Central America (Vucic et al., 2009)

C. Etiology

1. The cause of GBS is unknown, but there are several triggers that seem to relate to the autoimmune attack on the body.

   a. Most often the client may have had a respiratory or gastrointestinal virus in the days to weeks before onset. The viruses typically considered include the following:

      1) *Campylobacter jejuni*
      2) Cytomegalovirus
      3) Epstein-Barr virus
      4) *Mycoplasma pneumoniae*

   b. Less often surgery or a vaccination is believed to cause onset. The vaccines considered to be most frequently associated with GBS are as follows:

      1) Rabies
      2) Swine flu
      3) Poliovirus

   c. There is only minimal evidence of an association between influenza vaccine and GBS (Jefferson et al., 2010).

2. There is no clear understanding of why a person does or does not get GBS.

3. No specific disease-causing agent has been identified, and so it is called a syndrome.

D. Pathophysiology

1. Overview

   a. Immune-mediated cellular and humoral response that triggers antibody production

   b. An antimyelin antibody has been identified that causes antimyelination.

   c. Normal myelin will be attacked by macrophages; inflammatory lesions occur throughout the peripheral nervous system.

      1) Schwann cells and myelin sheath, located on segmental peripheral nerves and the anterior and posterior spinal nerve roots, are affected.

      2) Severe lesions can cause axonal degeneration.

   d. Remyelination occurs slowly.

2. Variations

   a. AIDP

      1) Most common
      2) Numbness and weakness begin in legs and progress upward, ending at cranial nerves.
      3) Loss of motor function is symmetric.
      4) Sensory loss occurs, typically as mild numbness, and is typically most severe in the toes.

      5) Approximtely 50% of clients will need respiratory support.

   b. AMAN

      1) Progression is the same as that of GBS, but no sensory loss occurs.
      2) Children and young adults are affected most often.
      3) Muscle pain does not generally occur.
      4) AMAN is often considered a milder form of GBS.

   c. AMSAN

      1) Adults are most typically affected.
      2) Downward progression begins with motor weakness in brainstem cranial nerves.
      3) Respiratory involvement occurs quickly.
      4) Sensory loss and numbness occur distally, and are more prominent in hands than in feet.

   d. Miller-Fisher syndrome

      1) Very rare, occurring in approximately 5% of GBS cases (adults and children)
      2) Ophthalmoplegia, ataxia, and areflexia occur.
      3) Sensory loss does not typically occur.

3. Clinical manifestations (vary in severity depending on the individual case)

   a. Ascending symmetric motor weakness occurs.

   b. Ascending flaccid paralysis is typical.

   c. Loss of neurologic function and deep-tendon reflexes occurs.

   d. Respiratory insufficiency and failure may result from weakness in the diaphragm and intercostal muscles and mechanical failure.

   e. In approximately 50% of cases, damage to the facial nerve (CN VII) causes facial diplegia (Polak et al., 2004).

   f. If involved, damage to glossopharyngeal (CN IX) and vagus (CN X) nerves will cause dysphagia and laryngeal paralysis.

   g. Autonomic dysfunction is highly likely because of changes in sympathetic and parasympathetic nervous systems and certain if vagus nerves (CN X) are involved.

      1) Paroxysmal hypertension
      2) Orthostatic hypotension
      3) Cardiac arrhythmias
      4) Paralytic ileus
      5) Urinary retention
      6) Syndrome of inappropriate antidiuretic hormone secretion

   h. High sensitivity to touch and paresthesia typically occur and may include numbness, most often in the hands and feet.

i. Pain management can be challenging because of the adverse effects of drugs. Pain management may include opioids, nonsteroidal anti-inflammatory drugs, antidepressants, anticonvulsants, muscle relaxants, benzodiazepines, intravenous magnesium, and local anesthetics.

j. Pain is sometimes reported as cramping in lower extremities followed by acute pain in the trunk and upper extremities (Haroutinunian, Lecht, Zur, Hoffman, & Davidson, 2009).

4. Diagnosis

a. Criteria based on clinical presentation
1) Progressive weakness in two or more limbs due to neuropathy
2) Areflexia
3) Disease course of less than 4 weeks
4) Exclusion of other causes of symptoms

b. History of recent viral infection

c. Electrophysiological study shows slowing of conduction or a block in motor or sensory nerves (test can help distinguish between variations of disease).

d. Lumbar puncture shows increase in protein.

E. Management Options

1. Medical management will probably be urgent because of the rapid onset of the disease (Polak et al., 2004).

a. Therapeutic plasma exchange may be performed every other day for 10–15 days to decrease the severity and duration of the disease.

b. Intravenous immunoglobulin administration (divided dose of 1–2 mg/kg over 3–5 days) helps to lessen the attack on the nervous system.

c. Medication is often needed to assist with complications such as cardiac arrhythmias, blood pressure changes, constipation, urinary retention, and depression.

d. Corticosteroids do not appear to hasten the course of the illness, and oral corticosteroids may delay recovery (Hughes, Swan, & van Doorn, 2010).

2. The disease most often has spontaneous recovery, so the goal is to manage complications that will involve numerous body systems and rehabilitative therapies.

a. Respiratory management and support, due to loss of function and loss of mobility causing the need for secretion management

b. Management of autonomic dysfunction
1) Management of cardiac arrhythmias
2) Blood pressure management
3) Bowel and bladder management

4) Management of electrolyte imbalances

c. Nutrition management

d. Management of complications from immobility
1) Deep vein thrombosis (DVT) and embolism monitoring and prevention
2) Muscle atrophy
3) Skin integrity

e. Psychological intervention for management of depression

F. Nursing Process

1. Assessment

a. Obtain a full health history, with emphasis on any recent illnesses or symptoms, vaccinations, and surgeries.

b. Obtain a list of current symptoms and onset, as well as an approximate timeline of deterioration of function to assess speed of progression.

c. Assess respiratory function.

d. Assess for pain, paresthesia, numbness, or paralysis.

e. Assess bowel and bladder function.

f. Evaluate cranial nerve involvement with neurological testing.

g. Evaluate swallowing.

h. Assess nutrition and weight.

i. Observe client and family interaction to assess for psychological and rehabilitative support.

2. Plan of care: Nursing diagnoses

a. Impaired physical mobility related to disease process

b. Ineffective breathing pattern related to neuromuscular weakness of respiratory muscles

c. Altered nutrition: Less than body requirements related to inability to swallow

d. High risk for aspiration related to dysphagia secondary to cranial nerve involvement

e. Impaired communication related to impairment of speech muscles secondary to cranial nerve involvement

f. Risk for impaired skin integrity related to immobility

g. Risk for DVT related to immobility

h. Risk for constipation related to paralytic ileus

i. Risk for urinary retention related to autonomic dysfunction

j. Acute pain related to disease process

k. Self-care deficit related to loss of function

l. Altered sensory perception due to disease process

m. Potential for anxiety related to lack of control within environment

n. Risk for depression related to loss of function and independence

3. Goals

    a. Limit pain and discomfort.

    b. Maintain function in unaffected limbs and limit extent of atrophy to affected limbs.

    c. Maintain oxygenation and an effective breathing pattern.

    d. Manage autonomic dysfunction.

    e. Provide nutritional support.

    f. Provide means for effective communication.

    g. Prevent skin breakdown.

    h. Prevent DVT formation.

    i. Maintain bowel and bladder elimination.

    j. Provide means of environmental control to lessen anxiety.

    k. Provide psychological and emotional support to the client and family.

4. Interventions

    a. Provide pain management.

        1) Assess pain and changes throughout the disease course and consult with the medical team.

        2) Administer medications as ordered for pain relief.

        3) Help the client to be positioned comfortably.

        4) Educate assistive personnel and family on managing the client's pain (i.e., placing socks on the client can cause a high level of pain, so they should adjust their care appropriately).

    b. Maintain function in unaffected limbs and limit the extent of atrophy to affected limbs.

        1) Teach active ROM to clients and passive ROM to caretakers.

        2) Consult with a physical therapy team.

    c. Maintain oxygenation and effective breathing patterns.

        1) Consult with a respiratory therapist and pulmonologist.

        2) Monitor pulse oximetry.

        3) Maintain a ventilator if needed.

        4) Provide tracheostomy care.

        5) Provide airway management.

        6) Administer oxygen as prescribed.

        7) Teach effective coughing to clear secretions.

        8) Teach and assist with respiratory adjuncts (e.g., incentive spirometer).

        9) Educate on energy conservation techniques.

    d. Manage autonomic dysfunction.

        1) Monitor blood pressure in lying and sitting positions.

        2) Provide supportive measures for orthostatic hypotension (e.g., abdominal binders, compression stockings).

        3) Monitor for cardiac arrhythmias.

        4) Monitor electrolyte balance.

    e. Provide nutritional support.

        1) Consult with a dietitian.

        2) Monitor patient weight.

        3) Provide safe gastrostomy or nasogastric tube feedings if needed.

    f. Provide a means for effective communication.

        1) Consult with a speech pathologist.

        2) Provide communication boards and establish an alternative way for the client to respond (e.g., blinking).

        3) Educate the healthcare team and family members on established communication techniques.

    g. Prevent skin breakdown.

        1) Assess skin regularly for signs of breakdown.

        2) Apply proper aids such as moisture barrier creams.

        3) Monitor serum protein levels.

        4) Assess fluid intake and monitor for skin turgor changes.

        5) Turn the client every 2 hours in bed and weight shift every 20 minutes when in a wheelchair.

        6) Educate the client and family on identifying signs of skin breakdown and preventive techniques.

        7) Educate the family on turning and weight shifting.

    h. Prevent DVT formation.

        1) Provide compression devices as ordered.

        2) Educate the client and family on signs and symptoms of DVT.

    i. Maintain bowel and bladder elimination.

        1) Insert a Foley catheter if needed and perform proper catheter care.

        2) Closely monitor intake and output and encourage increased fluid intake to assist with constipation management.

        3) If the client is voiding independently, monitor postvoid residuals.

        4) Monitor bowel movements.

        5) Assess activity of bowel sounds and distention and firmness of the abdomen.

        6) Administer bowel program as ordered, including medications and suppository administration.

j. Provide control and a comfortable environment for the client.
   1) Allow clients to make decisions about their environment, including lighting, sounds, open doors, and room temperature.
   2) Because changes occur in pain and paresthesia throughout the disease course, be sure to consistently ask the client what is comfortable while providing care.
   3) Provide an accessible nurse call bell (e.g., tent for head activation, sip and puff in case of complete paralysis).
k. Provide psychological and emotional support to the client and family.
   1) Consult with a psychologist on the healthcare team. Report changes in mood, attitude, affect, and family dynamics to the psychologist.
   2) Educate the client and family on the disease course.
   3) Offer community support group information and resources.

V. Myasthenia Gravis (MG)
A. Overview
   1. A chronic autoimmune disease involving the destruction of ACh receptors, resulting in fluctuating weakness of the voluntary muscle groups.
   2. Most common symptoms include muscle fatigue, drooping eyelids, difficulty with speech and swallowing, weakness in extremities, and respiratory difficulty.
   3. Weakness increases with activity and improves with rest.
   4. MG was first documented by an English clinician, Sir Thomas Willis, in 1672.
   5. Variations of the disease exist, including ocular, generalized, and bulbar.
   6. Onset can be subtle or fast, and a myasthenia crisis will necessitate emergent respiratory support for survival.
   7. Numerous treatments exist, with the goal of keeping the client symptom free and improving quality of life. No cure exists for MG.
   8. Typical clients can live in the community and will need acute care and rehabilitation only while in myasthenic or cholinergic crisis.
   9. Stages of MG and a Global Clinical Classification of Myasthenic Severity help classify the individual case.
B. Epidemiology
   1. Affects approximately 1 per 5,000 people in the United States (Myasthenia Gravis Foundation of America, 2010).
   2. Can affect all ages and races and both sexes, but the clinical course may vary by age and sex (Grob, Brunner, Namba, & Pagala, 2008)
      a. Highest incidence in women younger than 40 years of age and men older than 60 years of age
      b. Female-to-male ratio of 3:2 affected before age 50. Sex distribution is closer to equal after age 50, with more men affected.
      c. Neonatal myasthenia is seen in 12%–20% of babies born to mothers with MG because some of the mother's antibodies are passed to the child. The child does not produce its own antibodies. This is a transient condition, and the general weakness the baby experiences typically subsides in 3–5 weeks.
   3. Mortality rates and quality of life have improved due to thymectomy, use of steroids, use of immunoglobulins, and plasma exchange for MG crisis (Diaz-Manera, Rojas-Garcia, & Illa, 2009).
   4. The most severe weakness and highest mortality occur within the first and second year, with some improvement thereafter (Grob et al., 2008).
C. Etiology
   1. The cause of MG is unknown.
   2. Presence of a thymoma or an abnormal thymus gland is seen in approximately 75% of people with MG. The relationship is not fully understood, but it is believed that a malfunction in the thymus could cause an error in the production of immune cells, resulting in the production of ACh receptor antibodies.
   3. MG is not believed to be directly hereditary, although predisposition for autoimmune disease can be inherited.
   4. Disease can go into remission for long periods of time during which no treatment is needed.
D. Pathophysiology
   1. Overview
      a. For unknown reasons, the body does not recognize the ACh receptors as self and produces autoantibodies against these receptors.
      b. Autoimmune attack occurs on the ACh receptors by binding of the autoantibodies to the receptors, although the role of the autoantibodies is not fully understood.
      c. ACh can no longer be used in neurotransmission because of mechanical blockage of the receptor, resulting in muscle weakness and fatigue.

d. Cholinergic receptors of cardiac and smooth muscle have different antigenicity than skeletal muscle and so are not affected.

e. Weakness increases with activity throughout the day and improves with rest. As the disease progresses, fatigue occurs with less activity.

f. Two types of crisis can occur.

   1) Myasthenic crisis

     a) Involvement of respiratory and accessory muscles escalates, necessitating mechanical ventilation

     b) Infection, fever, adverse reaction to medication, and insufficient medication are causes for crisis for clients who have respiratory involvement.

   2) Cholinergic crisis

     a) Results from excessive dosage of cholinergic treatment medications

     b) Symptoms can mimic organophosphate poisoning (salivation, lacrimation, urinary incontinence, gastrointestinal upset, emesis, miosis).

     c) In some case, symptoms may include flaccid paralysis and respiratory failure, which are clinically indistinguishable from those of MG itself.

2. Clinical manifestations

a. Onset variable

   1) Most often gradual

   2) Reports of rapid onset when associated with emotional upset or respiratory infection

b. For all muscles involved, activity throughout the day increases symptoms and rest can help to relieve symptoms. With disease progression, the client will fatigue more easily.

c. Exacerbation can result from infection, illness, surgery, pregnancy, menses, changes in thyroid function, heat, or electrolyte imbalances (hypokalemia). Clients taking other medications must also be aware of side effects involving neurotransmission.

d. Variations of disease

   1) Ocular: Eye and lid muscles are affected

   2) Bulbar: Muscles of speech, swallowing, and breathing are affected

   3) Generalized: Proximal muscles of both upper and lower extremities are involved, with ocular or bulbar involvement

   4) Neonatal transient: Passes to baby from a mother with MG

e. Muscle groups tend to be affected in pattern.

f. Early findings include ptosis and diplopia.

   1) Ptosis may be unilateral or bilateral.

   2) Ptosis intensifies with upward gaze.

g. Secondary muscle groups involve facial, speech, neck, and masticator.

   1) Facial expressions become altered by weakness and fatigue of facial muscles.

   2) Chewing becomes tiresome quickly, and rest periods are needed.

   3) The voice becomes weak and fades after conversation and often sounds nasal.

h. Generalized weakness will involve larger muscle groups.

   1) Limb muscle and proximal muscle involvement

     a) Clients may have a hard time lifting their arms over their head and performing ADLs that require this motion (i.e., grooming hair).

     b) Difficulty in reaching for objects

   2) Neck extensor muscle involvement will cause the head to fall forward.

   3) Diaphragm and intercostal involvement will constitute myasthenic crisis and necessitate respiratory support, intubation, or mechanical ventilation.

3. Myasthenia Gravis Foundation of America, Inc. Classification System (**Table 10-5**)

4. Diagnosis

a. Tensilon testing: This anticholinesterase is administered to test for immediate improvement in muscle strength. If strength improves, the test is positive.

b. Blood test for elevation of ACh receptors (80%–90% of people with MG show antibody titer elevation)

c. Electrophysiology: Rapid reduction in nerve conduction studies is a positive result

d. Single-fiber electromyography: Tests neuromuscular transmission from a single nerve fiber to pairs of muscles. Detection of failure to transmit or delay indicates a positive test, and for MG a confirmation test proves to be approximately 99% sensitive.

e. Mediastinal MRI or computed tomography (CT) scan: Many people with MG have an enlarged thymus, and this test will show thymoma if existent.

E. Management Options

1. Treatment must be individualized for each client after the diagnosis of the specific type of MG.

2. In approximately 10% of cases, MG is associated with a thymoma and surgical removal is often indicated (Gold & Schneider-Gold, 2008).

3. The goal of treatment is to remain as symptom free as possible to achieve a good quality of life.
4. Myasthenic crisis is a life-threatening emergency necessitating early diagnosis and respiratory assistance and is typically treated with some combination of high-dose corticosteroids, plasma exchange, immunoglobulins, and respiratory support (Chaudhuri & Behan, 2009).
5. The use of bilevel positive airway pressure and other external respiratory supportive systems may prevent the need for intubation or reduce the duration of crises (Argov, 2009).
6. Statins may aggravate MG and are contraindicated (Argov, 2009).
7. Pharmacological management including cyclosporin (with or without corticosteroids) or cyclophosphamide (with corticosteroids) has been found to significantly improve MG (Hart, Sharshar, & Sathasivam, 2009).
   a. Anticholinesterase medication is usually the first approach.
      1) Symptom management does not treat the underlying cause.
      2) Most commonly used is pyridostigmine (Mestinon) and, occasionally, neostigmine (Prostigmin)
   b. Muscarinic side effects on smooth muscle and glands can occur.
      1) Bradycardia
      2) Bronchial constriction and spasms, increase in secretions, and wheezing
      3) Blurred vision and constricted pupils
      4) Involuntary micturition
      5) Gastrointestinal upset (e.g., abdominal cramping, diarrhea, vomiting)
      6) Diaphoresis
   c. Nicotinic side effects on skeletal muscle may occur, including facial twitching and spasms.
   d. Long-term corticosteroid therapy
      1) Prednisone is the most common choice.
      2) Seventy percent to 80% remission or improvement (Hickey, 2009).
   e. Immunosuppressant agents
      1) Azathioprine (Imuran) is often chosen if prednisone is contraindicated for a client.

Table 10-5. Myasthenia Gravis Foundation of America, Inc., Classification System

Class	Description
Class I	Any ocular muscle weakness May have weakness of eye closure All other muscle strength is normal
Class II	Mild weakness affecting other than ocular muscles May also have ocular muscle weakness of any severity
Class IIa	Predominantly affecting limb or axial muscles May also have lesser involvement of oropharyngeal muscle
Class IIb	Predominantly affecting oropharyngeal or respiratory muscles May also have lesser or equal involvement of limb or axial muscles
Class III	Moderate weakness affecting other than ocular muscles May also have ocular muscle weakness of any severity
Class IIIa	Predominantly affecting limb or axial muscles May also have lesser involvement of oropharyngeal muscles
Class IIIb	Predominantly affecting oropharyngeal or respiratory muscles May also have lesser or equal involvement of limb or axial
Class IV	Severe weakness affecting other than ocular muscles May also have ocular muscle weakness of any severity
Class IVa	Predominantly affecting limb or axial muscles May also have lesser involvement of oropharyngeal muscles
Class IVb	Predominantly affecting oropharyngeal or respiratory muscles May also have lesser or equal involvement of limb or axial muscles
Class V	Defined by intubation, with or without mechanical ventilation, except when used during routine postoperative management; the use of a feeding tube without intubation places a client in class IVb

From "Comparison of myasthenic crisis and cholinergic crisis" (p.433), by L. Neal Boylan, 2008. In S. P. Hoeman (Ed.), *Rehabilitation nursing: Prevention, Intervention, & outcomes* (4th ed.), St. Louis: Mosby. Copyright 2008 by Mosby. Reprinted with permission.

2) Cyclophosphamide (Cytoxan) is a possible choice but has high toxicity.
   f. Intravenous immunoglobulin
      1) Short-term treatment
      2) Known to improve autoimmune conditions
8. Plasmapheresis
   a. Short-term treatment to stabilize clients who may be in crisis
   b. Removes ACh receptor antibodies from blood
9. Surgical thymectomy for long-term improvement of disease
10. Nursing management
    a. Monitoring for crisis events
    b. Monitoring for side effects of treatments
    c. Monitoring for individual tolerance and weakness
    d. Communicating with medical team for treatment changes based on client response
    e. Assisting the client to remain as independent as possible with ADLs
F. Nursing Process
   1. Assessment
      a. Obtain a full health history and focus on the client's daily symptoms, including his or her weakest time of day.
      b. Assess and record baseline for the client to safely monitor for crisis (preferably during the client's strongest time of day).
         1) Respiratory function
         2) Cardiac function
         3) Bowel and bladder function
         4) Baseline gastrointestinal symptoms
         5) Visual acuity
         6) Strength and mobility
         7) Swallowing
         8) Speech
   2. Plan of care
      a. Nursing diagnoses
         1) Knowledge deficit relating to disease process and side effects of treatment
         2) Activity intolerance related to fatigue
         3) Risk for aspiration related to muscle weakness and increased secretions
         4) Risk for falls related to muscle weakness
         5) Risk for medical crisis (myasthenic or cholinergic)
      b. Goals
         1) The client and family will be able to identify signs and symptoms of disease and side effects of medical treatment.
         2) The client and family will be able to distinguish signs and symptoms of myasthenic

and cholinergic crisis and know to seek medical attention immediately.
         3) The client will learn and use energy-conservation techniques.
         4) Respiratory support will be provided.
         5) Nutritional support will be provided.
         6) Medication side effects will be managed.
         7) A safe environment and assistance to prevent falls will be provided.
         8) The client will be assisted to manage energy output and provided an appropriate schedule for therapy and activities based around fluctuations in strength throughout the day.
   3. Interventions
      a. Education for the client, family, caretaker
         1) Disease process
         2) Side effects of medications and treatments
         3) Myasthenic crisis
            a) Often precipitated by infection but can occur spontaneously
            b) Signs and symptoms
               (1) Sudden relapse of symptoms
               (2) Difficulty swallowing
               (3) Rapid decrease in respiratory function
            c) Seek immediate medical attention for life-saving treatment.
         4) Cholinergic crisis
            a) Caused by toxicity, overmedication with acetylcholinesterase inhibitors
            b) Signs and symptoms may present more slowly than myasthenic crisis.
               (1) Generalized profound weakness
               (2) Bradycardia
               (3) Bronchial constriction and spasms
               (4) Increase in secretions
               (5) Wheezing cough
               (6) Blurred vision and constricted pupils
               (7) Involuntary micturition
               (8) Gastrointestinal upset (e.g., abdominal cramping, diarrhea, vomiting)
               (9) Diaphoresis
               (10) Facial twitching
            c) Seek immediate medical attention for life-saving treatment.
         5) Importance of medic alert bracelet
         6) Energy-conservation techniques and need for rest periods throughout day
         7) Not to take any over-the-counter medications without consulting doctor

8) Diet choices that will require less work to chew and swallow

9) Causes of relapses (menstruation, infection, stress, extreme temperatures)

b. Provide respiratory support if needed.
1) Monitor oxygenation.
2) Provide tracheostomy care if needed.
3) Teach effective coughing to clear secretions.

c. Provide nutritional support.
1) Consult with a speech therapist for safe food choices and techniques for swallowing.
2) Consult with a dietitian to ensure that caloric intake is adequate.
3) Encourage a soft diet, which takes less energy to chew and swallow.

d. Manage side effects of medications.
1) Provide a private room and limited exposure for clients on immunosuppressive medications.
2) Monitor for effects of medications on all body systems, report untoward symptoms to the physician, and provide nursing interventions to mitigate any negative side effects.

e. Provide a safe environment to prevent falls.
1) Teach the client to request assistance when weak.
2) Provide essentials within reaching distance of bed.
3) Consult with a physical therapist to provide proper aids for ambulation.
4) Educate the client on wearing safe, comfortable footwear.

f. Provide an appropriate schedule for the client.
1) Consult with a medical team and therapy team.
   a) Individualize the client's medication schedule.
   b) Individualize the client's therapy schedule to allow for rest periods throughout day.
2) Monitor the client daily and record how he or she is managing with medications and activities and adjust accordingly.

VI. **Postpolio Syndrome (PPS)**
A. Overview
1. PPS affects survivors of polio decades after the acute illness.
2. Major symptoms are pain, fatigue, and weakness, with new weakness being the hallmark of PPS.
3. Clients may have sleep, breathing, and swallowing problems (Post-Polio Health International, 2010).

4. Clients may experience muscle atrophy or wasting (Post-Polio Health International, 2010).
5. PPS is rarely life-threatening.
6. The severity of initial acute polio illness predicts the severity of the PPS (National Institute of Neurological Disorders and Stroke [NINDS], 2010).

B. Epidemiology
1. Experienced by 25%–40% of polio survivors (Post-Polio Health International, 2010)
2. There are more than 440,000 polio survivors in the United States (NINDS, 2010).
3. More common in women than in men

C. Etiology
1. Criteria for diagnosing from the NINDS
   a. Prior paralytic poliomyelitis with lower motor neuron loss that is confirmed
   b. Period of partial or completed recovery for 15 years or more
   c. Gradual onset of progressive or persistent new muscle weakness or fatigue, often after surgery or a period of inactivity
   d. Symptoms that persist for 1 year
   e. Exclusion of other problems as a cause of the symptoms
2. There are no diagnostic tests for PPS, but MRI, CT, neuroimaging, and electrophysiological studies may be useful to investigate the course of decline in muscle strength.
3. People with PPS are at high risk for fracture (Mohammad, Khan, Galvin, Hardiman, & O'Connell, 2009).

D. Pathophysiology (Boyer et al., 2010)
1. Wechler theory
   a. New "sprouts" of nerve cells reconnect the nerve cell to the muscles during recovery from acute polio.
   b. New "sprouts" trigger contraction of the muscles and supply more muscle fibers with innervation.
   c. New "sprouts" are not stable and degenerate over time through "overexertion" and no longer contract muscle fibers, leading to the perception of new weakness or loss of function.
2. Associated with an inflammatory process in the CSF and overall inflammation (Boyer et al., 2010)

E. Management Options
1. The primary focus of treatment is energy conservation and lifestyle changes to reduce stress, avoiding both inactivity and overuse (Gonzalez, Olsson, & Borg, 2010).
2. Rehabilitation that is comprehensive and interdisciplinary can have a positive effect, including ability to perform ADLs, personal view of the

illness, and long-term outcomes (Larsson Lund & Lexell, 2010).

3. Bracing to support weak muscles
4. Canes or crutches to enhance safety and relieve weight on weak limbs
5. Orthotics to correct leg length discrepancy and gait disturbances
6. Weight loss
7. Select exercises to avoid disuse or overuse weakness
8. Use of a biphasic positive pressure ventilator at night to treat underventilation
9. Depression
   a. Depression in PPS is common.
   b. Highly correlated among those 65 and older with the resilience factor of spiritual growth (Pierini & Stuifbergen, 2010)
10. Training programs including warm water are helpful (Farbu, 2010).
11. Training programs that are low-level aerobic and that have low-level muscle strengthening are most effective (Tiffreau et al., 2010).
12. Pharmacology
    a. Steroids, amantadine, pyridostigmine, and coenzyme Q10 are of no benefit.
    b. Intravenous immunoglobulin has demonstrated some positive effect on the disease (Farbu, 2010).
13. Pain is a persistent and common problem in PPS (Stoelb et al., 2008).
    a. Nociceptive pain is more common than neuropathic pain (Werhagen & Borg, 2010).
    b. Pain is worse in younger people.
    c. Pain is worse in females.
    d. Pain is worse with a younger age of onset of the initial acute polio.
14. Adjustment and education
    a. Experience with initial polio as a child may influence adjustment to PPS.
    b. Late-onset deterioration is feared by many.
    c. Must consider individual experiences and the underlying components of fatigue and pain (Yelnik & Laffont, 2010)
15. Prevent pathological fracture and reduce the risk of falls.

F. Nursing Process
   1. Assessment
      a. Obtain a full health history, with emphasis on the initial acute polio illness, recovery, functional level, work history, and the onset of PPS symptoms.
      b. Obtain a list of current symptoms and onset and approximate timeline of deterioration of function.
      c. Obtain a history of the exacerbations of symptoms and associated factors, including things that improve symptoms and things that make symptoms worse.
      d. Assess for pain, paresthesia, numbness, and paralysis.
      e. Assess bowel and bladder function.
      f. Observe client and family interaction to assess for psychological and rehabilitative support.
   2. Plan of care: Nursing diagnosis
      a. Impaired physical mobility related to disease process
      b. Decreased activity tolerance related to muscle weakness, pain, and overuse syndrome
      c. Ineffective breathing pattern related to neuro-muscular weakness of respiratory muscles
      d. Altered nutrition: Less than body requirements
      e. Risk for DVT related to change in gait and mobility
      f. Risk for constipation related to change in activity and medication effect
      g. Acute pain related to disease process
      h. Self-care deficit related to loss of function
      i. Altered sensory perception due to disease process
      j. Potential for anxiety related to lack of control within environment and change in lifestyle
      k. Risk for depression related to loss of function and independence
   3. Goals
      a. Implement energy conservation strategies.
      b. Maintain function in unaffected limbs and limit extent of atrophy of affected limbs.
      c. Maintain breathing patterns and oxygenation.
      d. Provide nutritional support.
      e. Prevent DVT formation.
      f. Maintain bowel and bladder elimination.
      g. Provide psychological and emotional support to the client and family.
   4. Interventions
      a. Teach energy conservation strategies.
         1) Schedule activities with rest periods.
         2) Make environmental accommodations to decrease energy needs to perform ADLs.
         3) Teach strategies to identify activities and compensatory strategies focused on energy conservation.
      b. Maintain function in unaffected limbs and limit the extent of atrophy of affected limbs.
         1) Teach active ROM to clients and passive ROM to caretakers.
         2) Consult with a physical therapy team.
      c. Maintain oxygenation and effective breathing patterns.

1) Consult with a respiratory therapist and pulmonologist.
2) Monitor pulse oximetry and teach the client how to monitor at home.
3) Based on respiratory needs, teach the use of ventilator devices for home use.
4) Teach effective coughing to clear secretions.
5) Teach and assist with respiratory adjuncts (e.g., incentive spirometer).

d. Provide nutritional support.
1) Consult with a dietitian.
2) Monitor the client's weight.
3) Instruct the client in maximizing nutritional intake.

e. Prevent DVT formation.
1) Provide compression devices as ordered.
2) Educate the client and family on signs and symptoms of DVT.

f. Maintain bowel and bladder elimination.
1) Assess any urinary functional changes and develop a plan to address urinary dysfunction, including the use of assistive devices and equipment.
2) Teach the the client management strategies for home to achieve continence or manage incontinence.
3) Assess for any signs of constipation or diarrhea.
4) Develop a plan with the client that involves dietary intake, fluid intake, and the use of medications to achieve regular bowel movements.

g. Provide control and a comfortable environment for the client.
1) Allow clients to make decisions about their environment including lighting, sounds, open doors, and room temperature.
2) Due to changes in pain and paresthesia throughout the disease course, be sure to consistently ask the client what is comfortable while providing care and strategize with the client for his or her home environment.

h. Provide psychological and emotional support to the client and family.
1) Consult with a psychologist on the healthcare team. Report changes in mood, attitude, affect, and family dynamics to the psychologist.
2) Educate the client and family on the disease course.
3) Offer community support group information and resources.

References

ALS Association. (2010). *Facts you should know about ALS*. Retrieved August 6, 2010, from www.alsa.org/about-als/facts-you-should-know.html.

Argov, Z. (2009). Management of myasthenia conditions: Non-immune issues. *Current Opinions in Neurology, 22*(5), 493–497.

Beretich, B. D., & Beretich, T. M. (2009). Explaining multiple sclerosis prevalence by ultraviolet exposure: A geospatial analysis. *Multiple Sclerosis, 15*(8), 891–898.

Boyer, F. C., Tiffeau, V., Rapin, A., Laffont, I., Percebois-Macadre, L., Supper, C., et al. (2010). Post-polio syndrome: Pathophysiological hypotheses, diagnosis criteria, drug therapy. *Annals of Physical Rehabilitation Medicine, 53*(1), 34–41.

Brettschneider, J., Kurent, J., Ludolph, A., & Mitchell, J. D. (2008). Drug therapy for pain in amyotrophic lateral sclerosis or motor neuron disease. *Cochrane Database of Systematic Reviews, 16*(3), CD005226.

Brundin, P., Barker, R. A., & Parmar, M. (2010). Neural grafting in Parkinson's disease: Problems and possibilities. *Progress Brain Research, 184*, 265–294.

Chaudhuri, A., & Behan, P. O. (2009). Myasthenic crisis. *QJM, 102*(2), 97–107.

Cronin, S., Hardiman, O., & Trayor, B. J. (2007). Ethnic variation in the incidence of ALS: A systematic review. *Neurology, 68*(13), 1002–1007.

Deuschi, G., Schade-Brittinger, C., Krack, P., Volkmann, J., Schafer, H., Botzel, K., et al. (2006). A randomized trial of deep-brain stimulation for Parkinson's disease. *New England Journal of Medicine, 355*(9), 896–908.

Diaz-Manera, J., Rojas-Garcia, R., & Illa, I. (2009). Treatment strategies for myasthenia gravis. *Expert Opinion on Pharmacotherapy, 10*(8), 1329–1342.

Farbu, E. (2010). Update on current and emergency treatment options for post-polio syndrome. *Therapeutic Clinical Risk Management, 6*, 307–313.

Fujimoto, K. (2009). Management of non-motor complications in Parkinson's disease. *Journal of Neurology, 256*(Suppl. 3), 299–355.

Gagne, J. J., & Power, M. C. (2010). Anti-inflammatory drugs and risk of Parkinson disease: A meta-analysis. *Neurology, 74*(12), 995–1002.

Gold, R., & Schneider-Gold, C. (2008). Current and future standards in treatment of myasthenia gravis. *Neurotherapeutics, 5*(4), 535–541.

Gonzalez, H., Olsson, T., & Borg, K. (2010). Management of postpolio syndrome. *Lancet Neurology, 9*(6), 634–642.

Grob, D., Brunner, N., Namba, T., & Pagala, M. (2008). Lifetime course of myasthenia gravis. *Muscle and Nerve, 37*(2), 141–149.

Habek, M., Kami, A., Balash, Y., & Gurevich, T. (2010). The place of the botulinum toxin in the management of multiple sclerosis. *Clinical Neurology and Neurosurgery, 112*(7), 592–596.

Haroutinunian, S., Lecht, S., Zur, A. A., Hoffman, A., & Davidson, E. (2009). The challenge of pain management in patients with myasthenia gravis. *Journal of Pain, Palliative Care, and Pharmacotherapy, 23*(3), 242–260.

Hart, I. K., Sharshar, T., & Sathasivam, S. (2009). Immunosuppressant drugs for myasthenia gravis. *Journal of Neurology, Neurosurgery, and Psychiatry, 80*(1), 5–6.

Hayes, M. W., Fung, V .S., Kimber, T. E., & O'Sullivan, J. D. (2010). Current concepts in the management of Parkinson disease. *Medical Journal of Australia, 192*(3), 144–149.

Hickey, J. V. (2009). Neurodegenerative diseases. In J. Hickey (Ed.), *The practice of neurological and neurosurgical nursing* (6th ed.). New York: Lippincott Williams & Wilkins.

Hughes, R. A., Swan, A. V., & van Doorn, P. A. (2010). Corticosteroids for Guillain-Barré syndrome. *Cochrane Database of Systematic Reviews, 2,* CD001446.

Jefferson, T., DiPietrantonj, C., Rivetti, A., Bawazeer, G. A., Al-Ansary, L. A., & Ferroni, E. (2010). Vaccine for preventing influenza in healthy adults. *Cochrane Database of Systematic Reviews, 7,* CD001269.

Kerr, G. K., Worringham, C. J., Cole, M. H., Lacherez, P. F., Wood, J. M., & Silburn, P. A. (2010). Predictors of future falls in Parkinson disease. *Neurology, 72*(2), 116–124.

Lad, S. P., Chapman, C. H., Vaninetti, M., Steinman, L., Green, A., & Boakye, M. (2010). Socioeconomic trends in hospitalizations for multiple sclerosis. *Neuroepidemiology, 35*(2), 93–99.

Larsson Lund, M., & Lexell, J. (2010). A positive turning point in life: How persons with late effects of polio experience the influence of an interdisciplinary rehabilitation programme. *Journal of Rehabilitation Medicine, 42*(6), 559–565.

Lewis, S. M., Heitkemper, M. M., & Dirksen, S. R. (2004). *Medical-surgical nursing: Assessment and management of clinical problems* (6th ed.). St Louis: Mosby.

Logroscino, G., Traynor, B. J., Hardiman, O., Chio, A., Couratier, P., Mitchell, J. D., et al. (2008). Descriptive epidemiology of amyotrophic lateral sclerosis: New evidence and unsolved issues. *Journal of Neurology, Neurosurgery, and Psychiatry, 79*(1), 6–11.

Mattson, D. H. (2002). Update on the diagnosis of multiple sclerosis. *Expert Review in Neuro-Therapy, 2*(3), 319–328.

McGrogan, A., Madle, G. C., Seaman, H. E., & de Vries, C. S. (2009). The epidemiology of Guillain-Barré syndrome worldwide: A systematic literature review. *Neuroepidemiology, 32*(2), 150–163.

Miller, R. G., Jackson, C. E., Kasarskis, E. J., England, J. D., Forshew, D., Johnston, W., et al. (2009). Practice parameter update: The care of the patient with amyotrophic lateral sclerosis: Multidisciplinary care, symptom management, and cognitive/behavioral impairment (an evidence-based review). Report to the Quality Standards Subcommittee of the American Academy of Neurology. *Neurology, 73*(15), 1227–1233.

Mohammad, A. F., Khan, K. A., Galvin, L., Hardiman, O., & O'Connell, P. G. (2009). High incidence of osteoporosis and fractures in an aging post polio population. *Europe Neurology, 62*(6), 369–374.

Monahan, F. D., Sands, J. K., Neighbors, M., Marek, J. F., & Green, C. J. (2007). *Phipps' medical-surgical nursing: Health and illness perspectives* (8th ed.). St. Louis: Mosby Elsevier.

Multiple Sclerosis Foundation. (2009). *FAQs: What is multiple sclerosis?* Retrieved August 7, 2010, from http://msfacts.org/what-is-multiple-sclerosis.aspx.

Myasthenia Gravis Foundation of America. (2010). *What is myasthenia gravis?* Retrieved August 1, 2011, from http://myasthenia.org/WhatisMG.aspx.

National Institute of Neurological Disorders and Stroke. (2010). *Post polio syndrome fact sheet.* Retrieved August 7, 2010, from www.ninds.nih.gov/disorders/post_polio/detail_post_polio.htm.

National Multiple Sclerosis Society. (2010). *About MS: Who gets MS?* Retrieved August 6, 2010, from www.nationalmssociety.org/about-multiple-sclerosis/what-we-know-about-ms/who-gets-ms/index.aspx.

Parkinson's Disease Foundation. (2010). *What is Parkinson's disease?* Retrieved January 27, 2011, from www.pdf.org/en/about_pdf.

Pardo, G., Boutwell, C., Conner, J., Denney, D., & Loeen-Burkey, M. (2010). Effect of oral antihistamine on local injection site reactions with self-administered glatiramer acetate. *Journal of Neuroscience Nursing, 42*(1), 40–46.

Pfeiffer, R. F. (2010). Gastrointestinal, urological, and sexual dysfunction in Parkinson's disease. *Movement Disorders, 25*(Suppl. 1), S94–S97.

Pierini, D., & Stuifbergen, A. K. (2010). Psychological resilience and depressive symptoms in older adults diagnosed with post-polio syndrome. *Rehabilitation Nursing, 35*(4), 167–175.

Poewe, W. (2009). Treatments for Parkinson disease: Past achievements and current clinical needs. *Neurology, 72*(7 Suppl.), S65–S73.

Polak, M., Richman, J., Lorimer, M., Boynton-DeSepulveda, L., & Del Bene, M. (2004). Neuromuscular disorders of the nervous system. In M. K. Bader & L. R. Littlejohn (Eds.), *AANN core curriculum for neuroscience nursing* (4th ed.). Glenview, IL: American Association of Neuroscience Nursing.

Post-Polio Health International. (2010). *Post-polio syndrome: A new challenge for the survivors of polio.* Retrieved August 14, 2010, from www.post-polio.org/edu/pps.html.

Rowland, L. P., & Shineider, N. L. (2001). Amyotrophic lateral sclerosis. *New England Journal of Medicine, 344*(22), 1688–1700.

Schwarz, A. (2010, August 17). Study says brain trauma can mimic ALS. *New York Times, p.* A1.

Simmons, R. D., Tribe, K. L., & McDonald, E. A. (2010). Living with multiple sclerosis: Longitudinal changes in employment and the importance of symptom management. *Journal of Neurology, 257*(6), 926–936.

Sinclair, V. G., & Scroggie, J. (2005). Effects of a cognitive–behavioral program for women with multiple sclerosis. *Journal of Neuroscience Nursing, 37*(5), 249–257, 276.

Smolders, J. (2010). Vitamin D and multiple sclerosis: Correlations, causality, and controversy. *Autoimmune Disease,* Oct 5, 2011: 629538.

Solaro, C., & Messmer Uccelli, M. (2010). Pharmacological management of pain in patients with multiple sclerosis. *Drugs, 70*(10), 1245–1254.

Steefel, L. (2006, May 22). Not just for grown-ups: The number of children with multiple sclerosis is climbing at an alarming rate. *Nursing Spectrum,* 16–17.

Stoelb, B. L., Carter, G. T., Abresch, R. T., Purekal, S., McDonald, C. M., & Jensen, M. P. (2008). Pain in persons with postpolio syndrome: Frequency, intensity and impact. *Archives of Physical Medicine and Rehabilitation, 89*(10), 1933–1940.

Tiffreau, V., Rapin, A., Serafi, R., Percebolis-Macadre, L., Supper, C., Jolly, D., et al. (2010). Post-polio syndrome and rehabilitation. *Annals of Physical Rehabilitation Medicine, 53*(1), 42–50.

Tomik, B., & Gulloff, R. J. (2010). Dysarthria in amyotrophic lateral sclerosis: A review. *Amyotrophic Lateral Sclerosis, 11*(1–2), 4–15.

van Doorn, P. A. (2009). What's new in Guillain-Barré syndrome in 2007–2008. *Journal of Peripheral Nervous System, 14*(2), 72–74.

van Doorn, P. A., Ruts, L., & Jacobs, B. C. (2008). Clinical features, pathogenesis, and treatment of Guillain-Barre syndrome. *Lancet Neurology, 10,* 939–950.

Venkateswaran, S., & Banwell, B. (2010). Pediatric multiple sclerosis. *Neurologist, 16*(2), 92–105.

Vucic, S., Kiernan, M. C., & Cornblath, D. R. (2009). Guillain-Barré syndrome: An update. *Journal of Clinical Neuroscience, 16*(6), 733–741.

Werhagen, L., & Borg, K. (2010). Analysis of long-standing nociceptive and neuropathic pain in patient with post-polio syndrome. *Journal of Neurology, 257*(6), 1027–1031.

Woolley, S. C., & Katz, J. S. (2008). Cognitive and behavioral impairment in amyotrophic lateral sclerosis. *Physical Medicine and Rehabilitation Clinics of North America, 19*(3), 607–617.

Yelnik, A., & Laffont, I. (2010). The psychological aspects of polio survivors through their life experience. *Annals of Physician Rehabilitation Medicine, 53*(1), 60–67.

Zesewicz, T. A., Sullivan, K. L., Chaudhuri, D. R., Morgan, J. C., Gronseth, G. S., Miyasaki, J., et al. (2010). Practice parameter: Treatment of nonmotor symptoms of Parkinson's disease. *Neurology, 74,* 924.

CHAPTER 11
Stroke

Paddy Garvin-Higgins, MN CNS RN CRRN • Delilah Hall-Towarnicke, MSN CNS RN CRRN • Carla J. Howard, ACNP-BC CRRN

Stroke or "brain attack" (also called cerebrovascular or cerebral vascular accident [CVA]), affects hundreds of thousands of people each year. The effects of stroke may be slight or severe, temporary or permanent, and can be devastating to the client and family. Clients who have had a stroke must cope with numerous sensorimotor, visual, perceptual, and language deficits. Rehabilitation should begin when the person is admitted to care. Initially rehabilitation is focused on minimizing complications of the stroke. As the client stabilizes, he or she may be transferred to a rehabilitation unit as soon as 2 days after the stroke has occurred, and rehabilitation should be continued as necessary after the client leaves the hospital. Rehabilitation provides an interdisciplinary team effort that focuses on helping the person who has had a stroke regain as much functional independence as possible. Rehabilitation also plays a major role in helping to prevent secondary complications and minimize long-term disabilities after stroke. To intervene effectively as a member of the rehabilitation team, the nurse should have a good understanding of the physiological, perceptual, and psychological changes that occur after stroke. Nursing goals should focus on maintaining effective tissue perfusion, preventing complications, and enhancing adjustment and quality of life.

I. Overview of Stroke
A. Description
1. A stroke or CVA is a sudden onset of focal neurological deficit (cerebro) caused by a regional disruption of blood supply (vascular) and oxygen in the brain (Merck Sharp & Dohme Corporation, 2009–2010).
2. A stroke, or brain attack, should be treated as a medical emergency; delay of treatment can affect the amount and permanence of the brain damage.
3. There are two major types of stroke: ischemic and hemorrhagic.
   a. An *ischemic stroke* occurs when a blood clot blocks a blood vessel or artery.
   b. A *hemorrhagic stroke* occurs when a blood vessel breaks or bursts, interrupting blood flow to an area of the brain and causing bleeding in the brain (National Stroke Association [NSA], 2009g).
4. When a stroke occurs, blood flow to that part of the brain is disrupted, resulting in tissue anoxia and death of brain cells (infarction). As many as 2 million brain cells die every minute while blood flow is interrupted (NSA, 2009g).
   a. Neurons and other brain cells need oxygen and glucose delivered via the circulatory system to function.
   b. A few minutes of oxygen deprivation (ischemia) is enough to cause permanent damage.
   c. Cell death triggers a cascade of inflammation, edema, and energy depletion that can continue to cause damage for hours to days after the initial insult (National Institute of Neurological Disorders and Stroke [NINDS], 2009b).
5. A transient ischemic attack (TIA) is a "warning stroke" or "mini-stroke" that produces stroke-like symptoms but no lasting damage. Recognizing and treating TIAs can reduce the risk of a major stroke.
   a. TIA symptoms are the same as those of stroke but usually resolve within 24 hours, leaving no residual deficits (American Heart Association [AHA], 2010).
B. Epidemiology (AHA, 2009; NSA, 2009g; Schwamm et al., 2010)
1. Incidence
   a. At current rates, the number of strokes in the United States is projected to jump to 1 million per year by 2050 (Becker, Wira, & Arnold, 2010). On average, every 40 seconds someone in the United States has a stroke.
   b. Each year, 795,000 Americans have a stroke (NSA, 2009g).
      1) About 610,000 of these are first attacks and 185,000 are recurrent attacks.
      2) Approximately 55, 000 more women than men have a stroke each year.
      3) Men's stroke rates are higher than women's at younger ages but not older ages.
      4) Slightly more than 50% of all strokes occur in men, but more than 60% of deaths due to stroke occur in women, possibly because women are older on average when the stroke occurs (Merck Sharp and Dohme Corporation, 2009–2010).
   c. 137,000 people per year die as a result of a stroke. Between 1995 and 2005, the stroke death rate fell 29.7% and the actual number of stroke deaths declined 13.5%.

d. About 20% of people who experience a first stroke between ages 40 and 69 will have another stroke within 5 years (NINDS, 2009b).

1) Second strokes are twice as common in men as women, with 24% of women and 42% of men having a second stroke within 5 years.

2) Second strokes often have a higher rate of disability and death because parts of the brain that are already damaged by the original stroke may not be as able to withstand another insult.

e. TIA precedes approximately 15%–23% of strokes and carries a 90-day stroke risk of 9%–17%. An estimated 240,000 TIAs occur in the United States each year (Wu et al., 2007).

2. Severity: Stroke is the third-leading cause of death in the United States after heart disease and cancer.

3. Risk for stroke: Both modifiable and unmodifiable risk factors contribute to a person's risk of having a stroke.

a. The incidence of stroke occurring in children is low, about 6 cases per 100,000 children per year. Strokes are slightly more common in children younger than 2 years old. In all children, 55% of strokes are ischemic, and the remainder are hemorrhagic (NSA, 2009c; Roach et al., 2008). Boys have a 1.28-fold higher risk of stroke than girls. There are no ethnic differences in stroke severity or case fatality, but boys have a higher case fatality rate for ischemic stroke (Fullerton, Wu, Zhao, & Johnston, 2003).

b. Stroke occurs more often in people with risk factors that cannot be changed, such as being older than 55 years, being male or African American, having a family history of stroke, or having a history of diabetes. Others at risk include those who are of Hispanic or Asian/Pacific Islander origin.

c. The age-adjusted incidence of stroke is about twice as high in African Americans and Hispanic Americans as in Caucasians. The rate of first strokes in African Americans is almost twice the number of Caucasians, and African Americans are twice as likely to die from strokes as Caucasians and Hispanics. On average, African and Hispanic Americans tend to experience stroke at younger ages than Caucasians (NINDS, 2009a).

d. Stroke mortality is unusually high in people living in a cluster of Southeastern states—Alabama, Arkansas, Georgia, Louisiana, Mississippi, North Carolina, South Carolina, and Tennessee—known as the Stroke Belt. A recent study funded by the National Institutes of Health National Institute on Aging suggests that the "belt" is worn from childhood. Higher rates of diabetes and hypertension and possibly socioeconomic conditions for those, particularly African Americans, living in the Stroke Belt contribute to this mortality (NINDS, 2009b).

e. Risk factors for stroke are controllable (preventable) and uncontrollable. Controllable risk factors fall into two categories: lifestyle and medical. Uncontrollable risk factors include age, gender, ethnicity, and family history (NSA, 2009f).

1) Controllable
   a) Hypertension
   b) Obesity
   c) Smoking
   d) Diabetes
   e) Hypercholesteremia and hyperlipidemia
   f) Heavy ingestion of alcohol
   g) Substance abuse (e.g., cocaine, amphetamines, other illegal drugs; Buttaro, 2003; Graykoski, 2003)
   h) Sedentary lifestyle (lack of regular exercise)
   i) Cardiac disorders (e.g., atrial fibrillation)
   j) Carotid artery disease
   k) Blood disorders (e.g., sickle cell anemia, polycythemia)
   l) TIA or previous stroke

2) Uncontrollable
   a) Family history of stroke
   b) Older age: Approximately 72% of strokes occur in people who are at least 65 years of age or older (Hinkle, 2006).
   c) Gender: Stroke is most prevalent in men; however, women who use oral contraceptives, smoke, and have migraines are at a higher risk (Buttaro, 2003; Graykoski, 2003).
   d) Women who enter menopause before age 42 are at twice the risk for stroke (Salaycik et al., 2007).

e) In the Framingham Heart Study, among participants younger than age 65, the risk of stroke or TIA was 4.2 times higher in subjects with symptoms of depression (Salaycik et al., 2007).

f) Race: Stroke is more common in African Americans, Hispanics, and Pacific Islanders (NSA, 2009f).

4. Recovery: A wide range of morbidity is associated with stroke (NSA, 2009e).

a. Ten percent recover almost totally.

b. Twenty-five percent are left with minor disabilities.

c. Forty percent have moderate to severe problems that necessitate care.

d. Stroke is the leading cause of serious, long-term adult disability.

e. Ten percent need long-term facility care.

f. Fifteen percent die soon after having a stroke.

5. The direct and indirect costs of stroke are estimated to be $73.7 billion per year (NSA, 2009g).

C. Etiology of Stroke (AHA, 2009; Buttaro, 2003; Graykoski, 2003; NINDS, 2009b; NSA, 2009g; Patel, Jain, & Wagner, 2008; Sugerman, 2002)

1. Stroke is the result of an interruption in the blood supply to some part of the brain.

a. The arterial blood supply to the brain comes from the internal carotid arteries and the vertebral arteries.

1) The internal carotid arteries supply the anterior portion of the brain with a greater amount of blood flow and originate from the common carotid arteries. They enter the cranium through the base of the skull, passing through the cavernous sinus and then branching off into the anterior and middle cerebral arteries.

2) The vertebral arteries are posterior and originate as branches off the subclavian arteries. They pass through the foramen magnum and join at the junction of the pons and medulla oblongata to form the basilar artery. The basilar artery divides at the level of the midbrain to form the two posterior cerebral arteries (Sugerman, 2002).

3) The arterial circle (circle of Willis) is the structure in the brain with the ability to compensate for reduced blood flow from any of the major contributors (collateral blood flow). This circle is formed by the posterior cerebral arteries, posterior communicating arteries, internal carotid arteries, anterior cerebral arteries, and anterior communicating artery.

b. Ischemic stroke accounts for 87% of all strokes. It is occlusive in nature as the result of a cerebral embolism or cerebral thrombosis and it is categorized by vascular distribution or location (NINDS, 2009b).

c. Hemorrhagic stroke has a lower incidence (10%) than ischemic stroke but is associated with a higher mortality rate. A *subarachnoid stroke* is a rupture of a large vessel in the protective lining of the brain, and an *intracerebral stroke* is the rupture of a vessel in the brain itself (3%; NINDS, 2009b).

2. Metabolic needs of the brain

a. The brain needs constant circulation of approximately 20% of the body's blood supply to maintain adequate oxygen and nutrients.

b. Blood flow is autoregulated by the brain itself (Patel et al., 2008).

c. The physiological demands served by the blood supply of the brain are particularly significant because neurons are more sensitive to oxygen deprivation than other kinds of cells with lower rates of metabolism. In addition, the brain is at risk from circulating toxins and is specifically protected in this respect by the blood-brain barrier.

D. Signs and Symptoms of Stroke (NSA, 2009g)

1. Sudden numbness or weakness of face, arm, or leg, especially unilaterally

2. Sudden confusion, trouble speaking or understanding

3. Sudden trouble seeing in one or both eyes

4. Sudden ataxia, dizziness, or loss of balance or coordination

5. Sudden severe headache with no known cause

E. Pathophysiology

1. Ischemic stroke (approximately 85%–88% of all strokes; Buttaro, 2003; NINDS, 2009b; Sauerbeck, 2006)

a. Process (Adams et al., 2007; Boss, 2002a; Buttaro, 2003)

1) Acute ischemic stroke is stroke caused by thrombosis or embolism and is more common than hemorrhagic stroke. On the macroscopic level, ischemic stroke most often is caused by extracranial embolism or intracranial thrombosis, but it may also be caused by decreased cerebral blood flow. On the cellular level, any process that disrupts blood flow to a portion of the brain unleashes an ischemic

cascade, leading to the death of neurons and cerebral infarction (Becker et al., 2010).

2) Acute ischemic stroke often begins as a result of atherosclerotic disease and progresses slowly as the affected artery becomes narrowed and eventually occluded. It may also occur as a result of a rupture of an atherosclerotic plaque that travels as an embolus to the brain and blocks blood flow.

3) Atherosclerotic plaques (stenotic lesions) form at branches and curves in the cerebral circulation. The stenotic area degenerates, which forms an ulcerated vessel wall. Platelets and fibrin adhere to the damaged wall and form clots, which eventually occlude the artery.

4) The thrombus may enlarge in the vessel distally and proximally, or a portion of the clot may break off and travel up the vessel to a distant site, forming an embolus.

5) Focal areas of the brain and adjoining brain tissue are deprived of oxygen and glucose. When the deprivation is severe enough and lasts long enough, permanent damage occurs. The timing of the restoration of cerebral blood flow appears to be a critical factor. Time also may prove to be a key factor in neuronal protection (Becker et al., 2010).

6) Neurons near the ischemic or infarcted areas undergo changes that disrupt plasma membranes, causing cellular edema and further compression of capillaries. On the cellular level, the ischemic neuron becomes depolarized as adenosine triphosphate (ATP) is depleted and membrane ion transport systems fail. The resulting influx of calcium leads to the release of a number of neurotransmitters, including large quantities of glutamate, which activates N-methyl-D-aspartate (NMDA) and other excitatory receptors on other neurons. These neurons then become depolarized, causing further calcium influx, further glutamate release, and local amplification of the initial ischemic insult. This massive calcium influx also activates various degradative enzymes, leading to destruction of the cell membrane and other essential neuronal structures (Becker et al., 2010).

7) It is thought that some cortical reorganization and neuroplasticity occurs following a stroke. This has been described as a "rewiring" of brain cells in response to the environment and experience, including therapy. This change results in a different pattern of movement for the client (Caswell, 2008).

8) Most people survive an initial hemispheric ischemic stroke unless there is massive cerebral edema (Becker et al., 2010).

9) Massive brainstem infarcts from basilar thrombosis or embolism almost always are fatal.

b. Types of ischemic strokes
   1) TIA (Easton et al., 2009)
      a) Persists for several minutes or hours and then resolves
      b) Usually lasts 5–15 minutes, followed by full recovery of neurological function within 24 hours; the majority last less than 1 hour
      c) It has also been defined as "a brief episode of neurological dysfunction caused by focal brain or retinal ischemia, with clinical symptoms typically lasting less than one hour, and without evidence of acute infarction" (Easton et al., 2009, pp. 2276–2277).
      d) Roughly 80% resolve within 60 minutes. Tissue-based definitions are being proposed with magnetic resonance imaging (MRI; Becker et al., 2010).
      e) Resolution results in a negative neurological examination, and diagnosis may be based on history.
      f) People who experience TIA may have nine times the risk of a stroke, and often stroke occurs within 30 days of the TIA. (A valid estimate of the incidence of TIA is not available because many TIAs go unreported due to the subtle nature of the symptoms.) After a stroke many clients and families report episodes that were likely TIAs preceding the stroke.
      g) Vertebrobasilar TIA is the result of inadequate blood flow from the vertebral arteries, usually secondary to a partially obstructed subclavian artery, which supplies this area (Keiser, 1999).

h) Carotid TIA is the result of inadequate blood flow from the carotid artery, usually because of carotid stenosis.

2) Reversible ischemic neurological deficit is a TIA or signs of a stroke that persist more than 24 hours but eventually resolve completely, usually within 48 hours.

3) Embolic stroke

   a) A traveling clot, which typically originates from thrombi in the heart or from plaque in the aortic arch or carotid or vertebral arteries that becomes lodged and obstructs cerebral blood flow

   b) Commonly associated with a history of cardiac disease, especially atrial fibrillation in older people

   c) The sources of cardiogenic emboli include valvular thrombi (e.g., in mitral stenosis, endocarditis, prosthetic valve, mural thrombi, myocardial infarction [MI], atrial fibrillation, dilated cardiomyopathy, severe congestive heart failure, and atrial myxoma). MI is associated with a 2%–3% incidence of embolic stroke, of which 85% occur in the first month after MI (Becker et al., 2010).

4) Thrombotic stroke

   a) Most common cause of stroke

   b) A stationary clot in a large blood vessel, usually caused by atherosclerotic plaque

      i. Plaque forms when calcium and lipids collect and attach to the vessel wall, especially in bifurcations of a large artery. This produces narrowing that impedes or obstructs blood flow.

      ii. Atherosclerosis can produce degeneration of blood vessel walls. This can involve tearing or degeneration of a weakened vessel wall or plaque, which can trigger the normal clotting process, and this congestion further reduces circulation to the area.

      iii. Large-vessel thrombosis: Thrombotic strokes occur most often in large arteries and usually are caused by a combination of long-term atherosclerosis followed by rapid blood clot formation.

Clients with thrombotic stroke are likely to have coronary artery disease, and heart attack is a common cause of death in people who have had this type of stroke (NSA, 2006c).

5) Lacunar infarcts (small vessel disease; Becker et al., 2010; NSA, 2009g)

   a) Thrombotic strokes that affect the small arteries deep within the subcortical white matter of the brain (Becker et al., 2010)

   b) Are microinfarcts smaller than 1 cm in diameter (usually 2–20 mm) and involve the small perforating arteries, predominantly in the basal ganglia, internal capsules, and pons (Boss, 2002b)

   c) Are caused by atherosclerosis

   d) Often result in pure motor, pure sensory, or ataxic hemiparetic deficits

   e) Are closely linked to small-vessel disease found in hypertension or diabetes

6) Stroke caused by systemic hypoperfusion (Merck Sharp & Dohme Corporation, 2009–2010)

   a) Caused by inadequate cardiac output with system hypoperfusion

   b) Usually caused by MI, cardiac arrest, and life-threatening ventricular arrhythmias; less commonly caused by pulmonary emboli, acute gastrointestinal bleeding, and shock

   c) Symptoms include pallor, sweating, and hypotension. Neurological deficits are sudden and associated with systemic symptoms related to the underlying problem.

   d) Prominent signs include decreased level of consciousness and symmetric depression of hemispheric function.

   e) Also called a watershed stroke (Likosky et al., 2003)

c. Risk factors for ischemic stroke (Becker et al., 2010; Boss, 2002a; NINDS, 2009b)

1) Arterial hypertension; elevated systolic and diastolic blood pressures are independent risk factors

2) Smoking increases the risk by 50%.

3) Diabetes increases the risk by 2.5–3.5 times.

4) Insulin resistance is an independent risk factor.

5) Thrombocythemia and polycythemia increase the risk.

6) Impaired cardiac function (coronary artery disease, left ventricular hypertrophy, chronic atrial fibrillation)

7) Chronic atherosclerosis; elevated lipoprotein(a) is an independent risk factor.

8) Hyperhomocysteinemia is a strong and independent risk factor.

9) Estrogen deficiency in postmenopausal women increases the risk.

10) Advanced age (the risk doubles every decade)

11) Use of oral contraceptives places a person at a higher risk for an ischemic stroke.

12) Previous cerebrovascular disease can place a person at a higher risk for an ischemic stroke.

2. Hemorrhagic stroke: Intracerebral hemorrhage accounts for 10%–15% of all strokes and is associated with higher mortality rates than cerebral infarctions (Broderick et al., 2007).

a. Process (Boss, 2002a; Graykoski, 2003)

1) Spontaneous rupture of a cerebral vessel occurs; blood enters the brain tissue or subarachnoid space.

2) The most common causes of hemorrhagic stroke are hypertension (up to 60%), ruptured aneurysms, vascular malformations, vasculitis, bleeding into a tumor, hemorrhage from bleeding disorders or anticoagulation, head trauma, and illicit drug use (Nassisi, 2010).

3) The area around the injury dies within a few minutes from lack of oxygen and the failure of the oxygen-dependent ATP metabolic pathway. The broader area of injury is called the penumbra, and this damage is more dynamic, taking 12–24 hours to occur. The release of intracellular calcium initiates the programmed cell death or apoptosis (Graykoski, 2003).

4) With hemorrhagic strokes, focal neurological deficits are found in 80% of people, and altered consciousness occurs in 50% of people (Boss, 2002a).

5) People with hemorrhagic stroke present with similar focal neurologic deficits but tend to be more ill than people with ischemic stroke (Nassisi, 2010). Only 20% of

clients regain functional independence (Broderick et al., 2007).

b. Types of hemorrhagic stroke (Nassisi, 2010; Zebian & Kazzi, 2010)

1) Subarachnoid hemorrhage (SAH)

a) This is the rupture of a blood vessel located within the subarachnoid space, a fluid-filled space between layers of connective tissue (meninges) that surround the brain. It is caused by some pathologic process, usually rupture of a berry aneurysm or arteriovenous malformation (AVM; Sen, Webb, & Selph, 2010).

b) Annual incidence of nontraumatic aneurysmal SAH is 6–25 cases per 100,000. An estimated 10%–15% of people die before reaching the hospital. The mortality rate reaches as high as 40% within the first week. About half die in the first 6 months.

c) Presents clinically as a sudden onset of a severe headache ("the worst headache of my life"), nausea and vomiting, signs of meningeal irritation (neck stiffness, low back pain, bilateral leg pain), photophobia and visual disturbances, and varying degrees of neurological dysfunction

d) Can result in elevated intracranial pressure, vasospasms, and ischemia, which further reduces cerebral blood flow

e) Can also present as prodromal (warning) headaches from minor blood leakage; this is referred to as sentinel headache with a reported median of 2 weeks before the SAH may occur (30%–50% of aneurysmal SAHs)

f) More than 25% of people experience seizures close to the acute onset; the location of a seizure focus has no relationship to the location of the aneurysm.

2) Intracerebral (intraparenchymal) hemorrhage

a) Often caused by hypertension (blood pressure is elevated in almost all cases)

b) Involves small, deep-penetrating blood vessels that rupture and release blood directly into the brain tissue (parenchyma)

c) An intracerebral hemorrhage usually invades deep white matter first. Intracerebral hemorrhage has a predilection for certain sites in the brain, including the thalamus, putamen, cerebellum, and brainstem (Nassisi, 2010).

d) Neurological signs and symptoms vary with the site and size of the extravasation of blood (released blood puts pressure on surrounding tissue, which can cause small arterioles and capillaries to tear).

e) It may present clinically as an almost immediate lapse into stupor and coma, with hemiplegia and steady deterioration to death over several hours after initial presentation. More often it presents with a headache, followed within a few minutes by unilateral neurological deficits involving face and limbs.

f) In addition to the area of the brain injured by the hemorrhage, the surrounding brain can be damaged by pressure produced by the mass effect of the hematoma. A general increase in intracranial pressure may occur. This resulting hematoma acts as a space-occupying lesion that, if large enough, will cause brain shifting or herniation.

c. Risk factors for hemorrhagic stroke (NSA, 2009f; NINDS, 2009b)

1) High blood pressure is responsible for approximately 60% of intracerebral hemorrhages and is a controllable stroke risk factor.

2) Excessive alcohol and drug use are associated with higher incidences of intracerebral hemorrhage and SAH. Cocaine-related strokes are caused by an erosion of the vessel from the cocaine, which causes the vessel wall to become weaker and rupture (Boss, 2002a; NSA, 2009g). Cocaine has been linked to aneurysm formation (Boss, 2002a). About 85%–90% of drug-associated intracerebral hemorrhages occur in people 20–30 years old.

3) Anticoagulant medication may prevent ischemic stroke but may increase the risk of intracerebral hemorrhage if the amount taken exceeds the therapeutic range.

4) Blood clotting disorders such as hemophilia and sickle cell anemia can increase risk.

5) Advanced age

6) History of prior stroke

F. Clinical Manifestations of Stroke: The symptoms of stroke depend on the part of the brain that is damaged by a disruption in arterial blood flow. In some cases, a person may not even be aware that he or she has had a stroke (Boss, 2002a; Buttaro, 2003; Patel et al., 2008; **Figure 11-1**).

1. Each internal carotid artery ascends along one side of the neck and supplies the cerebral hemispheres and diencephalon. These arteries have many twists and turns where plaque can build up, causing a blockage. Such blockages can be identified by sonogram (noninvasive) or by angiogram (invasive). Also, a sound called a bruit can sometimes be heard via stethoscope when a blockage exists. Signs and symptoms of occlusion may include

a. Headaches
b. Altered level of responsiveness
c. Bruits over the carotid artery
d. Profound aphasia
e. Ptosis
f. Unilateral blindness or retinal emboli
g. Weakness, paralysis, numbness, sensory changes, and visual deficits on the affected side

2. The anterior cerebral artery (one of two main branches of the carotid artery) supplies medial surfaces and upper areas of the frontal and parietal lobes, including the medial aspect of the motor and sensory strip of the hemisphere. Signs and symptoms of occlusion may include

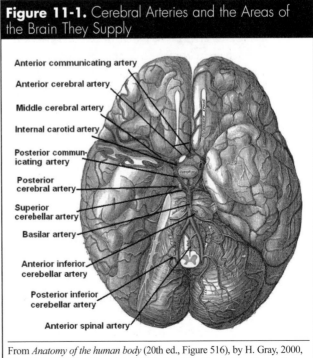

Figure 11-1. Cerebral Arteries and the Areas of the Brain They Supply

Anterior communicating artery
Anterior cerebral artery
Middle cerebral artery
Internal carotid artery
Posterior communicating artery
Posterior cerebral artery
Superior cerebellar artery
Basilar artery
Anterior inferior cerebellar artery
Posterior inferior cerebellar artery
Anterior spinal artery

From *Anatomy of the human body* (20th ed., Figure 516), by H. Gray, 2000, New York: Bartleby. Copyright 2000 by Bartleby. Reprinted with permission.

a. Confusion

b. Labile emotions, personality changes

c. Weakness or numbness on affected side

d. Paralysis of contralateral foot and leg

e. Impaired mobility, sensation greater in lower extremities than upper extremities, impaired sensory function

f. Urinary incontinence

g. Loss of coordination

3. The middle cerebral artery (the most commonly occluded vessel in stroke and the largest branch in the internal carotid artery) supplies part of the frontal lobe and lateral surface of the temporal and parietal lobes, including primary motor and sensory areas for the face, throat, hand, and arm and, in the dominant hemisphere, the areas for speech. Signs and symptoms of occlusion include

a. Altered level of responsiveness

b. Alterations in communication, including aphasia, dysphasia, reading difficulty (dyslexia), inability to write (dysgraphia)

c. Visual field deficits

d. Alterations in cognition, mobility, and sensation, including contralateral sensory deficit and hemiparesis (more severe in the upper than lower)

4. The anterior communicating artery joins the anterior cerebral arteries of both hemispheres together. Signs and symptoms of occlusion may include

a. Memory impairments, amnesia

b. Decreased executive functioning

5. The posterior cerebral artery joins the middle cerebral arteries to the posterior cerebral arteries, which are part of the basilar artery system. It supplies the medial and inferior temporal lobes, medial occipital lobe, thalamus, posterior hypothalamus, and visual receptive area. Signs and symptoms of occlusion may include

a. Hemiplegia

b. Receptive aphasia

c. Sensory impairment

d. Dyslexia

e. Visual field deficits (cortical blindness from ischemia)

f. Coma

6. Vertebral or basilar arteries supply the brainstem and cerebellum.

a. Signs and symptoms of incomplete occlusion

1) TIA

2) Unilateral or bilateral weakness of extremities

3) Visual deficits on affected side such as lack of depth perception, diplopia, or color blindness

4) Nausea, vertigo, tinnitus

5) Headache

6) Dysarthria

7) Numbness

8) Dysphagia

9) "Locked-in" syndrome: No movement except eyelids, sensation and consciousness preserved

b. Signs and symptoms of complete occlusion

1) Coma

2) Decerebrate rigidity

3) Respiratory and circulatory abnormalities

G. Residual Deficits of Stroke (**Table 11-1**; NSA, 2009e)

1. Significant alterations in many psychosocial areas

a. Diminished affect

b. Increased dependence in activities of daily living (ADLs)

c. Decreased self-esteem

d. Altered role performance

e. Sexual dysfunction

f. Change in leisure or social activity

g. Decreased financial earning or vocational capability

2. General sequelae (all of which can influence safety)

a. Hemiplegia: Weakness or paralysis on one side of the body contralateral to the lesion

b. Abnormal tone, including flaccidity initially and then hypertonicity or spasticity on the affected side

c. Sensorimotor problems, ataxia, imbalance

d. Language deficits if lesion is in the dominant hemisphere

e. Visuospatial perception impairments

f. Cognitive deficits

g. Memory changes

h. Emotional lability: inability to control emotions, especially crying and laughter (these may be expressed at inappropriate times)

i. Fatigue

j. Depression (may persist for months after the stroke)

k. Seizure activity

3. Left hemispheric stroke: Common impairments and deficits

a. Right hemiparesis (weakness) or hemiplegia (paralysis)

Table 11-1. Residual Deficits of Stroke and Interventions

Manifestations	Left Hemispheric Damage	Interventions
Paresis or paralysis	Right side	Involve affected side during therapy or activities of daily living (ADLs).
Major deficits	Right homonymous hemianopsia; language deficits (e.g., aphasia, expression, comprehension, word finding); confuses left and right; has trouble gesturing, reading, writing	Incorporate techniques used by the speech therapist when communicating with the client; use a communication board and tools; incorporate the affected side into ADLs and activities; use demonstration and positive feedback.
Thought processes	Has difficulty listening and understanding; cannot process incoming language normally	Be patient; work with clients in short time frames to reduce frustration; offer encouragement; have the same staff work with a client when possible; speak slowly.
Emotional style	Is easily frustrated or depressed; is aware of deficits	Be patient; offer encouragement; exhibit acceptance; educate family on realistic expectations for communication; have a rehabilitation psychologist work with the client.
Attention span	Usually normal	Limit sessions, care, or treatments based on individual need.
Behavioral style	Is slow and cautious; needs encouragement	Allow plenty of time to work with a client; don't appear rushed; don't fragment care.

Manifestations	Right Hemispheric Damage	Interventions
Paresis or paralysis	Left side	Involve the affected side during therapy or ADLs.
Major deficits	Left homonymous hemianopsia; displays visual, spatial, perceptual deficits (e.g., gets lost, cannot dress self correctly, misjudges distance and position in space, spills things, gets stuck in doorways); has distorted body image; may have agnosia	Use repetition and one-step commands; approach on the left side and place objects in view past midline (e.g., affected arm on table while eating); orient the client in the room so all people enter the room on the left side of the client.
Thought processes	Has poor judgment; may have unrealistic thoughts; has memory deficits; has difficulty with concrete thinking	Always be aware of safety for this client (the client will take risks and act impulsively); establish a routine and stick with it; use a memory book; mark the client's room so it can be easily found with cueing.
Emotional style	Is often cheerful or euphoric; will deny illness or deficits; is unaware of problems; neglects left side; exhibits socially inappropriate behavior	Cue to deficits; constant reminders to call for help; don't leave unattended in bathroom or shower; monitor for inappropriate behavior; educate the family on expectations and deficits (the client will try to convince the family that he or she is fine).
Attention span	Short; is highly distractible	Work with the client one to one in a quiet setting; minimize outside noise and distractions; keep sessions and treatments short.
Behavioral style	Is quick and impulsive; needs supervision to prevent injury	Do not leave clients unattended; may need to use bed and chair alarms or an enclosure bed to prevent injury (clients will not call for help)

b. Impaired ability to think analytically, shortened retention span, difficulty in learning new information, and problems in conceptualizing and generalizing

c. Inability to do mathematical computations or interpret symbols

d. Right homonymous hemianopsia

e. Behavioral changes (e.g., slow and cautious, hesitant)

f. Language difficulty, which includes not only the motor aspect of speech but also the ability to express and understand thoughts, ideas, and symbols in sequence

   1) Expressive (Broca's dysphasia or nonfluent; Boss, 2002a)

     a) Occurs with lesions in the posterior part of the dominant frontal lobe (precentral gyrus) and usually is on the left hemisphere

b) Is responsible for the motor aspects of speech

c) Damage in this area results in the inability to form or difficulty forming or finding words; difficulty writing (translating thoughts into symbols, not the physical act of writing); and impaired ability to read letters, numbers, or written material

d) May have speech that is slow, effortful to produce, and punctuated by long pauses between words; verbal comprehension is largely intact

e) Altered comprehension of language

f) May have intact automatic speech (e.g., may express a word, phrase, profanity, or song unexpectedly in a clear manner)

g) May have anomia (difficulty finding words and naming objects), perseveration (unintentional repetition of a word or phrase), conductive aphasia (repeating words or phrases on command), and difficulty with sentence construction

2) Receptive (Wernicke's dysphasia or fluent; Boss, 2002a)

a) Occurs with lesions in the posterior, superior temporal dominant lobe (superior temporal gyrus)

b) This area is responsible for reception and interpretation of speech.

c) Able to produce verbal language, but language content is meaningless; able to speak fluently, but words may be incorrect or inappropriate in context; unable to detect his or her own errors

d) Besides being impaired with verbal comprehension, is also impaired in naming, reading, and writing

3) Global dysphasia

a) Occurs with lesions in the frontal-temporal dominant lobes; anterior and posterior speech areas are extensively impaired

b) Exhibits comprehension and speaking problems (produces very little speech, a few words or phrases)

c) Impaired reading, naming, and writing skills

d) May have intact automatic speech only for routines such as counting, singing a song, or stating the days of the week

4) Transcortical dysphasias (transcortical sensory dysphasia, mixed transcortical dysphasia, isolated speech center; Boss, 2002a)

a) Occurs with lesions in anterior and posterior presylvian fissures

b) Have the ability to repeat (echolalia) and recite

c) Speech can be fluent but uses paraphrases

d) Inability to read and write

e) Comprehension is impaired

5) Apraxia of speech

a) Occurs when there is damage to the motor centers in the cortex that control speech

b) Inability to program the position of the speech muscles, and the sequence of the muscle movements is necessary to produce understandable speech.

c) Understanding of speech remains intact.

d) Speech may be clear at times and undecipherable the next.

e) Common for perseveration and inconsistency

6) Dysarthria

a) Occurs with damage to a central or peripheral motor nerve, brainstem, or cranial nerve

b) Exhibits poorly articulated speech, resulting from interference in the control and execution over the muscles of speech; muscle control of the palate and tongue may be abnormal

c) May have abnormal voice quality (too soft or loud); speech is slow, may be slurred and hard to understand

7) Anarthria

a) Total loss of articulation as a result of loss of control of the muscles of speech; inability to articulate words

b) Occurs with damage to a central or peripheral motor nerve or brainstem

4. Right hemispheric stroke: Common impairments and deficits

a. Left hemiparesis (weakness) or hemiplegia (paralysis)

b. Problems with depth perception and spatial relationships

c. Visual disturbances (including left homonymous hemianopsia)

d. Inability to distinguish directional concepts such as up-down, front-back, in-out

e. Difficulty distinguishing foreground from background information (figure-ground, spatial-temporal perception)

f. Decreased ability to distinguish between similar shapes and forms (form constancy, spatial-temporal perception)

g. Anosognosia: Lack of awareness or denial of a neurological deficit, especially paralysis, on one side of the body; reduced insight into the ramifications of the impairment

h. Lack of awareness of others' nonverbal communication (e.g., facial expressions, tone of voice, territorial space, gestures); display of a flat affect

i. Unilateral neglect: Inability to integrate sensory and perceptual stimuli from one side of the body or environment

j. Behavioral changes (e.g., impulsivity, egocentricity, quickness to try things, risk taking)

k. Social inappropriateness: Sexual disinhibition and inappropriate self-disclosure

l. Difficulty in finding locations, such as one's room, and understanding maps and objects (geographic-topographic memory)

5. Brainstem strokes

a. Result from ischemic or hemorrhagic process in the midbrain, pons, or medulla

b. Potential deficits: Many vital centers and nuclei of cranial nerves exist, so deficits can vary greatly, including dysarthria, dysphagia (chewing or swallowing difficulty), ataxia, quadriparesis or quadriplegia, poor balance or coordination, double or blurred vision, pinpoint pupils, horizontal gaze palsy (e.g., eye moves to the side, away from the cerebral lesion), vertigo with nausea, abnormal respiratory patterns, hyperthermia, coma or persistent vegetative state, locked-in syndrome (quadriplegia and facial paralysis, except for eye or eyelid movement; intact cognition; stroke is in the pons).

H. Children and Stroke (NINDS, 2009b; NSA, 2009c)

1. Etiology

a. Childhood stroke occurs between 1 month and 18 years of age.

b. The incidence of stroke in children younger than 15 years old is about 6 cases in every 100,000 children per year. Stroke and other cerebrovascular disorders are among the top 10 causes of death in children in the United States. Cerebrovascular disorders are among the top 10 causes of death in children, with rates highest in the first year of life. Stroke mortality in children younger than age 1 has remained the same during the last 40 years.

c. Approximately 55% are ischemic, and the remainder are hemorrhagic (Roach et al., 2008).

d. A perinatal stroke (before 28 days of age) encompasses a cerebrovascular event that occurs between 28 weeks of gestation and 1 month after birth. This may lead to a greater propensity to develop childhood epilepsy.

e. A stroke that occurs before birth may be called an in-utero stroke, fetal stroke, or prenatal stroke. Stroke occurs more frequently in the perinatal and prenatal age group than in older children.

f. Slightly more common in children under the age of 2

g. Babies who have strokes in the womb or within the first month of life are at risk of cerebral palsy.

h. Premature babies are at risk for stroke during or shortly after delivery if hypoxia occurs.

i. On average it takes 48–72 hours for children to get to a hospital after their caregivers recognize the first symptom of stroke (related to the widespread belief that strokes do not happen to children).

j. Children have a greater ability to heal because of the greater plasticity or flexibility of their nervous system and brain. The brain is still developing, so it may be more likely to repair itself (children usually recover function with the help of physical and speech therapy).

2. Causes of childhood stroke

a. Birth defects

b. Infections such as meningitis or encephalitis

c. Trauma

d. Blood disorders such as sickle cell disease

3. Childhood stroke symptoms are similar to those of adult stroke.

a. Severe headache (often the first complaint)

b. Speech difficulties

c. Problems with eye movement

d. Numbness

4. Stroke-related disabilities

a. Speech and communication from brain cell damage

b. Paralysis or weakness unilaterally from brain cell damage

c. Cerebral palsy (unique to children)

d. Mental retardation (unique to children)

e. Epilepsy (unique to children)

5. Stroke education for children
   a. NSA developed the Hip Hop Stroke Program in 2004.
   b. The program uses children to educate families about stroke, primarily in urban elementary schools.
   c. The program teaches children to develop life-long healthy habits to prevent stroke and to recognize symptoms of stroke.
   d. The program teaches children to identify stroke as an emergency and to call 911.

II. **Primary Prevention of Stroke**
A. Nonmodifiable Risk Factors
   1. Age: A stroke can happen at any age, but risk doubles every decade after age 55.
   2. Gender: A stroke is more common in men, but more women than men die from a stroke.
   3. Race and ethnicity: A stroke is more common in African Americans (twice the risk) and Hispanics, Asians, and Pacific Islanders.
   4. Family history (hereditary factors)
   5. Previous stroke or a TIA
   6. Fibromuscular dysplasia
   7. Hole in the heart: Patent foramen ovale
B. Modifiable or Treatable Risk Factors (NSA, 2009f; Sauerbeck, 2006)
   1. Hypertension (blood pressure 140/90 mm Hg or higher for an extended period of time, although >120/80 mm Hg is considered prehypertension)
   2. Heart disease (includes MI, atrial fibrillation, and heart failure)
   3. Diabetes mellitus (four times more likely to have a stroke; should have hemoglobin A1c lower than 6)
   4. High cholesterol level with hyperlipidemia (low-density lipoprotein of 160 mg/dl or more; control with statins)
   5. Carotid stenosis (carotid artery narrowed by 70% or more by atherosclerotic plaque doubles risk of stroke)
   6. TIA (treat with aspirin or antiplatelet drug)
C. Lifestyle Risk Factors (NSA, 2009f; Sauerbeck, 2006) 1.   May be independent of or contribute to medical risk factors that could cause stroke
   2. Smoking: Toxic compounds contribute to atherosclerosis, increasing clustering of platelets and increasing clotting time and viscosity.
   3. Physical inactivity: 30 minutes per day of moderate to vigorous exercise reduces risk of stroke; exercise controls obesity and diabetes, lowers blood pressure, and increases high-density lipoproteins, which also lowers risk.

4. Alcohol abuse increases triglycerides, can produce cardiac arrhythmias, and can cause heart failure.
5. Obesity: A body mass index higher than 30 increases risk; abdominal obesity (waist circumference greater than 40 inches in men, 35 inches in women) is an independent risk factor.
6. Stress reduction through lifestyle changes decreases release of stress hormones, which contribute to obesity.
7. The Stroke Risk Scorecard can be used to rate or score personal risk (www.stroke.org).

III. **Treatment of Stroke**
A. Early Recognition of Stroke
   1. A stroke is a "brain attack."
   2. Time is brain (i.e., early intervention is critical for preventing the loss of cerebral perfusion).
   3. Community education of emergency medical personnel and the general public is key.
   4. Any person experiencing signs and symptoms of a stroke should seek help immediately in a hospital setting. He or she should activate the emergency medical system (911) and preferably be transported to a primary stroke center.
   5. Consultation with a neurosurgeon or neurologist is preferred.
   6. Participation in stroke performance measures that improve client outcomes and save lives is essential.
B. Diagnostic Tests
   1. Brain computed tomography (CT) scan (to rule out hemorrhagic stroke to administer anticoagulants and recombinant tissue plasminogen activator [rt-PA])
   2. An MRI test may also be ordered with diffusion-weighted imaging. This is especially useful for detecting small infarcts and is superior to CT for diagnosing ischemic stroke.
   3. Blood tests: Complete blood cell count, electrolytes, liver and renal profiles, clotting studies, lipid panel
   4. Angiogram (may be needed for clients with a SAH to rule out an aneurysm or AVM)
   5. Other tests that may be ordered are electrocardiogram, chest X ray, echocardiogram, electroencephalogram, lumbar puncture, carotid studies, and magnetic resonance angiography.
C. Medications: Drug therapy is one of the newest ways to combat the damaging effects of a stroke and lessen a person's chance of a recurrent stroke if other lifestyle factors are maintained.

1. Thrombolytic therapy (ischemic strokes; The Brain Attack Coalition [BAC], 2002; NINDS, 2009b; NSA, 2009g)
   a. rt-PA
      1) Only systemic thrombolytic drug approved by the U.S. Food and Drug Administration (in 1996) for ischemic stroke
      2) Enzyme that targets a thrombus within a blood vessel (Lutsep & Clark, 2009)
      3) Must meet the inclusion criteria (arrival in the emergency department [ED] within 3 hours of symptom onset, CT rules out hemorrhage, exam consistent with symptoms of stroke)
      4) The client is assessed against exclusion criteria: platelet count <100,000, current use of anticoagulants or prothrombin time more than 15 seconds, use of heparin in past 48 hours and prolonged partial thromboplastin time (international normalized ratio 1.7 or higher), recent previous stroke (<3 months), major surgery within past 14 days, uncontrolled hypertension (blood pressure >185/110), recent MI, blood glucose lower than 50 mg/dL or higher than 400 mg/dL, neurological signs that are improving rapidly (BAC, 2002).
      5) The client is assessed using the National Institutes of Health Stroke Scale (the most widely accepted tool for neurological assessment of stroke; www.strokecenter.org/trials/scales/nihss.html).
      6) The Cincinnati Stroke Scale often is used for initial screening of stroke by emergency medical service staff and bedside clinicians (www.strokecenter.org/trials/scales/cincinnati.html).
      7) Intravenous rt-PA, 0.9 mg/kg (maximum of 90 mg) is given as a bolus (10% of dose given over 1 minute) and followed by the remaining 90% of the dose as an infusion over 60 minutes.
      8) The client is monitored closely for bleeding complications during and after infusion, which includes neurological assessments and control of blood pressure.
   b. Antiplatelet and anticoagulation (AHA, 2008; NSA, 2009g)
      1) Antiplatelet and anticoagulant drugs are the most common medications used to reduce risk of a secondary stroke.
      2) Aspirin is currently viewed as the gold standard antiplatelet drug because of its effectiveness and low cost. Other antiplatelet drugs used to treat heart disease and ischemic-type stroke include clopidogrel bisulfate (Plavix) and ticlopidine hydrochloride (Ticlid).
      3) The antiplatelet drug dipyridamole (Aggrenox), in combination with aspirin, reduced risk of recurrent stroke by 37% in clinical trials (NSA, 2009c).
      4) The antiplatelet drug ticlopidine (Ticlid) may be prescribed for those allergic to aspirin.
      5) Low-molecular weight heparin may be used in combination with aspirin and antiplatelet drugs for deep vein thrombosis (DVT) prevention in ischemic-type strokes only (NSA, 2009g).
      6) Low-molecular weight heparin may also be started as an anticoagulant (studies show no real benefit over aspirin) only for people with atrial fibrillation who have an ischemic stroke, and then the person is bridged over to warfarin (Coumadin) for a maintenance dose that may last 90 days to a lifetime (warfarin is commonly prescribed for patients with atrial fibrillation).
2. Anticonvulsants are controversial. Some physicians may prescribe prophylactically if the stroke involves the temporal lobe; others use it if seizures appear as a complication. Medication selection is based on type of seizure (may use lorazepam initially and phenytoin in the longer term).
3. Vasopressors are used as needed to maintain cerebral perfusion pressure. Nimodipine (Nimotop) may be used to reduce the deficit produced by cerebral ischemia (vasospasm).
4. Support and comfort: Analgesics, antipyretics, sedation, pain medication (for central pain syndrome; NINDS, 2008)
5. Statin drugs may be prescribed to treat and prevent hypercholesterolemia and hyperlipidemia (low-density lipoprotein 100 or lower with heart disease).
6. Nutripharmaceuticals such as an omega 3-6-9 fatty acid supplement along with a low-fat diet may be prescribed to treat and prevent hypercholesterolemia and hyperlipidemia.
7. Neurostimulant agents may be useful in the pharmacological management of neurobehavioral disorders following a stroke.

8. Citicoline, a supplement also known as cytidine diphosphate-choline (CDP-choline) and cytidine 5'-diphosphocholine, has also shown great promise as a psychostimulant or nootropic agent. Studies show that it may stimulate dopamine receptor densities and acetylcholine production, which can reduce memory impairment caused by stroke (Teather & Wurtman, 2005).

9. Neuroprotective agents may be useful in making the brain less susceptible to the damaging effects of a stroke. These agents attempt to save ischemic neurons in the brain from irreversible injury. They may prevent early ischemic injury or prevent reperfusion injury. Clinical trials are looking at the benefits of such agents (Lutsep & Clark, 2009).

   a. Agents that may help prevent early ischemic injury by preventing excitatory neurotransmitter release and reducing the deleterious effects of ischemia on cells under current clinical study include NMDA antagonists, magnesium, nalmefene, lubeluzole, clomethiazole, and calcium channel blockers (Lutsep & Clark, 2009).

   b. Agents under clinical study that may help prevent reperfusion injury by preventing white blood cells from adhering to vessel walls, limiting formation of free radicals, or promoting neuronal repair and possibly protecting the brain from additional injury include enlimomab, Hu23F2G, tetracycline antibiotics, citicoline, and fiblast (Lutsep & Clark, 2009).

10. All clients with an ischemic type of stroke should be maintained on a regimen of aspirin, statin therapy, and an antiplatelet or thrombolytic agent unless otherwise contraindicated.

D. Surgery

   1. Ruptured aneurysms are repaired using a clip or the aneurysm is treated from inside the vessel by embolization (a metal coil through the artery in the brain that fills the aneurysm and allows a clot to form and prevent more bleeding).

   2. AVMs can be treated the same way using interventional neuroradiologic procedures and a coil to clot off the AVM or instillation of glue during an angiogram (keeps blood from flowing through the AVM).

   3. An AVM may still warrant surgical excision.

   4. Surgical removal of an intracerebral hematoma may be performed through a craniotomy or through a CT- or MRI-guided aspiration procedure (Bogousslavsky, 2003).

5. Surgical treatment for ischemic strokes may include decompressive craniectomy, ventricular shunting, angioplasty, intra-arterial thrombolysis, stenting, and mechanical retrieval devices. An interventional neuroradiologist plays a key role on the surgical team (Bader & Palmer, 2006; Bogousslavsky, 2003).

E. Intensive Care Management (AHA, 2005)

   1. Onset to treatment time is critically associated with improved functional outcomes. The ability to identify and treat such events as hypotension, hypertension, and hypoxia is crucial in the first hours after a stroke. Elevated intracranial pressure is managed through monitors and catheters (ventriculostomy).

   2. Respiratory support with mechanical ventilation is provided if needed (supplemental oxygen and hyperventilation may be indicated for hypoxic clients).

   3. Cardiovascular support and management of blood pressure: Labetalol, nicardipine, or nitroprusside is recommended if blood pressure exceeds recommended levels.

   4. Nutritional support (enteral or parenteral feeding) is provided, and serum glucose is managed (hyperglycemia may increase neuronal damage, and hypoglycemia may extend infarct).

   5. Body temperature (hypothermia may be neuroprotective after ischemia) and fluids are managed (avoid aspiration, sustain cerebral perfusion, avoid cerebral edema or fluid overload). Fever reduction with appropriate cooling measures is an essential component in the care of the critically ill client. Isotonic intravenous fluids such as normal saline or Ringer's lactate are often the intravenous fluids of choice when dehydration and hypotension are present because these may exacerbate an infarction.

   6. Early rehabilitation should begin at the rail. Early identification of rehabilitation needs and an early start to rehabilitation can decrease healthcare costs by reducing dependence, nursing care, and length of stay and preventing disability (Stucki, Stier-Jarmer, Grill, & Melvin, 2005). Physical, occupational, and speech and language therapy; rehabilitation psychology; therapeutic recreation; and consultation with a physical medicine and rehabilitation physician or advanced practice nurse (APN) have been shown to be beneficial.

   7. Many hospitals have designated stroke units or are primary stroke centers that provide clients with the complex interventions they need, including medical, nursing, and therapy professionals

working as a team from the beginning toward stroke recovery. Early rehabilitation is the emphasis, and active participation by the client and family is encouraged.

F. Stroke Centers

1. Primary stroke centers (AHA, 2009; Bader & Palmer, 2006; The Joint Commission [JC], 2010)

   a. In 2000 a multidisciplinary group (BAC) conducted a literature search with the objectives of improving the level of care and standardization of rapid diagnosis, treatment, and care for stroke survivors.

   b. The BAC focused hospitals on prioritizing care with six connecting elements: identification of stroke and rapid transport to a stroke-receiving hospital by emergency medical personnel; ED prioritization of stroke care with rapid triage, protocols for management, and procedures for rt-PA administration; an organized acute stroke team for rapid response to the ED; written care protocols for the multidisciplinary team to follow using evidence-based literature; a designated stroke unit with highly skilled staff; and neurosurgeons available within 2 hours if neurosurgery is needed

   c. The BAC-recommended support services include a stroke center medical director; 24-hour, 7-days-a-week neuroimaging and laboratory services; outcome and quality improvement tracking for client outcomes; and educational programs for staff and the community.

   d. The goal of a primary stroke center is to provide the personnel and infrastructure to stabilize and treat the majority of clients.

   e. Development of primary stroke centers led to further recommendations by the BAC and the American Stroke Association (ASA) to work with the JC on establishing criteria for certification of primary stroke center programs (AHA, 2009).

   f. The ASA and the JC provide tools and resources to help hospitals become ready for certification (e.g., Acute Stroke Treatment Program toolkit, Get with the Guidelines/Stroke Quality Improvement program) and numerous professional education opportunities (online continuing medical education, International Stroke Conference; AHA, 2009; JC, 2010).

   g. For more information about the JC Primary Stroke Center Certification or Accreditation programs, visit www.jointcommission.org (AHA, 2009).

   h. A state-by-state list of stroke centers is available from the NSA website at www.stroke.org/site/PageServer?pagename=RESOUR or by calling 1.800.STROKE.

2. Comprehensive stroke centers (Bader & Palmer, 2006)

   a. The BAC met in late 2004 and 2005 and used an evidence-based approach to establish criteria for the development of comprehensive stroke center (CSC) models. Thirteen quality measures were identified.

   b. A CSC has the personnel and infrastructure to care for clients needing high-intensity care with specialized tests or neurointerventional therapies.

   c. A CSC is capable of taking care of clients with strokes involving larger areas of the brain (large ischemic strokes, complex hemorrhagic strokes).

   d. A CSC provides more advanced care and serves as a resource for a primary stroke center.

   e. A stroke registry is an important element of a CSC. CSCs are in the earliest stage of development at this time. Only a few exist in the United States today, primarily in Delaware, Florida, Massachusetts, and New York (NSA, 2011).

3. The Commission on Accreditation of Rehabilitation Facilities (CARF) also offers an additional certification for a stroke specialty program. Standards need to be met that address serving the person with a stroke with services that focus on prevention, minimizing impairment, reducing activity limitations, and maximizing the quality of life of people who have had a stroke (CARF, 2010).

G. Future Treatment for Strokes (Ginsburg, 2008; Ohio State University Medical Center, 2011; Seppa, 2003)

1. Vampire bat (*Desmodus rotundus*) saliva

   a. *Desmodus rotundus* salivary plasminogen activator (DSPA) or desmoteplase (recombinant form of potent bat saliva) has been trialed at Ohio State University Medical Center and approximately 80 centers around the world; studies include animals and humans.

   b. Vampire bats secrete an enzyme in the saliva that prevents the blood of their prey from clotting; in a study with mice DSPA targeted the protein fibrin without causing collateral damage to the brain from further bleeding.

c. DSPA has been used in studies with humans 9 hours after onset of stroke symptoms without evidence of neurotoxicity or bleeding into the brain.

2. Advantages over rt-PA
   a. Only about 3%–5% of clients arrive within the necessary 3-hour timeframe for this drug because their symptoms are too subtle.
   b. DSPA can be introduced into the circulatory system in 1–2 minutes, compared with the 60-minute infusion of rt-PA.
   c. DSPA has been studied up to 9 hours after onset of symptoms with good results and without negative side effects such as bleeding into the brain (occurs with rt-PA in about 6.4% of clients).
   d. The disadvantage of DSPA is that it is not approved by the U.S. Food and Drug Administration at this time but continues to be studied throughout the world.

3. Clinical trials are underway looking at advances in thrombolysis for ischemic strokes (Lutsep & Clark, 2009). One such trial involves the intravenous administration of anchrod (a defibrinogenating agent derived from the venom of the Malaysian pit viper snake; NSA, 2009g).

4. Clinical trials are underway investigating the influence of genetics and biological agents on prevention and treatment of strokes (Elkind & Carlino, 2010).

5. There will be continued advances in the development of neuroprotection agents, neurostimulants, and injection of neural stem cells in the treatment of strokes (Imitola & Khoury, 2008).

6. There will continue to be advances in neurointerventional radiology procedures, including the use of diagnostic procedures that study diffusion and perfusion differences in ischemic stroke (NSA, 2009g).

IV. **Family and Caregiver Support**
A. General Facts
1. A stroke changes life not only for the client but for the entire family, more than any other type of disability.
2. Strokes are the most common cause of adult disability, costing more than $68 billion in hospitalization and lost productivity in 2008 (Rosamond et al., 2008).
3. Stroke survivors are often left with major disabilities and loss of functional independence.
4. To ensure continuity of care between the hospital and the community setting, the best possible after-stroke care is a family-centered approach.

This will provide the emotional and psychological support clients and their families need (Hare, Rogers, Lester, McManus, & Mamt, 2006) and preserve the gains already made in rehabilitation.

5. Many stroke survivors are able to remain in the home or community when they have the support of a family member (Hare et al., 2006).

6. There is a need for stroke rehabilitation to shift focus away from the client and on to the family, but this has not occurred in most settings (Rochette, Korner-Bitensky, & Desrosiers, 2007).

7. Caregivers must meet an enormous challenge in caring for the physical and emotional needs of the stroke survivor without neglecting their own needs.

8. Caregivers must suspend their own feelings of grief, fear, and frustration to take care of the stroke survivor. The caregiver may be grieving the loss of companionship and may feel a lack of support.

B. Education
1. Caregivers need information about stroke, its impact, the expected prognosis, and the rehabilitation process. Caregivers are known to benefit significantly in physical and mental well-being from nurse-led support and educational programs (Larson et al., 2005).
2. Caregivers need to understand the physical and psychological needs of the stroke survivor. Psychosocial factors include grief at the loss of function, independence, and employment. Social isolation, decreased self-esteem, relationship or sexual difficulties, and difficulties in managing finances should also be considered as psychosocial factors that a caregiver may need to deal with (Pfeil, Gray, & Lindsay, 2009).
3. Caregivers need assistance improving their own caring and coping skills. Caring for a family member after a stroke is demanding. Caregivers of stroke survivors have a role in providing extensive and comprehensive care, along with their previous role as a family member. The pressure from these new roles might cause the caregiver to experience physical and emotional strain (Visser-Meily et al., 2006).
4. Caregivers need to understand their own role changes that evolve when they become the caregiver. They may need to take on roles they are not familiar with, such as shopping, cooking, finances, or home maintenance and repair.
5. Caregivers need to understand the changes that occur in the client, such as fatigue, frustration, egocentricity, or depression.

Poststroke depression is a comorbidity that has a negative effect on overall stroke outcomes (NINDS, 2009a). Poststroke depression peaks at 6 months after a stroke (Dafaer, Rao, Shareef, & Sharma, 2008).

6. Caregivers need support groups to share ideas, information, and coping, including peer counseling in which they can share methods with others in the same situation. Caring for a family member who survived a stroke has been shown to be strongly associated with depression in the caregiver (Berg et al., 2005). Poor motor function, impaired memory, and behavior changes in the stroke survivor seem to have the most profound impact on the caregiver's mental health (Visser-Meily et al., 2006).

7. Caregivers need to be aware of community services and resources available to them. Caregivers rely on the Internet more now than in the past; however, not all caregivers have Internet access, and not all Internet resources are reliable.

C. Considerations by Medical Professionals
1. The age and health of the caregiver and stroke survivor must be considered. As the average lifespan lengthens and medical care improves, there are more people living beyond the age of 80 years who have a high quality of life. Increases in life expectancy and advances in medical management of stroke have contributed to greater number of people surviving stroke or providing care for a family member (Sanossian & Ovbiagele, 2009).

2. Stroke affects more women than men because women live longer, and stroke rates increase dramatically with age (Reeves et al., 2008). Risk factor profiles differ between the sexes. Recent studies show that men more often have a history of MI or diabetes and are more likely to have a history of hypertension and prestroke dementia (Gall et al., 2010).

3. The culture of the client and caregiver (e.g., role of the "sick" person, role of the caregiver, sharing information with the client) may have an effect on stroke recovery as well as patient and family coping mechanisms. This might also include the client's and family's perspectives on diet and physical activity

4. The client and caregiver may have limited resources due to job loss.

5. Medical professionals must address safety concerns with caregivers (e.g., handling emergencies such as falls or safety in the bathroom; aspiration related to dysphagia).

6. Caregiver stress can lead to neglect or abuse of the stroke survivor.

7. Thirty-one percent of women are widowed at the time of stroke, compared with 7% of men; therefore, a spouse may not be available to act as caregiver (Foerch et al., 2007).

D. Problems Identified by Caregivers (Pierce, Steiner, Hicks, & Holzaepfel, 2006; www.caregivers.com)
1. Independence (not enough personal time or ability to maintain own role in society)
2. Emotions (anger, frustration, fear, isolation)
3. Balancing duties (e.g., caregiver role versus potentially new roles in taking care of a house and finances)
4. Having a partner with physical or emotional limitations (change in relationship between the stroke survivor and caregiver)
5. Changes in sleep and rest (increase in duties, worry, and physical exhaustion)
6. Lack of support (spiritual or emotional support present initially and decline after the acute phase of the stroke)

E. Resources for Caregivers and Families
1. American Stroke Association (888.4.STROKE; www.strokeassociation.org) provides information on signs and symptoms of stroke, provides information in English and Spanish about stroke, distributes *Stroke Connection* magazine, lists stroke-certified hospitals, and is a division of AHA.
2. The National Family Caregivers Association (www.thefamilycaregiver.org) is a national nonprofit organization dedicated to empowering family caregivers with concentration in the areas of education, community building, and advocacy.
3. The National Alliance for Caregiving (www.caregiving.org) helps family caregivers learn about videos, pamphlets, and other information sources that have been reviewed and approved as providing solid information.
4. The Friends' Health Connection (www.48friend.org) connects people with illness or disability and their family caregivers with others experiencing the same challenges.
5. The Well Spouse Association (www.wellspouse.org) is a national membership organization that gives support to husbands, wives, and partners of the chronically ill and disabled. Well Spouse has a network of support groups and a newsletter.
6. Disability.gov (www.disability.gov) is a federal government website that provides easy access to disability-related information and resources with

links to relevant programs and services offered by numerous government agencies.

7. The Centers for Medicare & Medicaid Services (www.medicare.gov/caregivers) "Ask Medicare" service helps family caregivers access and use valuable healthcare information about Medicare and other essential resources to help with family caregiving, including links to key partner organizations that assist caregivers and beneficiaries.

8. Lotsa Helping Hands (www.nfca.lotsahelping hands.com) is a volunteer coordination service using a Web calendar that organizes a community of family and friends to help with tasks, meals, rides, and other needs.

Figure 11-2. Assessment of a New Client with Stroke

- Obtain verbal report from a nurse on the unit that sent the client.

- Make an appropriate room assignment based on deficits (e.g., turn affected side toward the door for stimulation, place close to the nursing station if at high risk for falls).

- When the client arrives, assist with his or her transfer to bed. The nursing assessment begins now as the nurse observes how much the client can do during the transfer.

- Determine whether the client can answer questions and is cognitively aware. This can be determined in a short time with conversation while welcoming him or her to the unit. If the client is unable to provide his or her own history, ask a family member to attend the assessment.

- Assess general data (e.g., allergies, medications, identification band on).

- Obtain a complete medical history and complete a head-to-toe assessment, including neurological checks (e.g., for strength, orientation). During this time, also assess communication and cognition skills.

- Assess bowel and bladder function using information obtained from the report of other nurses, combined with information from the client and family. This assessment may not be complete until the nurse actually toilets the client during the first 24 hours.

- Obtain histories for sleep, nutrition, safety, and sex.

- Assess psychosocial history and educational wants, needs, and preferences for learning style.

- Assess leisure interests, community reentry needs, and discharge planning needs.

- Provide the client and family with verbal and written orientation information about the unit and the staff.

- Communicate pertinent information to team members as soon as possible.

- Provide the client with necessary safety equipment (e.g., bed alarm, wheelchair alarm) as soon as the assessment is complete.

- Follow the assessment pattern of the unit but keep in mind that the client may get tired or frustrated if several team members assess the same things at different times.

V. Nursing Process

A. Assessment by Nurses and the Interdisciplinary Rehabilitation Team (**Figures 11-2, 11-3,** and **11-4**) Administer stroke scale items in the order listed. The performance in each category is recorded after each subscale exam. Do not go back and change scores. Follow directions provided for each exam technique. Scores should reflect what the client does, not what the clinician thinks he or she can do. The clinician should record answers while administering the exam and work quickly. Except where indicated, the client should not be coached (i.e., repeating requests to the client to make a special effort).

1. Medical management: Assessed by the registered nurse (RN), physicians (e.g., rehabilitation physiatrist, primary physician, and consulting physicians), and licensed independent practitioner (e.g., APNs: nurse practitioners and clinical nurse specialists). The Functional Independence Measure (FIM) is highlighted in Chapter 22.

   a. Client's medical stability: The initial primary focus in rehabilitation. The client should be medically stable before admission to an inpatient rehabilitation facility (Miller et al., 2010).

   b. Assessment of medical needs that can impede rehabilitation progress if left unmanaged (e.g., comorbidities such as hypotension, hypertension, hyperglycemia, oxygen saturation, cardiac irregularities, or other chronic illnesses affecting medical stability)

2. Communication: Assessment by a speech-language pathologist (SLP), RN, and registered occupational therapist (OTR)

Figure 11-3. Modified Rankin Scale

Grade	Description
0	No symptoms at all.
1	No significant disability despite symptoms. Able to carry out all usual duties and activities.
2	Slight disability: Unable to carry out all previous activities but able to look after own affairs without assistance.
3	Moderate disability: Needs some help but able to walk without assistance.
4	Moderately severe disability: Unable to walk without assistance and unable to attend to own bodily needs without assistance.
5	Severe disability: Bedridden, incontinent, and needing constant nursing care and attention.

From "Interobserver agreement for the assessment of handicap in stroke patients," by J. C. van Swieten, P. J. Koudstaal, M. C. Visser, H. J. Schouten, and J. van Gijn, 1988, *Stroke, 19*(5), 604–607. Copyright 1988 by the American Heart Association. Reprinted with permission.

THE SPECIALTY PRACTICE OF REHABILITATION NURSING

Figure 11-4. National Institutes of Health (NIH) Stroke Scale

Category	Description	Score
1a. Level of Consciousness (LOC) Is the client alert, drowsy, etc.?	Alert Drowsy Stuporous Coma	0 1 2 3
1b. LOC questions Ask the client the month and his or her age. The answer must be exactly right.	Answers both correctly Answers one correctly Both incorrect	0 1 2
1c. LOC Commands Ask the client to open/close eyes and then grip/release nonparetic hand.	Obeys both correctly Obeys one correctly Both incorrect	0 1 2
2. Best Gaze Only horizontal movement tested. Oculocephalic reflex is OK, but no calorics. Eyes open—clilent follows finger or face.	Normal Partial gaze palsy Forced deviation	0 1 2
3. Visual Test by confrontation; introduce visual stimulus to the client's upper- and lower-field quadrants.	No visual loss Partial hemianopsia Complete hemianopsia Bilateral hemianopia	0 1 2 3
4. Facial Palsy Ask the client to show teeth/smile, raise eyebrows, and squeeze eye shut.	Normal Minor Partial Complete	0 1 2 3
5a. Motor Arm Left Extend the left arm, palm down, to 90 degrees if sitting or 45 degrees if supine.	No drift Drift Can't resist gravity No effort against gravity No movement Amputation, joint fusion	0 1 2 3 4 UN
5b. Motor Arm Right Extend the right arm, palm down, to 90 degrees if sitting or 45 degrees if supine.	No drift Drift Can't resist gravity No effort against gravity No movement Amputation, joint fusion	0 1 2 3 4 UN
6a. Motor Leg Left Elevate the left leg to 30 degrees and flex at hip, always supine.	No drift Drift Can't resist gravity No effort against gravity No movement Amputation, joint fusion	0 1 2 3 4 UN
6b. Motor Leg Right Elevate the right leg to 30 degrees and flex at hip, always supine.	No drift Drift Can't resist gravity No effort against gravity No movement Amputation, joint fusion	0 1 2 3 4 UN

continued

Figure 11-4. National Institutes of Health (NIH) Stroke Scale *continued*

7. Limb Ataxia Finger-nose, heel-shin tests done on both sides.	Absent	0
	Present in one limb	1
	Present in two limbs	2
8. Sensory Use a pinprick to face, arm, trunk, and leg; compare side to side. Assess the client's awareness of being touched.	Normal	0
	Partial loss	1
	Severe loss	2
9. Best Language Ask clients to name items, describe a picture, read a sentence; intubated clients should write responses.	No aphasia	0
	Mild-to-moderate aphasia	1
	Severe aphasia	2
	Mute	3
10. Dysarthria Evaluate speech clarity by asking the client to repeat listed words.	Normal articulation	0
	Mild to moderate dysarthria	1
	Near to unintelligible	2
	Intubated or other barrier	UN
11. Extinction and Inattention Use information from prior testing to identify neglect or double simultaneous stimuli testing.	No neglect	0
	Partial neglect	1
	Complete neglect	2

From NIH Stroke Scale, by National Institute of Neurological Disorders and Stroke, 2009a. Retrieved September 21, 2011, from www.ninds.nih.gov/doctors.

a. Request a consult with the SLP; do not ignore or dismiss language and speech errors.

b. Evaluation should include assessment of language, cognition, pragmatics, and speech.

c. Presence of aphasia; expressive or receptive communication

d. Other methods of communication (e.g., nodding, pointing, gesturing, using symbols)

e. Premorbid communication pattern: History from family or significant other and developmental level of client

f. Vocalization problems from motor inability; tracheostomy

g. Agnosia, apraxia, dysarthria

h. Hearing aid or glasses

3. Memory: Assessed by SLP, OTR, RN, and physical therapist (PT)

a. Premorbid ability

b. Short-term memory

c. Long-term memory

d. Memory problems involving auditory or visual information

4. Problem-solving ability: Assessed by RN, SLP, OTR, PT

a. Premorbid ability

b. Ability to make appropriate choices

c. Ability to find solutions

d. Presence of planning or organizational skills

5. Sensory and visual perception: Assessed by RN, OTR, PT

a. Premorbid use of hearing aid or glasses

b. Perceptual responses; acuity of senses (e.g., vision, hearing, touch, taste, smell)

c. Medications that may change sensation or perception

6. ADLs and self-care: Assessed by RN, OTR

a. Ability to bathe, dress, or toilet self

b. Premorbid abilities

c. How much help is needed

d. Ability to gather needed equipment, supplies, clothing

e. Mobility to carry out activities

f. Adaptive equipment needed (e.g., bath sponge, reacher, shoe horn)

7. Dysphagia and swallowing: Assessed by RN, SLP, OTR (Hinchey et al., 2005)

a. Must be assessed before any oral medication or food is given

b. Ability to feed self; amount of assistance needed

c. Ability to chew, drink, and swallow without difficulty

d. Correct diet and consistency ordered

e. Adequate caloric and fluid intake

f. Use of correct position for eating, alertness

g. Presence of drooling and pocketing, not swallowing

h. Presence of cough and gag reflex

i. Voice quality (e.g., wet, gurgling, nasal while eating)

j. Use and fit of dentures

k. Use of upper extremities (e.g., grip, able to lift utensils, able to cut and prepare food)

l. Ability to see food (e.g., hemianopsia)

8. Bowel management: Assessed by RN (Consortium for Spinal Cord Medicine, 1998)

   a. Neurogenic bowel (uninhibited or reflexive type; sudden, involuntary defecation)

   b. Continence history before stroke; bowel history (e.g., when, how often)

   c. Current pattern of elimination

   d. Assess diet and hydration.

   e. Review current medications.

   f. If necessary, assess sphincter tone.

   g. Cognitive ability: Awareness of need to defecate

   h. Medication use

   i. Bowel sounds, abdominal tenderness or distention, rigidity

   j. Transfer skills, sitting tolerance

   k. Ability to get to bathroom, ability to don and doff clothing

   l. Hygiene needs, assistance needed

   m. Positioning, privacy

9. Bladder management: Assessed by RN (Consortium for Spinal Cord Medicine, 2006)

   a. Neurogenic bladder: Decreased capacity and involuntary voiding as soon as urge is perceived; usually uninhibited type. Also noted some urinary retention in a small percentage of clients.

   b. Continence history before stroke

   c. Current pattern of elimination

   d. Review of current medications

   e. Premorbid history (e.g., nocturia, stress incontinence)

   f. Recent history (e.g., urgency, frequency, urinary tract infection)

   g. Cognitive ability: Awareness of need to urinate, cognition

   h. Transfer skills, sitting tolerance

   i. Ability to perform toileting and to ambulate or call for assistance or get to the bathroom

   j. Hygiene needs, assistance, privacy

   k. Catheter (e.g., intermittent, indwelling): Indwelling should be removed as soon as possible.

   l. Fluid intake

   m. Medication use

10. Mobility: Assessed by RN, PT, OTR

    a. Bed mobility: Moving up, down, side to side; bridging; sitting up; amount of assistance needed

    b. Transfers: Bed to chair, wheelchair to toilet, to bath bench or shower chair, to car; amount of assistance and type of lift equipment needed

    c. Wheelchair mobility: Type of wheelchair, ability to self-propel, amount of assistance needed

    d. Gait, sitting, standing; need for devices (e.g., walker, cane, crutches)

    e. Endurance, strength, balance, tone, and proprioception

    f. Environment (e.g., lighting, open space)

11. Sexual functioning: Assessed by RN, physician, licensed independent practitioner, psychologist

    a. Premorbid sexual history (e.g., preferences, frequency, initiation [partner or self])

    b. Sensory deficits

    c. Mobility

    d. Ability to communicate; visual or perceptual deficits

    e. Emotional status, fear

    f. Fatigue

    g. Knowledge

    h. Positioning

    i. Libido

    j. Need for birth control

    k. Bowel and bladder management before sex

12. Skin integrity: Assessed by RN, PT, OTR, skin care nursing consultant (if available)

    a. Immobility

    b. Loss of sensation

    c. Incontinence and hygiene

    d. Presence of pressure, friction, shearing

    e. Presence of any pressure ulcers or skin breakdown

    f. Poor circulation

    g. Risk of skin breakdown: Use of skin assessment scales such as Norton, Braden, or Risk Assessment Pressure Sore

    h. Hydration and nutrition: Nutrition consults

13. Equipment: Assessed by OTR, PT, RN, social worker (SW), discharge planner, case manager

    a. Need for assistance with mobility

    b. Need for assistance with ADLs

    c. Financial resources available

14. Psychosocial needs: Assessed by RN, SW, psychologist

    a. Role changes

    b. Relationships with family members

    c. Family and community support

    d. Coping skills and stressors

    e. Problems with self-image

    f. Depression

15. Leisure: Assessed by RN and certified therapeutic recreation specialist
    a. Premorbid leisure history
    b. Current physical ability and endurance related to leisure interest
    c. Cognitive status
16. Education: Assessed by each rehabilitation team member
    a. Cognitive status, intellectual capacity
    b. Attention span
    c. Premorbid learning needs (e.g., visual, auditory, kinesthetic, combination)
    d. Level of formal education
    e. Ability to read or write
    f. Language and cultural barriers
    g. Motivation and readiness to learn
    h. Environmental barriers
    i. Knowledge of disability and self-care needs
    j. Support and presence of caregivers
17. Safety: Assessed by each rehabilitation team member
    a. Cognition and awareness
    b. Risk for and history of falls
    c. Environment (e.g., hospital, home)
    d. Medication that changes level of consciousness
    e. Sensory impairments
18. Comfort and pain level: Assessed by RN
    a. Subluxation and shoulder pain: Subluxation (loss of normal muscle tone in supraspinatus and deltoid muscles) is painless; however, manipulation and improper positioning of a subluxed shoulder cause pain. Prevent through support of affected shoulder, proper positioning, and ROM.
    b. Shoulder-hand syndrome
    c. Pain and its location and frequency; use a different pain scale for nonverbal aphasic clients (e.g., Wong-Baker FACES Pain-Rating scale available at www.partnersagainstpain.com/printouts/A7012AS6.pdf).
    d. Pain related to activity or randomly occurring location and description of pain
    e. What relieves pain or makes it worse
    f. Effectiveness of pain medicine
    g. Alternatives to medication: Repositioning, visual imagery, music
    h. Changes in sleep pattern; may have reversal of sleep-wake cycle
    i. Sleep history (e.g., normal bedtime, need for white noise, lights)
    j. Sleep problems: onset, frequent awakenings, nocturia
    k. Environmental (e.g., hot, cold, comfortable bed)
19. Spiritual: Assessed by RN, SW, and chaplain
    a. Sources of hope and strength
    b. Religious practices
    c. Scheduled time for privacy
20. Discharge planning: Assessed by discharge planner, SW, case manager in conjunction with rehabilitation team
    a. Physical deficits and need for adaptive equipment
    b. Caregiver knowledge and support
    c. Financial resources available
    d. Need for community resources
    e. Adaptations needed for home environment with rehabilitation team input
B. Nursing Diagnoses (**Table 11-2**)

Table 11-2. Nursing Diagnoses, Desired Outcomes, and Interventions in the Care of the Client with Stroke

Nursing Diagnosis	Nursing Outcomes Classification (NOC)	Nursing Interventions Classification (NIC)
Transfer ability, impaired	0202 Balance; body positioning, self-initiated; 0208 Mobility	0200 Exercise promotion; 6490 Fall prevention; 0840 Positioning
Self-care deficit	0300 Self-care (ADL)	1801 Self-care assistance (SCA): bathing/hygiene; 1802 SCA: Dressing/grooming; 1803 SCA: Feeding; 1804 SCA: Toileting; 1806 SCA: Transfers
Communication, impaired	0902 Communication	4976 Communication enhancement-speech deficit
Knowledge deficit	1803 Knowledge of disease process	5602 Teaching: Disease process
Swallowing, impaired	1010 Swallowing status	1056 Enteral tube feeding; 1860 Swallowing therapy; 1710 Oral health maintenance
Urinary incontinence Urinary retention	0502 Urinary incontinence	0560 Pelvic muscle exercise; 0640 Prompted voiding; 0610 Urinary incontinence care; 0620 Urinary retention care
Caregiver role strain	2202 Caregiver homecare readiness; 2205 Caregiver performance: direct care; 2203 Caregiver lifestyle disruption	7040 Caregiver support; 5430 Support group

1. Impaired physical mobility
2. Self-care deficits (specify level)
3. Sensory-perceptual alteration
4. Impaired verbal communication or communication barrier
5. Altered elimination (bowel and bladder)
6. High risk of aspiration or impaired swallowing
7. Potential for injury or risk for falls
8. Impaired home maintenance management and discharge planning
9. Impaired thought processes
10. Disturbance in body image
11. Altered sexuality pattern
12. Caregiver distress
13. Ineffective coping
14. Ineffective family coping
15. Spiritual distress
16. Alteration in skin integrity
17. Knowledge deficit
18. Alteration in comfort with or without pain
19. Altered sleep patterns
20. Risk for impaired nutrition
21. Activity intolerance, fatigue

C. Planning and Client Goals: Nursing Outcomes Classification (NOC; University of Iowa, n.d.a; Table 11-2)
   1. Demonstrate maximal independence in mobility.
   2. Perform ADLs at the optimal level of independence with or without the use of assistive devices.
   3. Be free from falls or injury.
   4. Identify diversional activities to decrease stress (by caregivers).
   5. Verbalize level of satisfaction with sexuality.
   6. Identify negative feelings related to self-image.
   7. Verbalize understanding of the diagnosis and treatment of stroke or CVA.

D. Interventions: Nursing Interventions Classification (University of Iowa, n.d.b; Table 11-2)
   1. Medical management
      a. Monitor vital signs (more frequently during early rehabilitation); medication for hypertension as needed; intravenous fluids for hypotension (if the patient is hypotensive, hemoconcentration can occur and cerebral perfusion decreases, potentially worsening the infarct).
      b. Monitor blood glucose and regulate with insulin as needed.
      c. Use intravenous solutions of normal saline.
      d. Provide oxygen as ordered and titrate to 90% or more.
      e. Use telemetry monitoring or electrocardiogram for cardiac abnormalities.

f. Check lung sounds and risk of aspiration; perform dysphagia screening on all newly admitted patients.
      g. Check for fever (e.g., for possible urinary tract infection, pneumonia).
      h. Check lab values (e.g., activated partial thromboplastin time, hemoglobin and hematocrit, electrolytes).
      i. Measure legs daily for swelling; assess for DVT, implement DVT prophylaxis measures.
   2. Communication: "Language is the most human of mental skills" (Mace & Rabins, 1981, p. 29). Without language, the person with a stroke is lonely, depends on others, and loses self-confidence.
      a. Determine communication method: All disciplines should use consistent methods.
      b. Ensure that hearing aids and glasses are available if needed.
      c. Use symbols and communication boards.
      d. Provide a supportive environment; be patient and calm.
      e. Include the family when possible.
      f. Use music therapy: The person may be unable to speak but able to sing.
      g. Use pet therapy; it provides mental stimulation, outward focus, and psychological well-being and helps with physical mobility.
      h. Speak slowly and distinctly; use short, simple sentences; maintain eye contact.
      i. Establish yes-no reliability.
      j. Try cueing; prompt if the direction of verbalization is understood.
      k. Provide opportunities for success; offer praise.
   3. Memory
      a. Use memory books.
      b. Use cueing and repetition.
      c. Use memory games and allow the patient to reminisce.
      d. Work from simple to complex concepts and promote success.
      e. Present material in different ways (e.g., written, verbal, pictures, demonstration).
   4. Problem-solving ability
      a. Allow the client to make choices, beginning with safe and simple options.
      b. Help with planning.
      c. Organize and prioritize information.
      d. Break problems into steps and cue the client through the steps.
   5. Sensory and visual perception
      a. Provide adaptive equipment (e.g., glasses, hearing aids).
      b. Ensure appropriate lighting and color contrast.

c. Make large-print books and materials available.

d. Place items to allow for visual cuts (homonymous hemianopsia) and teach the client to visually scan the environment.

e. Reduce environmental noise (e.g., radio, television).

f. Adapt the environment to accommodate hearing loss (e.g., flashing light for phone).

g. Use aromatherapy.

h. Provide various textures and temperatures.

i. Ensure safety (e.g., hot or cold, especially with decreased sensation).

j. Serve foods of various colors, tastes, and smells.

k. Review medications (e.g., sedatives).

l. Set up the room to stimulate the neglected side.

m. Eliminate spatial difficulties (e.g., place colored food on a white plate).

6. ADLs and self-care

a. Ensure privacy and a safe environment (e.g., grab bars, tub bench).

b. Establish a bathing and toileting routine and provide adaptive equipment for bathing, dressing, and toileting.

c. Involve caregivers in ADL training.

d. Incorporate crossover neurodevelopmental techniques (NDTs; i.e., the client's uninvolved side helps the involved side during activity).

e. Provide an ongoing comprehensive history and assessment for ADL training and for determining the client's home care assistance needs (documentation of this may be required by the client's insurance company).

f. Adapt the home environment for a wheelchair, equipment, and accessibility.

g. Allow the client to choose his or her clothing; encourage use of clothing that is loose or easy to put on.

h. Allow time for activity and rest between self-care activities and promote energy-saving techniques, beginning in bed and progressing throughout the day.

i. Dress the client's affected side first.

7. Dysphagia and swallowing

a. Evaluate swallowing (via bedside or radiology) as identified by a video fluoroscopic swallow study.

b. Position the client upright for feeding and administering medication.

c. Ensure the correct level of dysphagia diet and consistency (e.g., thicken if needed); ensure that dentures fit properly; obtain a dental consult.

d. Observe during meals for pocketing, drooling, and swallowing.

e. Provide adaptive equipment (e.g., divided plate, cutout cup).

f. Crush medications into applesauce; turn the client's head to the affected side if he or she has difficulty swallowing medications.

g. Monitor weight changes and lab values.

h. Consult with a dietitian about the client's food preferences.

i. Monitor hydration: Clients on oral dysphagia diets need adequate fluids to avoid dehydration.

j. Use supplemental tube feedings: Check for residual and placement of the tube and position the client upright for feedings.

k. Use supplemental parental nutrition: Maintain the tube site and monitor labs. Evidence-based literature suggests that the Frazier water protocol helps prevent dehydration.

8. Bowel management

a. Verify the client's premorbid bowel evacuation routine and adapt a bowel program to accommodate the previous routine.

b. Increase fluid intake, bulk, and fiber; monitor intake and output.

c. Monitor bowel sounds and abdominal distention; avoid gas-forming foods.

d. Position the client upright; use a toilet or commode rather than a bedpan; allow time for complete evacuation.

e. Provide appropriate medications (e.g., stool softeners, enemas, and suppositories; laxatives and enemas should be used sparingly).

f. Encourage the client to wear loose clothing and use good hygiene after each stool.

9. Bladder management

a. Determine continence history and provide adequate lighting if the client has a history of nocturia.

b. Set up a bladder program to decrease or avoid incontinence.

c. Assess medications that contribute to incontinence (e.g., diuretics, sedatives, anticholinergics, antihypertensives).

d. Provide adequate hydration (i.e., fluid intake of 2,000–3,000 ml per day if tolerated or if not contraindicated due to comorbidity) and monitor intake and output.

e. Use a bladder scan and catheterize for postvoid residuals greater than 150 ml generally or greater than 300 ml if the client is unable to void.

f. Provide time, privacy, and adaptive equipment for hygiene.

g. Provide medication to facilitate bladder tone and emptying.

10. Mobility
    a. Work with the client on bed mobility, bridging, bracing lower extremities, sitting up, moving up and down, and increasing endurance.
    b. Use general concepts of neurodevelopmental treatment (e.g., normalizing muscle tone, integration versus compensation, meaningful activities versus simulated activities) to help with proprioception.
    c. Consider use of NDTs for transfers.
    d. Use general concepts of neurointegrative functional rehabilitation and habilitation (Neuro-IFRAH Organization, 2005).
    e. Provide a safe environment for mobility practice (space and lighting).
    f. Encourage the client to wear sturdy shoes to prevent foot drop.
    g. Ensure safety when the client attempts to sit or stand. According to clinical experience, more than one-third of falls in clients who have had a stroke occur during rising or sitting down.
    h. Use adaptive equipment as necessary, including lifts if needed.
11. Sexual functioning
    a. Encourage the use of times of day when the client is most rested.
    b. Provide education and support to the client's significant other.
    c. Teach positioning (e.g., supine or on affected side, use pillows for support).
    d. Discuss fear of another stroke.
    e. Instruct the client's partner on the emotional lability of the client.
    f. Encourage tactile stimulation to enhance communication, especially if the client is aphasic.
    g. Discuss birth control methods.
    h. Encourage the client to evacuate the bowel and bladder before sex.
12. Skin integrity
    a. Inspect skin regularly for friction, shearing, and pressure.
    b. Teach weight-shifting techniques.
    c. Use pressure-relieving devices.
    d. Keep the client clean and dry.
    e. Consult with a dietitian for nutritional needs to promote healing.
    f. If the client has sensory loss, guard against contact with extreme hot and cold temperatures (e.g., bath water).
    g. Assess for medications that may alter level of consciousness, sensation, or awareness.
13. Equipment
    a. Provide adaptive equipment as needed; attempt to increase the client's functional ability without equipment if possible.
    b. Verify insurance payment for durable medical equipment (usually done by the SW or case manager).
    c. Reinforce the use of equipment that therapists have obtained.
14. Psychosocial needs
    a. Provide time for verbalization and counseling for the client and family with a psychologist.
    b. Facilitate team and family conferences as needed.
    c. Provide socialization opportunities (e.g., eating meals in the dining room, group therapy, stroke support groups).
    d. Role changes occur and should be discussed with the client and family.
    e. Allow the client and family to grieve their losses (e.g., function, role, relationships).
    f. Reduce stress when possible and allow the client and family to have as much control over care as possible.
15. Leisure
    a. Incorporate the client's leisure interests into therapy (e.g., card games).
    b. Promote community reentry using adaptive equipment (e.g., outing to a wheelchair-accessible fishing dock using a mounted fishing rod holder).
    c. Use memory games to work on cognition in group therapy.
    d. Use NDTs during games (e.g., incorporate the hemiplegic side using the strong side hand over hand to hit a balloon or reach for cards).
    e. Try to adapt the client's leisure interests that use equipment (e.g., fasten an embroidery hoop to a wheelchair).
    f. Encourage pet therapy.
16. Education
    a. Determine readiness and motivation to learn.
    b. Provide information at the client's ability and intellectual level.
    c. Use a variety of teaching methods.
    d. Use an interpreter if language barriers exist.
    e. Plan family teaching sessions.
    f. Reduce distraction and noise when teaching.
    g. Make use of the time when the client is most alert, attentive, and rested.
    h. Test cognition and use return demonstration or verbalization.
    i. Check awareness of current status and build the knowledge base.
17. Safety

a. Ensure the environment is free of hazards.
b. Use bed alarms, electronic wristband monitors, and vest restraints as necessary. Use alternative measures whenever possible to decrease use of restraints (e.g., locate the client close to the nursing station, have a family member stay overnight, do hourly rounds, establish a timed voiding program).
c. Assess medications that may alter awareness.
d. Evaluate the client's home (e.g., handrails, throw rugs, wheelchair ramp) with assistance from an OTR, case manager, or SW and family or caregivers.
e. Ensure kitchen and bathroom safety for clients with sensory impairments (e.g., stove, hot and cold water) with assistance from an OTR, case manager, or SW and family or caregivers.
f. Teach postmorbid impulse control and fall-prevention techniques.

18. Comfort and pain level
a. Position the client comfortably, be aware of shoulder pain (subluxation possible), and position in bed so the client's shoulder is protracted (**Figure 11-5**).
b. Do not use the client's arms or shoulders to move the client up in bed. This can cause shoulder injury (torn rotator cuff).
c. Assess the intensity and location of pain and medicate as appropriate.
d. Watch for shoulder-hand syndrome: Reduce edema; maintain range of motion of metacarpal phalangeal, proximal interphalangeal, and distal interphalangeal joints; maintain wrist in slight extension; encourage movement of the involved shoulder; and maintain correct bed positioning.
e. Allow rest periods throughout the day, but decrease frequency if the client cannot sleep at night.
f. Provide night lighting and white noise if needed.
g. Monitor the room with cameras if the client is impulsive at night.

19. Spiritual
a. Notify the chaplain if requested.
b. Make spiritual readings available (e.g., scriptures, daily devotions).
c. Arrange for the client to attend chapel services if requested.

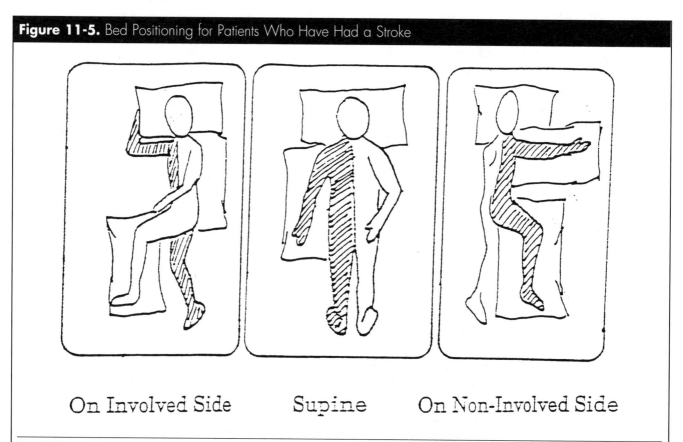

Figure 11-5. Bed Positioning for Patients Who Have Had a Stroke

On Involved Side   Supine   On Non-Involved Side

d. Schedule time for meditation and prayer.
20. Discharge planning (in conjunction with case manager or SW)
    a. Discharge planning starts at the time of admission.
    b. Discuss discharge goals and education with the client and family or caregiver at conferences.
    c. Set up follow-up appointments.
    d. Arrange home health care, outpatient therapy, or long-term care placement.
    e. Obtain durable medical equipment.
    f. Arrange for prescriptions.
    g. Provide discharge instructions and explain medications (e.g., side effects, administration).
    h. Assist with financial and community resource information.
E. Evaluation and Expected Outcomes
    1. Evaluate the client's optimal level of functioning.
    2. Individualize each client's outcomes based on goals related to nursing diagnoses.
F. Posthospitalization Follow-Up
    1. Education about stroke prevention is essential because stroke can be a recurring disorder.
    2. Stroke survivors may go through a predictable recovery process (Easton, 2001). If so, nursing interventions may be targeted to the client's unique needs throughout the rehabilitation process and after discharge to the home setting (Mauk, 2006).

3. Stroke recovery may be facilitated by several controllable and uncontrollable factors such as age, life experience, knowledge of the cause of stroke, expectations, social support, and faith (Mauk, 2006; **Figure 11-6**).
4. Rehabilitation nurses can gain insight into the concerns and challenges facing stroke survivors who have returned to the community by assessing their learning needs and making referrals for follow-up care.
5. Many people who have had a stroke experience depression, lack of concentration, anxiety, fatigue that continues even years after stroke, and memory loss (Easton, 2001).
6. Quality of life is also affected by stroke (Secrest, 2002).
7. It is important to refer the client and family for counseling if needed.
G. Future Reimbursement
    1. In this time of chronic disease management, rehabilitation plays an important role in the clinical management of stroke survivors.
    2. According to the AHA (2009), the estimated direct and indirect cost of stroke for 2009 was nearly $73.1 billion.
    3. Reimbursement changes affect the length of stay in rehabilitation units.
    4. Rehabilitation nurses will be challenged to meet clients' needs more rapidly and with fewer resources available.

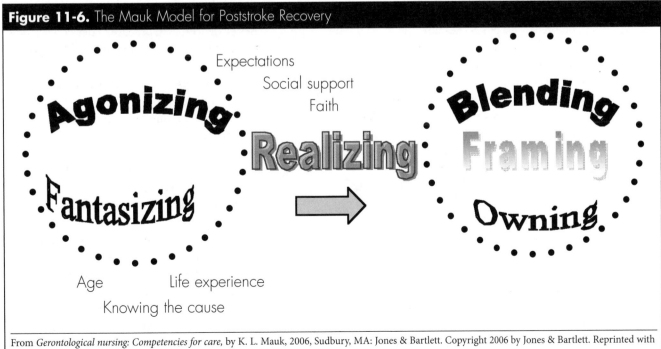

Figure 11-6. The Mauk Model for Poststroke Recovery

Expectations
Social support
Faith

Agonizing
Fantasizing

Realizing

Blending
Framing
Owning

Age   Life experience
Knowing the cause

From *Gerontological nursing: Competencies for care,* by K. L. Mauk, 2006, Sudbury, MA: Jones & Bartlett. Copyright 2006 by Jones & Bartlett. Reprinted with permission.

VI. Advanced Practice (Lemke, 2006)

APNs, whether clinical nurse specialists or nurse practitioners, can play a significant role in the care of stroke survivors. In many situations, APNs may engage in several role components of advanced practice simultaneously. Whether as direct care providers, educators, consultants, researchers, theorists, or leaders, APNs should be at the forefront in improving the quality of life for stroke survivors.

A. Clinician: The APN possesses advanced assessment skills. APNs should be knowledgeable about current best practices for care of stroke survivors. Specifically, the APN specializing in stroke could reasonably be expected to have mastered knowledge related to the content of this chapter but with greater depth and expertise (Newland, 2009).

  1. Practice settings may include

    a. ED

    b. Acute care hospital

    c. Acute rehabilitation

    d. Transitional care

    e. Skilled care

    f. Long-term care facility

      1) Intermediate or skilled care

      2) Independent living

      3) Assisted living

    g. Home care

    h. Community (living in a home or residential setting after stroke)

    i. Private practice

  2. Additional skills as a direct care provider (clinical nurse specialist or nurse practitioner) may include

    a. Comprehensive physical exam

    b. Thorough history

    c. Screening for dysphagia, risk for skin breakdown, DVT risk

    d. Identification of risk factors for stroke

    e. Assessment of stroke severity using standardized scales

    f. Assessment of cranial nerve function

    g. Clinical management of acute stroke

    h. Knowledge of stroke rehabilitation principles and concepts

    i. Appropriate referrals to stroke service and initiation of rehabilitation

    j. Outpatient follow-up visits with survivor and family

    k. Coordination of stroke support groups

    l. Staff, client, and family education about treatment plan and discharge plans, including ordering of appropriate adaptive equipment

    m. Care management or coordination

    n. Home care supervision

    o. Management of potential common complications

      1) Skin breakdown

      2) Dysphagia

      3) DVT

      4) Aphasia

      5) Ongoing functional limitations including gait disorders, hemiplegia

      6) Depression and anxiety

      7) Sleep disorders

      8) Shoulder subluxation

      9) Altered nutrition or dehydration

    p. Prescribing and managing medications

B. Educator: The APN as educator focuses on identifying areas of need; providing essential knowledge of stroke prevention, treatment, and rehabilitation to the target audience; and fostering a positive learning environment.

  1. Educates various populations in all levels of stroke prevention

    a. Nursing staff

    b. Clients and families

    c. Interdisciplinary team members

    d. Communities

    e. Students

  2. Educates in various settings

    a. Hospitals

    b. Acute rehabilitation units

    c. Transitional care

    d. Long-term care facilities

    e. Academia, universities and colleges of nursing

    f. Communities

  3. Uses evidence-based practice to develop teaching strategies in areas of need to improve the quality of care

    a. Promotes use of evidence-based practice in the clinical setting

    b. Reviews literature for current evidence-based practice

    c. Develops interventions

    d. Educates staff regarding best practice

    e. Implements best practice

    f. Nursing follow-up after patient discharge shows positive results.

    g. Nursing interventions related to education have both short- and long-term effects on a variety of variables (Nir, Zolotogorsky, & Sugarman, 2004).

    h. Web-based teaching interventions have shown positive outcomes with stroke survivors and caregivers (Pierce, Steiner, & Govoni, 2002; Pierce et al., 2004).

i. Female stroke survivors may have unique needs related to body image and self-perception that are infrequently addressed by rehabilitation nurses (Kvigne, Kirkevold, & Gjengedal, 2005).

C. Leader: The APN as leader may also be active in organizations at the local, regional, state, national, and international levels. The APN may also demonstrate leadership through civic and professional involvement, presentations at conferences, publications, consulting work, and research programs.
   1. Tasks as leader
      a. Advocate for social reform.
      b. Act as a change agent by holding office in professional organizations.
      c. Assist with the development of clinical practice and policy guidelines.
      d. Participate on committees within professional organizations and interdisciplinary national organizations of interest.
      e. Hold positions of influence or lobby within appropriate political arenas to support the rights of those with disabilities.
      f. Write grants for funding of stroke research.
      g. Become a fellow in a national organization such as the AHA.
   2. Organizations for involvement
      a. AHA and ASA
      b. NSA
      c. Association of Rehabilitation Nurses
      d. American Geriatrics Society
      e. American Association of Neuroscience Nurses

D. Consultant: As a consultant, the APN may engage in a variety of activities. The role of consultant is continually redefined as nurses increase their expertise in areas related to rehabilitation. These areas may include the following:
   1. Legal consulting
      a. Expert opinion
      b. Expert testimony, written and in court
      c. Clinical expert in law practice
      d. For attorneys, insurance companies, private clients, companies
   2. Educational consulting
      a. For academic institutions, on site
      b. For private clients needing one-on-one teaching
      c. For rehabilitation units providing educational seminars related to stroke
      d. For rehabilitation facilities or private companies that provide outreach in different parts of the country

   3. Clinical consulting
      a. Expert clinician on research team
      b. Expert consultant for grant applications and funding
      c. Expert on complex cases (in a variety of settings)
      d. Share expertise with other team members
      e. Author or reviewer of publications (books, articles, case studies)
   4. Guardianship: Generally court appointed; often complex cases that do not have appropriate family involvement or that require involvement of a healthcare expert
   5. Advocacy: Care planning and mediation for those in care settings; interacting with the interdisciplinary team to ensure quality of care and continuity
   6. Life care planning
      a. "A life care plan is a comprehensive document designed to help meet the long-term financial and health needs of a person who has experienced a catastrophic injury" (Mauk & Mauk, 2006, p. 818).
      b. "A Life Care Plan is a dynamic document based upon published standards of practice, comprehensive assessment, data analysis and research, which provides an organized, concise plan for current and future needs with associated costs, for individuals who have experienced catastrophic injury or have chronic health care needs" (Weed & Berens, 2009, p. 3).
      c. Advanced practice status is not needed, but APNs generally have more credibility when involved in legal matters where credentialing and advanced education are important; a background in case management is helpful.
      d. Life care planning for stroke survivors could involve
         1) Estimating the lifetime cost of care and other needs related to medical malpractice in a lawsuit (e.g., in which the injured party had a stroke)
         2) Predicting lifetime care costs in relation to care coordination or management over time

E. Researcher: The APN as researcher will discover and facilitate the use of evidence-based practice for stroke survivors. Some APNs may hold positions with a major emphasis on research related to stroke.
   1. Examples of APN involvement in stroke research
      a. Stroke program coordinator
         1) In acute care hospital (including those with primary or comprehensive stroke centers)
         2) In acute rehabilitation
         3) In freestanding rehabilitation facilities

b. Researcher in research institutions or academic settings

c. Research scientist in large rehabilitation institutes

d. Writer of grants to seek funding for stroke research

2. Examples of current areas of stroke research by rehabilitation APNs

   a. Continuity and Discontinuity of Self Scale (Secrest & Zeller, 2007), which relates to quality of life after stroke

   b. Mauk model for poststroke recovery (Mauk, 2006), a grounded theory that suggests targeting of nursing interventions to each phase of stroke recovery

   c. Adaptation to stroke (Ch'Ng, French, & Mclean, 2008)

   d. Caregivers of stroke survivors

     1) Web-based nursing interventions for caregivers of stroke survivors (Pierce et al., 2004; Pierce, Steiner, Havens, & Tormoehlen, 2008)

     2) New caregivers of stroke survivors (Pierce et al., 2006)

     3) Problems of stroke caregivers (King, Ainsworth, Ronen, & Hartke, 2010)

     4) Efficacy of evidence-based urinary guidelines in the management of poststroke incontinence (Vaughn, 2009)

3. Evidence-based practice example

   a. Background on evidence-based practice related to dysphagia screening for stroke survivors

     1) More than 700,000 strokes occur per year in America, with more than two-thirds of people surviving.

     2) The prevalence of dysphagia after stroke is 40%–70% (Nishiwaki et al., 2005), although more than 80% of people recover the ability to swallow 2–4 weeks after stroke (Ramsey, Smithard, & Kalra, 2003).

     3) Dysphagia is one of the most serious complications resulting from stroke and can lead to dehydration, aspiration, pneumonia, and death.

     4) The most reliable screening tool is radiography (video fluoroscopy [VFS]), but researchers have been working on developing a reliable bedside screening tool that is safe and efficient in predicting dysphagia. Most hospitals and rehabilitation facilities use bedside screening and will consult speech therapy for the VFS if needed.

b. The clinical question: What is the best screening tool for dysphagia in the stroke survivor?

c. Appraisal of evidence: Eight relevant sources provide good evidence to address the question but with conflicting results. No qualitative studies have been found. The review is limited to clients with stroke and excludes dysphagic clients with other diagnoses.

     1) One Level 1 source with good evidence (Scottish Intercollegiate Guidelines Network, 2004)

     2) One Level 1 source with fair and poor evidence (Veterans Health Administration, 2003)

     3) Three Level 3 articles with good evidence (Hinds & Wiles, 1998; McCullough, 1997; Smith, Lee, O'Neill, & Connolly, 2000)

     4) One Level 4 article with good evidence (Nishiwaki et al., 2005)

     5) One Level 4 article with good evidence (DePippo, Holas, & Reding, 1994)

     6) One Level 5 article with good evidence (Ramsey et al., 2003)

d. Recommendations for best rehabilitation nursing practice

     1) The evidence cited here provides conflicting results about recommendations for best practice.

     2) All studies agree that early screening tools for dysphagia in stroke survivors are important and that VFS, though the standard, is not practical in all situations.

     3) Most researchers agree that a reliable bedside tool for screening those at risk for dysphagia and its complications would be useful. The Veterans Health Administration (2003) recommended that the SLP perform a simple bedside screening on all stroke survivors and that those with abnormal findings receive a comprehensive bedside exam. Those assessed to have swallowing problems would then undergo VFS. However, these recommendations are supported by only fair evidence.

     4) The major methods studied for screening of dysphagia include the following:

       a) VFS, the gold standard and reliable

       b) Clinical observation of wet voice and spontaneous cough during swallow or dysarthria and poor speech intelligibility (McCullough, 1997)

       c) 30-ml water swallowing tests were found to be highly accurate in one study

(DePippo et al., 1994) but had variable sensitivity and were poor at detecting silent aspiration (Ramsey et al., 2003).

    d) Oxygen saturation was found to detect 86% of aspirators and was most accurate in combination with bedside swallowing assessment with a 10-ml water swallow screening (Smith et al., 2000).

5) The practice guidelines examined recommend that the water swallow test be used as part of the screening for aspiration risk in stroke survivors.

6) VFS is still the most reliable and accurate screening tool for dysphagia, but the water test, clinical observation for signs and symptoms of dysphagia, and oxygen saturation all show promise as screening tools for stroke survivors.

7) More level 1 evidence is needed to determine other evidence-based practice for screening for dysphagia in stroke survivors.

8) Evidence-based practice suggests the use of free water between meals to prevent dehydration.

References

Adams, H. P., Jr., del Zoppo, G., Alberts, M. J., Bhatt, D. L., Brass, L., Furlan, A., et al. (2007). Guidelines for the early management of adults with ischemic stroke: A guideline from the American Hearth Association/American Stroke Association Stroke Council, Clinical Cardiology Council, Cardiovascular Radiology and Intervention Council, and the Atherosclerotic Peripheral Vascular Disease and Quality of Care Outcomes in Research Interdisciplinary Working Groups: The American Academy of Neurology affirms the value of this guideline as an educational tool for neurologists. *Stroke, 38*(5), 1655–1711.

American Heart Association. (2005). Critical care and emergency medicine neurology in stroke. *Stroke, 36,* 205.

American Heart Association. (2008). *Get with the guidelines: Stroke.* Retrieved September 13, 2010, from www.americanheart.org/downloadable/heart/1203521452783StrokeFactSheet.pdf.

American Heart Association. (2009). *Primary stroke center certification program.* Retrieved June 17, 2010, from www.heart.org/idc/groups/heart-public/@wcm/@mwa/documents/downloadable/ucm_315542.pdf.

American Heart Association. (2010). Heart disease and stroke statistics: 2010 update. *Circulation, 121*(7), e46.

Bader, M., & Palmer, S. (2006). What's the "hyper" in hyperacute stroke? *AACN Advanced Critical Care, 17*(2), 194–214.

Becker, J., Wira, C., & Arnold, J. (2010). Ischemic stroke. *Medscape Emedicine.* Retrieved June 15, 2010, from http://emedicine.medscape.com/article/793904-overview.

Berg, A., Palomaki, H., Lonnaqvist, J., Lethihalmes, M., Phil, L., & Kaste, M. (2005). Depression among caregivers of stroke survivors. *Stroke, 36*(3), 639–643.

Bogousslavsky, J. (Ed.). (2003). *Acute stroke treatment.* New York: Martine and Dunitz.

Boss, B. J. (2002a). Alterations of neurologic function. In K. L. McCance & S. E. Huether (Eds.), *Pathophysiology: The biologic basis for disease in adults & children* (4th ed., pp. 487–549). St. Louis: Mosby.

Boss, B. J. (2002b). Concepts of neurologic dysfunction. In K. L. McCance & S. E. Huether (Eds.), *Pathophysiology: The biologic basis for disease in adults & children* (4th ed., pp. 438–486). St. Louis: Mosby.

The Brain Attack Coalition. (2002). *TPA Stroke Study Group guidelines.* Retrieved August 20, 2010, from www.stroke-site.org/guidelines/tpa_guidelines.html.

Broderick, J., Connolly, S., Feldmann, E., Hanley, D., Kase, C., Krieger, D., et al. (2007). Guidelines for the management of spontaneous intracerebral hemorrhage in adults: 2007 update: A guideline from the American Heart Association/American Stroke Association Stroke Council, High Blood Pressure Research Council, and the Quality of Care and Outcomes in Research Interdisciplinary Working Group. *Circulation, 116*(16), e391–e413.

Buttaro, T. M. (2003). Cerebrovascular accident. In T. M. Buttaro, J. Trybulski, P. P. Bailey, & J. Sandberg-Cook (Eds.), *Primary care: A collaborative practice* (2nd ed., pp. 150–153). St. Louis: Mosby.

Caswell, J. (2008). New developments in rehab. *Stroke Connection,* July–August, 16–17. Retrieved November 12, 2010, from www.nxtbook.com/nxtbooks/aha/strokeconnection_20080708/index.php?startid=16#/18.

Ch'Ng, A., French, D., & Mclean, N. (2008). Coping with the challenges of recovery from stroke: Long term perspectives of stroke group members. *Journal of Health Psychology, 13,* 1136.

Commission on Accreditation of Rehabilitation Facilities. (2010). *2010 medical rehabilitation program descriptions.* Retrieved November 12, 2010, from www.carf.org/Programs/.

Consortium for Spinal Cord Medicine. (1998). *Clinical practice guidelines: Neurogenic bowel management in adults wih spinal cord injury.* Washington, DC: Paralyzed Veterans of America.

Consortium for Spinal Cord Medicine. (2006). *Clinical practice guidelines: Bladder management for adults with spinal cord injury.* Washington, DC: Paralyzed Veterans of America.

Dafaer, R. M., Rao, M., Shareef, A., & Sharma, A. (2008). Post-stroke depression. *Stroke Rehabilitation, 15*(1), 13–21.

Davis, J. (1997). *NDT course for nursing.* Port Townsend, WA: Inernational Clinical Educators, Inc.

DePippo, K. L., Holas, M. A., & Reding, M. J. (1994). The Burke dysphagia screening test: Validation of its use in patients with stroke. *Archives of Physical Medicine & Rehabilitation, 75*(12), 1284–1286.

Easton, K. L. (2001). *The post-stroke journey: From agonizing to owning.* Doctoral dissertation, Wayne State University, Detroit, MI.

Easton, J. D., Saver, J., Albers, G., Alberts, M., Chaturvedi, E., Feldmann, E., et al. (2009). Definition and evaluation of transient ischemic attack: A scientific statement for healthcare professionals from the American Heart Association/American Stroke Association Stroke Council; Council on Cardiovascular Surgery and Anesthesia; Council on Cardiovascular Radiology and Intervention; Council on Cardiovascular Nursing; and the Interdisciplinary Council on Peripheral Vascular Disease. *Stroke, 40,* 2276–2293.

Elkind, M., & Carlino, R. (2010). Genetic and inflammatory mechanisms in stroke. *Medscape Emedicine.* Retrieved August 20, 2010, from http://emedicine.medscape.com/article/1163331-overview.

Foerch, C., Misselwitz, B., Humpich, M., Steinmetz, H., Neumann-Haefelin, T., & Sitzer, M. (2007). Sex disparity in the access of elderly patients to acute stroke care. *Stroke, 38,* 2123–2126.

Fullerton, H., Wu, Y., Zhao, S., & Johnston, S. C. (2003). Risk of stroke in children: Ethnic and gender disparities. Neurology, 61, 189–194.

Gall, S. L., Donnan, G., Dewey, H. M., Macdonell, R., Sturm, J., Gilligan, A., et al. (2010). Sex differences in presentation, severity, and management of stroke in a population-based study. *Neurology, 74*(12), 975–981.

Ginsburg, M. (2008). Neuroprotection for ischemic stroke. *Neuropharmacology,* 55(3), 363–389.

Graykoski, J. J. (2003). Cerebrovascular events. In T. M. Buttaro, J. Trybulski, P. P. Bailey, & J. Sandberg-Cook (Eds.), *Primary care: A collaborative practice* (2nd ed., pp. 929–934). St. Louis: Mosby.

Hare, R., Rogers, H., Lester, H., McManus, R. J., & Mamt, J. (2006). What do stroke patients and their carers want from community services? *Family Practice, 23*(1), 131–136.

Hinchey, J. A., Shepherd, T., Furie, K., Smith, D., Wang, D., Tonn, S., et al. (2005). Formal dysphagia screening protocols prevent pneumonia. *Stroke, 36,* 1972–1976.

Hinds, N. P., & Wiles, C. M. (1998). Assessment of swallowing and referral to speech and language therapists in acute stroke. *QJM: An International Journal of Medicine, 91,* 829–835.

Hinkle, J. L. (2006). Variables explaining functional recovery following motor stroke. *Journal of Neuroscience Nursing, 38*(1), 6–12.

Imitola, J., & Khoury, S. (2008). *Neural stem cells and the future treatment for neurological diseases.* Springer Science and Business Media. Retrieved June 4, 2010, from www.ncbi.nlm.nih.gov/pubmed/18369745.

The Joint Commission. (2010). *Primary stroke centers.* Retrieved September 13, 2010, from www.jointcommission.org/assets/1/18/stroke_pm_implementation_guide_ver_2a.pdf.

Keiser, M. M. (1999). Neurologic disorders. In A. Gawlinski & D. Hamwi (Eds.), *Acute care nurse practitioner: Clinical curriculum and certification review* (pp. 295–384). Philadelphia: W. B. Saunders.

King, R., Ainsworth, C. R., Ronen, M., & Hartke, R. (2010). Stroke caregivers: Pressing problems reported during the first months of caregiving. *Journal of Neuroscience Nursing, 42*(6), 302–311.

Kvigne, K., Kirkevold, M., & Gjengedal, E. (2005). The nature of nursing care and rehabilitation of female stroke survivors: The perspective of hospital nurses. *Journal of Clinical Nursing, 14*(7), 897–905.

Larson, J., Franzen-Dahlin, A., Billing, E., von Arbin, M., Murray, V., & Wredling, R. (2005). The impact of a nurse-led support and education program for spouses of stroke patients: A randomized controlled trial. *Journal of Clinical Nursing, 14*(8), 995–1003.

Lemke, D. (2006). Advancing nursing practice: The role of the nurse practitioner in an acute stroke program. *Journal of Neuroscience Nursing, 38*(4), 328.

Likosky, D., Marrin, C. A., Caplan, L. R., Baribeau, Y. R., Morton, J. R., Weintraub, R. M., et al. (2003). Determination of etiologic mechanisms of strokes secondary to coronary artery bypass graft surgery. *Stroke, 34,* 2830.

Lutsep, H., & Clark, W. (2009). Neuroprotective agents in stroke. *Medscape Emedicine.* Retrieved August 20, 2010, from http://emedicine.medscape.com/article/1161422-overview.

Mace, N. L., & Rabins, P. V. (1981). *The 36-hour day.* Baltimore: Johns Hopkins University Press.

Mauk, K. L. (2006). Nursing interventions within the Mauk model of poststroke recovery. *Rehabilitation Nursing, 31*(6), 267–263.

Mauk, K. L., & Mauk, J. M. (2006). Future trends in gerontological nursing. In K. Mauk (Ed.), *Gerontological nursing: Competencies for care* (pp. 815–828). Sudbury, MA: Jones & Bartlett.

McCullough, G. H. (1997). *Sensitivity and specificity of a clinical/bedside examination of swallowing for detecting dysphagia in adults subsequent to stroke.* Doctoral dissertation, Vanderbilt University, Nashville, TN.

Merck Sharp & Dohme Corporation. (2009–2010). *Introduction to cerebrovascular accident.* Retrieved June 5, 2010, from www.merck.com/mmpe/sec16/ch211/ch211a.html.

Miller, E., Murray, L., Richard, L., Zorowitz, R. D., Bakas, T., Clark, P., et al. (2010). Stroke: Comprehensive overview of nursing and interdisciplinary rehabilitation care of the stroke patient. *Council on Cardiovascular Nursing and the Stroke Council, 41,* 2402–2448.

Nassisi, D. (2010). Hemorrhagic stroke. *Medscape Emedicine.* Retrieved June 17, 2010, from http://emedicine.medscape.com/article/1916662-overview.

National Institute of Neurological Disorders and Stroke. (2008). *NINDS central pain syndrome page.* Retrieved September 13, 2010, from www.ninds.nih.gov/disorders/central_pain/central_pain.htm.

National Institute of Neurological Disorders and Stroke. (2009a). *NIH stroke scale.* Retrieved August 20, 2010, from www.strokecenter.org/trials/scales/nihss.html.

National Institute of Neurological Disorders and Stroke. (2009b). *Stroke information page.* Retrieved June 17, 2010, from www.ninds.nih.gov/disorders/stroke/stroke.htm.

National Stroke Association. (2009a). *African Americans and stroke.* Retrieved June 30, 2010, from www.stroke.org/site/PageServer?pagename=AAMER.

National Stroke Association. (2009b). *Caregivers and families.* Retrieved June 30, 2010, from www.stroke.org/site/PageServer?pagename=care.

National Stroke Association. (2009c). *Kids and stroke.* Retrieved June 30, 2010, from www.stroke.org/site/PageServer?pagename=kids.

National Stroke Association. (2009e). *Recovery.* Retrieved June 30, 2010, from www.stroke.org/site/PageServer?pagename=recov.

National Stroke Association. (2009f). *Stroke risk factors.* Retrieved June 30, 2010, from www.stroke.org/site/PageServer?pagename=risk.

National Stroke Association. (2009g). *What is stroke?* Retrieved June 30, 2010, from www.stroke.org/site/DocServer/STROKE_101_Fact_Sheet.pdf?docID=4541.

National Stroke Association. (2011). *Resources.* Retrieved July 15, 2011, from www.stroke.org/site/PageServer?pagename=RESOUR.

Neuro-IFRAH Organization. (2005). *What is Neuro-IFRAH?* Retrieved August 20, 2010, from www.neuro-ifrah.org/faq.aspx.

Nir, Z., Zolotogorsky, Z., & Sugarman, H. (2004). Structured nursing intervention versus routine rehabilitation after stroke. *American Journal of Physical Medicine & Rehabilitation, 83,* 522–529.

Nishiwaki, K., Tsuji, T., Liu, M., Hase, K., Tanaka, N., & Fujiwara, T. (2005). Identification of a simple screening tool for dysphagia in patients with stroke using factor analysis of multiple dysphagia variables. *Journal of Rehabilitation Medicine, 37,* 247–251.

Ohio State University Medical Center. (2011, May 5). *Bat saliva drug may extend window for stroke treatment.* Retrieved July 18, 2011, from from www.healthnewsdigest.com/news/Stroke0/Bat_Saliva_Drug_May_Extend_Window_for_Stroke_Treatment.shtml.

Patel, S., Jain, R., & Wagner, S. (2008). The vasculature of the human brain. In *Neuroscience in medicine* (pp. 147–166). Totowa, NJ: Humana Press.

Pfeil, M., Gray, R., & Lindsay, B. (2009). Depression and stroke: A common but often unrecognized combination. *British Journal of Nursing, 18*(6), 365–369.

Pierce, L., Steiner, V., & Govoni, A. L. (2002). In-home online support for caregivers of survivors of stoke. *CIN & Computers Information Nursing, 20*(4), 154–164.

Pierce, L., Steiner, V., Govoni, A., Hicks, B., Thompson, T., & Friedemann, M. (2004). Caring-Web: Internet-based support for rural caregivers of persons with stroke show promise. *Rehabilitation Nursing, 29*(3), 95–99, 103.

Pierce, L. L., Steiner, V., Hicks, B., & Holzaepfel, A. L. (2006). Problems of new caregivers of persons with stroke. *Rehabilitation Nursing, 31*(4), 166–172.

Pierce, L., Steiner, V., Havens, H., & Tormoehlen, K. (2008). Spirituality expressed by caregivers of stroke survivors. *Western Journal of Nursing Research, 30*(5), 606–619.

Ramsey, D. J. C., Smithard, D. G., & Kalra, L. (2003). Early assessments of dysphagia and aspiration risk in acute stroke patients. *Stroke, 34,* 1252–1257.

Reeves, M. J., Bushnell, C. D., Howard, G., Gargano, J. W., Duncan, P. W., Lynch, G., et al. (2008). Sex differences in stroke: Epidemiology, clinical presentation, medical care, & outcomes. *Lancet Neurology, 7,* 915–926.

Roach, E. S., Golomb, M., Adams, R., Biller, J., Daniels, S., deVeber, G., et al. (2008). Management of stroke in infants and children: A scientific statement from a special writing group of the American Heart Association Stroke Council and the Council on Cardiovascular Disease in the Young. *Stroke, 39*(9), 2644–2691.

Rochette, A., Korner-Bitensky, N., & Desrosiers, J. (2007). Actual versus best practice for families post-stroke according to three rehabilitation disciplines. *Journal Rehabilitation Medicine, 39*(7), 513–519.

Rosamond, W., Flegal, K., Furie, K., Go, A., Greenlund, K., Haase, N., et al. (2008). Heart disease and stroke statistics—2008 update: A report from the American Heart Association Statistics Committee and Stroke Statistics Subcommittee. *Circulation, 117,* e25–e146.

Salaycik, K., Kelly-Hayes, M., Beiser, A., Nguyen, A. H., Brady, S., Kase, C., et al. (2007). The Framingham Study: Depressive symptoms and risk of stroke. American Heart Association. *Stroke, 38,* 16–21.

Sanossian, N., & Ovbiagele, B. (2009). Prevention and management of stroke in very elderly patients. *Lancet Neurology, 8,* 1031–1041.

Sauerbeck, L. R. (2006). Primary stroke prevention. *American Journal of Nursing, 106*(11), 40–41, 43–45, 48–49.

Schwamm, L., Fayad, P., Acker, J., Duncan, P., Fonarow, G., Girgus, M., et al. (2010). Translating evidence into practice: A decade of efforts by the American Heart Association/American Stroke Association to reduce death and disability due to stroke. *Stroke, 41*(5), 1051–1065.

Scottish Intercollegiate Guidelines Network. (2004). *Management of patients with stroke: Identification and management of dysphagia. A national clinical guideline.* Edinburgh: Author.

Secrest, J. S. (2002). How stroke survivors and primary support persons experience nurses in rehabilitation. *Rehabilitation Nursing, 24*(6), 240–246.

Secrest, J., & Zeller, R. (2007). The relationship of continuity and discontinuity, functional ability, depression and quality of life over time in stroke survivors. *Rehabilitation Nursing, 32*(4), 158–164.

Sen, S., Webb, S., & Selph, J. (2010). *E-medicine neurology.* Retrieved June 30, 2010, from http://emedicine.medscape.com/article/1160167-media.

Seppa, N. (2003, January 18). *Nifty spittle: Compound in bat saliva may aid stroke patients.* Retrieved October 24, 2006, from http://sciencenews.org/view/generic/id/3508/title/Nifty_Spittle_Compound_in_bat_saliva_may_aid_stroke_patients.

Smith, H. A., Lee, S. H., O'Neill, P. A., & Connolly, M. J. (2000). The combination of bedside swallowing assessment and oxygen saturation monitoring of swallowing in acute stroke: A safe and humane screening tool. *Age and Ageing, 29,* 495–499.

Stucki, G., Stier-Jarmer, M., Grill, E., & Melvin, J. (2005). Rationale and principles of early rehabilitation care after an acute injury or illness. *Disability and Rehabilitation, 27*(7–8), 353–359.

Sugerman, R. A. (2002). Structure and function of the neurologic system. In K .L. McCance & S. E. Huether (Eds.), *Pathophysiology: The biologic basis for disease in adults & children* (4th ed., pp. 363–396). St. Louis: Mosby.

Teather, L., & Wurtman, R. (2005). Dietary CDP-choline supplementation prevents memory impairment caused by impoverished environmental conditions in rats. *Learning & Memory, 12*(1), 39–43.

University of Iowa (n.d.a). Nursing outcomes classification (NOC). Retrieved July 18, 2011, from www.nursing.uiowa.edu/excellence/nursing_knowledge/clinical_effectiveness/noc.htm.

University of Iowa (n.d.b). Nursing interventions classification (NIC), 5th edition interventions labels & definitions. Retrieved July 18, 2011, from www.nursing.uiowa.edu/excellence/nursing_knowledge/clinical_effectiveness/documents/LabelDefinitionsNIC5.pdf.

van Swieten, J. C., Koudstaal, P. J., Visser, M. C., Schouten, H. J., & van Gijn, J. (1988). Interobserver agreement for the assessment of handicap in stroke patients. *Stroke, 19*(5), 604–607.

Vaughn, S. (2009). Efficacy of urinary guidelines in the management of post-stroke incontinence. *International Journal of Urological Nursing, 3*(1), 4–12.

Veterans Health Administration, Department of Defense. (2003). *VA/DoD clinical practice guideline for the management of stroke rehabilitation in the primary care setting.* Washington, DC: Author.

Visser-Meily, A., Post, M., Gorter, J., Berlekom, S. B. V., van den Bos, T., & Lindeman, E. (2006). Rehabilitation of stroke patients needs a family-centered approach. *Disability Rehabilitation, 28*(24), 1557–1561.

Weed, R., & Berens, D. (Eds.). (2009). *Life care planning and case management handbook* (3rd ed.). Boca Raton, FL: CRC Press.

Wu, C. M., McLaughlin, K., Lorenzetti, D. L., Hill, M. D., Manns, B. J., & Ghali, W. A. (2007). Early risk of stroke after transient ischemic attack: A systematic review and meta-analysis. *Archives of Internal Medicine, 167,* 2417–2422.

Zebian, R., & Kazzi, A. (2010). Subarachnoid hemorrhage. *Medscape Emedicine.* Retrieved June 4, 2010, from http://emedicine.medscape.com/article/794076-overview.

Suggested Resources

Hickey, J. (2009). *The clinical practice of neurological & neurosurgical nursing* (6th ed.). Philadelphia: Lippincott Williams & Wilkins.

Hinkle, J. L. (2010). Outcome three years after motor stroke. *Rehabilitation Nursing, 35*(1), 23–30.

Hoeman, P. (2008). *Rehabilitation nursing prevention, intervention, & outcomes* (4th ed.). St. Louis: Mosby.

Kliewer, K. L. (2008). Nutrition and ischemic stroke. *Archives of Neurology, 65*(9), 1257–1258.

National Stroke Association. (2004). *Lotsa Helping Hands* Retrieved December 28, 2006, from http://stroke.lotsahelpinghands.com.

National Stroke Association. (2009). *Public stroke prevention guidelines.* Retrieved June 30, 2010, from www.stroke.org/site/PageServer?pagename=PREVENT.

Ordway, C. (2009). Mild cognitive impairment: Routine screening can slow the course. *Advance for Nurse Practitioners, 11,* 37–40.

Ostwald, S. K., Godwin, K. M., & Cron, S. G. (2009). Predictors of life satisfaction in stroke survivors and spousal caregivers after inpatient rehabilitation. *Rehabilitation Nursing, 34*(4), 160–167, 174.

Panther, K. (n.d.). *Frazier water protocol summary.* Retrieved November 19, 2010, from www.vitalstim.com/uploadedFiles/Health_Professionals/Certified_Provider_Resources/Dysphagia_Treatment_Resources/VitalStim_Frazier_Water_Protocol.pdf.

Perry, A. G., & Potter, P. A. (2010). *Clinical nursing skills and techniques* (7th ed.). St. Louis: Mosby.

Yeager, S. (2009). The neuroscience acute care nurse practitioner: Role development, implement, and improvement. *Critical Care Nursing Clinics of North America, 21,* 561–593.

CHAPTER 12

Traumatic Injuries: Traumatic Brain Injury and Spinal Cord Injury

Paula Martinkewiz, MS RN CRRN • Betty J. Furr, PhD RN CRRN • Catharine Farnan, MS CRRN CBIS • Patricia G. Martinez, BSN RN CRRN

Catastrophic injuries of the brain and spinal cord affect millions of people each year. Falls, motor vehicle accidents, violence, and sporting and recreational injuries are the major causes. Annually, about 12,000 new spinal cord injuries (SCIs) occur (National Spinal Cord Injury Statistical Center [NSCISC], 2010a), and an estimated 1.4 million people sustain a traumatic brain injury (TBI; National Center for Injury Prevention and Control [NCIPC], 2007). Both injuries affect primarily the younger population and tend to occur more often in males. Both types of injuries have effects that vary according to the specific location and severity of injury. These injuries usually necessitate rehabilitation.

Victims of catastrophic injuries need assistance from healthcare professionals to improve health function and learn to adapt to changes in their functional status in the community. Rehabilitation nurses play a vital role in improving client outcomes through astute assessment, timely interventions, and thorough evaluation and they help clients and families with the transition to work and community. The rehabilitation process is interdisciplinary and works to improve all aspects of the client's life. Often, technology is used to improve function after catastrophic injuries.

I. TBI
   A. Overview
      1. Definitions
         a. Refers to a blow or a jolt to the head or a penetrating injury to the head that disrupts the function of the brain (Brain Injury Association of America, 2006)
         b. May produce altered levels of consciousness, changes in cognition and behavior, and physical limitations (Brain Injury Association of America, 2006)
         c. The severity of brain injury may range from mild to moderate or severe (Brain Injury Association of America, 2006).
         d. The result may be long-term or short-term problems with independent function (Brain Injury Association of America, 2006).
      2. Impact
         a. Affects roles and relationships for the client and family (Baggerly & Le, 2001)
         b. Often affects employment, finances, and leisure activities (Baggerly & Le, 2001)

         c. Brain damage from external injuries can be immediate or secondary to a variety of pathophysiological changes and it leads to long-term or lifelong needs for assistance from others (Lunney, MaGuire, Endozo, & McIntosh-Waddy, 2010).
      3. General symptoms (**Table 12-1**)
   B. Types of Injuries
      1. Concussion
         a. Definition: An immediate, temporary loss of consciousness resulting from a mechanical force to the brain (Hickey, 2003b)
         b. Symptoms: May or may not report unconsciousness (Evans, 2003), momentary loss of reflexes or memory, headache, confusion, dizziness, irritability, and visual and gait disturbances (Hickey, 2003b)
      2. Contusion: Bruising to the brain cortex; may be moderate or severe; associated with a loss of consciousness, stupor, and confusion; outcomes vary according to location and severity of injury (Blank-Reid & Barker, 2002)
      3. Hemorrhagic injuries
         a. Subdural hematoma
            1) Results from bleeding between the dura and arachnoid interface
            2) May be acute, subacute, or chronic
            3) Occurs in 5%–22% of people with intracranial injuries and is more common in older adults
            4) Changes in level of consciousness, elevated intracranial pressure and associated symptoms, seizure, paresis
            5) Surgical evacuation may be needed for larger sizes (more than 1 cm in adult); smaller sizes may benefit from medical management (Chanda & Nanda, 2003).
         b. Epidural hematoma
            1) Develops as a rapid arterial or venous bleed, often associated with skull fracture or a lacerated meningeal artery (most common cause)
            2) More common in young adults and adults older than age 60
            3) Accounts for approximately 2% of traumatic intracranial insults

Table 12-1. General Symptoms of Traumatic Brain Injury

Physical	Cognitive and Behavioral
Paresis	Poor initiation
Dysphagia	Disinhibition
Dysarthria	Agitation
Cerebrospinal fluid leaks	Restlessness
Balance and coordination impairments	Impulsivity
Visual impairments	Aphasias
Loss of bowel control	Memory and thinking deficits
Loss of bladder control	Sequencing difficulties
Spasticity and loss of tone	Attention and concentration deficits
Seizures	Problem solving and reasoning deficits
Dysautonomia ("storming")	Anxiety
Sleep–wake disturbance	Depression
Pain	Emotional lability
Metabolic effects (higher nutritional needs)	Loss of social competence

Baggerly, J., & Le, N. (2001). Nursing management of the patient with head trauma. In J. B. Derstine & S. D. Hargrove (Eds.), *Comprehensive rehabilitation nursing* (pp. 331–367). Philadelphia: W. B. Saunders.

Hickey, J. (2003b).Craniocerebral trauma. In J. Hickey (Ed.), *Clinical practice of neurological and neurosurgical nursing* (5th ed., pp. 373–406). Philadelphia: Lippincott.

Hickey, J. (2003c). Overview of neuroanatomy and neurophysiology. In J. Hickey (Ed.), *Clinical practice of neurological and neurosurgical nursing* (5th ed., pp. 45–92). Philadelphia: Lippincott.

4) Changes in level of consciousness, elevated intracranial pressure and associated symptoms, seizure, paresis

5) Usually warrants surgical management (Chanda & Nanda, 2003)

   c. Intracerebral hemorrhage

1) Develops from bleeding into the cerebral tissue and is associated with contusions

2) May act as a space-occupying lesion compressing brain tissue; poor prognosis

3) Headache, deteriorating consciousness, coma, contralateral paresis, ipsilateral dilated pupil, signs of herniation (Hickey, 2003b)

   d. Subarachnoid hemorrhage

1) Develops from bleeding into the subarachnoid space

2) Is associated with severe head injury and aneurysmal ruptures

3) Symptoms related to elevated intracranial pressure and meningeal irritation (Hickey, 2003b)

  4. Penetrating injuries

   a. Missile injuries (high-velocity trauma)

1) Caused by gunshots, nail guns, or other types of missiles; the location, path of injury, and depth of penetration directly affect the severity of the injury

2) May be associated with infection caused by bone fragments, hair, and skin entering the brain with the missile (Blank-Reid & Barker, 2002)

3) Herniation of brain tissue is possible.

   b. Missile injuries (low-velocity trauma): Local parenchymal damage, most commonly caused by a bullet or sharp object, is the most important factor in determining the extent of injury (Blank-Reid & Barker, 2002).

   c. Stab wounds

1) Refers to the piercing of the scalp, skull, or brain by a foreign object (e.g., knife, ice pick, pencil, scissors)

2) May cause severe neurologic impairment depending on the location of the insult (Vinas et al., 2006)

C. Epidemiology

  1. It is estimated that at least 5.3 million people have a need for extended or permanent assistance in activities of daily living (ADLs) because of a TBI. Annually 80,000–90,000 people experience the onset of long-term or permanent disability caused by TBI.

  2. Based on 2002–2006 data about emergency department visits, hospitalizations, and deaths, the Centers for Disease Control and Prevention (CDC; 2010b) reported that each year

   a. 1.7 million people sustain a TBI in the United States.

b. 80.7% of reports were for emergency department visits, 16.3% were for hospitalizations, and 3.0% were for deaths.

c. 1.365 million people are treated for TBI and released from hospital emergency departments.

d. 275,000 people are hospitalized and survive TBI, and 50,000 do not survive.

e. It is estimated that more than 3.17 million Americans lived with disabilities resulting from TBI-related injuries in 2000 (Brain Injury Association of America, 2010).

f. Direct medical costs and indirect costs of TBI, such as lost productivity, totaled an estimated $60 billion in the United States (CDC, 2010a).

3. The CDC (2010a) also reported the following 2002–2006 data:

a. Males age 0–4 years had the highest rates of TBI-related emergency department visits, hospitalizations, and deaths combined (1,451 per 100,000).

b. Rates were also high for females age 0–4 (1,218 per 100,000), and for both males and females age 15–19 years (896 per 100,000) and 75 years and older (932 per 100,000).

D. Etiology and Causes of TBI (CDC, 2010a; Faul, Waid, & Coronado, 2010)

1. In all age groups, falls are the leading cause of TBI (35.2% of all TBIs, or 595,095 per year). Falls cause approximately half (50.2%) of the TBIs among children age 0–14, compared with 60.7% among adults age 64 years and older.

2. 17.3% (292,202) of TBIs are related to motor vehicle accidents, with the highest rates among adults age 20–24 years.

3. 16.5% (279,882) are struck by objects or thrown against objects.

4. 10.0% (169,625) of TBIs are related to assaults.

5. 21% (199,447) of TBIs have other or unknown causes.

6. Blasts are a leading cause of brain injury in military personnel active in war zones (Department of Defense and Veterans Brain Injury Center, unpublished data, 2005).

7. A 62% increase in fall-related TBI was seen in emergency departments among children age 14 years and younger between 2002 and 2006 (Faul et al., 2010).

E. Pathophysiology

1. Although some degree of irreversible damage occurs at the moment of impact (the primary injury), TBI is a process in which additional and progressive secondary injury evolves over minutes, hours, and days after the injury (Blank-Reid & Barker, 2002).

2. Primary injuries

a. *Primary injury* is damage to the brain that occurs at the moment of impact (Gennarelli & Graham, 2005).

b. *Acceleration and deceleration injuries* are caused by changes in velocity, when the head moves rapidly and then stops abruptly, which causes strain on the brain tissue in the form of compression, tension, or shearing (Hickey, 2003b). They are associated with motor vehicle crashes, falls, and objects striking the head (Blank-Reid & Barker, 2002).

c. Diffuse axonal injuries (DAIs)

1) DAIs are caused by microscopic damage to neuronal axons; microscopic lesions are not seen on traditional computed tomography (CT) and conventional magnetic resonance imaging (MRI) scans; they may appear as small areas of hemorrhage (Flanagan, Cantor, & Ashman, 2008; Meythaler, Peduzzi, Eleftheriou, & Novack, 2001; Wasserman & Koenigsberg, 2004).

2) Diffusion tensor imaging, a newer MRI technique, produces in vivo images of white matter tracts, allowing visualization of neural pathways to determine connectivity and assist in establishing the presence of DAI (Xu, Rasmussen, Lagopoulos, & Haberg, 2007).

3) Destruction occurs in the cerebral hemispheres, corpus callosum, and brainstem; it is often seen in areas where brain densities differ, such as the junctions of gray and white matter.

4) Severity depends on the magnitude of the acceleration forces involved in the traumatic event and usually is worse than what is noted on imaging studies (Wasserman & Koenigsberg, 2004).

5) Classified as mild, moderate, or severe; about 45% of clients fall into the moderate category, with incomplete recovery in those who survive (Hickey, 2003b).

d. *Focal injuries* are damage resulting from a localized trauma, involving consolidated areas of tissue destruction such as contusions, lacerations, hematomas, and intracranial hemorrhages; symptoms vary according to type, extent, and location of injury (Hickey, 2003b).

3. Secondary injuries
   a. Complications after a primary event (Gennarelli & Graham, 2005)
   b. Causes (Blank-Reid & Barker, 2002; Povlishock & Katz, 2005)
      1) Cerebral edema
      2) Elevated intracranial pressure
      3) Hypoxia and ischemia
      4) Infection and inflammatory response
      5) Hypotension
      6) Electrolyte imbalance, hypocapnia
      7) Hyperthermia
      8) Vasospasm
   c. Postinjury complications (National Institute of Neurological Disorders and Stroke [NINDS], 2010)
      1) Pain
      2) Infections
      3) Seizures
      4) Pressure ulcers
      5) Hydrocephalus
      6) Cerebrospinal fluid leaks
      7) Vascular injuries
      8) Cranial nerve injuries
      9) Multiple organ system failure
      10) Polytrauma
      11) Elevated intercranial pressure
      12) Altered hemodynamic states
      13) Herniation
      14) Respiratory complications
      15) Stress ulcers
      16) Deep vein thrombosis
F. Assessment
   1. Classification
      a. Mild brain injury
         1) Description
            a) May result in a loss of consciousness for 30 or fewer minutes (NCIPC, 2003)
            b) Glasgow Coma Scale (GCS) scores of 13–15 (NCIPC, 2003) and negative neuroimaging (**Table 12-2**)
            c) A complicated mild brain injury has the same GCS score but with positive CT findings (Kennedy et al., 2006).
            d) About 75% of TBIs are classified as mild (NCIPC, 2006).
         2) Symptoms may include dizziness, headache, insomnia, fatigue, decreased memory, irritability, confusion, vision changes, tinnitus, unpleasant taste, decreased concentration, and attention deficits (NCIPC, 2006; NINDS, 2010).
      b. Moderate brain injury
         1) Description
            a) GCS scores ranging from 9–12 (Department of Defense [DOD] and Veteran's Head Injury Program & Brain Injury Association of America, 1999; van Baalen et al., 2003)
            b) Abnormal CT findings
         2) Consists of coma lasting less than 24 hours with incomplete recovery (Barker, 2002)
         3) May have a good recovery or learn to compensate for neurological deficits with proper treatment (Barker, 2002)
      c. Severe brain injury
         1) Description
            a) Loss of consciousness lasting hours, days, months, or years (DOD and Veteran's Head Injury Program & Brain Injury Association of America, 1999).
            b) GCS scores lower than 8 (van Baalen et al., 2003).
            c) May make significant improvements but often are left with permanent residual neurological deficits (DOD and Veteran's Head Injury Program & Brain Injury Association of America, 1999)
         2) Severe disorders of consciousness (subcategories of severe brain injury; Giacino & Whyte, 2005; Giacino et al., 2002)
            a) Coma: Complete absence of arousal or responsiveness
               (1) The eyes do not open spontaneously or in response to stimulation.
               (2) Absent sleep-wake cycle
               (3) No purposeful motor activity, distinct defensive movements, or localization to noxious stimuli
               (4) No ability to follow commands or intelligible verbalization
               (5) No conscious awareness of self or environment
            b) Vegetative state: No distinct evidence of conscious awareness of self or environment
               (1) Eyes open spontaneously.
               (2) The sleep-wake cycle resumes; arousal is sluggish, poorly sustained.
               (3) No signs of intentional, purposeful, or reproducible behavioral responses to stimuli

THE SPECIALTY PRACTICE OF REHABILITATION NURSING

Table 12-2. Glasgow Coma Scale Categories

Category	Response	Score
Eye opening	Spontaneous: Eyes open spontaneously without verbal or noxious stimulation.	4
	To speech: Eyes open with verbal stimuli but not necessarily to command.	3
	To pain: Eyes open with various forms of noxious stimuli.	2
	None: No eye opening with any type of stimulation.	1
Verbal response	Oriented: Aware of person, place, time, reason for hospitalization, and personal data.	5
	Confused: Answers not appropriate to question but correct use of language.	4
	Inappropriate words: Disorganized, random speech, no sustained conversation.	3
	Incomprehensible sounds: Moans, groans, and mumbles incomprehensibly.	2
	None: No verbalization, even to noxious stimuli.	1
Best motor response	Obeys commands: Performs simple tasks on command and able to repeat task on command.	6
	Localizes to pain: Organized attempt to localize and remove painful stimuli.	5
	Withdraws from pain: Withdraws extremity from source of painful stimuli.	4
	Abnormal flexion: Decorticate posturing that occurs spontaneously or in response to noxious stimuli.	3
	Extension: Decerebrate posturing that occurs spontaneously or in response to noxious stimuli.	2
	None: No response to noxious stimuli; flaccid.	1

From *Clinical practice of neurological and neurosurgical nursing* (4th ed.), by J. Hickey, 1997, Philadelphia: Lippincott Williams & Wilkins. Copyright 1997 by Lippincott WIlliams & Wilkins. Reprinted with permission.

(4) No signs of language perception or communication

c) Minimally conscious state: Distinct behavioral signs of conscious awareness as evidenced by at least one of the following:
   (1) Basic command following
   (2) Intelligible verbalization
   (3) Yes-no responses, whether verbal or by gesture
   (4) Nonreflexive emotional or motor behavior that occurs in response to related environmental stimuli (e.g., affective responses to emotional content, object manipulation, pursuit eye movements)

d) Locked-in syndrome
   (1) Eye opening is present; eye movement is the primary mode of communication.
   (2) Basic cognitive function is evident on exam.
   (3) Clinical evidence of quadriplegia
   (4) Often occurs as a result of a lesion in the pons

e) Akinetic mutism: Condition characterized by diminished neurologic drive or inattention; movement and speech are extremely deficient
   (1) Eye opening and spontaneous visual tracking are present.

   (2) Can be considered a subcategory of minimally conscious state because purposeful responses often are inconsistent but can be elicited after application of stimulation

2. Assessment instruments and tools
   a. Agitated Behavior Scale
      1) Used for ongoing assessment of presence and intensity of agitation during the acute phase of recovery (Bogner, Corrigan, Bode, & Heinemann, 2000)
      2) Composed of 14 items that are each rated from 1 (*absent*) to 4 (*present to an extreme degree*)
      3) The best overall indicator for agitation is the total score, although subscales for disinhibition, aggression, and lability can be calculated (Corrigan & Bogner, 1994).
   b. Coma/Near Coma (Rappaport, 2000, 2005)
      1) Designed to expand the upper range of the Disability Rating Scale
      2) Measures clinical changes in vegetative and persistent vegetative state
      3) Has eight items grouped into five categories, ranging from *extreme coma* to *no coma*
   c. Coma Recovery Scale Revised (Giacino, Kalmar, & Whyte, 2004; Kalmar & Giacino, 2005)
      1) Designed to assess subtle changes in cognitive status and predict outcome in clients with severe disorders of consciousness

2) Differentiates between vegetative and minimally conscious state

d. Disability Rating Scale
   1) Designed to quantitatively assess moderate to severe brain injury along a wide continuum of recovery, from severe vegetative state to no disability (Wright, 2000)
   2) Composed of eight items that are divided into four categories: arousability, cognitive ability for self-care, degree of dependence, and employability (Rappaport, 2005; van Baalen et al., 2003)

e. FIM™ (Grosswasser, Schwab, & Salazar, 1997; van Baalen et al., 2003)
   1) Constructed to provide a uniform measure of function across rehabilitation settings
   2) Measures items of self-care, sphincter control, mobility, locomotion, communication, and social cognition

f. Galveston Orientation and Amnesia Test: Used to measure the duration of posttraumatic amnesia after a brain injury (Levin, O'Donald, & Grossman, 1975; van Baalen et al., 2003)

g. GCS (see Table 12-2)
   1) Used to assess the level of consciousness and neurological functioning after a brain injury
   2) Categorized into three main assessment areas: motor, verbal, and eye-opening responses
   3) Is very useful in the acute care setting (Rosebrough, 1998)

h. Glasgow Outcome Scale: Developed to assess general outcome after brain injury; categories include *good recovery, moderate disability, severe disability, persistent vegetative state,* and *death* (van Baalen et al., 2003)

i. Neurobehavioral Functioning Inventory (Kreutzer, Seel, & Marwitz, 1999; Marwitz, 2000)
   1) Used to assess the frequency of a variety of behaviors and symptoms that may occur after brain injury
   2) Composed of 76 items divided into six categories: depression, somatic, memory and attention, communication, aggression, and motor

j. Neuropsychological testing
   1) Refers to a variety of tests and test batteries that are used to measure cognitive function

2) May include measures of attention, memory, concentration, reasoning, processing speed, and executive function (Girard et al., 1996)

k. Rancho Los Amigos Levels of Cognitive Functioning Scale: Used to interpret the cognitive recovery process after a brain injury (Rancho Los Amigos National Rehabilitation Center, 2006; **Table 12-3**)
   1) Levels range from 1–10; lower scores indicate a more severe impairment of consciousness
   2) Hagen (personal communication, October 25, 2006) states that the Rancho Los Amigos Levels of Cognitive Function Scale was created as a team treatment scale.
   3) After level I, clients may fluctuate between three levels, with the middle level being the most common.
   4) All members of the team determine the factors that help the client remain at his or her most common level of cognitive functioning, the factors that facilitate movement to higher levels, and the factors that cause regression.

l. Sensory Stimulation Assessment Measure: Designed to expand the GCS and used to standardize sensory presentation (Duff & Wells, 1997; O'Dell & Riggs, 1996; Rader, Alston, & Ellis, 1989)

m. Western Neuro Sensory Stimulation Profile
   1) Used to assess auditory and visual comprehension; tracking; object manipulation; and attention, arousal, tactile, and olfactory function
   2) Contains 33 items in six areas (Ansell & Keenan, 1989)

3. Physical assessment
   a. General: Determine location of brain injury and corresponding symptoms (**Tables 12-4** and **12-5**)
   b. Neurologic
      1) Assess cognitive, motor, and sensory status, reflexes, and cranial nerves.
      2) Monitor anticonvulsant levels.
      3) Monitor for signs and symptoms of elevated intracranial pressure.
      4) Monitor changes in behavior (excesses and deficits).
      5) Monitor changes in level of consciousness.
      6) Monitor effects of medications prescribed for cognition and behavior (at present most of these are often used off label).

Table 12-3. Rancho Los Amigos Levels of Cognitive Functioning Scale—Revised

Cognitive Level	Expected Behavior
Level II Generalized response: Total assistance	Demonstrates generalized reflex response to painful stimuli
	Responds to repeated auditory stimuli with increased or decreased activity
	Responds to external stimuli with physiological changes generalized, gross body movement and/or not purposeful vocalization
	Responses noted above may be the same regardless of type and location of stimulation
	Responses may be significantly delayed
Level III Localized response: Total assistance	Demonstrates withdrawal or vocalization to painful stimuli
	Turns toward or away from auditory stimuli
	Blinks when strong light crosses the visual field
	Follows a moving object passed within visual field
	Responds to discomfort by pulling tubes or restraints
	Responds inconsistently to simple commands
	Responses directly related to type of stimulus
	May respond to some people (especially family and friends) but not to others
Level IV Confused/agitated: Maximal assistance	Alert and in heightened state of activity
	Purposeful attempts to remove restraints or tubes or crawl out of bed
	May perform motor activities such as sitting, reaching and walking, but without any apparent purpose or upon another's request
	Very brief and usually nonpurposeful moments of sustained alternatives and divided attention
	Absent short-term memory
	May cry out or scream out of proportion to stimulus even after its removal
	May exhibit aggressive or flight behavior
	Mood may swing from euphoric to hostile with no apparent relationship to environmental events
	Unable to cooperate with treatment efforts
	Verbalizations are frequently incoherent and/or inappropriate to activity or environment
Level V Confused, inappropriate non-agitated: Maximal assistance	Alert, not agitated, but may wander randomly or with a vague intention of going home
	May become agitated in response to external stimulation and/or lack of environmental structure
	Not oriented to person, place, or time
	Frequent, brief periods, nonpurposeful sustained attention
	Severely impaired recent memory, with confusion of past and present in reaction to ongoing activity
	Absent goal-directed, problem-solving, self-monitoring behavior
	Often demonstrates inappropriate use of objects without external direction
	May be able to perform previously learned tasks when structured and cues provided
	Unable to learn new information
	Able to respond appropriately to simple commands fairly consistently with external structures and cues
	Responses to simple commands without external structure are random and nonpurposeful in relation to the command
	Able to converse on a social, automatic level for brief periods of time when provided external structure and cues
	Verbalizations about present events become inappropriate and confabulatory when external structure and cues are not provided

continued

Table 12-3. Rancho Los Amigos Levels of Cognitive Functioning Scale—Revised *continued*

Cognitive Level	Expected Behavior
Level VI Confused, appropriate: Moderate assistance	Inconsistently oriented to person, time, and place Able to attend to highly familiar tasks in nondistracting environment for 30 minutes with moderate redirection Remote memory has more depth and detail than recent memory Vague recognition of some staff Able to use assistive memory aid with maximum assistance Emerging awareness of appropriate response to self, family, and basic needs Moderate assist to problem solve barriers to task completion Supervised for old learning (e.g., self-care) Shows carryover for relearned familiar tasks (e.g., self-care) Maximum assistance for new learning with little or no carryover Unaware of impairments, disabilities, and safety risks Consistently follows simple directions Verbal expressions are appropriate in highly familiar and structured situations
Level VII Automatic, appropriate: Minimal assistance for daily living skills	Consistently oriented to person and place within highly familiar environments; moderate assistance for orientation to time Able to attend to highly familiar tasks in a nondistraction environment for at least 30 minutes with minimal assist to complete tasks Minimal supervision for new learning Demonstrates carryover of new learning Initiates and carries out steps to complete familiar personal and household routine but has shallow recall of what he/she has been doing Able to monitor accuracy and completeness of each step in routine personal and household activities of daily living (ADLs) and modify plan with minimal assistance Superficial awareness of his/her condition but unaware of specific impairments and disabilities and the limits they place on his/her ability to safely, accurately, and completely carry out his/her household, community, work, and leisure ADLs Minimal supervision for safety in routine home and community activities Unrealistic planning for the future Unable to think about consequences of a decision or action Overestimates abilities Unaware of others' needs and feelings Oppositional/uncooperative Unable to recognize inappropriate social interaction behavior

continued

Table 12-3. Rancho Los Amigos Levels of Cognitive Functioning Scale—Revised *continued*

Cognitive Level	Expected Behavior
Level VIII Purposeful, appropriate: Stand-by assistance	Consistently oriented to person, place, and time
	Independently attends to and completes familiar tasks for 1 hour in distracting environments
	Able to recall and integrate past and recent events
	Uses assistive memory devices to recall daily schedule and "to do" lists and record critical information for later use with stand-by assistance
	Initiates and carries out steps to complete familiar personal, household, community, work, and leisure routines with stand-by assistance and can modify the plan when needed with minimal assistance
	Requires no assistance once new tasks/activities are learned
	Aware of and acknowledges impairments and disabilities when they interfere with task completion, but requires stand-by assistance to take appropriate corrective action
	Thinks about consequences of a decision or action with minimal assistance
	Overestimates or underestimates abilities
	Acknowledges others' needs and feelings and responds appropriately with minimal assistance
	Depressed
	Irritable
	Low frustration tolerance/easily angered
	Argumentative
	Self-centered
	Uncharacteristically dependent/independent
	Able to recognize and acknowledge inappropriate social interaction behavior while it is occurring and takes corrective action with minimal assistance
Level IX Purposeful, appropriate: Stand-by assistance on request	Independently shifts back and forth between tasks and completes them accurately for at least two consecutive hours
	Uses assistive memory devices to recall daily schedule and "to do" lists and record critical information for later use with assistance when requested
	Initiates and carries out steps to complete familiar personal, household, work, and leisure tasks independently and unfamiliar personal, household, work, and leisure tasks with assistance when requested
	Aware of and acknowledges impairments and disabilities when they interfere with task completion and takes appropriate corrective action, but requires stand-by assist to anticipate a problem before it occurs and take action to avoid it
	Able to think about consequences of decisions or actions with assistance when requested
	Accurately estimates abilities but requires stand-by assistance to adjust to task demands
	Acknowledges others' needs and feelings and responds appropriately with stand-by assistance
	Depression may continue
	May be easily irritable
	May have low frustration tolerance
	Able to self monitor appropriateness of social interaction with stand-by assistance

continued

Table 12-3. Rancho Los Amigos Levels of Cognitive Functioning Scale—Revised *continued*

Cognitive Level	Expected Behavior
Level X Purposeful, appropriate: Modified independent	Able to handle multiple tasks simultaneously in all environments but may require periodic breaks
	Able to independently procure, create, and maintain own assistive memory devices
	Independently initiates and carries out steps to complete familiar and unfamiliar personal, household, community, work, and leisure tasks, but may require more than usual amount of time and/or compensatory strategies to complete them
	Anticipates impact of impairments and disabilities on ability to complete daily living tasks and takes action to avoid problems before they occur, but may require more than usual amount of time and/or compensatory strategies
	Able to independently think about consequences of decisions or actions but may require more than usual amount of time and/or compensatory strategies to select the appropriate decision or action
	Accurately estimates abilities and independently adjusts to task demands
	Able to recognize the needs and feelings of others and automatically respond in appropriate manner
	Periodic periods of depression may occur
	Irritability and low frustration tolerance when sick, fatigued, and/or under emotional stress
	Social interaction behavior is consistently appropriate

Rancho Los Amigos Levels of Cognitive Functioning Scale—Revised. Reprinted with permission. Original scale coauthored by Hagen, C., Malkmus D., Durham P. (2006).

Communication Disorders Service, Rancho Los Amigos Hospital, 1972. Revised 1974 by Hagen, C., Malkmus, D. & Stenderup, K. Revised scale 1997 by Hagen, C.

Table 12-4. Location of Injury and Associated Symptoms

Region of Brain	Symptoms
Frontal lobe	Impaired judgment, reasoning, concentration, abstraction, executive functions, behavior, and impulse control; expressive aphasia in dominant hemisphere (usually the left hemisphere); impaired voluntary motor function
Temporal lobe	Impaired somatic, auditory, olfactory, and visual association; receptive aphasia in dominant hemisphere (usually the left hemisphere); impaired learning and detailed memories such as past experiences, conversations, art, music, and taste
Parietal lobes	Impaired sensory association; impaired ability to recognize size, shape, texture, presence of touch, pressure, and body position; impaired recognition of own body parts (often called neglect)
Occipital lobe	Impaired visual perception and visual reflexes
Cerebellum	Impaired fine motor movement, balance, coordination
Brainstem	Abnormalities of cranial nerve function depending on location in brainstem; impaired cardiac, respiratory, and vasomotor function; wakefulness

Barker, E. (2002). Neuroanatomy and physiology of the nervous system. In E. Barker (Ed.), *Neuroscience nursing: A spectrum of care* (pp. 3–50). St. Louis: Mosby.
Hickey, J. (2003c). Overview of neuroanatomy and neurophysiology. In J. Hickey (Ed.), *Clinical practice of neurological and neurosurgical nursing* (5th ed., pp. 45–92). Philadelphia: Lippincott.

c. Respiratory: Assess airway patency, oxygen saturation, nature of sputum, lung fields, and potential for aspiration.

d. Cardiovascular: Assess blood pressure, pulse, heart rate, rhythm, risk for or existence of deep vein thrombosis, and risk factors for emboli (atrial fibrillation); presence of dysautonomia.

e. Nutritional: Assess weekly weights, intake and output, daily hydration status, and dietary intake; anticipate the client will have higher metabolic demands; modify the diet if dysphagia is present (e.g., use of thickener).

f. Sensory and perceptual: Assess responses to various types of stimuli, sleep-wake cycles, level of consciousness, and presence of neglect.

g. Elimination

1) Assess bowel sounds and premorbid bowel patterns.

2) Assess premorbid elimination history, urinary output, and bowel movements.

3) Assess bowel and bladder continence and effectiveness of bowel and bladder programs (e.g., scheduled toileting programs, medications).

4) Monitor for potential alterations in elimination (e.g., constipation, diarrhea, urinary tract infection, and retention).

h. Musculoskeletal

1) Assess for heterotopic ossification, orthopedic injuries, premorbid history of joint

Table 12-5. Cerebral Hemispheres and Symptoms

Right Hemisphere	Left Hemisphere
Motor impairment on left side of body	Motor impairments on right side of body
Impulsivity	Impaired speech and language; aphasias
Impaired judgment	Impaired comprehension
Impaired insight into condition (may not realize that deficits exist)	Cautious, slow to perform
Left-sided neglect	Aware of deficits, depression, anxiety
Spatial-perceptual deficits	Impaired right-left discrimination

Barker, E. (2002). Neuroanatomy and physiology of the nervous system. In E. Barker (Ed.), *Neuroscience nursing: A spectrum of care* (pp. 3–50). St. Louis: Mosby.

disease, contractures, tone, spasticity, range of motion (ROM), and need for adaptive equipment.
2) Observe safety with transfers, gait, and mobility as appropriate.
3) Assess handedness.
4) Assess padding and positioning needs to maintain ROM.

i. Integumentary: Assess skin condition (turgor, color, wounds, and high-risk places under pressure such as areas with orthotic devices).

j. Communication: Assess for expressive, receptive, and global aphasias, dysarthria, and alternative communication strategies (e.g., augmentative communication devices).

k. Behavior: Assess for behavior excesses (e.g., agitation, disinhibition, impulsivity, poor judgment, motor restlessness, perseveration, emotional lability) and deficits (e.g., apathy, poor initiation).

l. Safety
1) Assess for risk of falls, wandering, impulsivity, balance, strength, judgment, and insight.
2) Assess need for least restrictive restraint or 1:1 sitter if necessary.

m. Psychosocial: Assess family support, coping mechanisms, and potential response to fear and anxiety.

n. Sexual: Assess function issues and related physical, cognitive, and behavioral alterations.
1) Last menstrual period
2) Pregnancy at time of admission
3) Premorbid sexual problems
4) Developmental stage

o. Educational needs of client and caregiver
1) Physical, psychosocial, safety care
2) Preferred learning style
3) Barriers to learning
4) Readiness to learn

p. Vocational: Assess potential for returning to work, school, or other purposeful activity (e.g., volunteering).

G. Planning: Client and Family Goals
1. Set individualized goals upon admission.
a. Bowel and bladder continence or established elimination schedules depending on cognition and level of consciousness
b. Improved cognition
c. Improved mobility
d. Improved functional independence
e. Improved safety (**Table 12-6**)
f. Improved judgment
g. Manageable behavior
h. Increased knowledge to care for self or client
i. Resolution of medical problems
j. Adequate nutritional status or plan to achieve such
k. Community reintegration skills
2. Meet at regular intervals to evaluate status of goal achievement.
3. Coordinate the plan with a highly structured interdisciplinary team.
a. Ensure consistency between providers (nurses, therapists, allied health professionals).
b. Set mutual goals.
c. Monitor functional progress and performance.
d. Use predicted goal attainment to guide readiness for discharge and maximize performance.
e. Document coordination of team members and comprehensive care plan daily.

H. Nursing Plan of Care and Interventions for Cognitive Rehabilitation (**Table 12-7**)

I. Evaluation
1. Evaluate progress toward client and family goals listed in Section G.
2. Use instruments described in Section F.2.

J. Discharge Planning and Community Resources
1. Discharge planning should begin before admission to the rehabilitation facility.
2. Discharge planning should incorporate extensive exploration of community resources for a lifetime of disability management.
a. Financial resources
1) Private insurance
2) Auto insurance

Table 12-6. Safety Tips

Don't	Do
Leave sharp objects within reach.	Provide the recommended supervision levels at home (as suggested by the rehabilitation team).
Leave poisons, chemicals, and household cleaners within reach.	Communicate with the client as an adult.
Leave car keys or keys to heavy equipment within reach.	Speak to the client in a regular tone of voice.
Leave the client alone near fire or heat sources (stove, barbecue, matches, lighters, cigarettes).	Praise small accomplishments and do so at the time of occurrence.
Assume the client has the same preinjury abilities or can resume his or her previous roles at home, at work, or in society.	Provide brain injury awareness information to the client's neighbors and fire and police departments.
Leave the client alone near bodies of water (ocean, lakes, swimming pools).	Provide structure and consistency of schedules.
Leave the client unattended and at risk for wandering, falls, or other injuries.	Provide a balance of stimulation and quiet time; recognize signs of impending escalation or fatigue.
Leave the client alone with heavy machinery.	Provide information on positive coping strategies regarding changes in family, work, and social roles.
Leave the client alone or in charge of small children until level of supervision or assistance is known.	Maintain a safe physical environment related to cognitive, behavioral, and physical changes.
Provide meal types or diet textures that are outside the prescribed plan of care.	Reintegrate the client into community activities as appropriate for his or her cognitive and behavioral level.
Overstimulate the client with a multitude of schedule changes, activities, or visitors.	Maintain diet type and texture to prevent aspiration.

Dufour, L., Williams, J., & Coleman, K. (2000). Traumatic injuries: TBI and SCI. In P. A. Edwards (Ed.), *The specialty practice of rehabilitation nursing: A core curriculum* (4th ed., p. 194). Glenview, IL: Association of Rehabilitation Nurses.

3) Medicare and Medicaid
4) Social Security Disability Insurance
5) Litigation awards
6) Donations

b. Continuum of care options
1) Home
2) Skilled nursing facilities
3) Long-term care facilities
4) Residential programs
5) Day therapy programs
6) Assisted living facilities
7) Clubhouse programs
8) Cognitive-based centers and neurobehavioral units

c. Healthcare resources
1) Home health services
2) Outpatient programs
3) Local hospital network
4) Primary care provider
5) Durable medical equipment (DME) supplier
6) Telehealth programs
7) State-level brain and spinal cord injury trust funds

d. Community resources (for information)
1) Brain Injury Association
2) American Heart Association
3) National Stroke Association
4) Epilepsy Foundation of America
5) Local library
6) Centers for Disease Control and Prevention
7) Department of Defense and Veterans Brain Injury Center
8) National Association of State Head Injury Administrators
9) National Center for Medical Rehabilitation Research, National Institute of Child Health and Human Development, National Institutes of Health
10) National Institute on Disability and Rehabilitation Research
11) North American Brain Injury Society
12) Social Security Administration
13) State Department of Rehabilitation Services
14) Technology recycled equipment exchange programs
15) United Disabilities Services

e. Technology assistance
1) Can come in many different forms, ranging from simple homemade devices such as ramps to complex computer-integrated systems
2) Pill holders with timed alarms
3) Alarmed wrist watches
4) Noise reduction headphones
5) Light switch dimmers
6) Augmentative communication device
7) Speed dial and memory options on communication devices
8) Voice recognition computer software programs

Table 12-7. Plan of Care for Cognitive Rehabilitation

Cognitive Level	Description	Nursing Management for Levels I, II, and III
I: No response	Unresponsive to touch, pain, or auditory or verbal stimuli	Orient client.
		Encourage family to bring in favorite music, pictures, blankets.
		Begin to talk to the client about family members and friends.
II: Generalized response	Displays inconsistent, nonpurposeful, reflexic responses to stimuli or pain	Talk in a normal tone of voice and use short, simple phrases, explaining all nursing tasks.
		Be careful what you say in front of the client.
		Guide client to follow simple commands (wink, wiggle fingers).
III: Localized response	Responds in a more focused manner to certain types of stimuli (e.g., turns to sound, withdraws from pain, tracks); may follow simple commands inconsistently	Allow extra time for a response.
		Introduce smells and tactile, auditory, and visual stimulation.
		Engage in familiar activities.
		Nursing assessments and physical care
		Monitor cardiovascular effects of pharmacological management (neurostimulants).
		Offer emotional support to family members.
		Talk to the client about familiar topics of interest, family, and close friends.
		Schedule nursing tasks to promote sleep-wake cycles.
		Begin family education; provide materials related to injury.
		Show family how to interact with the client; model behaviors; teach them not to overstimulate.
		Provide emotional support.
		Nursing Management for Level IV
IV: Confused agitated	Alert and in heightened state of activity; possibly aggressive; may display inappropriate behavior in response to internal confusion; short attention span	Limit the number of visitors to two or three.
		Provide a quiet, calm, environment; eliminate "noise clutter" from the environment.
		Reorient frequently.
		Reassure the client that he or she is safe.
		Monitor sleep-wake cycles.
		Provide familiar objects or photos from home.
		Allow as much freedom of movement as is safe.
		Do nursing care in short blocks; take a break, then start the next task.
		Have a helper for safety.
		Low stimulation during care; explain care in simple terms, avoiding "chatter"
		Consider 1:1 supervision rather than restraints during certain times of day.
		Use quiet, low-traffic areas for activities that require attention (e.g., eating).
		Remove items that might be frightening to the client (TV or news).
		Use closed-circuit cameras for additional monitoring.
		Consider an enclosure bed.
		Do not force the client to do things. Instead, listen to what he or she wants to do and follow his or her lead, within safety limits.
		Give breaks to prevent agitation or restlessness. Look for patterns. Work with team on this.
		Change activities frequently; redirect as needed.
		Consider that the client has no short-term memory, so behavior plans with "consequences" typically don't work.
		Preventing agitation through control of the external environment and therapeutic use of self is key.
		Monitor pharmacological management, which may include antianxiety agents.
		Use structure; same staff, same routing, same way of doing things.
		Prevention is better than intervention.

continued

Table 12-7. Plan of Care for Cognitive Rehabilitation *continued*

Cognitive Level	Description	Nursing Management for Levels V and VI
V: Confused inappropriate (nonagitated)	Alert, easily distracted, responsive to commands; pays gross attention to environment; displays absent carryover from one situation to another	Use repetition. Reorient frequently to person, place, and time. Use short and simple comments and questions. Assist with activity initiation; set up. Show the client pictures and objects that were of interest before the injury.
VI: Confused appropriate	Follows commands consistently but is inconsistently oriented to time and place; has short-term memory deficits; begins to participate in self-care	Provide frequent rest periods; collaborate with the therapy team on schedule. Limit the number of visitors. Monitor nutrition with increased activity. Establish bowel and bladder continence; start toileting programs. Provide tasks appropriate to level (e.g. hygiene, simple meal preparation—cold cereal). Identify areas of motivation for self-care tasks. Schedule rest and quiet time; fatigue or stress is common. Introduce memory aids (i.e. calendars, schedules); help with the schedule. Discuss events of the day to help improve memory. Monitor medication regimen; report sleep-wake, lethargy, agitation patterns to a physician. Begin to incorporate the client in the education process with family. Provide education to the client regarding injury and outcomes. Monitor for safety; it is still an important concern. Structure activities; staff should use a lot of cueing; the goal is for the client to "figure it out" with your help. Provide daily structure. Encourage participation in all therapies. Give immediate positive feedback. May start to use behavior plans with simple rewards.

Cognitive Level	Description	Nursing Management for Levels VII and VIII
VII: Automatic– appropriate	May perform tasks in familiar environment but in a robot-like manner; begins to have insight into deficits; continues to have poor judgment and problem-solving skills	The main goal is to promote reintegration into the community. Ask the client to remember more difficult things from day to day. Reduce environmental structure as necessary. Ask the client to solve problems he or she might encounter at home (e.g., "What would you do if you lost your keys to the house?"). Treat the client as an adult.
VIII: Purposeful– appropriate	Consistently oriented; has correct responses; intact memory; needs supervision; has realistic planning skills	Provide guidance and assistance in decision making. Encourage and allow the client to use his or her judgment, reasoning, and problem-solving skills within the home and safe community settings. Provide community outings to integrate client back into the social environment. Refer the client to community-based programs that support his or her condition. Encourage the use of memory aids such as note taking, calendars and schedules. Encourage independent functioning. Help the client to set reasonable goals for the future regarding education and employment. Discourage the use of alcohol and drugs. Help the client with conversations relating to social interaction and sexuality. Identify situations that make the client frustrated and discuss strategies for handling these situations. Help the client identify new roles within the family. Decrease barriers that contribute to isolation; transportation and esthetics.

continued

Table 12-7. Plan of Care for Cognitive Rehabilitation *continued*

Cognitive Level	Description	Nursing Management for Levels IX and X
IX: Purposeful–appropriate (standby assistance)	Client is aware and acknowledges impairments and disabilities when they interfere with tasks; initiates and carries out steps to complete familiar personal, household, work, and leisure tasks independently and unfamiliar personal, household, work, and leisure tasks with assistance when requested	Provide breaks with multiple tasks. Continue to provide memory aids with "to do" lists for use with assistance on request. Standby assistance is needed to anticipate a problem before it occurs and to take action to avoid it. Stand-by assistance to adjust to task demands Monitor for depression, irritability, and frustration; counsel as needed; may recommend a neuropsychologist. Stand-by assist to monitor for appropriateness of social interaction Discuss consequences of decision making; the client may take more time than usual or use compensatory strategies to select the appropriate decision. Discuss feelings and needs of others and how to respond to them appropriately. Discourage drugs and alcohol. Discuss difficulties of living with brain injury; provide counseling, resources, and information about support organizations.
X: Purposeful–appropriate (modified independent)	Independently initiates and carries out steps to complete familiar and unfamiliar personal, household, community, work, and leisure tasks, but may need more than the usual amount of time or compensatory strategies to complete them	Client is independent Monitor for depression. Monitor for irritability and low frustration tolerance when sick, fatigued, or under emotional stress. Encourage/support client and family. Encourage participation in a support group. Encourage counseling as needed. Follow up with a physician as needed (medications, outpatient therapy).

Brain Injury Association of America. (2006). *Scales and measurements of function.* Retrieved June 11, 2006, from www.biausa.org/Pages/what_is_the_rehab_process.html#ways

Brain injury.com. (2006a). Recovery and rehabilitation. Retrieved August 19, 2011, from www.braininjury.com/recovery.shtml.

Brain injury.com. (2006b). Symptoms of brain injury. Retrieved August 19, 2011, from www.braininjury.com/symptoms.shtml.

Dufour, L., Williams, J., & Coleman, K. (2000). Traumatic injuries: TBI and SCI. In P. A. Edwards (Ed.), *The specialty practice of rehabilitation nursing: A core curriculum* (4th ed., pp. 196–198). Glenview, IL: Association of Rehabilitation Nurses.

Gatens, C., & Hebert, A. R. (2001). Cognition and behavior. In S. Hoeman (Ed.), *Rehabilitation nursing: Process, application and outcomes* (pp. 599–630). St. Louis: Mosby.

Rancho Los Amigos National Rehabilitation Center. (2006). *Family guide to the levels of cognitive functioning.* Retrieved June 11, 2006, from www.rancho.org/patient_education/bi_cognition.pdf-88k-2006-01-06.

Rosebrough, A. (1998). Traumatic brain injury. In P. A. Chin, D. Finocchiaro, & A. Rosebrough (Eds.), *Rehabilitation nursing practice, major neurological deficits and common rehabilitation disorders* (pp. 223–244). New York: McGraw-Hill.

9) Screen readers or special computer screens, keyboards

K. Preventing TBI
1. Follow safety tips.
   a. Always wear a seatbelt when driving or riding in a car.
   b. Buckle children in an age-appropriate safety seat every time.
   c. Wear headgear when indicated and ensure that children do so (e.g., during contact sports, horseback riding, skateboarding, skiing).
2. Avoid injuries in and around the home.
   a. Eliminate slips and falls; use precautions and safety aids (e.g., step stools, grab bars, handrails, window guards, safety gates, nonslip mats, shock-absorbing material).
   b. Store firearms and bullets in different locked cabinets or safes (CDC, 2010a; NINDS, 2010).

L. TBI Research
1. Aims of research efforts
   a. Identify measures to reduce TBI-related morbidity.
   b. Improve outcomes.
2. Recent studies focus on new treatment approaches designed to address the different physiological, behavioral, emotional, and cognitive needs of TBI populations (Flanagan, Cantor, & Ashman, 2008; Zitnay et al., 2008).
   a. Assessment instruments
      1) Newer neuropsychological measurement focuses on evaluating functional abilities,

which supports the rehabilitative goal of treatment planning. Numerous examples of these assessment instruments are being evaluated (Chaytor & Schmitter-Edgecombe, 2003; Rabin, Burton, & Barr, 2007; Standen & Brown, 2005).

2) The Brief Objective Neurobehavioral Detector (BOND), a 16-item neurobehavioral task tool found to correlate with radiologic and cognitive findings, may be useful to detect mild TBI (Chapman, Andersen, Roselli, Meyers, & Pincus, 2010).

b. Structural, chemical, and functional neuroimaging

1) Diffusion tensor imaging is used to investigate white matter integrity and identify mild TBI (mTBI; Benson et al., 2010; Lo, Shifteh, Gold, Bello, & Lipton, 2009; Mayer et al., 2010; Perlbarg et al., 2009; Van Boven et al., 2009; Wang et al., 2008; Wu et al., 2009; Xu et al., 2007).

2) Functional magnetic resonance imaging (fMRI) assesses regional blood flow and local metabolic activity in the brain. fMRI is primarily a research tool that shows promise as a treatment modality to identify brain regions responsible for cognitive processes, which could result in improved dosing and timing of treatments (Flanagan et al., 2008; Provenzale, 2010).

3) Magnetic resonance spectroscopy (MRS) differs from standard MRI. MRS has additional software for analysis and imaging, which can be used to establish the presence of neuronal loss or abnormal changes in cellular function (Demougeot et al., 2001; Marino et al., 2007).

4) Magnetoencephalography (MEG) tracks neuronal brain activity using electrically generated magnetic fields. With MEG, spatial and temporal precision analysis of regional brain activation is possible. MEG abnormalities correlate with neural changes present in mTBI (Lewine et al., 2007).

c. Neuropsychology techniques (Bryant et al., 2010; Cicerone et al., 2008; McCrea et al., 2009).

d. Cell-based therapies

1) Stem cell research in adults shows that neural cells can differentiate into phenotypically diverse cell types under certain conditions, maintain the ability to generate neurons, and repair throughout life (Garbuzova-Davis et al., 2006). Stem cell rodent models have been used to replace neurons in central nervous system damage (Richardson et al., 2010).

2) Kinase inhibitors are used in regulation of cellular signaling and have emerged as a therapeutic strategy for the treatment of acute and chronic neurodegenerative disease (Cuny, 2009).

e. Genetics is becoming important in determining cognitive outcomes after TBI. Genetic factors are implicated in the regulation of catecholamine metabolism (Diaz-Arrastia & Baxter, 2006).

f. Cognitive rehabilitation

1) Cognitive remediation is well documented as improving cognitive functions such as attention, participation in ADLs, and self-regulation. Research efforts in this area continue (Cicerone, Levin, Malec, Struss, & Whyte, 2006).

2) Further research is recommended to optimize treatment and outcomes (Cicerone et al., 2005, 2006).

g. Electronic technologies

1) Assistive devices provide cues and memory aids for people with brain injury; several studies report gains in this area (Wilson, Emslie, Quirk, Evans, & Watson, 2005).

2) Additional well-designed clinical trials on technologically driven cognitive rehabilitation approaches are needed.

h. Computer simulation

1) Recent virtual reality (VR) studies evaluate the use of VR in people with TBI to assess cognitive abilities and simulate real-world scenarios for individualized rehabilitation training strategies (Flanagan et al., 2008).

2) Research findings support the use of VR rehabilitation as a training tool; it is anticipated that VR will become an integral assessment tool and rehabilitation model (Mumford & Wilson, 2009; Rose, Brooks, & Rizzo, 2005).

i. Pharmacologic management

1) Results of growth hormone therapy studies suggest that some of the cognitive impairments observed in people who experience growth hormone deficiencies after TBI may be partially reversible (High et al., 2010; Kelestimur, 2009).

2) Progesterone studies reveal that the hormone reduces cerebral edema,

inflammation, and tissue necrosis when given shortly after traumatic brain injury (MacNevin, Atif, Sayeed, Stein, & Liotta, 2009; Sayeed & Stein, 2009).

   3) Pharmacologic management (Chew & Zafonte, 2009; Francisco, Walker, Zasler, & Bouffard, 2007; McAllister, 2009).

   4) Melatonin is reported to be an antioxidative and antinitrosative agent. It acts as a unique neuroprotectant in traumatic central nervous system injuries (Samantaray et al., 2009).

   5) Simvastatin reduces postinjury beta-amyloid load and minimizes pathological conditions related to brain injury (Abrahamson, Ikonomovic, Dixon, & DeKosky, 2009).

   6) Antiepileptic drugs (AEDs) are given to manage impulsive aggressive behavior. Research findings show the positive anti-aggressive effects of AEDs to be specific to only impulsive forms of aggression (Stanford, Anderson, Lake, & Baldridge, 2009).

j. Pain

   1) Posttraumatic headache in mTBI is very common in Western societies, affecting approximately 1.8 million people in the United States. Recent investigations have found that a minority of people with mTBI develop chronic posttraumatic headache in combination with serious neurological and neuropsychological deficits (Obermann, Holle, & Katsarava, 2009).

   2) In a number of studies acupuncture has been found to be effective for treating TBI-related pain and spasticity (Tamai et al., 2007).

   3) Managing TBI-related pain (Hoffman et al., 2007; Lew et al., 2009; Sherman, Goldberg, & Bell, 2006): Pain is a common co-occurrence with TBI. One study found that 76% of people with TBI reported having chronic moderate to severe pain (Hoffman et al., 2007). Biologic (trauma, changes in sensory and motor function), psychological, and social factors (perception, emotional and cognitive function) influence the client's experience of pain. Regular, consistent evaluation of the client's response to pain medications appropriate for people with TBI, physical therapy, and cognitive and behavioral therapies assist in establishing the effectiveness of these therapeutic interventions (Sherman et al., 2006).

k. Complementary and alternative therapies

   1) Complementary and alternative medicine (CAM) includes a group of medical and healthcare therapies and practices that are generally not part of conventional, allopathic, or Western medicine (National Center for Complementary and Alternative Medicine, 2010).

   2) Oxygen therapies may offer a simple and effective therapeutic strategy for ischemic brain injuries in severe TBI (Rockswold, Rockswold, & Defillo, 2007; Zhou et al., 2007). Therapeutic effects of hyperoxia (both normobaric and hyperbaric) include mitochondrial rescue, stabilization of intracranial pressure, attenuation of cortical spreading depression, and inducing favorable endothelial-leukocyte interactions, all of which are postulated to decrease secondary injury. A neuroprotective role of normobaric hyperoxia is extremely promising, and further studies are warranted (Kumaria & Tolias, 2009).

   3) Few studies have reported the use of CAM in TBI. The popularity of CAM in the general population bolsters the need for more research in this area (Flanagan et al., 2008).

II. **Advanced Practice Considerations: Role of the Advanced Practice Nurse in TBI**

A. Educator

   1. Design a client and family caregiver education curriculum to be used by rehabilitation nurses in inpatient and outpatient settings (e.g., behavior, safety, cognition and memory, seizures, medications, bowel and bladder, community reentry).

   2. Present professional papers and posters at national and international brain injury meetings.

   3. Coordinate or teach certification review material to facility staff to increase the numbers of certified rehabilitation nurses.

   4. Collaborate with academic institutions to place nursing students in brain injury rehabilitation practicums.

   5. Collaborate with community agencies and academic institutions to teach rehabilitation nursing care for the client with TBI.

B. Leader

   1. Collaborate with local and national legislators to advocate for people with TBI regarding rehabilitation benefit coverage, accessibility, community resources, and other funding issues.

   2. Participate on local and state committees such as

TBI trust funds (check your local state).

3. Participate in your local chapter of the Association of Rehabilitation Nurses (ARN).

4. Participate in national ARN committees; run for office.

C. Consultant

1. Serve as a resource for clinical staff in inpatient and outpatient settings for complex client care problems (assist with treating a complex wound, assess a client's bowel problems, assist with strategies to facilitate cognitive and behavioral function, assist the case manager with discharge planning supplies related to nursing and medical care).

2. Attend team conferences and offer information; collaborate with the rehabilitation team.

3. Collaborate with external case managers regarding funding issues for brain injury rehabilitation stays.

4. Collaborate with community service agencies serving people with TBI (and their caregivers) for the purpose of providing information and additional resources.

5. Consult with community-based physicians about the care of their clients with TBI (for questions related to behavior, cognition, spasticity, and nutrition).

D. Researcher

1. Research question: What is the standard of practice for pharmacological management of agitation after TBI?

2. There have been many clinical studies evaluating pharmacology in TBI.

3. Many of the studies have been found to lack a rigorous method, limiting evidence for the prescribing clinician (Levy et al., 2005).

4. Case study reports usually are not generalizable (Pachet, Friesen, Winkelaar, & Gray, 2003; Sugden, Kile, Farrimond, Hilty, & Bourgeois, 2006; Wroblewski, Joseph, Kupfer, & Kalliel, 1997) even though the researchers achieved favorable or interesting results.

5. Several true experiments were reviewed with varied results ranging from inconclusive evidence to "general support," but most suggest further study with larger samples. See Levy and colleagues (2005) and Deb and Crownshaw (2004) for comprehensive analyses of the relevant literature.

6. Based on a critical review of the scientific literature, there is no established practice standard for the management of agitation after TBI. Many new studies are in progress, and it is important for the advanced practice nurse to design

well-controlled randomized clinical trials or to continually appraise the literature in this particular area for new and efficacious evidenced-based practices.

III. SCI

A. Definitions

1. SCI: Traumatic insult to the spinal cord resulting in alterations or complete disruption of normal motor, sensory, and autonomic function

2. Tetraplegia (replaced the term *quadriplegia*)

a. Injury to one of the eight cervical segments of the spinal cord

b. Impairment or loss of motor or sensory function in cervical segments causing loss of function in all four extremities

3. Paraplegia

a. Impairment or loss of motor or sensory function in the thoracic, lumbar, or sacral segments causing impairment in trunk, legs, and pelvic organs

b. Usually occurs as a result of injuries at T2 or below

4. Use of the terms *quadriparesis* and *paraparesis* is discouraged because they describe incomplete lesions imprecisely.

B. The Vertebral Segments (Refer to Chapter 9 for a discussion of neuroanatomy.)

1. Cervical vertebrae (7)

2. Thoracic vertebrae (12)

3. Lumbar vertebrae (5)

4. Sacral vertebrae (5)

5. Spinal cord segments correspond to muscles and associated movements.

C. Epidemiology (NSCISC, 2010b)

1. Incidence of SCI

a. Approximately 40 cases per million occur in the United States, or approximately 12,000 new cases per year.

b. No new overall incidence studies have been done in America since the 1970s.

c. In the 1970s SCI occurred primarily in young adults 16–30 years of age.

d. Over time, the median age of people with SCI in the United States has increased.

e. Since 2005 the median age at injury has been 40.2 years (NSCISC, 2010b).

f. 11.5% of injuries are in those older than 60.

g. 80.8% of those with SCI are male.

h. Since 2005 more than 67.3% of SCI injuries have been among Caucasians, 22.7% among African Americans, 7.9% among Hispanics, 1.6% among Asians, and 0.5% among others.

2. Prognosis
    a. Life expectancy after SCI is slightly shorter than normal with paraplegia, and for those with tetraplegia, life expectancy is shorter than that of people with paraplegia.
    b. Mortality rates are significantly higher in the first year after injury and among those who are older at the time of injury. For older clients (approximately 40%) they are higher still in more complete injuries (Fassett et al., 2007). Mortality rates are higher for those older than 65 years who are ventilator dependent (Pickett, Campos-Benitez, Keller, & Duggal, 2006).
    c. 10%–20% of people with SCI do not survive.
    d. The higher the injury, the more negative the effect on life expectancy.
    e. Leading causes of death are pneumonia, pulmonary emboli, and septicemia.
    f. Poor functional outcomes are associated with cervical cord injuries in people older than 50 years of age (Alander, Parker, Stauffer, & Shannon, 1997).
    g. Recovery of ambulation is significantly lower when injury occurs in those who are older than 50 years of age (Burns, Golding, Rolle, Graziani, & Ditunno, 1997).

D. Etiology (NSCISC, 2010b)
    1. Motor vehicle accidents account for 44.5% of SCI.
    2. Falls account for 18.1% of SCI; they are more common in those older than age 45.
        a. The rate of SCI from falls continues to increase steadily as the U.S. population ages.
        b. More than 50% of cervical fractures in those older than 65 years old are caused by low-impact mechanisms such as a fall from standing (Pickett et al., 2006).
    3. Violence accounts for 16.6%, or 15% of SCI since 2005, after peaking in the 1990s.
    4. Sports and recreational injuries account for 12.7%; diving is the most common sport associated with SCI.
    5. Other
        a. Tumors
        b. Abscess and infection
        c. Injuries after procedures such as spinal injections or epidural catheter placement
        d. Vertebral fractures
        e. Infarct

E. SCI and Aging (Pickett et al., 2006): Risk factors associated with aging include the following:
    1. Bone changes or arthritis
    2. Higher rate of spinal stenosis
    3. Higher risk for falls
    4. Higher risk of car accidents per miles driven

F. Mechanisms of Injury and Associated Common Abnormalities
    1. Direct trauma
        a. Flexion
            1) Occurs when head is thrown violently forward
            2) Occurs when head is struck from behind
            3) Occurs commonly in motor vehicle accidents and falls
        b. Flexion with rotation: Occurs when the combination of forces causes severe twisting, resulting in ruptured ligaments and dislocation
        c. Hyperextension: Occurs in forward falls in which the face or chin is struck
        d. Penetration: Injuries that directly pierce the spinal cord (e.g., gunshot wound, knife wound)
    2. Compression
        a. Flexion: Axial
            1) Occurs when vertebral bodies are wedged and compressed
            2) Occurs in the thoracic and lumbar region
            3) Caused by a fall onto the buttocks
        b. Vertical
            1) Occurs when vertebral bodies are shattered and burst into the spinal cord
            2) Typically occurs in the cervical region
            3) Caused by a high-velocity blow to the top of the head (e.g., diving)
    3. Ischemia: Injury as a result of damage or blockage, such as clots, in spinal arteries (Dawodu, 2007)

G. Pathophysiology
    1. Varying degrees of damage associated with SCI
        a. Severity of bony injury does not always correspond to the extent of neurological impairment.
        b. Common sites of injury—the cervical and thoracolumbar junctures—are the most mobile parts of the spine.
        c. The spinal cord itself may sustain contusion without vertebral fractures or dislocations.
        d. The most common levels of injury are C4 and C5 (Dawodu, 2007).
        e. Progressive tissue destruction occurs in the cord within hours and may involve several responses.
            1) Decrease of microperfusion at site of injury
            2) Hemorrhage in the gray matter
            3) Development of hematoma and edema

4) Release of biochemicals at site of injury
5) Ischemia and necrosis in the cord, secondary chemical cascade causing neurological damage

f. Clinical presentations related to edema and tissue damage
1) Spinal shock
   a) Temporary state of reflex depression of cord function occurring after injury
   b) Initial increase in blood pressure
   c) Flaccid paralysis, including bowel and bladder
   d) Lasts several hours to days
2) Neurogenic shock
   a) Characterized by hypotension, bradycardia, hypothermia
   b) More common in injuries above T6
   c) Need to differentiate between spinal and hypovolemic shock
3) Autonomic dysreflexia or hyperreflexia (Campagnolo, 2006)
   a) A medical emergency
   b) Occurs in 48%–90% of those with injuries at or above T6, especially cervical injuries; rare occurrences in injuries as low as T10
   c) More common in males than females (4:1)
   d) Caused by stimulation below the level of injury, often in the area of the sacral segments or lower, such as overdistended bladder, fecal impaction, decubitus ulcers, urological procedures, pregnancy and delivery, gynecological procedures, ingrown toenails, fractures, restrictive shoes or clothing, deep vein thrombosis, sexual activity, and kidney stones
   e) Characterized by hypertension, bradycardia, flushing and perspiration above the level of the lesion, gooseflesh above the level of the lesion, nasal congestion, and an impending sense of doom
   f) Blood pressure 20–40 mm Hg above the client's normal baseline may indicate autonomic dysreflexia.
   g) Treatment involves reducing the causing stimulus (e.g., empty the bladder) and lowering blood pressure by raising the head of the bed and administering appropriate medications.
   h) Untreated, can result in stroke, coma, or death
   i) Many episodes can be prevented with good bowel and bladder care and prevention of pressure ulcers.

2. Levels of SCI
   a. Upper motor neuron (UMN) injury
      1) Is evident in lesions above T12–L1 vertebrae
      2) Causes loss of cerebral control over all reflex activity below the level of lesion
      3) Causes spastic paralysis
      4) UMNs lie within the spinal cord.
   b. Lower motor neuron (LMN) injury
      1) Is evident in lesions below T12–L1 level (i.e., conus medullaris, cauda equina)
      2) Causes destruction of the reflex arc
      3) Causes flaccid paralysis
      4) LMNs branch off from the spinal cord.

3. Clinical syndromes
   a. Central cord syndrome
      1) Caused by damage to the central part of the cord
      2) Usually is in the cervical region
      3) Produces loss of motor power and sensation that affects upper limbs more than lower limbs
      4) Produces sacral sparing (American Spinal Injury Association [ASIA], 2008)
   b. Brown-Séquard syndrome
      1) Caused by damage to one side (hemisection) of the cord
      2) Produces loss of motor function and position sense on the same side as the damage and a loss of pain, temperature sensation, and light touch on the opposite side
   c. Anterior cord syndrome
      1) Caused by damage to the anterior artery, affecting the anterior two-thirds of the cord
      2) Produces paralysis and loss of pain and temperature sensation below the lesion with preservation of position sense
   d. Conus medullaris syndrome
      1) Caused by damage to the conus and lumbar nerve roots
      2) May produce areflexia (flaccidity) in bladder, bowel, and lower limbs
   e. Cauda equina syndrome
      1) Caused by damage below conus to lumbar-sacral nerve roots
      2) May produce areflexia in bladder, bowel, and lower limbs

H. Assessment
1. Classification: To be motor incomplete, an SCI must be incomplete (sacral sparing) and have either voluntary anal sphincter contraction or motor function preserved more than three levels below the motor level (ASIA, 2008).
    a. Skeletal level of injury: The level at which, by radiographic examination, the greatest vertebral damage is found
        1) Stable injury: Occurs when the bone or ligaments support the injured cord area, preventing progression of neurological deficit
        2) Unstable injury: Occurs when the bone and ligaments are disrupted and unable to support and protect the injured cord area, possibly causing further neurological deficit
    b. Neurological level of injury: The most caudal segment of the spinal cord with normal sensory and motor function on each side of the body (ASIA, 1996)
        1) Sensory level
            a) Refers to the most caudal segment of the spinal cord with normal sensory function on each side of the body
            b) Evaluated at a key sensory point within each of 28 dermatomes on the right and 28 dermatomes on the left side of the body
        2) Motor level (**Table 12-8**)
            a) Best predictor of a person's functional abilities (McKinley & Silver, 2006)
            b) Refers to the most caudal segment of the spinal cord with normal motor function on each side of the body
            c) Evaluated at a key muscle within each of 10 myotomes on the right and 10 myotomes on the left side of the body
    c. Complete injury: An absence of motor and sensory function in the lowest sacral segment
    d. Incomplete injury
        1) Results in partial preservation of sensory or motor function below the neurological level and includes the lowest sacral segment
        2) Includes sacral sensation at the anal mucocutaneous junction and deep anal sensation
        3) Includes motor function of voluntary contraction of the external anal sphincter upon digital examination
    e. Zone of partial preservation (ASIA, 2008)
        1) Consists of the dermatomes and myotomes that are caudal to the neurological level and remain partially innervated
        2) Term used only with complete injuries (e.g., a person with a complete C5 injury may have patchy sensation at C6 or C7 but not have any anal reflexes, such as sacral sparing, and thus still be classified as a complete C5 injury)
2. Assessment instruments and tools
    a. Assessing impairment: ASIA Impairment Scale (1996)
        1) Frequently used scale that reflects severity of impairment
        2) Modified version of Frankel Grading System for SCI
        3) Levels of ASIA scale
            A = Complete: No sensory or motor function preserved in S4–S5.
            B = Incomplete: Sensory function (but not motor function) preserved below the neurological level and extends through S4–S5.
            C = Incomplete: Motor function preserved below the neurological level; the majority of muscles below the level are grade 3 or lower.
            D = Incomplete: Motor function preserved below the neurological level; the majority of muscles below the level are grade 3 or higher.
            E = Normal: Normal sensory and motor function.
    b. Motor grading scale (ASIA, 2008): The strength of each muscle is graded on a six-point scale.
        0 = Total paralysis
        1 = Palpable or visible contraction of the muscle
        2 = Active movement < full range of motion with gravity eliminated
        3 = Active movement < full range of motion against gravity
        4 = Active movement < full range of motion against moderate resistance
        5 = Normal active movement < full range of motion against full resistance
    c. Sensory impairment scale scores: 0 = *absent*, 1 = *impaired*, 2 = *normal*, NT = *not tested*.
    d. Other: Spinal Cord Independence Measure assesses 16 categories of self-care, mobility, and respiratory and sphincteric function; Quadriplegic Index of Function detects slight changes in ADLs among those

Table 12-8. Neurological Levels and Functional Potential

Level	Abilities	Functional Goals
C1–C3	Limited movement of head and neck	Breathing: Depends on a ventilator or implant to control breathing.
		Communication: Talking is sometimes difficult, very limited or impossible. If ability to talk is limited, communication can be accomplished independently with a mouth stick and assistive technologies like a computer for speech or typing. Effective verbal communication allows the individual with SCI to direct caregivers in the person's daily activities, like bathing, dressing, personal hygiene, transferring as well as bladder and bowel management.
		Daily tasks: Assistive technology allows for independence in tasks such as turning pages, using a telephone and operating lights and appliances.
		Mobility: Can operate an electric wheelchair by using a head control, mouth stick, or chin control. A power tilt wheelchair also for independent pressure relief.
C4	Usually has head and neck control. Individuals at C4 level may shrug their shoulders.	Breathing: May initially require a ventilator for breathing; usually adjust to breathing full time without ventilator assistance.
		Communication: Normal, may have weaker voice projection
		Daily tasks: With specialized equipment, some may have limited independence in feeding and independently operate an adjustable bed with an adapted controller.
C5	Typically has head and neck control, can shrug shoulder and has shoulder control. Can bend his/her elbows and turn palms face up.	Daily tasks: Independence with eating, drinking, face washing, brushing of teeth, face shaving and hair care after assistance in setting up specialized equipment.
		Health care: Can manage their own health care by doing self-assist coughs and pressure relief's by leaning forward or side -to-side.
		Mobility: May have strength to push a manual wheelchair for short distances over smooth surfaces. A power wheelchair with hand controls is typically used for daily activities. Driving may be possible after being evaluated by a qualified professional to determine special equipment needs.
C6	Has movement in head, neck, shoulders, arms and wrists. Can shrug shoulders, bend elbows, turn palms up and down and extend wrists.	Daily tasks: With help of some specialized equipment, can perform with greater ease and independence, daily tasks of feeding, bathing, grooming, personal hygiene and dressing. May independently perform light housekeeping duties.
		Health care: Can independently do pressure reliefs, skin checks and turn in bed.
		Mobility: Some individuals can independently do transfers but often require a sliding board. Can use a manual wheelchair for daily activities but may use power wheelchair for greater ease of independence.
C7	Has similar movement as an individual with C6, with added ability to straighten his/her elbows.	Daily tasks: Able to perform household duties. Need fewer adaptive aids in independent living.
		Health care: Able to do wheelchair push-ups for pressure reliefs.
		Mobility: Daily use of manual wheelchair. Can transfer with greater ease.

continued

with tetraplegia; Modified Barthel Index is a 15-item measure of self-care and mobility (McKinley & Silver, 2006).

3. Physical assessment
   a. Neurologic
      1) Assess cognitive, motor, and sensory status, reflexes, and cranial nerves.
      2) Monitor for signs and symptoms of increase or decrease in function, pain, and abnormal sensations.
   b. Respiratory: Assess breath sounds, airway patency, oxygen saturation, diaphragm movement, nature of sputum and potential for aspiration, and potential for pulmonary emboli.
   c. Cardiovascular: Assess blood pressure, pulse, heart rate, rhythm, edema, deep vein thrombosis, and signs and symptoms of orthostatic hypotension.
   d. Nutritional
      1) Assess weekly weight, daily hydration status, and dietary intake.
      2) Monitor complete blood cell count, electrolytes, albumin and prealbumin levels for anemia, electrolyte imbalance, and nutritional status.
   e. Elimination
      1) Assess abdomen for tenderness, distention, masses, and bowel sounds,

Table 12-8. Neurological Levels and Functional Potential *continued*

C8–T1	Has added strength and precision of fingers that result in limited or natural hand function.	Daily tasks: Can live independently without assistive devices in feeding, bathing, grooming, oral and facial hygiene, dressing, bladder management and bowel management. Mobility: Uses manual wheelchair. Can transfer independently.
T2–T6	Has normal motor function in head, neck, shoulders, arms, hands and fingers. Has increased use of rib and chest muscles, or trunk control.	Daily tasks: Should be totally independent with all activities. Mobility: A few individuals are capable of limited walking with extensive bracing. This requires extremely high energy and puts stress on the upper body, offering no functional advantage. Can lead to damage of upper joints.
T7–T12	Has added motor function from increased abdominal control.	Daily tasks: Able to perform unsupported seated activities.
L1–L5	Has additional return of motor movement in the hips and knees.	Mobility: Walking can be a viable function, with the help of specialized leg and ankle braces. Lower levels walk with greater ease with the help of assistive devices.
S1–S5	Depending on level of injury, there are various degrees of return of voluntary bladder, bowel and sexual functions.	Mobility: Increased ability to walk with fewer or no support devices.

From *Rehabilitation functional goals*, by Spinal Injury Network. (n.d.). Retrieved September 15, 2011, from www.spinal-injury.net. Copyright by Spinal Injury Network. Reprinted with permission.

premorbid and current bowel patterns, current bladder program; assess urine for color, odor, clarity, and amount.

   2) Review effectiveness of bowel and bladder programs. Modify programs as patterns become evident.

  f. Musculoskeletal: Assess for swelling, spasticity, ROM, tone, contractures, orthopedic injuries, and heterotopic ossification.

  g. Integumentary

   1) Assess the entire body for skin breakdown, especially bony prominences for redness, warmth, and blanching.

   2) Assess and record size, appearance, and location of any skin breakdown.

   3) Assess knowledge and practices to prevent skin breakdown. Staging of a wound should be based on National Data of Nursing Quality Indicator Standards (www.ndnqi.org).

  h. Psychosocial: Assess family support, coping mechanisms, adjustment to disability, and potential response to fear and anxiety; monitor for suicidal ideation.

  i. Sexual

   1) Assess level of injury in relation to physical capabilities; emotional state; and behavior consistent with denial, anger, or depression.

   2) Assess the current home situation including presence of significant other or spouse, children, history of birth control practices (if applicable).

I. Planning

  1. Setting goals (Hoeman, 2002)

   a. Goals should be developed with the client's strengths and limitations in mind, with consideration of access and resources.

   b. Rehabilitation goals should be directed toward helping the client achieve and maintain maximum independence and safe performance of self-care activities.

   c. Goals should focus on the person, not the disability.

   d. Family involvement with goals from the beginning can influence the success of the client's rehabilitation.

   e. Support and instructions from rehabilitation team members can help the family assist the client in achieving maximum independence throughout life.

  2. Functional outcomes of SCI (see Table 12-8)

J. Interventions (Hoeman, 2002; Mahoney, 2001)

  1. In the acute phase, interventions emphasize spinal stability, preservation of life, and prevention of complications.

   a. Spinal stability

   1) Use log rolling; avoid twisting.

   2) Surgery may be needed to stabilize the spine (i.e., spinal fusion).

3) Various orthotics are used depending on the level of the injury; the name of the brace indicates the part of the spine it immobilizes (Kulkarni & Sam, 2005).

a) Halo brace or cervical tongs immobilize the cervical spine; the halo brace is skeletal traction that provides maximal restriction of movement for those with cervical or high thoracic injuries (to T3).

b) Cervical collars are used commonly during surgical treatments. However, clients must still observe spinal precautions.

c) A sternal occipital mandibular immobilizer brace is used in minimally unstable fractures; it allows greater movement than the halo brace but must be fitted correctly; it is ideal for bedridden clients.

d) Thoracic lumbar sacral orthosis

e) Thoracolumbar orthosis is used to treat T10–L2 fractures.

f) Lumbar sacral orthosis stabilizes L1–L4.

4) Instruct the client that the immobilizer is to remain on at all times.

5) Immobilizers often are worn for about 3 months to allow the spine to heal.

6) Emphasize the importance of immobilization to allow time for healing and prevent further injury that could result in more damage to the spinal cord.

b. Prevention of secondary complications, especially common in older adults (Krassioukov, Furlan, & Fehlings, 2003)

1) Infections

2) Psychiatric disorders

3) Pressure sores

4) Cardiovascular problems

2. Interventions are determined with the client's and family's input to promote maximum health, independence, and safety.

3. Interventions may involve teaching the client and family about the problem-solving process, providing adaptive devices as necessary, and educating the client and family about safe and effective performance of skills.

4. Rehabilitation nurses must encourage the client and family to work toward achieving goals and to continue to perform goals that have already been accomplished.

5. Little research has been done on the unique needs of women experiencing spinal cord injury, and women have specific needs to be addressed (Newman, 2006).

6. Additional suggestions for client care (Hickey, 2003a)

a. Establish a therapeutic nurse-client relationship.

b. Cultivate a climate of trust.

c. Allow the client to verbalize feelings.

d. Accept the client's behavior without being judgmental.

e. Let the client know it will take time to adjust to the disability.

f. Answer questions, referring those you are unable to answer to the appropriate source.

g. Include written reports of the client's emotional and psychological reactions in the chart.

h. Incorporate steps for meeting the emotional and psychological needs of the client into the care plan.

i. Promote a good self-concept and body image by encouraging the client to use good grooming habits.

j. Use team conferences to discuss the client's emotional and psychological status.

k. Involve the client in the decision-making process related to his or her care to foster a feeling of self-control.

l. Address common concerns expressed by people with SCI (Lindsey, 1998).

1) Wanting to walk again

2) Sexual dysfunction

3) Pain

4) Impaired bowel and bladder function

5) Financial difficulties

6) Loss of independence

7) Anxiety

m. Adapt strategies for older clients with SCI that optimize the length of stay and provide resources after discharge (Scivoletto, Morganti, Ditunno, Ditunno, & Molinari, 2003).

n. Address the needs of the family caregiver, particularly in the following areas (Lindsey, 1998):

1) Negative attitudes toward the person with SCI

2) Feelings of guilt

3) Frustration at lack of appreciation from the client

4) Loss of alone time

5) Feeling overwhelmed

6) Setting boundaries in the relationship of caregiving

7. Nursing plan of care (**Table 12-9**).
K. Evaluation
   1. ASIA Impairment Scale
   2. FIM instrument
   3. Residual deficits and systemic dysfunction that may occur after SCI (Mahoney, 2001; NINDS, 2007)
      a. Neurological manifestations
         1) Loss or decrease of voluntary motor function below level of injury
         2) Loss or decrease of sensation
         3) Loss of normal reflex activity
         4) Autonomic dysfunction caused by loss of normal sympathetic nervous system functioning
            a) Autonomic dysreflexia
            b) Hypotension
            c) Loss of thermoregulation
            d) Loss of vasomotor tone or control
      b. Cardiovascular manifestations
         1) Hypotension and vasodilation, causing decreased cardiac output
            a) Orthostatic hypotension: Rapid drop in blood pressure when the erect position is assumed; clients with cervical or high thoracic injury have poor vasomotor control, so there is difficulty getting blood out of the lower extremities and back to the heart
            b) Vasodilation: Results from loss of sympathetically induced vasoconstriction, which triggers pooling of blood in abdomen and lower extremities
         2) Bradycardia is caused by unopposed vagal tone (10th cranial nerve)
         3) Impaired temperature regulation manifested by poikilothermia, a condition in which the body assumes the environmental temperature because of the inability to sweat or shiver below the injury
         4) Cardiac dysrhythmias, which usually appear in the first few weeks and are more common in severe injuries
         5) Blood clots (risk is three times higher than in a person without SCI)
      c. Respiratory manifestations
         1) Injury above C4: Results in paralysis of respiratory muscles, including the diaphragm; the client is dependent on a ventilator. Avoid saline installation into ventilated clients without a working diaphragm; evidence shows this is a harmful and outdated intervention.
         2) Injury between C4 and T6: Results in

paralysis of the intercostal and abdominal muscles; the client usually is weaned from the ventilator but needs aggressive pulmonary management.
         3) Injury between T6 and T12: Results in paralysis of some abdominal muscles; the client does not need a daily respiratory program unless an upper respiratory infection is present.
         4) Pneumonia is a common complication; intubation increases the risk of ventilator-acquired pneumonia (VAP), which accounts for about 25% of deaths (NINDS, 2007). Oral hygiene minimizes VAP.
      d. Metabolic and musculoskeletal manifestations
         1) Negative nitrogen balance
         2) Decreased basal metabolic rate and expenditure of energy
         3) Hypercalcemia or hypercalciuria
         4) Altered secretion of pituitary-derived hormones
         5) Heterotopic ossification
         6) Contractures
         7) Muscle spasms
      e. Gastrointestinal manifestations
         1) Peristaltic slowing, causing paralytic ileus
         2) Increased acidity, causing gastrointestinal bleeding
         3) Pancreatitis after injury (Sugarman, 1985)
         4) Abnormal liver function caused by trauma
         5) Neurogenic bowel (Refer to Chapter 7.)
         6) Constipation and hemorrhoids
      f. Genitourinary manifestations
         1) Neurogenic bladder (Refer to Chapter 7.)
            a) Reflexic (UMN dysfunction)
            b) Areflexic (LMN dysfunction)
         2) Urinary outlet sphincter dysfunction
         3) Autonomic dysreflexia
      g. Sexual manifestations (Refer to Chapter 7.)
         1) Males
            a) Reflexogenic erection
            b) Psychogenic erection
            c) Variability in sperm production, penile erection, fertility, or ejaculation, depending on level of injury
         2) Females
            a) Menses cease and then resume within 6 months to a year.
            b) May still conceive and bear children but should be under the care of a physician specializing in women with SCI

Table 12-9. Plan of Care for Patients with Spinal Cord Injury

System-Specific Considerations	Nursing Diagnosis and Collaborative Problems	Nursing Management	Level of Injury
Respiratory system If possible, wean the client from the ventilator. If weaning is not possible, plan for long-term ventilation management options (discharge home on ventilator, diaphragmatic pacer, or other options). Clients with cervical injuries usually have decreased volumes of air exchange in tidal volumes, movement of the chest with each respiration, forced expiration volume, and responsiveness to chemical stimuli for respirations, resulting in chronic alveolar hypoventilation.	Ineffective airway clearance High risk for aspiration Ineffective breathing pattern High risk for respiratory infection Impaired gas exchange Risk of altered respiratory function Hypoxemia Atelectasis, pneumonia	Continue with the pulmonary program initiated in the acute phase (e.g., chest physical therapy, deep breathing and assistive coughing, use of incentive spirometer). Begin a client and family teaching program (e.g., respiratory care, breathing exercises, assisted coughing, suction technique, oxygen, intermittent positive pressure breathing, and other therapy treatments).	Cervical injuries
Cardiovascular system Bradycardia and orthostatic hypotension may occur. Orthostatic hypotension may be a problem when the head of the bed is raised or when the client is in a wheelchair.	Risk of peripheral neurovascular dysfunction Impaired gas exchange Dysrhythmias Deep vein thrombosis Pulmonary embolus Hypovolemia Orthostatic hypotension	Apply abdominal binder and thigh-high elastic stockings. Continue with air boots. Slowly position the client from supine to sitting (e.g., first sit the client upright in bed, then sit the client on edge of bed with support; if the client becomes hypotensive in wheelchair, tilt wheelchair into recline position and elevate legs)	Cervical injuries High-thoracic injuries May occur in low-thoracic injuries
Nervous system Autonomic hyperreflexia can occur with injuries at the level of T6 or above. Initially, pain may be experienced at the level of injury. Some sensation (ranging from mild tingling to severe pain) may return if the lesion is incomplete. Pain may be caused by scar tissue or posttraumatic sympathetic dystrophy. Parathesias and hyperthesias may be noted.	Dysreflexia Pain Knowledge deficit Impaired physical mobility Self-care deficit Sensory and perceptual alterations Sexual dysfunction Sleep pattern disturbance Risk of injury	Manage autonomic hyperreflexia. Assess pain and use pain control strategies. Provide information to client and family. Provide for total care needs of client. Begin client and family teaching related to prevention and treatment of dysreflexia, comfort measures, and prevention of injury to tissue.	Autonomic dysreflexia (T6 and above) Pain (all levels of injury) Parathesias and hyperthesias (all levels of injury)
Integumentary system Skin pressure problems are a concern, although there is decreased sensation below the level of injury.	Impaired skin integrity Risk of peripheral neurovascular dysfunction Impaired tissue integrity Altered tissue perfusion peripheral Pressure ulcers Osteomyelitis	Provide skin care and turn the client every 2 hours. Inspect skin, especially bony prominences, twice a day. Provide for weight shifts in the wheelchair every 15–30 minutes. Provide for range-of-motion exercises once daily. Begin client and family education about the potential for and prevention of skin breakdown.	Skin breakdown (all levels of injury)

continued

THE SPECIALTY PRACTICE OF REHABILITATION NURSING

System-Specific Considerations	Nursing Diagnosis and Collaborative Problems	Nursing Management	Level of Injury
Musculoskeletal system Prolonged immobility and paralysis have significant effects on bone, joints, and muscles. Spasticity may be present.	Impaired physical mobility Disuse syndrome Contractures Ankylosis Muscle atrophy Osteoporosis Spasticity		
Gastrointestinal (GI) system Neurogenic bowel may be present. Peristalsis returns but is sluggish. Other GI reflexes are sluggish. The development of gastric ulcers or hemorrhage remains a concern.	Altered bowel elimination Paralytic ileus GI bleeding Constipation	Implement an aggressive physical therapy program. Provide for range-of-motion exercises once daily. Position the client's extremities in proper body alignment. Monitor spasticity.	Bones, joints, and muscles (all levels of injuries can have significant effects) Spasticity (T12 and above)
Genitourinary system Neurogenic bladder may be present. Altered sexual function may be present.	Altered urinary elimination High risk for infection Sexual dysfunction Renal calculi Kidney disease	Initiate a bowel program.	Neurogenic bowel (potentially all levels of injury)
Metabolic system A high-fluid, high-carbohydrate, and high-protein diet is still needed for energy and tissue repair.	Fluid volume deficit Altered nutrition, less than body needs Electrolyte imbalances	Initiate a bladder program.	Neurogenic bladder (potentially all levels of injury)
Psychological and emotional responses The effect of the injury on the client's previous functional level and lifestyle begins to be realized.	Impaired adjustment Body image disturbance Ineffective denial Grieving	Provide adequate fluid and nutritional intake.	Altered nutrition (all levels of injury)
System-Specific Considerations The client begins the loss, grief, and bereavement process. The effect of the injury on the family and significant others begins to be realized.	Anxiety Fear Depression Altered family processes Hopelessness Powerlessness Impaired social interaction Social isolation Spiritual distress High risk for self-directed violence	Communicate with the client and the family. Be supportive. Set realistic goals.	Altered psychological and emotional response (all levels of injury)

From *Clinical practice of neurological and neurosurgical nursing* (5th ed., pp. 407–408), by J. Hickey, 1997, Philadelphia: Lippincott. Copyright 1997 by Lippincott Williams & Wilkins. Reprinted with permission.

c) Autonomic dysreflexia may be a problem during delivery.
d) Discuss contraception practices.

h. Psychosocial manifestations
1) Stressors and losses
   a) Stressors
      (i) Survival
      (ii) Quality of life
      (iii) Lifestyle changes
      (iv) Occupational changes
      (v) Participation in recreational activities
      (vi) Change in relationships and roles
      (vii) Neurogenic pain
   b) Losses
      (i) Sensation
      (ii) Mobility
      (iii) Bowel and bladder control
      (iv) Sexual function
      (v) Control and independence
      (vi) Former roles
      (vii) Self-esteem
2) Emotions and behaviors
   a) Anxiety
   b) Frustration
   c) Anger
   d) Hostility
   e) Fear
   f) Sarcasm
   g) Regression
   h) Denial
   i) Guilt
   j) Depression
   k) Sensory overload
   l) Pain manifestations with neuropathic pain

L. Discharge Planning
1. Begins before admission to rehabilitation
2. Is a collaborative effort between the client, family, and interdisciplinary team
3. Includes the following considerations:
   a. Identify key family members who will be learning or performing care.
   b. Provide education using return demonstration by the client and family throughout the rehabilitation stay; teach the client and family members about the prevention of complications, including bladder infections, pressure sores, respiratory problems, fatigue, and constipation (Blackwell, Krause, Winkler, & Stiens, 2001).
   c. Identify the location or setting to which the client is being discharged.
   d. Perform a home evaluation.
   e. Identify and order necessary DME.
   f. Identify funding sources.
4. Ensure the client is discharged to a safe environment.
5. Make referrals to a life care planner if needed.

M. Research on Aging with SCI (Charlifue, 2007a, 2007b, 2007c; Charlifue & Gerhart, 2004; Charlifue, Lammertse, & Adkins, 2004; Gerhart, Charlifue, Menter, Weitzenkamp, & Whiteneck, 1999; Gerhart, Weitzenkamp, Kennedy, Glass, & Charlifue, 1999; McColl, Arnold, Charlifue, & Gerhart, 2001; Northwest Regional Spinal Cord Injury System, 2009; Winkler, 2007).
1. Krause and Broderick (2005) demonstrated that psychological adjustment improved over time in people aging with SCI. Studies indicate that older adults use better coping strategies and have more realistic expectations.
2. Typically, the greater the number of years since the injury, the better the psychological adaptation to the injury, up to 30 years.
3. A longitudinal study began in 1990 in Great Britain to track more than 800 people with SCI (Gerhart, Charlifue, et al., 1999).
   a. Three phases: 1990, 1993, and 1996
   b. Results of this study were published beginning in the late 1990s.
      1) Death rates and causes of death
         a) SCI survivors have a higher death rate than the general population.
         b) Causes of death include cardiovascular disease, pneumonia, septicemia, cancer, and suicide.
         c) The rate of cardiovascular disease is more than 200% higher in people with SCI than people the same age without spinal injury (Winkler, 2007).
      2) Morbidity (illnesses and complications)
         a) Urinary tract infections
         b) Pressure sores
         c) Chest infections, spasticity, perceived abdominal pain, and general malaise (more likely in people with tetraplegia)
         d) Musculoskeletal problems such as joint pain, stiffness, pressure sores, diarrhea, and constipation (especially in people with paraplegia)
         e) Increased fractures, cystitis, and motor and sensory changes (especially in people with incomplete injuries)
         f) Functional decline or decreasing physical independence

g) Gastrointestinal problems are common and worsen with age, including hemorrhoids and difficulty with bowel evacuation (Winkler, 2007).

3) General health, life satisfaction, stress

    a) More than 75% reported feeling generally healthy.

    b) Seventy-four percent were generally satisfied with their lives.

    c) Stress and depression seemed to decrease as more years passed since the injury.

    d) Stress was related to adaptation and coping but unrelated to injury severity or physician independence.

4) Risk factors

    a) Pressure sores

        (i) More likely in people with paraplegia

        (ii) More likely in people who have already developed one pressure sore

        (iii) Higher risk for those with abnormal pulses in feet and lower extremities

        (iv) Higher risk with unemployment

        (v) The number of pressure ulcers increased with time according to data from the National Spinal Cord Injury Database in one study of those 5–25 years after injury (Charlifue et al., 2004).

    b) Upper-extremity pain

        (i) Decreased psychosocial well-being coincided with an increase in upper-extremity pain.

        (ii) Limitations in ROM increased the risk of upper-extremity pain.

    c) Life satisfaction

        (i) Younger participants who had greater psychosocial well-being and financial resources reported greater life satisfaction.

        (ii) Participants who reported social involvement had less fatigue and were less likely to be overweight.

        (iii) Declined over time (Charlifue & Gerhart, 2004)

        (iv) Less life satisfaction was associated with less community reintegration.

    d) Factors related to decreased physical independence

        (i) Advanced age, especially among people with paraplegia

        (ii) Changes in DME

        (iii) Changes in bladder management program

        (iv) Increased fatigue over time

    e) Fatigue: Those with a poor self-perception of health had more fatigue.

    f) Community integration and social support (Charlifue & Gerhart, 2004)

        (i) A general decline in community integration over time related to decreased physical independence, decreased mobility, and a lack of social integration.

        (ii) Life satisfaction was related to community reintegration.

        (iii) In a study of 132 Canadians and 158 Britons with SCI (mean age of 57 and length of time since injury averaged 33 years) (McColl et al., 2001)

            (a) Informational support was less available than emotional support.

            (b) Age had a negative effect on satisfaction with social support.

    g) Spirituality and depression (Charlifue, 2007a)

        (1) No significant relationship between spiritual well-being and age

        (ii) No significant relationship between spiritual well-being and length of time since injury

        (iii) People reporting better spiritual well-being were less depressed and reported better quality of life.

4. Conclusions

    a. Pressure sores and respiratory problems appear to be more common with age.

    b. Musculoskeletal problems are associated more with longer durations of injury.

    c. Life satisfaction and quality of life are vital concepts, neither of which is totally dependent on the level or severity of the disability or on the number of medical complications; however, each seems to be very important as a predictor of future outcomes.

    d. Fatigue appears to be an important predictor of future problems.

    e. Fatigue, depression, and decreased life satisfaction should not go unaddressed because they may lead to costly and compromising complications.

f. There is a general decline in community integration based on a variety of factors.

N. Other Research and Advanced Adaptive Equipment

1. Clinical and rehabilitative research focusing on understanding the nature of SCI and defining the nervous system's response to injury (The Miami Project, 1999a, 1999b; NINDS, 2007)

   a. Technology innovation

     1) Can require significant fiscal resources, but evidence for efficiency outcomes can be challenging

     2) LiteGait treadmills

     3) Diaphragmatic pacer device

     4) Tracheal suctioning (*American Journal of Critical Care*)

   b. Neuroplasticity revolution

     1) Body weight support systems

       a) The navigator

       b) Zero G

       c) LiteGait

       d) Smart Step

     2) Biofeedback and monitoring system for the lower extremities

     3) Auto Ambulator

   c. Improving upper-extremity movement (DME and adaptive equipment)

     1) Computerized robotic systems

     2) Robot technology used in spinal cord and stroke recovery (ReoGO)

     3) Mass repetition of functional arm movements to gain cortical stimulation

     4) Transcranial magnetic stimulation

     5) The Hand Mentor: An exercise device that uses biofeedback to involve the client in his or her rehabilitation

2. Research and stem cell studies

   a. Oligodendrocyte progenitor research may prove to be promising for SCI.

   b. The FDA approved the first test in humans in July 2010. Testing derived from human embryonic stem cells. The trial began testing cells developed by the Geron Corp and University of California–Irvine in patients with a new diagnosis of SCI (Geron, 2009).

   c. Study of the pathology of human SCI: A detailed analysis of postmortem human spinal cords is underway to compare actual spinal cord anatomy with diagnostic radiography (e.g., MRIs) and define the nature of the cellular damage that results from SCI.

   d. Electrophysiology of the spinal cord: Researchers have identified the appearance of a newly formed reflex, which demonstrates that nerve circuits may be altered and new connections formed after injury in humans.

   e. Spasticity and fatigue in paralyzed muscle: These factors provide essential information for designing exercise programs that optimize function in muscles that have lost some or all of their nerve supply.

   f. Central pattern generator: This group of nerve cells synchronizes muscle activity during alternating stepping of the legs.

   g. Pain research group: This group is evaluating the effect of SCI pain on quality of life.

   h. Neural prostheses: Bioengineers are trying to restore functional connections through computers and functional electrical stimulation systems to control the muscles of the arms and legs, especially to stimulate walking, reaching, and gripping.

   i. Surgery to relieve pressure: Some research has shown improvement with early decompression surgery in animals but has not been replicated reliably in humans.

   j. Pain treatment: Chronic pain syndromes are thought to continually trigger functional changes in neurons; drugs that interfere with neurotransmitters related to pain syndromes are being investigated.

   k. Spasticity: Drug interventions, surgery, and electrical stimulation below the injury may decrease spasms.

   l. Bladder control: Electrical stimulation, surgical procedures, and root stimulator implants (or combinations thereof) may be helpful for those with reflex incontinence.

3. Basic science research (NINDS, 2007) concentrating on techniques that hold the promise of repairing different types of spinal cord damage

   a. Stopping excitotoxicity: When nerve cells are damaged, they release the neurotransmitter glutamate, which can cause secondary damage. Researchers are examining receptor antagonists that may block a specific type of glutamate receptor.

   b. Controlling inflammation

     1) Cooling the body immediately after injury protects tissue and nerve cells.

     2) Boosting T-cell response may reduce secondary damage.

     3) More studies of induced hypothermia are needed.

   c. Preventing apoptosis

     1) Research is aimed at understanding cellular mechanisms that cause damage after SCI.

2) Research is exploring how to promote axonal regrowth and repair.
 d. Promoting regeneration
  1) Cell grafts show some promise.
  2) Fetal spinal cord tissue implants have had some success in animal trials.
  3) Stem cells are still under investigation, and more research must be done.
 e. Axonal regrowth research is focusing on
  1) Encouraging growth
  2) Clearing away debris
  3) Examining axon connections to reconnect to the spinal cord

4. General notes
 a. No one theory or approach will encompass all the effects of SCI.
 b. Many scientists believe that significant new treatments will be found not in a single approach but rather in a combination of techniques.
 c. The Christopher and Dana Reeve Foundation Neuro Recovery Network (CDRF NRN) provides body weight support treadmill training for clients with SCI. This treatment program gathers data about the use of a specialized treadmill. The treadmill training is intended to promote a focus of neurorecovery of signals that are being affected through physical training. It is believed that neuro pathways are affected by physical training.
  1) The treadmill is a special piece of machinery for the CDRF NRN program, of which there are only seven in the United States. Each CDRF NRN program must provide rigorous training to each staff member for proper and safe handling of each client. The client is helped to stretch before beginning the treadmill training. The client is harnessed in the treadmill, and several specially trained staff members provide maximum assistance for the 1 hour of trunk-strengthening forced-use program, a technique that is thought to foster regeneration. The entire treatment session is about 2 hours.
  2) This treatment is generally covered by insurance. The insurance will normally cover about 40 visits. The wait time to begin the program is about 9 months. Each of the seven facilities has different wait times, and each program treats only six clients at a time.

O. Advocacy Organizations
 1. Christopher & Dana Reeve Foundation: www.crpf.org
 2. Professional nursing organization: Academy of Spinal Cord Injury Professionals: http://academyscipro.org

P. Advanced Practice Considerations: Role of the Advanced Practice Nurse in SCI Rehabilitation
 1. Educator
  a. Work alongside the rehabilitation team as a clinical nurse specialist to develop education platforms for clients and families in both inpatient and postacute care settings. This would include addressing community reintegration challenges.
  b. Present professional papers and posters at national and international symposiums and professional educational events.
  c. Coordinate or teach certification review material to rehabilitation staff to increase the numbers of certified rehabilitation brain injury nurses.
  d. Assist with the placement of nursing students in the spinal cord clinical setting to increase the overall understanding of the care of the client with SCI.
  e. Advocate by education of the community, related healthcare agencies, and academia to increase the knowledge base of healthcare professionals who care for the client and family.
 2. Advocate and leader
  a. Collaborate with local and national legislators to advocate for people with SCI regarding rehabilitation benefit coverage, accessibility, community resources, and other funding issues.
  b. Participate on local and state committees.
  c. Participate with the local chapter of ARN while providing education and advocacy for people with SCI.
  d. Participate in ARN on a national level.
 3. Consultant
  a. Provide direct rehabilitation nursing services to clients with SCI and their families who help care for them, actively addressing the often complicated issues that arise from complex neurological deficits.
  b. Serve as a vital component of the rehabilitation team by providing expert knowledge in the treatment and complex care of the client with SCI.
  c. Collaborate with all rehabilitation team disciplines to ensure receipt of coordinated care

throughout the healthcare continuum and beyond into the community.

d. Advocate financial assistance by providing guidance and sharing knowledge of assistive organizations to care managers, social workers, family, and the client with SCI.

4. Researcher and catalyst of change

a. Remain active in the field of research for SCI as a reviewer, assisting in active research, serving as pilot or test sites for new innovative strategies.

b. Address areas of complications, client challenges, and creative ideas as an opportunity to further support clinical education and services.

c. Develop and maintain facility procedures based on evidence-based clinical practice.

References

Abrahamson, E. E., Ikonomovic, M. D., Dixon, C. E., & DeKosky, S. T. (2009). Simvastatin therapy prevents brain trauma-induced increases in beta-amyloid peptide levels. *Annals of Neurology, 66*(3), 407–414.

Alander, D., Parker, J., Stauffer, E., & Shannon, M. D. (1997). Intermediate-term outcome of cervical spinal cord-injured patients older than 50 years of age. *Spine, 22*(11), 1189–1192.

American Association for Respiratory Care. (2004). Clinical practice guidelines. *Respiratory Care, 49*(9), 1080–1084.

American Spinal Injury Association. (1996). *International standards for neurological and functional classification of spinal injury patients* (Rev. ed.). Atlanta, GA: Author.

American Spinal Injury Association. (2008). *International standards for neurological and functional classification of spinal injury patients* (Rev. ed.). Atlanta, GA: Author.

Ansell, B., & Keenan, J. (1989). The Western Neuro Sensory Stimulation Profile: A tool for assessing slow-to-recover head injured patients. *Archives of Physical Medicine and Rehabilitation, 70,* 104–108.

Baggerly, J., & Le, N. (2001). Nursing management of the patient with head trauma. In J. B. Derstine & S. D. Hargrove (Eds.), *Comprehensive rehabilitation nursing* (pp. 331–367). Philadelphia: W. B. Saunders.

Barker, E. (2002). Neuroanatomy and physiology of the nervous system. In E. Barker (Ed.), *Neuroscience nursing: A spectrum of care* (pp. 3–50). St. Louis: Mosby.

Benson, R. R., Meda, S. A., Vasudevan, S., Kou, Z., Govindarajan, K. A., Hanks, R. A., et al. (2007). Global white matter analysis of diffusion tensor images is predictive of injury severity in traumatic brain injury. *Journal of Neurotrauma, 24,* 446–459.

Blackwell, T. L., Krause, J. S., Winkler, T., & Stiens, S. A. (2001). *Spinal cord injury desk reference.* New York: Demos Medical Publishing.

Blank-Reid, C., & Barker, E. (2002). Neurotrauma: Traumatic brain injury. In E. Barker (Ed.), *Neuroscience nursing: A spectrum of care* (pp. 409–437). St. Louis: Mosby.

Bogner, J. A., Corrigan, J. D., Bode R. K., & Heinemann A. W. (2000). Rating scale analysis of the Agitated Behavior Scale. *The Journal of Head Trauma Rehabilitation, 15*(1), 656–669.

Brain Injury Association of America. (2006). *Scales and measurements of function.* Retrieved June 11, 2006, from www.biausa.org/Pages/what_is_the_rehab_process.html#ways.

Brain Injury Association of America. (2010). *Scales and measurements of function.* Retrieved August 19, 2011, www.biausa.org/brain-injury-treatment.htm#Scales and Measurement.

Brain injury.com. (2006a). *Recovery and rehabilitation.* Retrieved August 19, 2011, from www.braininjury.com/recovery.shtml.

Brain injury.com. (2006b). *Symptoms of brain injury.* Retrieved August 19, 2011, from www.braininjury.com/symptoms.shtml.

Bryant, R. A., O'Donnell, M. L., Creamer, M., McFarlane, A. C., Clark, C. R., & Silove, D. (2010). The psychiatric sequelae of traumatic injury. *American Journal of Psychiatry, 167*(3), 312–320.

Burns, S. P., Golding, D. G., Rolle, W. A., Graziani, V., & Ditunno, J. F. (1997). Recovery of ambulation in motor-incomplete tetraplegia. *Archives of Physical Medicine and Rehabilitation, 78*(11), 1169–1172.

Campagnolo, D. I. (2006). *Autonomic dysreflexia in spinal cord injury.* Retrieved May 1, 2007, from www.emedicine.com/pmr/topic217.htm.

Centers for Disease Control and Prevention. (2010a). Heads up: Preventing brain injuries. Retrieved June 29, 2010, from www.cdc.gov/ncipc/pub-res/tbi_toolkit/patients/preventing.htm.

Centers for Disease Control and Prevention. (2010b). *Injury prevention and control: Traumatic brain injury.* Retrieved Augsut 19, 2011, from http://cdc.gov/traumaticbraininjury/statistics.html.

Chanda, A., & Nanda, A. (2003). Subdural and epidural hematomas. In R. W. Evans (Ed.), *Saunders manual of neurologic practice* (pp. 500–506). Philadelphia: Saunders.

Chapman, J. C., Andersen, A. M., Roselli, L. A., Meyers, N. M., & Pincus, J. H. (2010) . Screening for mild traumatic brain injury in the presence of psychiatric comorbidities. *Archives of Physical Medicine and Rehabilitation, 91*(7), 1082–1086.

Charlifue, S. (2007a). A collaborative longitudinal study of aging with spinal cord injury: Overview of the background and methodology. *Topics in Spinal Cord Injury Rehabilitation, 12*(3), 1–14.

Charlifue, S. (2007b). Effects of aging on individuals with chronic SCI. *Topics in Spinal Cord Injury Rehabilitation, 12*(3), 1–96.

Charlifue, S. (2007c). Living well: Aging and SCI: Some good news. *PN/Paraplegia News, 61*(1), 12–13.

Charlifue, S., & Gerhart, K. (2004). Community integration in spinal cord injury of long duration. *NeuroRehabilitation, 19*(2), 91–101.

Charlifue, S., Lammertse, D. P., & Adkins, R. J. (2004). Aging with spinal cord injury: Changes in selected health indices and life satisfaction. *Archives of Physical Medicine and Rehabilitation, 85*(11), 1848–1853.

Chaytor, N., & Schmitter-Edgecombe, M. (2003). The ecological validity of neuropsychological tests: A review of the literature on everyday cognitive skills. *Neuropsychology Review, 13,* 181–197.

Chew, E., & Zafonte, R. D. (2009). Pharmacological management of neurobehavioral disorders following traumatic brain injury: A state-of-the-art review. *Journal of Rehabilitation Research and Development, 46*(6), 851–879.

Cicerone, K. D., Dahlberg, C., Malec, J. F., Langenbahn, D. M., Felicetti, T., Kneipp, S., et al. (2005). Evidence-based cognitive rehabilitation: Updated review of the literature from 1998 through 2002. *Archives of Physical Medicine and Rehabilitation, 86,* 1681–1692.

Cicerone, K., Levin, H., Malec, J., Struss, D., & Whyte, J. (2006). Cognitive rehabilitation interventions for executive function: Moving from bench to bedside in patients with traumatic brain injury. *Journal of Cognitive Neuroscience, 18,* 1212–1222.

Cicerone, K. D., Mott, T., Azulay, J., Sharlow-Galella, M., Ellmo, W. J., Paradise, S., et al. (2008). A randomized controlled trial of holistic neuropsychological rehabilitation. *Archives of Physical Medicine & Rehabilitation, 89*(12), 2239–2249.

Corrigan, J. D., & Bogner, J. A. (1994). Factor structure of the Agitated Behavior Scale. *Journal of Clinical and Experimental Neuropsychology, 16*(3), 386–392.

Cuny, G. D. (2009). Kinase inhibitors as potential therapeutics for acute and chronic neurodegenerative conditions. *Current Pharmaceutical Design, 15*(34), 3919–3939.

Dawodu, S. T. (2007). *Spinal cord injury: Definition, epidemiology, pathophysiology.* Retrieved April 30, 2007, from www.emedicine.com/pmr/topic185.htm.

Deb, S., & Crownshaw, T. (2004). The role of pharmacotherapy in the management of behavior disorders in traumatic brain injury. *Brain Injury, 18*(1), 1–31.

Demougeot, C., Garnier, P., Mossiat, C., Betrand, N., Giroud, M., Beley, A., et al. (2001). N-acetylaspartate, a marker of both cellular dysfunction and neuronal loss: Its relevance to studies of acute brain injury. *Journal of Neurochemistry, 77,* 408–415.

Department of Defense (DOD) and Veteran's Head Injury Program & Brain Injury Association of America. (1999). *Brain injury and you.* Washington, DC: Author.

Diaz-Arrastia, R., & Baxter, V. K. (2006). Genetic factors in outcome after traumatic brain injury: What the Human Genome Project can teach us about brain trauma. *Journal of Head Trauma Rehabilitation, 21*(4), 361–374.

Duff, D., & Wells, D. (1997). Postcomatose unawareness/vegetative state following severe brain injury: A content methodology. *Journal of Neuroscience Nursing, 29*(5), 305–317.

Dufour, L., Williams, J., & Coleman, K. (2000). Traumatic injuries: TBI and SCI. In P. A. Edwards (Ed.), *The specialty practice of rehabilitation nursing: A core curriculum* (4th ed., pp. 196–198). Glenview, IL: Association of Rehabilitation Nurses.

Evans, R. W. (2003). Mild head injury and postconcussion syndrome. In R. W. Evans (Ed.), *Saunders manual of neurologic practice* (pp. 488–493). Philadelphia: Saunders.

Fassett, D. R., Harrop, J. S., Maltenfort, M., Jeyamohan, S. B., Ratcliff, J. D., Anderson, D. G., et al. (2007). Mortality rates in geriatric patients with spinal cord injuries. *Journal of Neurosurgery Spine, 7*(3), 277–281.

Faul, M. X. L., Waid, M. M., & Coronado, V. G. (2010). *Traumatic brain injury in the United States: Emergency department visits, hospitalizations and deaths 2002–2006.* Atlanta, GA: Centers for Disease Control and Prevention, National Center for Injury Prevention and Control.

Flanagan, S. R., Cantor, J. B., & Ashman, T. A. (2008). Traumatic brain injury: Future assessment tools and treatment prospects. *Neuropsychiatric Disease and Treatment, 4*(5), 877–892.

Francisco, G. E., Walker, W. C., Zasler, N. D., & Bouffard, M. H. (2007). Pharmacological management of neurobehavioral sequelae of traumatic brain injury: A survey of current physiatric practice. *Brain Injury, 21*(10), 1007–1014.

Garbuzova-Davis, S., Willing, A. E., Saporta, S., Bickford, P. C., Gemma, C., Chen, N., et al. (2006). Novel cell therapy approaches for brain repair. *Progress in Brain Research, 157,* 207–222.

Gatens, C., & Hebert, A. R. (2001). Cognition and behavior. In S. Hoeman (Ed.), *Rehabilitation nursing: Process, application and outcomes* (pp. 599–630). St. Louis: Mosby.

Gennarelli, T. A., & Graham, D. I. (2005). Neuropathology. In J. M. Silver, T. W. McAllister, & S. C. Yudofsky (Eds.), *Textbook of traumatic brain injury* (pp. 27–50). Washington, DC: American Psychiatric Publishing.

Gerhart, K., Charlifue, S., Menter, R., Weitzenkamp, D., & Whiteneck, G. (1999, August 10). *Aging with spinal cord injury.* Retrieved July 1, 2007, from www.ed.gov/pubs/American Rehab/spring97/sp9706.html.

Gerhart, K. A., Weitzenkamp, D. A., Kennedy, P., Glass, C. A., & Charlifue, S. (1999). Correlates of stress in long-term spinal cord injury. *Spinal Cord, 37*(3), 183–190.

Geron. (2009, January 23). *Geron receives FDA clearance to begin world's first human clinical trial of embryonic stem cell-based therapy.* Retrieved August 19, 2011, from www.geron.com/media/pressview.aspx?id=1148.

Giacino, J. T., Ashwal, S., Childs, N., Cranford, R., Jennett, B., Katz, D. I., et al. (2002). The minimally conscious state: Definition and diagnostic criteria. *Neurology, 58*(3), 1–11.

Giacino, J., Kalmar, K., & Whyte, J. (2004). The JFK Coma Recovery Scale—Revised: Measurement characteristics and diagnostic utility. *Archives of Physical Medicine and Rehabilitation, 85*(12), 2020–2029.

Giacino, J., & Whyte, J. (2005). The vegetative and minimally conscious states. *Journal of Head Trauma Rehab, 20*(1), 30–50.

Girard, D., Brown, J., Burnett-Stolnack, M., Hashimoto, N., Hier-Wellmer, S., Perlman, O. Z., et al. (1996). The relationship of neuropsychological status and productive outcomes following traumatic brain injury. *Brain Injury, 10,* 663–676.

Grosswasser, Z., Schwab, K., & Salazar, A. (1997). Assessment of outcome following traumatic brain injury in adults. In R. Herndon (Ed.), *Handbook of neurologic rating scales* (pp. 187–208). New York: Demos Vermande.

Hanak, M. (1993). *Spinal cord injury: An illustrated guide for health care professionals* (2nd ed.). New York: Springer.

Hickey, J. (1997). *Clinical practice of neurological and neurosurgical nursing* (4th ed.). Philadelphia: Lippincott.

Hickey, J. (2003a). *Clinical practice of neurological and neurosurgical nursing* (5th ed.). Philadelphia: Lippincott.

Hickey, J. (2003b).Craniocerebral trauma. In J. Hickey (Ed.), *Clinical practice of neurological and neurosurgical nursing* (5th ed., pp. 373–406). Philadelphia: Lippincott.

Hickey, J. (2003c). Overview of neuroanatomy and neurophysiology. In J. Hickey (Ed.), *Clinical practice of neurological and neurosurgical nursing* (5th ed., pp. 45–92). Philadelphia: Lippincott.

High, W. M., Briones-Galang, M., Clark, J. A., Gilkison, C., Mossberg, K. A., Zgaljardic, D. J., et al. (2010). Effect of growth hormone replacement therapy on cognition after traumatic brain injury. *Journal of Neurotrauma, 19,* 293–301.

Hoeman, S. P. (2002). *Rehabilitation nursing: Process, applications, and outcomes.* Philadelphia: Mosby.

Hoffman, J. M., Pagulayan, K. F., Zawaideh, N., Dikmen, S., Temkin, N., & Bell, K. R. (2007). Understanding pain after traumatic brain injury and its impact on community participation. *American Journal of Physical Medicine and Rehabilitation, 86*(12), 962–969.

Kalmar, K., & Giacino, J. T. (2005). The JFK Coma Recovery Scale—Revised. *Neuropsychological Rehabilitation, 15*(3–4), 454–460.

Kelestimur, F. (2009). Growth hormone deficiency after traumatic brain injury in adults: When to test and how to treat? *Pediatric Endocrinology Reviews, 6*(Suppl. 4), 534–539.

Kennedy, R. E., Livingston, L., Marwitz, J. H., Gueck, S., Kreutzer, J. S., & Sander, A. M. (2006). Complicated mild traumatic brain injury on the inpatient rehabilitation unit: A multicenter analysis. *Journal of Head Trauma Rehabilitation, 21*(3), 260–271.

Krassioukov, A. V., Furlan, J. C., & Fehlings, M. G. (2003). Medical co-morbidities, secondary complications, and mortality in elderly with acute spinal cord injury. *Journal of Neurotrauma, 29*(4), 391–399.

Krause, J. S., & Broderick, L. (2005). 25 year longitudinal study of the natural course of aging after spinal cord injury. *Spinal Cord, 43*(6), 349–356.

Kreutzer, J. S., Seel, R. T., & Marwitz, J. H. (1999). *Neurobehavioral Functioning Inventory (NFI).* San Antonio, TX: The Psychological Corporation, Harcourt Brace & Company.

Kulkarni, S., & Sam, H. (2005). *Spinal orthotic.* Retrieved July 17, 2007, from www.emedicine.com/pmr/topic173.htm.

Kumaria, A., & Tolias, C. M. (2009). Normobaric hyperoxia therapy for traumatic brain injury and stroke: A review. *British Journal of Neurosurgery, 23*(6), 576–584.

Levin, H., O'Donald, V., & Grossman, R. (1975). The Galveston orientation and amnesia test: A practical scale to assess cognition after head injury. *Journal of Nervous and Mental Disease, 167,* 675–686.

Levy, M., Berson, A., Cook, T., Bollegala, N., Seto, E., Turanski, S., et al. (2005). Treatment of agitation following traumatic brain injury: A review of the literature. *Neurorehabilitation, 20,* 279–306.

Lew, H. L., Otis, J. D., Tun, C., Kerns, R. D., Clark, M. E., & Cifu, D. X. (2009). Prevalence of chronic pain, posttraumatic stress disorder, and persistent postconcussive symptoms in OIF/OEF veterans: Polytrauma clinical triad. *Clinical Guidelines on TBI from VA and Department of Defense, 46*(6), v–vi.

Lewine, J. D., Davis, J. T., Bigler, E. D., Thomas, R., Hill, D., Funke, M., et al. (2007). Objective documentation of traumatic brain injury subsequent to mild head injury: Multimodal brain imaging with MEG, SPECT, and MRI. *Journal of Head Trauma Rehabilitation, 22,* 141–155.

Lindsey, L. (1998). *Caring for caregivers—SCI InfoSheet #17.* Spinal Cord Injury Information Network. Retrieved May 21, 2007, from www.spinalcord.uab.edu/show.asp?durki=22479.

Lo, C., Shifteh, K., Gold, T., Bello, J. A., & Lipton, M. L. (2009). Diffusion tensor imaging abnormalities in patients with mild traumatic brain injury and neurocognitive impairment. *Journal of Computer Assisted Tomography, 33*(2), 293–297.

Lunney, M., MaGuire, M., Endozo, N., & McIntosh-Waddy, D. (2010). Consensus-validation study identifies relevant nursing diagnoses, nursing interventions, and health outcomes for people with traumatic brain injuries. *Rehabilitation Nursing, 35*(4), 161–165.

MacNevin, C. J., Atif, F., Sayeed, I., Stein, D. G., & Liotta, D. C. (2009). Development and screening of water-soluble analogues of progesterone and allopregnanolone in models of brain injury. *Journal of Medicinal Chemistry, 52*(19), 6012–6023.

Mahoney, D. (2001). Nursing management of the patient with spinal cord injury. In J. B. Derstine & S. D. Hargrove (Eds.), *Comprehensive rehabilitation nursing* (pp. 368–423). Philadelphia: W. B. Saunders.

Marino, S., Zei, E., Battaglini, M., Vittori, C., Buscalferri, A., Bramanti, P., et al. (2007). Acute metabolic brain changes following traumatic brain injury and their relevance to clinical severity and outcome. *Journal of Neurology Neurosurgery and Psychiatry, 78,* 501–507.

Marwitz, J. (2000). *NFI background.* The Center for Outcome Measurement in Brain Injury. Retrieved October 23, 2006, from www.tbims.org/combi/nfibg.html.

Mayer, A. R., Ling, J., Mannell, M. V., Gasparovic, C., Phillips, J. P., Doezema, D., et al. (2010). A prospective diffusion tensor imaging study in mild traumatic brain injury. *Neurology, 74,* 643–650.

McAllister, T. W. (2009). Psychopharmacological issues in the treatment of TBI and PTSD. *Archives of Clinical Neuropsychology, 23*(8), 1338–1367.

McColl, M. A., Arnold, R., Charlifue, S., & Gerhart, K. (2001). Social support and aging with a spinal cord injury: Canadian and British experiences. *Topics in Spinal Cord Injury Rehabilitation, 6*(3), 83–101.

McCrea, M., Iverson, G. L., McAllister, T. W., Hammeke, T. A., Powell, M. R., Barr, W. B., et al. (2009). An integrated review of recovery after mild traumatic brain injury (MTBI): Implications for clinical management. *Archives of Clinical Neuropsychology, 23*(8), 1368–1390.

McKinley, W., & Silver, T. M. (2006). Functional outcomes per level of spinal cord injury. Retrieved May 8, 2007, from www.emedicine.com/pmr/topic183.htm.

Meythaler, J. M., Peduzzi, J. D., Eleftheriou, E., & Novack, T. A. (2001). Current concepts: Diffuse axonal injury-associated traumatic brain injury. *Archives of Physical Medicine and Rehabilitation, 82*(10), 1461–1471.

The Miami Project. (1999a). *Basic science research* [Brochure]. Miami, FL: Author.

The Miami Project. (1999b). *Clinical and rehabilitative research* [Brochure]. Miami, FL: Author.

Mumford, N., & Wilson, P. H. (2009). Virtual reality in acquired brain injury upper limb rehabilitation: Evidence-based evaluation of clinical research. *Brain Injury, 23*(3), 179–191.

National Center for Complementary and Alternative Medicine. (2010). *What is CAM?* Retrieved July 6, 2010, from http://nccam.nih.gov/.

National Center for Injury Prevention and Control. (2003). *Report to Congress on mild traumatic brain injury in the United States: Steps to prevent a serious health problem.* Atlanta, GA: Centers for Disease Control and Prevention.

National Center for Injury Prevention and Control. (2006). *Heads up: Brain injury in your practice tool kit.* Retrieved September 7, 2006, from www.cdc.gov/ncipc/pub-res/tbi_toolkit/toolkit.htm.

National Center for Injury Prevention and Control. (2007). *What is traumatic brain injury?* Retrieved July 18, 2007, from www.cdc.gov/ncipc/tbi/TBI.htm.

National Institute of Neurological Disorders and Stroke. (2007). *Spinal cord injury: Hope through research.* Retrieved May 21, 2007, from www.ninds.nih.gov/disorders/sci/detail_sci.htm.

National Institute of Neurological Disorders and Stroke. (2010). *Traumatic brain injury: Hope through research.* Retrieved June 29, 2010, from www.ninds.nih.gov/disorders/tbi/detail_tbi.htm.

National Spinal Cord Injury Statistical Center. (2010a). *Annual report for the spinal cord injury model systems.* Retrieved August 19, 2011, from www.nscisc.uab.edu/public_content/pdf/2010%20NSCISC%20Annual%20Statistical%20Report%20-%20Complete%20Public%20Version.pdf.

National Spinal Cord Injury Statistical Center. (2010b). *Facts and figures at a glance.* Retrieved July 2011, from www.nscisc.uab.edu/public_content/pdf/2010%20NSCISC%20Annual%20Statistical%20Report%20-%20Complete%20Public%20Version.pdf.

Newman, S. D. (2006). Community integration of women with spinal cord injury: A case for participatory research. *SCI Nursing.* Retrieved May 21, 2007, from www.unitedspinal.org/publications/nursing/2006/08/27/community-integration-of-women-with-spinal-cord-injury-a-case-for-participatory-research/.

Northwest Regional Spinal Cord Injury System. (2009). *Aging with a spinal cord injury.* Retrieved August 10, 2011, from http://sci.washington.edu/info/forums/reports/aging_6.09.asp.

Obermann, M., Holle, D., & Katsarava, Z. (2009). Post-traumatic headache. *Expert Review of Neurotherapeutics, 9*(9), 1361–1370.

O'Dell, M., & Riggs, R. (1996). Management of the minimally responsive patient. In L. Horn & N. Zasler (Eds.), *Medical rehabilitation of traumatic brain injury* (pp. 103–132). Philadelphia: Hanley & Belfus.

Pachet, A., Friesen, S., Winkelaar, D., & Gray, S. (2003). Beneficial behavioral effects of lamotrigine in traumatic brain injury. *Brain Injury, 17*(8), 715–722.

Perlbarg, V., Puybasset, L., Tollard, E., Lehéricy, S., Benali, H., & Galanaud, D. (2009). Relation between brain lesion location and clinical outcome in patients with severe traumatic brain injury: A diffusion tensor imaging study using voxel-based approaches. *Human Brain Mapping, 30*(12), 3924–3933.

Pickett, G. E., Campos-Benitez, M., Keller, J. L., & Duggal, N. (2006). Epidemiology of traumatic spinal cord injury in Canada. *Spine, 31*(7), 799–805.

Povlishock, J. T., & Katz, D. I. (2005). Update of neuropathology and neurological recovery after traumatic brain injury. *Journal of Head Trauma Rehabilitation, 20*(1), 76–94.

Provenzale, J. M. (2010). Imaging of traumatic brain injury: A review of the recent medical literature. *American Journal of Roentgenology, 194*(1), 16–19.

Rabin, L. A., Burton, L. A., & Barr, W. B. (2007). Utilization rates of ecologically oriented instruments among clinical neuropsychologists. *Archives of Clinical Neuropsychology, 21,* 727–743.

Rader, M., Alston, J., & Ellis, D. (1989). Sensory stimulation of severely brain injured patients. *Brain Injury, 3,* 141–147.

Rancho Los Amigos National Rehabilitation Center. (2006). *Family guide to the levels of cognitive functioning.* Retrieved August 29, 2011, from http://rancho.org/research/bi_cognition.pdf.

Rappaport, M. (2000). *The Coma/Near Coma Scale.* The Center for Outcome Measurement in Brain Injury. Retrieved October 22, 2006 from www.tbims.org/combi/cnc.

Rappaport, M. (2005). The Disability Rating and Coma/Near-Coma scales in evaluating severe head injury. *Neuropsychological Rehabilitation, 15*(3–4), 442–453.

Richardson, R. M., Singh, A., Sun, D., Fillmore, H. L., Dietrich, D. W., & Bullock, M. R. (2010). Stem cell biology in traumatic brain injury: Effects of injury and strategies for repair. *Journal of Neurosurgery, 112*(5), 1125–1138.

Rockswold, S. B., Rockswold, G .L., & Defillo, A. (2007). Hyperbaric oxygen in traumatic brain injury. *Neurological Research, 29,* 162–172.

Rose, F. D., Brooks, B. M., & Rizzo, A. A. (2005). Virtual reality in brain damage rehabilitation: Review. *Cyberpsychology and Behavior, 8,* 241–262.

Rosebrough, A. (1998). Traumatic brain injury. In P. A. Chin, D. Finocchiaro, & A. Rosebrough (Eds.), *Rehabilitation nursing practice, major neurological deficits and common rehabilitation disorders* (pp. 223–244). New York: McGraw-Hill.

Samantaray, S., Das, A., Thakore, N. P., Matzelle, D. D., Reiter, R. J., Ray, S. K., et al. (2009). Therapeutic potential of melatonin in traumatic central nervous system injury. *Journal of Pineal Research, 47*(2), 134–142.

Sayeed, I., & Stein, D. G. (2009). Progesterone as a neuroprotective factor in traumatic and ischemic brain injury. *Progress in Brain Research, 175,* 219–237.

Scivoletto, G., Morganti, B., Ditunno, P., Ditunno, J. F., & Molinari, M. (2003). Effects on age on spinal cord lesion patients' rehabilitation. *Spinal Cord, 41*(8), 457–464.

Sherman, K. B., Goldberg, M., & Bell, K. R. (2006). Traumatic brain injury and pain. *Physical Medicine and Rehabilitation Clinics of North America, 17*(2), 473–490, viii.

Standen, P. J., & Brown, D. J. (2005). Virtual reality in the rehabilitation of people with intellectual disabilities: Review. *Cyberpsychology and Behavior, 8,* 272–282.

Stanford, M. S., Anderson, N. E., Lake, S. L., & Baldridge, R. M. (2009). Pharmacologic treatment of impulsive aggression with antiepileptic drugs. *Current Treatment Options in Neurology, 11*(5), 383–390.

Sugarman, B. (1985). Medical complications of spinal cord injury. *Quarterly Journal of Medicine, 54*(213), 3–18.

Sugden, S. G., Kile, S. J., Farrimond, D. D., Hilty, D. M., & Bourgeois, J. A. (2006). Pharmacological intervention for cognitive deficits and aggression in frontal lobe injury. *Neurorehabilitation, 21,* 3–7.

Tamai, H., Yamaguchi, T., Watanabe, E., Salito, K., Hyodo, A., & Seo, N. (2007). Acupuncture treatment for a patient with diffuse axonal injury. *Masui, 56,* 203–206.

van Baalen, B., Odding, E., Maas, A. I. R., Ribbers, G. M., Bergen, M. P., & Stam, H. J. (2003). Traumatic brain injury: Classification of initial severity and determination of functional outcome. *Disability and Rehabilitation, 25*(1), 9–18.

Van Boven, R. W., Harrington, G. S., Hackney, D. B., Ebel, A., Gauger, G., Bremner, J. D., et al. (2009). Advances in neuroimaging of traumatic brain injury and posttraumatic stress disorder. *Clinical Guidelines on TBI from VA and Department of Defense, 46*(6), v–vi.

Vinas, F. C., Pilitsis, J., Nosko, M. G., Talavera, F., Pluta, R. M., Zamboni, P., et al. (2006). *Penetrating head trauma.* Retrieved October 18, 2006, from www.emedicine.com/med/topic2888.htm.

Wang, J., Bakhadirov, K., Devous, M., Abdi, H., McColl, R., Moore, C., et al. (2008). Diffusion tensor tractography in traumatic diffuse axonal injury. *Archives of Neurology, 65*(5), 619–626.

Wasserman, J. R., & Koenigsberg, R. A. (2004). *Diffuse axonal injury imaging.* Retrieved October 18, 2006, from www.emedicine.com/radio/topic216.htm.

Wilson, B. A., Emslie, H., Quirk, K., Evans, J., & Watson, P. (2005). A randomized control trial to evaluate a paging system for people with traumatic brain injury. *Brain Injury, 19,* 891–894.

Winkler, T. (2007). *Spinal cord injury and aging.* Retrieved May 18, 2007, from www.emedicine.com/pmr/topic185.htm.

Wright, J. (2000). *Introduction to the Disability Rating Scale.* The Center for Outcome Measurement in Brain Injury. Retrieved October 17, 2006, from www.tbims.org/combi/drs.

Wroblewski, B. A., Joseph, A. B., Kupfer, J., & Kalliel, K. (1997). Effectiveness of valproic acid on destructive and aggressive behaviors in patients with acquired brain injury. *Brain Injury, 11*(1), 37–47.

Wu, T., Wilde, E. A., Bigler, E. D., Yallampalli, R., McCauley, S. R., Troyanskaya, M., et al. (2009). Evaluating the relation between memory functioning and cingulum bundles in acute mild traumatic brain injury using diffusion tensor imaging. *Journal of Neurotrauma, 27*(2), 303–307.

Xu, J., Rasmussen, I. A., Lagopoulos, J., & Haberg, A. (2007). Diffuse axonal injury in severe traumatic brain injury visualized using high-resolution diffusion tensor imaging. *Journal of Neurotrauma, 24,* 753–765.

Zhou, Z., Daugherty, W. P., Sun, D., Levasseur, J. E., Altememi, N., Hamm, R. J., et al. (2007). Protection of mitochondrial function and improvement in cognitive recovery in rats treated with hyperbaric oxygen following lateral fluid-percussion injury. *Journal of Neurosurgery, 106,* 687–694.

Zitnay, G. A., Zitnay, K. M., Povlishock, J. T., Hall, E. D., Marion, D. W., Trudel, T., et al. (2008). Traumatic brain injury research priorities: The Conemaugh International Brain Injury Symposium. *Journal of Neurotrauma, 25*(10), 35–52.

Suggested Reading

Azouvi, P., Jokic, C., Attals, N., Denys, P., Markabi, S., & Bussel, B. (1999). Carbamazepine in agitation and aggressive behavior following severe closed-head injury: Results of an open trial. *Brain Injury, 13*(10), 797–804.

Baguley, I. J., Cameron, I. D., Gree, A. M., Slewayounan, S., Marosszeky, J. E., & Gurka, J. A. (2004). Pharmacological management of dysautonomia following traumatic brain injury. *Brain Injury, 18*(5), 409–417.

Bell, K. R., & Williams, F. (2003). Use of botulinum toxin type A and type B for spasticity in upper and lower limbs. *Physical Medicine and Rehabilitation Clinics of North America, 14,* 821–835.

Brooke, M. M., Patterson, D. R., Questad, K. A., Cardenas, D., & Farrel-Roberts, L. (1992). The treatment of agitation during initial hospitalization after traumatic brain injury. *Archives of Physical Medicine and Rehabilitation, 73,* 917–921.

Brooke, M. M., Questad, K. A., Patterson, D. R., & Bashak, K. J. (1992). Agitation and restlessness after closed head injury: A prospective study of 100 consecutive admissions. *Archives of Physical Medicine and Rehabilitation, 73,* 320–323.

Burnett, M. D., Kennedy, R. E., Cifu, D. X., & Levenson, J. (2003). Using atypical neuroleptic drugs to treat agitation in patients with a brain injury: A review. *Neurorehabilitation, 13,* 165–172.

Cicerone, K. D., Dahlberg, C., Malec, J. F., Langenbahn, D. M., Felicetti, T., Kneipp, S. S., et al. (2005). Evidence-based cognitive rehabilitation: Updated review of the literature from 1998 through 2002. *Archives of Physical Medicine and Rehabilitation, 86,* 1681–1692.

Demark, J., & Gemeinhardt, M. (2002). Anger and its management for survivors of acquired brain injury. *Brain Injury, 16*(2), 91–108.

Francisco, G. E., Hu, M. M., Boake, C., & Ivanhoe, C. B. (2005). Efficacy of early use of intrathecal baclofen therapy for treating spastic hypertonia due to acquired brain injury. *Brain Injury, 19*(5), 359–364.

Giacino, J. T., Ashwal, S., Childs, N., Cranford, R., Jennett, B., Katz, D. I., et al. (2002). The minimally conscious state: Definition and diagnostic criteria. *Neurology, 58*(3), 1–11.

Giacino, J., & Whyte, J. (2005). The vegetative and minimally conscious states: Current knowledge and remaining questions. *Journal of Head Trauma Rehabilitation, 20,* 30–50.

Glen, M. B. (1998). Methylphenidate for cognitive and behavioral dysfunction after traumatic brain injury. *Journal of Head Trauma Rehabilitation, 13*(5), 87–90.

Harvey, C. V. (2005). Spinal surgery patient care. *Orthopaedic Nursing, 24*(6), 426–440.

Hughes, S., Colantonio, A., Santaguida, P. L., & Paton, T. (2005). Amantadine to enhance readiness for rehabilitation following severe traumatic brain injury. *Brain Injury, 19*(14), 1197–1206.

Kajs-Wyllie, M. (2002). Ritalin revisited: Does it really help in neurological injury? *Journal of Neuroscience Nursing, 43*(6), 303–313.

Kraus, M. F., Smith, G. S., Butters, M., Donnell, A. J., Dixon, E., Yilong, C., et al. (2005). Effects of dopaminergic agent and NMDA receptor antagonist amantadine on cognitive function, cerebral glucose metabolism and D2 receptor availability in chronic traumatic brain injury: A study using positron emission tomography. *Brain Injury, 19*(7), 471–479.

Leone, H., & Polsonetti, B. W. (2005). Amantadine for traumatic brain injury: Does it improve cognition and reduce agitation? *Journal of Clinical Pharmacy and Therapeutics, 30,* 101–104.

Llemke, D. M. (2004). Riding out the storm: Sympathetic storming after traumatic brain injury. *Journal of Neuroscience Nursing, 36*(1), 4–7.

Maryniak, O., Manchanda, R., & Velani, A. (2001). Methotrimeprazine in the treatment of agitation in acquired brain injury patients. *Brain Injury, 15*(2), 167–174.

Meythaler, J., Brunner, R., Johnson, A., & Novack, T. (2002). Amantadine to improve neurorecovery in traumatic brain injury–associated diffuse axonal injury: A pilot double-blind randomized trial. *Journal of Head Trauma Rehabilitation, 17*(4), 300–313.

Meythaler, J. M., Clayton, W., Davis, L. K., Guin-Renfroe, S., & Brunner, R. C. (2004). Orally delivered baclofen to control spastic hypertonia in acquired brain injury. *Journal of Head Trauma Rehabilitation, 19*(2), 101–108.

Meythaler, J. M., Depalma, L., Devivo, M. J., Guin-Renfroe, S., & Novack, T. A. (2001). Sertraline to improve arousal and alertness in severe traumatic brain injury secondary to motor vehicle crashes. *Brain Injury, 15*(4), 321–331.

Mooney, G. F., & Haas, L. J. (1993). Effect of methylphenidate on brain injury–related anger. *Archives of Physical Medicine and Rehabilitation, 74,* 153–160.

Pachet, A., Friesen, S., Winkelaar, D., & Gray, S. (2003). Beneficial behavioral effects of lamotrigine in traumatic brain injury. *Brain Injury, 17*(8), 715–722.

Pena, C. G. (2003). Seizure emergency. *American Journal of Nursing, 103,* 73–81.

Port, A., Willmott, C., & Charlton, J. (2002). Self-awareness following traumatic brain injury and implications for rehabilitation. *Brain Injury, 16*(4), 277–289.

Povlishock, J.T ., & Katz, D. J. (2005). Update on neuropathology and neuronal recovery after traumatic brain injury. *Journal of Head Trauma Rehabilitation, 20*(1), 76–94.

Rao, V., & Lyketsos, C. G. (2002). Psychiatric aspects of traumatic brain injury. *Psychiatric Clinics of North America, 25*(1), 1–24.

Rhijn, J. V., Molenaers, G., & Ceulemans, B. (2005). Botulinum toxin type A in the treatment of children and adolescents with an acquired brain injury. *Brain Injury, 19*(5), 331–335.

Schiff, N. D., Rodriguez-Moreno, D., Kamal, A., Kim, K. H. S., Giacino, J. T., Plum, F., et al. (2005). fMRI reveals large-scale network activation in minimally conscious patients. *Neurology, 64,* 514–523.

Schneider, W. N., Drew-Cates, J., Wong, T. M., & Dombovy, M. L. (1999). Cognitive and behavioral efficacy of amantadine in acute traumatic brain injury: An initial double-blind placebo-controlled study. *Brain Injury, 13*(11), 863–872.

Shoumitro, D., & Crownshaw, T. (2004). The role of pharmacotherapy in the management of behavior disorders in traumatic brain injury patients. *Brain Injury, 18*(1), 1–31.

Silver, J. M., Kourmara, B., Chen, M., Mirski, D., Potkin, S. G., Reyes, P., et al. (2006). Effects of rivastigmine on cognitive function in patients with traumatic brain injury. *Neurology, 67,* 748–755.

Stanislav, S. W., & Childs, A. (2000). Evaluating the usage of droperidol in acutely agitated persons with brain injury. *Brain Injury, 14*(3), 261–265.

Sugden, S. G., Kile, S. J., Farrimond, D. D., Hilty, D. M., & Bourgeois, J. A. (2006). Pharmacological intervention for cognitive deficits and aggression in frontal lobe injury. *Neurorehabilitation, 21,* 3–7.

Thorley, R. R., Wertsch, J. J., & Klingbeil, G. E. (2001). Acute hypothalamic instability in traumatic brain injury: A case report. *Archives of Physical Medicine and Rehabilitation, 82,* 246–249.

Whiteneck, G. (Ed.). (1993). *Aging with spinal cord injury.* New York: Demos.

Wiercisiewski, D. R. (2001). Pharmacologic management of behavior in traumatic brain injury. *Physical Medicine and Rehabilitation: State of the Art Review, 15*(2), 267–281.

Wroblewski, B. A., Joseph, A. B., Kupfer, J., & Kalliel, K. (1997). Effectiveness of valproic acid on destructive and aggressive behaviors in patients with acquired brain injury. *Brain Injury, 11*(1), 37–47.

Zafonte, R. D., Lexell, J., & Cullen, N. (2001a). Possible applications for dopaminergic agents following traumatic brain injury: Part 1. *Journal of Head Trauma Rehabilitation, 16*(1), 1179–1182.

Zafonte, R. D., Lexell, J., & Cullen, N. (2001b). Possible applications for dopaminergic agents following traumatic brain injury: Part 2. *Journal of Head Trauma Rehabilitation, 16*(1), 112–116.

CHAPTER 13
Orthopedic Disorders, Burns, Blasts, and Posttraumatic Stress Disorder

Cheryl A. Lehman, PhD RN CNS-BC RN-BC CRRN • Ann Gutierrez, MSN RN CRRN CBIS

Rehabilitation nurses often care for clients with orthopedic conditions such as osteoporosis, arthritis, and amputation. Less common but also seen in the rehabilitation setting are clients with burns and injuries related to blasts. Rehabilitation clients with traumatic injuries are also frequently diagnosed with posttraumatic stress disorder (PTSD) and related psychological disorders. Rehabilitation nurses must assume the essential roles of care provider, educator, care coordinator, and counselor to achieve a well-rounded plan of care for clients with these diagnoses.

Osteoporosis is a silent illness that is often not diagnosed until after a fracture. Osteoporosis has been deemed a major public health threat in the United States for more than half the population 50 years of age and older. Ten million people in the United States are estimated to already have the disease, and almost 34 million more are estimated to have low bone mass, placing them at higher risk for osteoporosis (National Osteoporosis Foundation [NOF], 2010c). Osteoporosis-related fractures are a major threat to many Americans, with the potential for significant morbidity and mortality.

Arthritis is also highly prevalent among American adults. It is the leading cause of disability and is associated with substantial activity limitation, work disability, reduced quality of life, and high healthcare costs. Arthritis is expected to affect an estimated 67 million adults in the United States by 2030 (Cheng, Hootman, Murphy, Langmaid, & Helmick, 2010). "Research shows that pain, fear of pain, fear of worsening symptoms or damaging joints, and lack of information on how to exercise safely prevent people with arthritis from being physically active. To manage chronic conditions such as diabetes, heart disease, and obesity effectively, people with arthritis need help finding ways to overcome arthritis-specific barriers to physical activity" (Centers for Disease Control & Prevention [CDC], 2010a, p. 2).

Approximately 1.7 million people are living with limb loss in the United States. It is estimated that one out of every 200 people in the United States has had an amputation. The majority of new amputations result from complications of the vascular system caused by diabetes: As many as 82% of amputations are due to vascular disease (National Limb Loss Information Center, 2008). A national healthcare goal is to reduce the rate of lower extremity amputations in people with diabetes. Progress is being made toward this goal, and it is being continued in the 2020 Healthy People objectives (Healthy People 2020, 2009).

The recent wars in Iraq and Afghanistan have brought other conditions to the forefront of national attention. These include blast injuries, burns, and PTSD. Traumatic brain injury (TBI) related to blasts is emerging as the signature injury of these wars, as is traumatic amputation, being seen with increasing frequency among our service members. Blast research is in the early stages, but it is hoped that research will help determine whether and how disability related to blasts differs from disability attributable to other causes. Burns have become more prevalent since the wars, and research into burn treatment is accelerating.

Anyone who has endured a life-threatening event can have PTSD. These events can include motor vehicle accidents, sexual or physical abuse, natural disasters, and military combat. "Strong emotions caused by the event create changes in the brain that may result in PTSD" (National Center for PTSD, 2010). People with PTSD often have the disorder for years, reliving the event, avoiding similar situations, and having other physical and psychological reactions that interfere with quality of life. An estimated 5.2 million Americans ages 18–54 are estimated to have PTSD, including many rehabilitation clients and military service members.

Rehabilitation nurses have a great deal to offer clients with disability due to orthopedic origins, blast injuries, burns, and PTSD. Using excellent assessment skills, rehabilitation nurses can monitor chronic illnesses and injuries such as these over time and adjust treatments to meet each client's needs. Client and family education are also essential elements of care. This chapter discusses rehabilitation nursing care of clients with osteoporosis, arthritis, and amputation, as well as blast injuries, burns, and PTSD. Rehabilitation nurses play many roles in the treatment plans for clients with these diagnoses, which are designed to return the client to functional independence with successful community reintegration.

I. **Osteoporosis**
   A. Overview (International Osteoporosis Foundation [IOF], 2009h; NOF, 2010c)
      1. A degenerative disease that causes bones to become fragile and break with little or no trauma. A fragility fracture is the clinical expression of osteoporosis; however, bone loss is asymptomatic, which has led to it being described as a "silent thief" (Saag & Geusens, 2009).
      2. Affects more than 10 million people in the United States (8 million women and 2 million men) and is estimated to affect more than 200 million people worldwide

a. 30% of postmenopausal women in the United States and Europe

b. 40% of women and 15%–30% of men affected will have one or more fragility fracture (IOF, 2009h).

3. Approximately 44 million Americans and 55% of people 50 years of age and older are at risk for osteoporosis because of low bone mass.

4. A major health problem for more than half of Americans older than 50 years: The aging of the population worldwide has caused a major increase in osteoporosis in postmenopausal women (IOF, 2009h).

5. Osteoporosis increases with age (Joint Commission & National Pharmaceutical Council, 2008).

   a. Affects 37% of women age 50–57

   b. Affects 50% of women age 70–79

   c. Affects 87% of women older than age 80 (IOF, 2009h)

   d. In 2001 5% of men on Medicare were diagnosed with osteoporosis (Tucci, 2006).

6. Leads to 1.5 million fractures at an annual cost of $18 billion per year to the U.S. healthcare system (NOF, 2010c)

7. A leading cause of disability in the aging population. It is estimated that by 2020 half of all Americans older than 50 years will have osteoporosis or will be at a high risk for developing it (U.S. Department of Health and Human Services [HHS], 2004).

8. Affects not only the ability to perform activities of daily living (ADLs) but also social and psychological functioning (HHS, 2004)

9. Leads to a decrease in quality of life. Because osteoporosis causes back pain and loss of height, the prevention of osteoporosis and associated fractures is important for the maintenance of quality of life, health, and independence in older adults (Chan, Anderson, & Lau, 2003; World Health Organization [WHO], 2004b).

10. Osteoporsis is characterized by low bone mass and structural deterioration of bone tissue, leading to bone fragility and greater susceptibility to fractures, especially of the hip, spine, and wrist, although any bone can be affected (Meiner & Lueckenotte, 2006; NOF, 2010c).

11. Occurs when bone resorption exceeds bone formation

12. Often is not diagnosed until a fracture is sustained

B. Etiology

1. Cause remains unknown

2. Risk factors (WHO, 2003; Swearingen, 2007a; IOF, 2009j; NOF, 2010a, 2010c)

a. Genetic

   1) Female

   2) Hispanic, Asian, or Caucasian, especially northern European ancestry

   3) Family history of hip fracture, kyphosis (dowager's hump), osteoporosis

   4) Red or blond hair

   5) Fair skin

   6) Scoliosis

   7) Rheumatoid arthritis (RA)

   8) Small-framed body (low body mass index; IOF, 2009j)

b. Advanced age

c. Nutritional problems

   1) Low calcium and vitamin D intake (Saag & Geusens, 2009; IOF, 2009j; NOF, 2010c)

   2) Excessive intake of protein (IOF, 2009j)

   3) Poor gastrointestinal (GI) absorption

   4) Eating disorders (e.g., anorexia, bulimia)

   5) Heavy alcohol use (Kanis, Johansson, et al., 2005; Tucker et al., 2009)

   6) High caffeine intake

d. Lifestyle factors

   1) Low level of activity

   2) Prolonged immobilization

   3) Previous falls

   4) Heavy cigarette smoking (Kanis, Johnell, et al., 2005; Law & Hackshaw, 1997; Supervía et al., 2006).

e. Endocrine disorders (Rosen, 2007)

   1) Hyperthyroidism

   2) Diabetes mellitus

   3) Gonadal dysfunction in men, low testosterone levels in men

   4) Normal, early, or surgically induced menopause (Swearingen, 2007a)

   5) Exercise-induced amenorrhea

   6) Nulliparity

   7) Abnormally low weight or leanness

   8) Female hypogonadism

   9) Low bone density

f. Pharmacological factors

   1) Antacids containing aluminum cause calcium loss in stool.

   2) Antiseizure medications (e.g., phenytoin, phenobarbital, primidone) interfere with vitamin D metabolism and decrease calcium absorption.

   3) Tetracycline, isoniazid, and furosemide cause increased calcium loss in urine.

   4) Vitamin A: More than 5,000 IU/day increases calcium loss in the urine.

5) Corticosteroids (e.g., prednisone, dexamethasone): Long-term use results in severe osteoporosis.
6) Thyroid hormones in excessive dosages
7) Heparin
8) Lithium
9) Selected chemotherapy agents
g. Other risk factors
1) Hyperparathyroidism
2) Neoplasm
3) Renal dysfunction
4) High vitamin D intake
5) High calcium carbonate intake (Kanis et al., 2004)
6) Previous fracture (Swearingen, 2007a)
7) Family history of fractures (Kanis et al., 2004)
8) Osteomalacia
9) Neuromuscular disease (IOF, 2009k)
3. Incidence (NOF, 2010c)
a. It is estimated that osteoporosis affects more than 200 million people worldwide.
1) Of those affected, 40% of women and 15%–30% of men will sustain more than one fragility fracture.
2) The aging of the population worldwide will cause a major increase in incidence in postmenopausal women (Reginster & Burlet, 2006).
b. Osteoporosis was reported to be responsible for more than 2 million fractures in 2005.
1) 297,000 hip fractures
2) 547,000 vertebral fractures
3) 387,000 wrist fractures
4) 135,000 pelvic fractures
5) 675,000 fractures in other bones
c. Osteoporotic fractures most often involve the hip, vertebra, or wrist, but any bone can be affected.
d. Worldwide incidence of hip fractures each year is about 1.7 million (IOF, 2009g).
e. 61% of fractures related to osteoporosis occur in women with a ratio of maie to female of 1:6 (IOF, 2009h).
f. 90% of hip fractures occur in people 50 years of age or older (Sambrook & Cooper, 2006).
g. Women with hip fracture have a four times higher risk of having a second hip fracture.
h. One in three women and one in five men older than age 50 will sustain a related fracture sometime before the end of life (IOF, 2009h).
i. Approximately 24% of people age 50 and older die in the year after a hip fracture (IOF, 2009h).
j. One in five people who were ambulatory before a hip fracture will need long-term care afterward.
k. The risk of osteoporosis is significant among people of all ethnic backgrounds 50 years of age and older (NOF, 2010c).
1) Of non-Hispanic Caucasian and Asian women, 20% are estimated to have osteoporosis, and another 52% are estimated to have low bone mass.
2) Of non-Hispanic Caucasian and Asian men, 7% are estimated to have osteoporosis, and another 35% are estimated to have low bone mass.
3) Of non-Hispanic African-American women, 5% are estimated to have osteoporosis, and an additional 35% are estimated to have low bone mass.
4) Of non-Hispanic African-American men, 4% are estimated to have osteoporosis, and another 19% are estimated to have low bone mass.
5) Of Hispanic women who are age 50 and older, 10% are estimated to have osteoporosis, and another 49% are estimated to have low bone mass.
6) Of Hispanic men, 3% are estimated to have osteoporosis, and another 23% are estimated to have low bone mass.
7) When compared with other ethnic and racial groups, the risk of osteoporosis is increasing most rapidly among Hispanic women.
l. It is predicted that the costs related to osteoporotic fractures among people of Hispanic origin will increase from an estimated $754 million in 2005 to $2 billion per year in 2025 (NOF, 2010c).
m. Hip fractures account for a significant number of nursing home admissions.
4. Classification of osteoporosis (Meiner & Lueckenotte, 2006; NYU Hospital for Joint Diseases Spine Center, 2005)
a. Primary osteoporosis
1) Type I (postmenopausal): Related to rapid drop in estrogen production around the time of menopause. Estrogen is essential for normal calcium absorption.
a) Type I is seen in women between the ages of 51 and 75.
b) It is six times more prevalent in women than men.

c) It produces a gradual loss of cortical bone. Because cortical bone provides support to the body, weakening results in hip fracture.
d) Diet low in calcium and vitamin D
2) Type II (senile or age-related)
a) Occurs in men and women older than age 70
b) Is the result of the normal aging process and chronic lack of calcium
c) May be caused by renal dysfunction, which affects the conversion of vitamin D to a form usable for calcium absorption
b. Secondary osteoporosis
1) Seen in 15% of osteoporosis cases
2) Result from diseases such as hyperthyroidism, hyperparathyroidism, GI disorders, neoplasms, and alcoholism
3) In women it is seen after bilateral oophorectomy.
4) Prolonged use of such medications such as corticosteroids, methotrexate, antacids that contain aluminum, phenytoin, and heparin may also result in secondary osteoporosis.
c. Disuse osteoporosis
1) Neurogenic osteoporosis in paralyzed extremities (Dudley-Javoroski & Shields, 2008)
a) Spinal cord injury (SCI)
(i) Contributing factors that influence a decrease in bone mass (Dudley-Javoroski & Shields, 2008; Jiang, Dai, & Jiang, 2006)
(a) People with SCI and flaccid paralysis and women show lower bone mineral density (BMD) and bone mineral content (BMC) than men with SCI and those with thoracic injuries (Coupaud, McLean, & Allan, 2009).
(b) Muscle spasticity
(c) Severity and level of injury
(d) Age
(e) Sex
(f) Loss of routine gravitational and muscular loads removes an important stimulation for the maintenance of BMD.
(g) Amount of time since the injury occurred

(ii) Involvement
(a) Tetraplegia involves the pelvis, upper and lower extremities.
(b) Paraplegia involves the pelvis and lower extremities.
(iii) Treatment
(a) Calcium contributes to the homeostasis of serum calcium after SCI but does not prevent osteoporosis.
(b) Phosphate reduces serum calcium excretion but does not prevent bone loss.
(c) Vitamin D assists in the absorption of calcium.
(d) Calcitonin has been shown in people with SCI to prevent the early increase of resorption of bone.
(e) Bisphosphonates strongly inhibit bone resorption.
(f) Functional electrical stimulation–induced cycling; Ragnarsson, 2008)
b) Stroke (Carda, Cisari, Invernizzi, & Bevilacqua, 2009; Pang, Ashe, & Eng, 2007)
(i) Contributing factors that influence a decrease in bone mass
(a) The degree of paresis
(b) Inability to walk
(c) The length of time the client was immobile
(d) Difference in muscle strength
(e) Spasticity
(f) Chronic disuse
(ii) Involvement
(a) Involves the paretic side
(b) Upper extremities usually more than the lower extremities
(iii) Treatment
(a) Adequate calcium intake
(b) Vitamin D
(c) Vitamin B_{12} and folate
(d) Bisphosphonates
(e) Risedronate, the only drug that has been shown to not only prevent bone loss but to also reduce hip fracture (Carda et al., 2009)
2) Other forms of disuse osteoporosis

a) Disuse in people who have been bed-fast for a period of time or have been unable to bear weight on an extremity

b) BMD has been found to be low in people who have lacked gravitational and muscular loads, such as astronauts (Traon, Heer, Narici, Rutweger, & Vernikos, 2007).

  (i) Contributing factors that influence a decrease in bone mass

    (a) Calcium excretion is increased from the beginning of bed rest.

    (b) Calcium absorption is reduced.

    (c) Body weight and muscle mass are decreased.

    (d) Bone stiffness of the lower extremities and spinal cord and bone architecture are changed.

  (ii) Ways to improve bone mass

    (a) Aerobic exercise

    (b) Resistive exercises

    (c) Vibration

C. Pathophysiology (Post, Cremers, Kerbusch, & Danhof, 2010; Rosen, 2007)

1. Skeletal system influence

  a. The normal bone remodeling cycle is constant and is governed by resorption activities of osteoclasts and bone-forming osteoblasts and deeply imbedded osteoclasts that sense gravitational forces (Kessenich, 1997; The North American Menopause Society [NAMS], 2010).

    1) There are two basic types of bone.

      a) Cortical bone: Makes up 80% of bone mass. It is dense, is less metabolically active, and forms the outer shell of the bone

      b) Trabecular bone: Makes up 20% of bone mass but 80% of bone surface. It is metabolically active and is concentrated in the flat bones of the pelvis, vertebrae, forearms, and ribs (Post et al., 2010).

    2) All bones are made of both types, but the proportions differ.

  b. Normally, 10% of bone is undergoing remodeling at a given time (Kessenich, 1997).

    1) In adults, bone remodeling is balanced (resorption equals bone formation). This process lasts approximately 90–130 days.

2) Maintenance of bone mass during remodeling ensures an available source of calcium for use by the body and maintenance of a reservoir of stored calcium (Rosen, 2007).

c. The cycle is balanced until approximately age 30, when bone loss outweighs bone growth at a rate of 3%–5% per decade (Kessenich, 1997).

  1) Imbalances of the remodeling units can occur, which can result in significant bone loss.

  2) These imbalances can be a result of changes in hormone levels systemically, a decrease of intake of calcium, or a decrease in mechanical loading (Rosen, 2007).

d. Signal communication between osteoblast and osteoclast cells begins the process of resorption (Post et al., 2010; Rosen, 2007; HHS, 2004).

  1) Osteoblasts produce macrophage colony-stimulating factor and receptor activator of nuclear factor kappa B ligand (RANKL) proteins that attach to receptors on the osteoclast precursors. They stimulate proliferation and differentiation and increase the activity of osteoclasts.

  2) Osteoblasts also produce the hormone osteoprotegerin (OPG), which can bind RANKL and prevent it from interacting with osteoclasts.

  3) The balance between RANKL and OPG production is critical in determining the rate at which bone breaks down.

2. Endocrine system involvement

  a. Bone reabsorption is affected by parathyroid hormone (PTH), 1,25-dihydroxyvitamin D, and calcitonin.

  b. Each affects the regulation of serum calcium (**Figure 13-1**)

  c. PTH increases the reabsorption of bone by increasing osteoclast activity and, ultimately, bone breakdown.

  d. Release of PTH activates vitamin D to 1,25-dihydroxyvitamin D3 and allows calcium to be absorbed in the GI tract (HHS, 2004).

  e. Release of calcitonin inhibits osteoclasts, decreasing bone resorption and causing a decrease in serum calcium levels.

  f. Estrogen may affect these hormones and has been noted to increase the osteoblastic cells

Figure 13-1. Hypocalcemia and Hypercalcemia

Hypocalcemia

⇓ Calcium blood level

⇓

Release of parathyroid hormone from parathyroid gland

⇓

⇑ Release of calcium from bones

⇑ Calcium reabsorption from kidneys

⇑ Calcium absorption from the gut
(requires presence of vitamin D)

⇓

⇑ Blood calcium levels normal

Signs and symptoms
- Nerve excitability
- Paresthesias
- Muscle cramping
- Muscle spasm
- Tetany
- Death

Hypercalcemia

⇑ Calcium blood levels

⇓

Release of calcitonin from thyroid gland

⇓

⇓ Release of calcium from bones

⇓ Calcium reabsorption from kidneys and gut

⇓

⇓ Blood calcium levels normal

Signs and symptoms
- Muscle weakness
- Ataxia, coma
- Arrhythmia, cardiac arrest
- Fractures
- Extreme polyuria

available for new bone growth (Crowley, 2004).

3. Menopausal influence (Watts, 2010)
   a. Menopause begins a marked acceleration in bone loss—as much as 15% during the peri-menopausal period.
      1) Bone loss begins approximately 1.5 years before the last menstrual period.
      2) Continued rapid bone loss continues until about 1.5 years after the last menstrual period.
   b. Bone loss is caused by a decrease in natural estrogen.
   c. Estrogen replacement decreases the effects of menopause on bone loss.

D. Diagnosis (Institute for Clinical Systems Improvement [ICSI], 2008; Nelson, Haney, Dana, Bougatsos, & Chou, 2010; NOF, 2010b)
   1. Thorough history (Mauck & Clarke, 2006; Yurkow & Yudin, 2002)
      a. Family history
      b. Excessive height loss (more than 2 in.)
      c. Fractures from minimal trauma before age 40
      d. Complaints of bone pain, particularly in the back
      e. Onset of menopause and estrogen deficiency, the single most common cause of osteoporosis (Yurkow & Yudin, 2002)
      f. Low intake of calcium, lactose intolerance
      g. Steroid use
      h. Northern European heritage
      i. Gum disease or tooth decay
      j. Excessive caffeine use
      k. Cigarette use
      l. High alcohol intake
      m. Sedentary lifestyle or long-term immobilization
      n. History of specific conditions
         1) Thyroid problems
         2) Liver problems
         3) Diabetes mellitus
         4) Renal failure
         5) Malignancies (Watts, 1997)
         6) Other endocrine disorders
         7) RA (Rosen, 2007)
      o. Medication history
         1) Corticosteroids
         2) Isoniazid
         3) Heparin
         4) Tetracycline
         5) Anticonvulsants
         6) Thyroid supplements
   2. Physical examination (Swearingen, 2007a; Yurkow & Yudin, 2002)
      a. Fracture of wrist or femur, vertebral compression fractures
      b. Marked kyphosis, dowager's hump
      c. Shortened status
      d. Muscle atrophy
      e. Muscle spasms in back
      f. Difficulty bending forward
      g. Impaired breathing
      h. Poor dentition
   3. Laboratory tests (NOF, 2010b; Yurkow & Yudin, 2002)
      a. 24-hour urine calcium level
      b. Serum calcium
      c. Phosphorus levels (elevated)

d. Alkaline phosphatase levels (elevated with severe bone loss)
e. Serum osteocalcin
f. Thyroid function studies
g. PTH level
h. Testosterone levels in men
i. Serum 25 hydroxyvitamin D measurement (Binkley & Krueger, 2005; NOF, 2010b; Rosen, 2007).
j. Biochemical marker tests of bone resorption mediated by osteoclasts (IOF, 2009f; NOF, 2010b)
   1) Urine pyridinoline and deoxypyridinoline
   2) NTX (N-terminal peptides of type 1 collagen formation; serum or urine)
   3) CTX (C-terminal peptides of type 1 collagen formation; serum or urine)
4. Standard X ray: Anteroposterior and lateral X ray of the spine to rule out fractures (Swearingen, 2007a)
5. BMD evaluation, which is assessed by dual-energy X-ray absorptiometry (DXA), is the gold standard used to diagnose osteoporosis (American Association of Clinical Endocrinologists, 2003; IOF, 2009f; NOF, 2008, 2010b).
   a. A BMD scan should be performed using a DXA measurement of the hip and spine scan to
      1) Establish or confirm a diagnosis of osteoporosis
      2) Determine whether a person has a decrease in bone density after a fracture
      3) Predict future fracture risk
      4) Monitor clients by performing serial assessments (determine whether bone density is staying the same or decreasing when scans are performed at intervals of 1 year or more).
      5) A BMD scan should be repeated 2 years after treatment is initiated to determine the effectiveness of the treatment (NOF, 2010a; Rahmani & Morin, 2009).
   b. Results are measured against two standard norms.
      1) Age- and sex-matched readings (the z-score): Compare a patient's results (the t-score) with what is expected in someone of the same age and sex.
      2) BMD t-scores: This represents a client's BMD, expressed as the number of standard deviations (SD) above or below the mean BMD value for a normal young adult.

c. WHO has established diagnostic criteria for women who have not experienced fractures, based on the BMD t-scores (WHO, 1994).
   1) Normal: BMD within 1 SD of the young adult mean
   2) Osteopenia or low bone mass: BMD between 1.5 and 2.5 SD below the young adult mean
   3) Osteoporosis: BMD at least 2.5 SD below the young adult mean
d. Medicare reimburses for a BMD scan every 2 years.
e. May be recommended for the following (NOF, 2010b):
   1) A woman who is younger than age 65 who has one or more osteoporosis risk factors
   2) A man who is age 50–70 who has one or more osteoporosis risk factors
   3) A woman who is age 65 or older who has no risk factors
   4) A man whose is age 70 years or older who has no risk factors
   5) A woman or man age 50 or older who has fractured a bone
   6) A woman going through menopause who has certain risk factors
   7) A woman who has stopped taking estrogen therapy or hormone therapy and is postmenopausal
f. Other reasons to recommend a BMD test (NOF, 2010a)
   1) Long-term use of certain medications, including steroids (e.g., prednisone and cortisone), some antiseizure medications, Depo-Provera, and aromatase inhibitors (e.g., anastrozole)
   2) A man being treated with certain treatments for prostate cancer
   3) A woman being treated with certain treatments for breast cancer
   4) A person with overactive thyroid gland (hyperthyroidism) or taking high doses of thyroid hormone medication
   5) A person with an overactive parathyroid gland (hyperparathyroidism)
   6) A person who has had a spinal X ray that showed a spinal fracture or bone loss
   7) A person complaining of back pain with a possible fracture
   8) A person stating that he or she has had a significant loss of height
   9) A person with a loss of sex hormones at an early age, which includes early menopause

10) A person with a disease or condition that can cause bone loss (e.g., RA or anorexia nervosa)

6. Other radiographic studies (Engelke et al., 2008; IOF, 2009f; NOF, 2010b)

  a. Quantitative computed tomography measures true volumetric BMC by separately measuring three-dimensional trabecular and cortical bone density of the spine and the hip (NOF, 2010b), detecting early changes in the spinal vertebrae and the hip (Kebicz, 2007).

  b. Quantitative ultrasound densitometry (IOF, 2009f; WHO, 2003)

    1) Does not measure BMD directly but measures the speed of sound or measures broadband ultrasound attenuation at the tibia, heel, patella, and other peripheral skeletal sites

    2) Provides information on structural organization of bone mass without exposing the person to ionizing radiation (IOF, 2009f)

  c. Radiographic absorptiometry

  d. Single-energy X-ray absorptiometry

7. WHO Fracture Risk Algorithm (FRAX; IOF, 2009i; NOF, 2010b)

  a. Developed to calculate the 10-year probability of the person having a hip fracture and also the 10-year probability of a major osteoporotic fracture (vertebral, hip, forearm, or proximal humerus fracture)

  b. The FRAX can be used to guide decisions about treatment under the following conditions:

    1) Postmenopausal women or men age 50 and older

    2) People with low bone density (osteopenia)

    3) People who have not taken an osteoporosis medicine

  c. The FRAX algorithm for the United States is available at www.nof.org.

E. Resulting Disabilities

1. Hip fracture (NOF, 2010a)

  a. In 2001 more than 300,000 Americans older than age 45 sustained hip fracture necessitating hospitalization, with an underlying cause of osteoporosis.

  b. Caucasian women older than age 65 are twice as likely to sustain a hip fracture as African-American women.

  c. The incidence of hip fracture is two to three times higher in women than in men worldwide; however, the 1-year mortality of hip fracture in men is nearly twice that of women.

  d. The incidence of hip fracture is higher in older adults who are institutionalized.

  e. A woman's risk for hip fracture is equal to her combined risk of breast, uterine, and ovarian cancer.

  f. Prompt surgical fixation allows earlier ambulation, which helps to decrease the complications of immobility.

  g. The cause of the hip fracture must be investigated; it may be a sign of an underlying medical problem (e.g., cardiac, neurological, oncological).

  h. Deep vein thrombosis (DVT) is a potential major complication after hip replacement (Brandes, Stulberg, & Chang, 1994).

    1) Pneumatic compression boots should be placed on the client postoperatively and followed by compression stockings.

    2) Prophylactic anticoagulation therapy should be initiated postoperatively (Richter & Deporto, 2005).

2. Vertebral compression fracture (VCF; Tanner, 2003–2004)

  a. Most common complication of osteoporosis

  b. Every year 750,000 VCFs occur in the United States. One-third of these are painful, and the rest are subclinical.

  c. Occurs most often in the midthoracic or thoracolumbar spine

  d. After the first fracture, there is a fivefold higher risk of another vertebral compression fracture.

3. Wrist fracture, usually seen in younger postmenopausal women

4. Balance disturbances as a result of kyphosis and scoliosis

5. Falls resulting from balance disturbances

6. Thoracic fractures

  a. Restrict lung function

  b. Cause digestive problems (Silverman et al., 2001).

F. Client Education (IOF, 2009d, 2009e, 2009l; NOF, 2010a)

1. Ensure a balanced diet with calcium-rich foods and vitamin D and calcium supplements when indicated (IOF, 2009d, 2009e, 2009l).

2. Promote a regular weight-bearing exercise program. Include information on the importance of avoiding activities that twist or compress the spine (Swearingen, 2007a).

3. Decrease or eliminate risk factors (e.g., smoking, consuming caffeine or alcohol).

4. Instruct in home and community safety measures.

5. Evaluate BMD.
6. Maintain a record of the client's height.
7. Discuss with the physician hormone replacement therapy or other osteoporosis medication.
8. Instruct about medications and their management.
9. Inform about community resources such as local osteoporosis support groups and the National Osteoporosis Foundation (www.nof.org).

G. Interventions After Diagnosis
1. Pharmacological management (Alexander, 2009; ICSI, 2008; IOF, 2010d; NAMS, 2010; Oaseem et al., 2008; Post et al., 2010)
   a. Calcium (IOF, 2009d, 2009e)
      1) Adequate calcium intake is essential to achieving optimal peak bone mass (Mayes, 2007; NIH Consensus Development Panel, 1994; NOF, 2010a, 2010b).
      2) Most Americans do not get the recommended daily allowance (RDA) of calcium based on their age and physiological need (Mayes, 2007; Joint Commission & National Pharmaceutical Council, 2008).
      3) Most women do not consume adequate amounts of calcium in their diets after menopause, and therefore their calcium intake must be supplemented (Sweet, Sweet, Jeremiah, & Galazka, 2009).
      4) The absorption of some medications when taken with calcium can be significantly decreased (e.g., levothyroxine, fluoroquinolones, tetracycline, phenytoin, angiotensin-converting inhibitors, iron, and bisphosphonates). They should be taken several hours before or after calcium supplements.
      5) In a prospective study, intake of dietary calcium in children was found to have a positive relationship to BMD in young women (Kanis, 1999; Maunier, 1999).
      6) In several meta-analyses and randomized controlled trials, an association was found between calcium supplementation and a reduction in the risk of fractures among healthy people (Bischoff-Ferrari et al., 2008; Reid, Ames, Evans, Gamble, & Sharpe, 1995; Shea et al., 2002; Tang, Eslick, & Nowson, 2007).
      7) According to the WHO (2003), the relationship between calcium intake and the rate of fractures is still under investigation. However, one study reported that for each additional gram of calcium in the diet, there was a 25% reduction in hip fracture risk (Cumming & Nevitt, 1997).
      8) Calcium and vitamin D are considered the foundation of any prevention or treatment regimen for osteoporosis (Boonen et al., 2006; Larsen, Mosekilde, & Foldspang, 2004; Heaney & Weaver, 2003).
      9) There are many sources of dietary calcium.
         a) Milk, yogurt, cheese, cottage cheese, ice cream, tofu, salmon, broccoli, spinach, kale, eggs, beans, sardines, clams, oysters
         b) Calcium-fortified foods (e.g., cereal)
         c) Supplements (Joint Commission & National Pharmaceutical Council, 2008)
            (i) Calcium carbonate (e.g., Tums), inexpensive and efficient
            (ii) Tricalcium phosphate or calcium citrate (e.g., Os-Cal): Effective alternatives if GI symptoms occur (McClung, 1999)
            (iii) Alkali antacids
         d) Calcium supplementation bioavailability is affected by meals, size of dose, and disintegration of the tablet.
         e) Calcium absorption decreases when doses greater than 600 mg are taken. Therefore calcium supplementation should be taken in divided doses (ICSI, 2008).
   b. Vitamin D is needed for adequate calcium absorption (Dawson-Hughes et al., 2010; IOF, 2009l , 2009m, 2010d; Kimball, Fuleihan, & Vieth, 2008).
      1) Vitamin D plays a major role in
         a) Assisting with the absorption of calcium from food
         b) Ensuring the renewal and mineralization of bone tissue
         c) Promoting a healthy immune system
         d) Promoting muscle strength and health (IOF, 2009e)
         e) Prevention of fractures (Zhu, Austin, Devine, Bruce, & Prince, 2010)
      2) Deficiency occurs when there is inadequate exposure to the sun, inadequate dietary intake, and acquired resistance to vitamin D (NIH Consensus Development Panel, 1994).
      3) As the body ages, a person's skin has less ability to manufacture vitamin D. Therefore, when older adults are exposed to

sunlight, they produce less vitamin D (Joint Commission & National Pharmaceutical Council, 2008).

4) Sensible exposure to sun can provide adequate amounts of vitamin D, which can be stored in body fat and then released in the winter. This can be accomplished with exposure of the arms and legs to sunlight 5–10 minutes daily or 5–30 minutes two times per week between 10 am and 3 pm (Holick, 2007).

5) Deficiency can be corrected by eating foods that are fortified with vitamin D and taking vitamin D supplements (NIH Consensus Development Panel, 1994; NOF, 2010a, 2010b).

6) The NOF (2010a) recommends an intake of 800–1,000 IU of vitamin D per day for adults 50 years of age and older.

7) Studies have shown that treatment with vitamin D reduces the risk of falls in older adults (Bischoff-Ferrari et al., 2004, 2009; Bischoff-Ferrari, Willett, Wong, Giovannucci, Dietrich, & Dawson-Hughes, 2005; IOF, 2010e; Kalyani et al., 2010).

c. Recommended intake of calcium and vitamin D: The Institute of Medicine (2010) has updated the Dietary Recommended Intake of calcium and vitamin D. This recommendation was supported by the NIH Office of Dietary Supplements (NIH, 2011a, 2011b); **Table 13-1**).

d. Bisphosphonates (Bock & Felsenberg, 2008; IOF, 2009b; McClung, 2003; NAMS, 2010; NOF 2010a)

1) Have become the preferred treatment for reducing fractures of the hip and spine in both men and women with involution and glucocorticoid osteoporosis (McClung, 2003)

2) Work by inhibiting the activity of osteoclasts and decreasing their lifespan, which reduces bone resorption (Mayes, 2007; McClung, 2003)

3) The most common side effects are related to upper GI disorders such as esophageal and gastric irritation and dysphagia. Neither of the IV forms has been shown to cause upper GI events in randomized trials.

4) Contraindicated in the oral form for people with a history of esophageal

Table 13-1. Dietary Reference Intake for Calcium and Vitamin D

Life Stage Group	Calcium Estimated Average Requirement (mg/day)	Recommended Dietary Allowance (mg/day)	Upper Level Intake (mg/day)	Vitamin D Estimated Average Requirement (IU/day)	Recommended Dietary Allowance (IU/day)	Upper Level Intake (IU/day)
Infants 0–6 months	*	*	1,000	**	**	1,000
Infants 6–12 months	*	*	1,500	**	**	1,500
1–3 years old	500	700	2,500	400	600	2,500
4–8 years old	800	1,000	2,500	400	600	3,000
9–13 years old	1,100	1,300	3,000	400	600	4,000
14–18 years old	1,100	1,300	3,000	400	600	4,000
19–30 years old	800	1,000	2,500	400	600	4,000
31–50 years old	800	1,000	2,500	400	600	4,000
51–70 year old males	800	1,000	2,000	400	600	4,000
51–70 year old females	1,000	1,200	2,000	400	600	4,000
>70 years old	1,000	1,200	2,000	400	800	4,000
14–18 years old, pregnant/lactating	1,100	1,300	3,000	400	600	4,000
19–50 years old, pregnant/lactating	800	1,000	2,500	400	600	4,000

*For infants, adequate intake is 200 mg/day for 0–6 months of age and 260 mg/day for 6–12 months of age.
**For infants, adequate intake is 400 IU/day for 0–6 months of age and 400 IU/day for 6–12 months of age.
From *Dietary reference intakes for calcium and vitamin D*, by the Institute of Medicine, 2010. Retrieved July 26, 2011, from www.iom.edu/Reports/2010/Dietary-Reference-Intakes-for-Calcium-and-Vitamin-D.aspx. Copyright 2010 by the Institute of Medicine.

THE SPECIALTY PRACTICE OF REHABILITATION NURSING

abnormalities that delay esophageal emptying or in people who are unable to sit or stand upright for at least 30 minutes after taking the oral medication

5) A transient flulike illness referred to as a transient phase reaction has occurred with some people who were taking large doses of oral or intravenous bisphosphonates.

6) Oral tablets are absorbed poorly, with only about 0.5% of the oral dose being absorbed.

7) The oral form must be taken first thing in the morning on an empty stomach with plain water.

8) The person must avoid food, drink, and medications (including supplements) for 30 minutes after taking alendronate and risedronate and for 60 minutes after taking ibandronate.

   a) Alendronate (Fosamax; NOF, 2010a; Saag & Geusens, 2009)

     (i) Approved orally in tablet form for

       (a) Postmenopausal osteoporosis prevention (dosage 5 mg/day or 35 mg/week)

       (b) Treatment of osteoporosis (dosage 10 mg/day or 70 mg/week; Mayes, 2007)

     (ii) Effectiveness of decreasing fracture risk has been validated only in postmenopausal women who have osteoporosis. It has been found to have lesser effects in women without osteoporosis (NAMS, 2010).

     (iii) A significant increase in bone mass has been shown in the lumbar spine, hip, and total body after treatment (Pitocco et al., 2005).

     (iv) Proven to prevent bone resorption, reduce the risk of fractures, and slow the course of disease (Spratto & Woods, 1998; Wells et al., 2008a)

     (v) Special precautions for ingestion are needed (**Figure 13-2**).

   b) Risedronate (Actonel and Actonel with Calcium; NOF, 2010c; Saag & Geusens, 2009)

     (i) Approved in oral form for doses of 5 mg/day, 35 mg/week, 75 mg taken on 2 consecutive days

one time a month, and 150 mg monthly

     (ii) Absorbed in the upper GI tract and reaches maximum absorption within 60 minutes (Mayes, 2007)

     (iii) Approved for the prevention and treatment of osteoporosis in postmenopausal women.

     (iv) Reduction of fracture risk has been shown in several randomized trials (Harris et al., 1999; Wells et al., 2008b).

   c) Ibandronate (Boniva; Chesnut et al., 2000; Delmas et al., 2004; NOF 2010a; Saag & Geusens, 2009)

     (i) Approved in the oral tablet form for 2.5 mg/day or 150 mg/month

     (ii) Approved in the oral form for the prevention and treatment of osteoporosis in women after menopause

     (iii) Also approved for intravenous administration at 3 mg every 3 months for treatment of osteoporosis in women after menopause

   d) Zoledronic acid (Reclast; NOF, 2010a; Saag & Geusens, 2009)

     (i) Approved for the treatment of osteoporosis in women after menopause.

     (ii) Given annually as 5 mg intravenous infusion administered over a period of no fewer than 15 minutes.

     (iii) Intravenous administration every 2 years has been approved in

---

Figure 13-2. Client Education: Precautions for Fosamax Therapy

Instruct the client to take the medication correctly.
- Take on an empty stomach first thing in the morning.
- Take with a full 8 ounces of tap water (not bottled water, coffee, or juice).
- Take with 1,200–1,500 mg of calcium and 400 IU of vitamin D.
- Wait at least 30 minutes before eating or drinking anything, including taking any other medication.
- If possible, wait 60 minutes before eating or drinking to ensure an enhanced absorption of the medication.
- Do not lie down after taking the medication.

Provide information about therapeutic side effects of the medication.

Explain the safety issues for proper storage of the medication.

---

the United States for the prevention of osteoporosis in women after menopause.

e. Selective estrogen receptor modulators (SERMs; nonsteroidal agents that act as estrogen agonists or antagonists and prevent bone loss throughout the body; Gennari, Merlotti, Valleggi, Martini, & Nuti, 2007; IOF, 2010c). SERMs include raloxifene (Evista; Eli Lilly, 2007).

   1) Approved for the prevention and treatment of osteoporosis (Mayes, 2007)

   2) Dosage: 60 mg/day

   3) Has been shown to have beneficial effects on BMD and to decrease bone loss throughout the body

   4) Side effects noted in trials were

      a) Increased risk for venous thromboembolism

      b) Increased risk for stroke in women with a baseline cerebrovascular risk

      c) Increase in vasomotor symptoms and leg cramps

   5) Special precaution: Avoid use in sedentary clients because of blood clot formation risk.

   6) Risk of breast cancer and heart attacks in clients taking raloxifene is under investigation (Mayes, 2007).

f. PTH: An anabolic agent that directly stimulates the osteoblasts' formation of bone, which results in trabecular bone density and connectivity in women with osteoporosis after menopause (IOF, 2010a)

   1) Teriparatide (recombinant human PTH 1-34; FORTEO; Blick, Dhillon, & Keum, 2008; Eli Lily, 2008; NOF, 2010a; Saag & Geusens, 2009) is a synthetic form of PTH.

   2) Recommended daily dose: 20 mcg subcutaneously for a maximum duration of 2 years (Blick, Dhillon, & Keam, 2008; Mauck & Clarke, 2006)

   3) In women with osteoporosis after menopause, it increases BMD and reduces the risk of vertebral and nonvertebral fractures.

   4) Indicated for the treatment of certain postmenopausal women with osteoporosis who are at high risk for fracture (Mauck & Clarke, 2006)

      a) Women with a history of osteoporotic fracture

      b) Women who have multiple risk factors for fracture

      c) Women who have failed or are intolerant of previous osteoporosis therapy, based on physician assessment

g. Calcitonin (Miacalcin) nasal spray (IOF, 2009c; Silverman, 2003)

   1) Indicated for women who are 5 or more years postmenopausal

   2) Has been shown to increase spinal bone mass and reduce the risk of new vertebral fractures (Chesnut et al., 2000; Cranney et al., 2002)

   3) Dosage of 200 IU given by nasal spray in alternating nostrils daily or subcutaneously (Gass & Dawson-Hughes, 2006; Mauck & Clarke, 2006). It should not be given orally because it is a polypeptide hormone that is destroyed in the GI tract (Meiner & Lueckenotte, 2006).

   4) Must be taken with 1,200–1,500 mg calcium and 400 IU of vitamin D (Heaney, 1998; Solomon, 1998)

h. Estrogen replacement therapy (IOF, 2010b)

   1) May consist of estrogen therapy alone or in conjunction with progestin.

   2) Slows the rate of bone turnover, and in all skeletal sites it increases the BMD in postmenopausal women

   3) Is surrounded by controversy related to increased risk for cardiovascular events and endometrial and breast cancer. Should be used only after other treatments have been considered and risks fully explained to the client (Rossouw et al., 2002).

i. Antiresorptive agent: Denosumab (Prolia) is a fully human monoclonal antibody directed against receptor activator for nuclear factor k b ligand (RANKL; Cummings et al., 2009; American College of Rheumatology [ACR], 2010b).

   1) Approved for use in the United States in June 2010 by the FDA for the treatment of postmenopausal women with osteoporosis that are at a high risk for fracture

   2) Interferes with the formation, activation, and survival of osteoclasts

   3) Dosage: 60 mg subcutaneously every 6 months given by a health professional

2. Treatment in men (IOF, 2010e)

a. Treatment for osteoporosis in men is based on the identification of the underlying cause, and treatment is with drugs that are also used in women.

  b. Hypogonadism has been treated with androgen replacement. (Caution should be taken with the use of androgen in older men because of the possible risk of prostate cancer.)

  c. Hydrochlorothiazide has been used to decrease hypercalciuria and may also increase bone density in men.

  d. In men with idiopathic osteoporosis or osteoporosis that is the result of an androgen deficiency, alendronate has demonstrated prevention of bone loss and reduction of fractures.

  e. PTH also increases bone density and reduces bone loss in male osteoporosis.

  f. FORTEO is used to increase bone mass in men who have primary or hypogonadal osteoporosis and are at a high risk for fracture.

    1) Includes men

      a) With a history of osteoporotic fracture

      b) Who have multiple risk factors for fracture

      c) Who have failed or are intolerant to previous osteoporosis therapy, based on physician assessment

    2) The effects of FORTEO on the prevention of fracture risk in men have not been studied (Eli Lilly, 2008).

  g. Selective androgen receptor modulators are being studied and are thought to possibly offer effective treatment for male osteoporosis.

3. Weight-bearing exercise (Gass & Dawson-Hughes, 2006; NOF, 2010a; World Orthopedic Osteoporotic Organization, 2002)

  a. Walk, jog, use a stationary bike, or do progressive or aerobic exercise on a regular basis to promote bone remodeling and increase bone density.

  b. Engage in weight-bearing activities daily and muscle-strengthening activities two to three times a week (Rawlins, 2009).

  c. Limit, as much as possible, any event that may cause prolonged immobilization.

4. Pain management: Manage pain resulting from changes in the musculoskeletal system and compression fractures to allow early and progressive activity.

5. Surgical interventions (HHS, 2004; Lemke, 2005)

  a. Vertebroplasty (Buchbinder et al., 2009; Oshima, Matsuzaki, Tokuhashi, & Okawa, 2010; Shin, Chin, & Yoon, 2009)

    1) Started in 1997 in North America

    2) Transpedicle approach to the vertebral body with the client in the prone position

    3) Small incision with an injection of polymethylmethacrylate, a low-viscosity bone cement, under radiographic guidance

    4) Restoration of vertebral height occurs in 30% of patients.

  b. Kyphoplasty (Chen et al., 2010; Gan et al., 2010; HHS, 2004; Song, Eun, & Oh, 2009)

    1) Similar to vertebroplasty except that a balloon is inserted into the vertebral body to reestablish height of vertebral body

    2) Cement is then injected when the balloon is withdrawn.

    3) Multiple levels can be done, but usually only one or two vertebral bodies are done at one time.

    4) Has ability to restore some vertebral height with deformity correction (Lemke, 2005)

  c. Joint replacements (Bren, 2004; Dheerebdra, Khan, Saeed, & Goddard, 2010)

    1) Hip replacement (AAOS, 2009a)

      a) Total hip replacement

        (i) Cemented total hip replacement: Used to obtain a better fixation of the femoral prosthesis

        (ii) Uncemented total hip replacement: Cementless implants are thought to reduce the chance for infection.

      b) Hip resurfacing: An alternative surgery to total hip replacement for younger patients

    2) Knee replacement

      a) Total knee replacement: Damaged areas of the thighbone, shinbone, and kneecap are removed

      b) Partial knee replacement: Only the damaged parts of the knee are replaced

  d. Complications after surgery (Mudano et al., 2009)

    1) The complication rate after kyphoplasty is 0.4% per patient, compared with 1.2% per patient for vertebroplasty.

    2) The major concern is cement leakage onto the nerve root or into spinal canal.

    3) Some clients have fever and pain related to a reaction to the cement.

    4) These clients are at high risk for future fracture because of the hardness of the

cemented vertebrae compared with the surrounding osteoporotic vertebrae. A 6-month follow-up X ray is recommended to check for additional fractures.

6. Rehabilitation after vertebral fractures (American Medical Association, 2004; Bonner et al., 2003; Pratelli, Cinotti, & Pasquetti, 2010)
    a. Rehabilitation measures are important after vertebral fractures to
        1) Prevent additional fractures
        2) Reduce falls
        3) Improve quality of life
        4) Decrease pain
        5) Decrease risk of DVT
        6) Prevent pressure ulcers
    b. Rehabilitation measures provided
        1) Muscle reeducation
        2) Resistance exercises for strengthening
        3) Exercises to prevent kyphosis

7. Safety issues: Conduct a fall prevention safety assessment, asking the following questions (Mosby Great Performance, 1995, pp. 6–7):
    a. Is there adequate lighting in each room?
    b. Are nightlights placed throughout the house where they are needed?
    c. Are stairways adequately lighted?
    d. Are light switches within reach and easy to use?
    e. If the person uses a wheelchair, can he or she still reach the light switches?
    f. Are you using lights that produce glare?
    g. Have you removed throw rugs that might cause falls?
    h. Do carpets have worn areas or places that have come loose or untacked?
    i. Are floors free of phone and extension cords?
    j. Are walkways clear of clutter, boxes, or low furniture that might cause a fall?
    k. Are there nonskid strips in potentially dangerous areas such as on stairs, on bathroom floors, in front of the toilet, and in the bath or shower?
    l. Are the stairs free of cracks and sagging carpeting?
    m. Are there sturdy railings on both sides of the stairway?
    n. Are carpets low-pile monotone rather than shag?
    o. Does the bathroom have grab bars around the toilet and in the tub or shower, capable of supporting a 250-pound load?
    p. Does the house have heat sources such as radiators and space heaters that may be obstacles for a person using a cane?
    q. Is there a possibility that the person's medications may affect his or her movement, balance, or consciousness?

H. Prevention Strategies (IOF, 2009d, 2009e, 2009l, 2009m; Michigan Quality Improvement Consortium, 2010; NOF, 2010a; Woodhead & Moss, 1988)
    1. Set a goal to have the optimal level of bone mass by the time menopause begins.
    2. Manage diet to take in the RDA of calcium and vitamin D throughout the lifespan.
    3. Exercise and continue an active, healthy lifestyle.
    4. Decrease or eliminate risk factors.
        a. Stop smoking.
        b. Decrease caffeine intake.
        c. Decrease alcohol intake.
        d. Maintain a balanced diet that includes calcium-rich foods and foods fortified with vitamin D.
        e. Limit medications that reduce bone mass.
        f. Maintain an ideal weight.
        g. Prevent falling episodes.
        h. Seek opportunities for daily exposure to sunlight if possible.

I. Research Topics (Siminoski, O'Keeffe, Levesque, Henley, & Brown, 2011; University of Minnesota Research, 2006)
    1. The role of hip protectors in decreasing the risk of hip fracture
    2. Risk factors associated with fractures in postmenopausal women
    3. Recommendations for BMD reporting
    4. Study of osteoporotic fractures and treatment in both men and women
    5. Outcomes of various drug studies, including alendronate, PTH, and raloxifene
    6. Estrogen replacement therapy
    7. Further studies to determine the importance of fracture risk with supplemental calcium intake alone or with vitamin D (Shea et al., 2002)
    8. Effective strategies for interdisciplinary collaboration and research are needed to study exercise in combination with pharmacologic therapy and its effect on BMD and prevention of falls in older adults (Rahmani & Morin, 2009).

II. Arthritis
A. Overview: Arthritis and other rheumatic diseases are the leading cause of disability in the United States (HHS, 2006).
    1. The inflammation of a joint (CDC, 2009a)
    2. Affects connective tissues (e.g., muscle, tendons, bursa, fibrous tissue)

3. A term the public uses to describe pain and stiffness of the musculoskeletal system (sometimes called rheumatism)
4. A medical term that is restricted to rheumatic diseases that involve inflammatory conditions affecting the joints
5. It is most common in adults age 65 years or older; however, people of all ages, including children, are affected, with about two-thirds of the people affected being younger than age 65 (CDC, 2010).
6. Approximately 50 million adults in the United States (22%) reported they have been informed by their doctor that they have some form of arthritis (Arthritis Foundation, 2010b; Cheng et al., 2010). In 2005 50% of adults 65 years of age or older reported having some type of arthritis (Hootman, Bolen, Helmick, & Langmaid, 2006; MMWR, 2006).
7. As a result of the aging of the U.S. population, it is projected that by 2030, 67 million Americans 18 years of age or older will have been diagnosed with arthritis by a doctor and that one in two people will develop knee osteoarthritis (OA) in their lifetime (CDC, 2010).
8. In the United States, arthritis affects
   a. More than 34 million Caucasians
   b. More than 4.5 million African Americans
   c. Approximately 3.1 million Hispanics
   d. An estimated 667,000 Asian/Pacific Islanders
   e. 280,000 American Indians/Alaskan Natives (Hootman & Helmick, 2006)
9. An estimated 28.3 million women and 18.1 million men reported being diagnosed with some form of arthritis (a prevalence for women of 28.3% and men of 18.2%; Hootman et al., 2006).
10. Approximately 294,000 children younger than age 18 have been diagnosed with some form of arthritis, a ratio of 1 in 250 children (Sacks, Helmick, Luo, Ilowik, & Bowyers, 2007).
11. The second leading cause of movement limitation (after heart disease; Benson & Mariano, 1998)
12. The leading cause of absenteeism in the workplace and the second leading reason for disability payments (after mental illness)
13. The total cost attributed to arthritis and other rheumatic conditions in 2003 in the United States was estimated to be $128 billion—1.2% of the gross domestic product—of which $80.8 billion was attributed to direct costs such as medical expenditures and $47 billion to indirect costs such as lost earnings (Yelin et al., 2007).
14. An increasing problem for the aging population in the United States that is putting an increased strain on Medicare
15. Each year arthritis in the United States results in
    a. 36 million visits to ambulatory care
    b. 744,000 hospitalizations
    c. 9,367 deaths
    d. 19 million people with activity limitations (Helmick et al., 2008)

B. Disorders
  1. The term *arthritis* is used to describe more than 100 different diseases and conditions that involve joints, tissues that surround the joints, and connective tissues.
  2. These diseases include RA, OA, fibromyalgia, gouty (metabolic) arthritis, Reiter's syndrome, ankylosing spondylitis, systemic lupus erythematosus, psoriatic arthritis, and many more.
  3. This chapter discusses the following arthritic diseases:
     a. RA
     b. OA
     c. Metabolic arthritis

C. RA
  1. Definition
     a. RA is chronic progressive inflammatory systemic condition that affects and destroys primarily synovial tissue of joints but can also damage muscles, lungs, skin, blood vessels, nerves, and eyes (Kebicz, 2007).
     b. Inflammation is associated with progressive deterioration of the extracellular matrices of bone and cartilage.
     c. Joints affected typically include the following (Walsh, Crotti, Goldring, & Gravallese, 2005):
        1) The metacarpophalangeal and proximal interphalangeal joints of hands and small joints of the feet
        2) Wrists, elbows, shoulders, knees, and ankles
     d. Associated with a symmetric involvement of the peripheral joints
     e. Common symptoms: Fatigue and weight loss
  2. Etiology
     a. Cause remains unknown
     b. Theories
        1) A genetically controlled host immune response to an unknown stimulus (Mercier, 2010b; O'Dell, 2007; Thalgott, LaRocca, & Gardner, 1993)
        2) An infectious microorganism (which has not been isolated)
        3) Genetic predisposition

a) Affects more women than men by a 3:1 ratio

b) Tends to be seen in families with a history of RA

4) Trauma

5) Alteration of the normal peripheral vascular bed by an autonomic influence (Schoen, 2001)

6) Increased stress (emotional and physical), known to cause acute exacerbations

7) Long-term use of steroids (Grossman et al., 2010)

3. Pathophysiology

a. Involvement (O'Dell, 2007; Thalgot et al., 1993)

1) Involves synovial proliferation, joint effusion, and inflammation in the small joints

a) During the inflammation process, immune system cells (i.e., monocytes, T-lymphocytes, B-lymphocytes, and neutrophils) become activated to secrete a variety of chemical substances.

b) The chemicals secreted into the joints stimulate synovial proliferation, which causes fluid accumulation in the joints, cartilage destruction, and bone erosion (Lee & Abramson, 2005).

2) Causes cartilage to erode and be destroyed

3) Pannus is the membrane of inflammatory cells and granulation tissue that covers and erodes the articular cartilage (Schoen, 2001). Ultimately pannus becomes converted to bony tissue, which results in the loss of movement in the joint.

4) Also affected are ligaments, tendons, and the joint capsule, making it impossible to maintain proper alignment and position, which causes deformity.

5) When a generalized osteoporosis develops in these areas, this makes surgical stabilization difficult.

6) Produces fibrous adhesions, bony ankylosis, and uniting of opposing joint surfaces, in the later stages of RA

7) Involves irreversible effects

b. Events involved in pathogenesis of RA (O'Dell, 2007)

1) Synovial tissues are the primary target of the autoimmune response of RA. The reason this happens is unknown.

2) After RA has been initiated, synovial tissues throughout the body become the target of a complex interaction of T cells (lymphocytes that play a role in cell-mediated immunity), B cells (lymphocytes that play a role in humoral immune response), macrophages (white blood cells that engulf foreign substances in response to an attack), and synovial cells.

3) Synovitis (the result of proliferation of the synovial tissues) results in excessive amounts of synovial fluid being produced and, together with pannus (inflamed synovial granulation tissue), infiltrates into the joint and causes destruction of bone and cartilage and stretches or ruptures the joint capsule, tendons, and ligaments.

4) In response, scar tissue forms that occludes the joint spaces, and as a result the fibrous tissue calcifies, which causes alkalosis and immobility of the joint (Sommers, Johnson, & Beery, 2007).

c. Effects of RA on the joint (O'Dell, 2007)

1) Joint destruction

2) Joint inflammation and effusion, particularly in the feet, hands, fingers, wrists, and elbows

3) Redness, swelling, and pain with motion

d. Effects of RA on the body (Arthritis Foundation, 2010d)

1) General: Fatigue, anorexia, weight loss, aching, and stiffness in the morning for >1 hour.

2) Lymph: Enlarged glands.

3) Pulmonary

a) Caplan's syndrome (i.e., rheumatic nodules with cavitation), seen in men (must perform an extensive diagnostic evaluation to distinguish nodules from cancer; Sommers et al., 2007)

b) Pleuritis

c) Interstitial fibrosis

d) Pleural effusion, common in men and usually asymptomatic

e) Interstitial pneumonia

4) Neurologic: Localized neuropathy

a) Foot drop as a result of nerve injury secondary to ischemia, compression, or obstruction of the nerves going to the ankle

b) Peripheral entrapment neuropathy

c) Spinal cord compression, more commonly subluxation of C1–C2

THE SPECIALTY PRACTICE OF REHABILITATION NURSING

5) Ocular: Uveitis, Sjögren's syndrome, scleritis, keratoconjunctivitis sicca (dry eye)
6) Cardiovascular
   a) Fibrous pericarditis in 10% of cases
   b) Cardiomyopathy
   c) Vasculitis, usually in small vessels
   d) Valve disease and valve ring nodules
7) Skin: Thinning
8) Rheumatic nodules may occur.
   a) Present in 20% of cases
   b) Presence is associated with a poor prognosis.
   c) Firm, nontender, oval mass up to 2 cm in diameter
   d) Found in subcutaneous tissue over pressure points (e.g., elbows, sacrum, dorsal surface of the hand)
   e) Found in other areas (e.g., lungs, heart valves, vocal cords, eyes)
9) Bone: Osteopenia
10) Kidney
   a) Amyloidosis
   b) Vasculitis
11) Hematopoietic
   a) Anemia
   b) Thrombocytosis
e. Effects of RA on costs (both direct and indirect)
   1) Direct (Gabriel, Crowson, Campion, & O'Fallon, 1997b)
      a) A study by the Mayo Clinic in 1987 found costs for people with RA averaged $3,802.05 per person/year ($5,753.32 in U.S. 2000 dollars).
      b) Also reported was that people with RA were approximately six times more likely to incur medical expenses than people without RA.
   2) Indirect (Gabriel, Crowson, Campion, & O'Fallon, 1997a)
      a) In 1992 a study of indirect costs and nonmedical expenses showed that for a person with RA the expenses were $2,269/year ($2,784.90 in U.S. 2000 dollars).
      b) Typical work experiences for people with RA and people without tended to result in the following due to illness:
         (1) Change in occupation (3.3% vs. 0%)
         (2) Decreased work hours (12.2% vs. 1.7%)
         (3) Lost job (3.3% vs. 0%)
         (4) Early retirement (26.3% vs. 5.2%)
         (5) Unable to find a job (15.3% vs. 5.2%)
4. Incidence (Arthritis Foundation, 2010d)
   a. About 1.3 million people, or 1% of the U.S. population, have RA (Arthritis Foundation, 2011).
   b. 85%–90% of people with RA have a positive rheumatoid factor (RF).
   c. Affects women more frequently than men, a ratio of 3:1 (Mercier, 2010b)
   d. Affects people of all races
   e. Is not affected by climate
   f. Onset usually occurs between 20 and 50 years of age. Most cases are diagnosed when people are in their 40s.
   g. Can affect older adults: 25% of older adults develop RA with sudden onset when they are affected by another severe disease. In these clients RA is best managed aggressively with disease-modifying antirheumatic drugs.
5. Types of RA
   a. Juvenile idiopathic arthritis (JIA; Beukelman et al., 2011; Jones & Higgins, 2009; Jordan & McDonagh, 2006; National Institute of Arthritis and Musculoskeletal and Skin Diseases [NIAMS], 2008; Southwood, 2008; **Table 13-2**)
      1) A chronic inflammatory condition that has an onset before age 16 years.
      2) Approximately 294,000 children younger than age 18 years are affected by juvenile arthritis (Helmick et al., 2008).
      3) Includes three types of onset, which are classified during the first 6 months of the illness (Cassidy, Petty, Lindsley, & Laxer, 2005; Youngblood & Edwards, 1999)
         a) Systemic onset: 10% of cases with variable number of joints involved
         b) Pauciarticular arthritis: 60% of cases with ≤4 joints involved
         c) Polyarticular onset: 30% of cases with ≥5 joints involved
            (1) RF negative
            (2) RF positive
      4) Clinical aspects vary with onset type.
      5) Affects approximately 1 in 1,000 children
      6) Affects slightly more girls than boys
      7) Is generally mild
   b. Adult RA
6. Classification of RA is based on the 2010 ACR/European League Against Rheumatism (EULAR) criteria (**Table 13**-3; Aletaha et al., 2010).

Table 13-2. Juvenile Arthritis: Onset Types and Clinical Aspects

Systemic onset	Any age; female = male; about 20% of cases
	Recurrent, intermittent fever greater than 103 °F, usually high once or twice each day
	Rheumatoid rash—pale red, nonpruritic, macular on trunk and extremities
	Joint manifestations vary and lag behind systemic symptoms
	Internal organ involvement—liver, spleen, heart
Polyarticular onset RF negative	Females 4:1, any age but peaks 1–3 years and 8–10 years
	Involves four joints or more—wrists, knees, ankles, elbows, feet
	Insidious or precipitated by infection—progression early, tends to get worse over time
	Morning sickness—systemic distribution
Polyarticular onset RF positive	Female, younger than 10 years of age
	Family history
	Clinical features as adult form—more likely to develop severe chronic arthritis
	Fever usually less than 103 °F, rash, anemia, fatigue, anorexia, failure to gain weight
Pauciarticular arthritis	Most common type, females younger than 4 years of age
	Four or less joints; knee most common, also ankles and hips
	Painless swelling, child is walking "funny"
	Few systemic signs—irritable, tired, poor weight gain, chronic eye inflammation

From "Autoimmune and endocrine conditions" (p. 414), by N. M. Youngblood and P. A. Edwards, 1999. In P. A. Edwards, D. L. Hertzberg, S. R. Hays, & N. M. Youngblood (Eds.), *Pediatric rehabilitation nursing*, Philadelphia: W. B. Saunders. Copyright 1999 by P. A. Edwards and N. M. Youngblood. Reprinted with permission. For more information about the onset types and clinical aspects of juvenile arthritis, please visit www.niams.nih.gov/Health_Info/Juv_Arthritis/default.asp#2.

The new ACR/EULAR criteria for the classification of RA have an approach with a specific emphasis on the identification of clients who have a short duration of symptoms that might possibly benefit from early therapy with disease-modifying antirheumatic drugs or might benefit from clinical trials of other new and promising agents that may halt or prevent the development of the disease (Aletaha et al., 2010).

7. Diagnosis (Yurkow & Yudin, 2002; Swearingen, 2007a; Sommers, Johnson, & Beery, 2007)

  a. Thorough history and physical assessment

    1) Assess for fatigue, malaise, and weakness.

    2) Note reports of vague arthralgias, myalgias, joint pain and stiffness, and decreased range of motion (ROM).

    3) Stiffness usually becomes more localized as the disease progresses. Morning stiffness usually last about 1 hour but may last as long as 6 hours.

    4) Note joint size, shape, color, and symmetry.

    5) Assess for presence and history of joint swelling, redness, cyanosis, warmth, tenderness, and a family history of arthritis.

    6) Note shiny, taut skin over the joint.

    7) Assess for muscle atrophy and flexion contractures.

    8) Subluxation in the metatarsal head and hallux valgus (bunion) of the feet may cause a walking disability and pain.

    9) Ulnar deviation; A "zigzag" deformity of the wrist is often noted.

    10) Assess for deformities or fibrous or bony ankylosis.

      a) Spindle-shaped fingers

      b) "Swan neck" deformity, caused by distal interphalangeal joint contracture

      c) "Boutonniere" deformity, caused by contractures of the distal and proximal joints

      d) "Cock-up toes" deformity of the metatarsophalangeal joint

      e) Broadening of the forefoot, clawing of the toes, plantar calluses

    11) Assess for side effects of steroid therapy.

      a) Buffalo hump, moon face

      b) Abdominal distention

      c) Ecchymosis after minimal trauma

      d) Impotence

      e) Amenorrhea

      f) Hypertension

      g) Generalized weakness

      h) Muscle atrophy

    12) Cutaneous nodules over bony prominences

    13) Assess for vascular deficits.

    14) Assess muscle strength and presence of muscle spasm and sensation.

Table 13-3. 2010 ACR/EULAR Classification Criteria for Rheumatoid Arthritis

	Score
Target population (Who should be tested?): Patients who have at least one joint with definite clinical synovitis (swelling)* with the synovitis not better explained by another disease[†]	
Classification criteria for RA (score-based algorithm: Add score of categories A–D; a score of ≥6/10 is needed for classification of a patient as having definite RA)[‡]	
A. Joint involvement[§]	
1 large joint[¶]	0
2–10 large joints	1
1–3 small joints (with or without involvement of large joints)[#]	2
4–10 small joints (with or without involvement of large joints)	3
>10 joints (at least 1 small joint)**	5
B. Serology (at least 1 test result is needed for classification)[††]	
Negative RF **and** negative ACPA	0
Low-positive RF **or** low-positive ACPA	2
High-positive RF **or** high-positive ACPA	3
C. Acute-phase reactants (at least 1 test result is needed for classification)[‡‡]	
Normal CRP **and** normal ESR	0
Abnormal CRP **or** abnormal ESR	1
D. Duration of symptoms[§§]	
<6 weeks	0
≥6 weeks	1

*The criteria are aimed at classification of newly presenting clients. In addition, clients with erosive disease typical of rheumatoid arthritis (RA) with a history compatible with prior fulfillment of the 2010 criteria should be classified as having RA. Clients with long-standing disease, including those whose disease is inactive (with or without treatment) who, based on retrospectively available data, have previously fulfilled the 2010 criteria, should be classified as having RA.

†Differential diagnoses vary between clients with different presentations but may include conditions such as systemic lupus erythematosus, psoriatic arthritis, and gout. If it is unclear which relevant differential diagnoses to consider, an expert rheumatologist should be consulted.

‡Although clients with a score of <6/10 are not classifiable as having RA, their status can be reassessed and the criteria might be fulfilled cumulatively over time.

§Joint involvement refers to any swollen or tender joint on examination, which may be confirmed by imaging evidence of synovitis. Distal interphalangeal joints, first carpometacarpal joints, and first metatarsophalangeal joints are excluded from assessment. Categories of joint distribution are classified according to the location and number of involved joints, with placement into the highest category possible based on the pattern of joint involvement.

¶"Large joints" refers to shoulders, elbows, hips, knees, and ankles.

#"Small joints" refers to the metacarpophalangeal joints, proximal interphalangeal joints, second through fifth metatarsophalangeal joints, thumb interphalangeal joints, and wrists.

**In this category at least one of the involved joints must be a small joint; the other joints can include any combination of large and additional small joints, as well as other joints not specifically listed elsewhere (e.g., temporomandibular, acromioclavicular, sternoclavicular).

††Negative refers to IU values that are less than or equal to the upper limit of normal (ULN) for the laboratory and assay; low-positive refers to IU values that are higher than the ULN but ≤3 times the ULN for the laboratory and assay; high-positive refers to IU values that are >3 times the ULN for the laboratory and assay. Where rheumatoid factor (RF) information is available only as positive or negative, a positive result should be scored as low-positive for RF. ACPA = anti-citrullinated protein antibody.

‡‡Normal/abnormal is determined by local laboratory standards. CRP = C-reactive protein; ESR = erythrocyte sedimentation rate.

§§Duration of symptoms refers to client self-report of the duration of signs or symptoms of synovitis (e.g., pain, swelling, tenderness) of joints that are clinically involved at the time of assessment, regardless of treatment status.

15) Note joint mobility, crepitus, function, and sensation.
16) In children, look for longer, shorter, or larger bones than normal. Inflammation can affect the growth plates in the bones.
17) In children, behavioral and physical changes (Youngblood & Edwards, 1999; Jones & Higgins, 2009)
 a) Irritability

b) Morning stiffness
c) Pain
d) Limping, walking "funny", refusing to walk, or complaining of hip pain when walking
e) Heat and swelling in a joint
f) Unexplained or intermittent rash
g) Muscle weakness associated with rash
h) Altered posture

18) Prolonged or cyclical fevers, unexplained rash or fevers, muscle weakness associated with rash

19) Many children present with painless joint effusions; because these children are able to continue with their normal activities, the diagnosis of JIA may be delayed (Weiss & Ilowite, 2005).

20) Delay in diagnosis has been found to have significant consequences for the child that may include a permanent discrepancy in leg length (Iesaka, Kubiak, Bong, Su, & DiCesare, 2006).

21) Recent trauma or infection

22) In children, changes in facial appearance and dental problems

b. Laboratory studies (Mercier, 2010b; Swearingen, 2007a)

1) Complete blood cell count (CBC): Decreased hemoglobin and hematocrit; elevated white blood cells, especially leukocytes

2) Elevated erythrocyte sedimentation rate: Measures inflammatory process

3) Protein electrophoresis

4) RF: Usually positive

5) Antinuclear antibodies: Elevated titers seen in 10%–20% of clients

6) Increased C-reactive protein (CRP): Increased during acute phase; indicates acute inflammatory process

7) Anticyclic citrullinated peptide auto antibodies: Specific for RA and better predict erosive disease (Mercier, 2010b); seen in 70% of people with RA (O'Dell, 2007)

8) Urinalysis

c. Radiologic studies

1) Early signs

a) Soft-tissue swelling

b) Periarticular osteoporosis

c) New bone formation

d) Subchondral cyst formation

2) Late signs

a) Subchondral erosions

b) Cartilage destruction

c) Narrowing of joint spaces

d) Diffuse osteoporosis

e) Joint deformity

d. Other

1) Arthroscopy: Pale synovium that is hypertrophic

2) Thermograph and bone scan: Bone scan demonstrates changes in synovium

3) Joint aspirations: Synovial fluid is usually opaque with a cloudy yellow appearance, elevated white blood cells are in the range of 5,000–100,000 mm^3, with two-thirds of the cells being polymorphonuclear leukocytes (Mercier, 2010b; O'Dell, 2007). Glucose level is usually lower than serum glucose.

8. Resulting disabilities

a. Deforming contractures of joints

b. Joint instability

c. Spinal cord compression, usually cervical

d. Depression and anxiety

e. Deficits in ADLs and instrumental activities of daily living (IADLs)

f. Mobility deficits

g. Chronic pain

h. Health-related quality of life is significantly impaired due to loss of physical function, pain, and fatigue (Strand & Singh, 2010).

i. JIA is the primary cause of disability in children.

9. Client education (Mäkeläines, Vehviläinen-Julkenen, & Pietilä, 2009; Olubumma, 2009; Sierakowska et al., 2005)

a. What does RA or JIA mean?

b. How will it affect the body?

c. Why me?

d. How is it diagnosed?

e. What causes RA or JIA?

f. Instruct about resources in the community to help the client cope with the effects of RA.

g. Teach coping strategies to deal with pain and limitations of RA.

h. Instruct in techniques and adaptive aids to perform ADLs and other activities.

i. Teach about lifestyle modifications to conserve energy.

j. Instruct the client about medications and the importance of following prescribed regimens.

10. Interventions after diagnosis for early arrest of the disease process

a. Goal: To maintain joint function, prevent deformities, and improve quality of life (Neal-Boylan, 2009)

b. Pharmacologic management (**Table 13-4;** Diaz-Barjon, 2009; Finckh et al., 2009; Gafeo, Saag, & Curtis, 2006; Villa-Blanco & Calvo-Alen, 2009). Baseline blood and urine studies should be performed before these medications are initiated (Mercier, 2010b; Neal-Boylan, 2009; Swearingen, 2007a).

1) Anti-inflammatory agents (Mercier, 2010b)

Table 13-4. Commonly Used Medications to Treat Arthritis Pain

Medication	Brand name	Nursing implication
Traditional NSAIDs	**Prescription:** Anaprox (naproxen sodium) Clinoril (sulindac) Indocin (indomethacin) Lodine (etodolac) Relafen (nabumetone) Voltaren (diclofenac sodium) **OTC:** Advil, Motrin IB, Nuprin (ibuprofen) Aleve (naproxyn sodium) Actron (ketoprofen)	**Side effects:** Gastrointestinal (GI) upset, stomach ulcers; cardiovascular complications; blood counts and liver enzymes; do not take with alcohol or blood thinners; take with food or antacids to reduce GI upset or heartburn
COX-2 inhibitors	Celebrex (celecoxib)	**Most common side effects:** Stomach pain, diarrhea, indigestion, headache; less risk of GI bleeding than with other NSAIDs; do not take with other NSAIDs; may be taken with low-dose aspirin; does not interfere with blood clotting; primary treatment option for patients at risk of GI complications; careful monitoring needed when taken with warfarin, fluconazole, and lithium; risk of stomach ulcers may be increased in those drinking more than three alcoholic beverages per day
OTC Salicylates		
Aspirin	Bayer, Ecotrin, Ascriptin, Excedrin	Take with food; do not take with other NSAIDs; confusion, dizziness, tinnitus are signs of toxicity; with high doses, monitor blood levels; may increase risk of bleeding and stomach ulcers

OTC = over the counter; nonprescription
From "Medications to treat arthritis," by K. L. Mauk, 2006, Oct/Nov, *ARN Network, 23*(5), pp. 7–8. Copyright 2006 by the Association of Rehabilitation Nurses.

a) Salicylates: 1,000–5,000 mg/day (adjusted based on serum salicylate levels)
b) Nonsteroidal anti-inflammatory drugs (NSAIDs; valuable for symptomatic relief of pain; American College of Rheumatology [ACR], 2007): 400–800 mg TID/QID
c) Phenylbutazone (ACR, 2007)
d) Cyclooxygenase-2 inhibitors (e.g., celecoxib; Nakamura et al., 2007): 200–400 mg daily
2) Glucocorticoids: Infrequently used in JA because of their effects on growth (ACR, 2010a)
3) Intraarticular steroids (remission-inducing agents)
   a) Gold salts (Myochrysine; ACR, 2009d): Used to treat RA for more than 70 years
      (i) Decreases pain and swelling and helps to prevent joint damage and disability
      (ii) Two injectable forms of gold, usually given as an intramuscular (IM) weekly injection
         (a) Aurothioglucose (Solganal): The starting dose is usually 10 mg IM the first week, increasing to 25 mg the second week for 2 weeks and then 25–50 mg weekly.
         (b) Sodium thiomalate: The first dose is 10 mg IM weekly, and the following doses are 1 mg/kg of body weight, but not more than 50 mg/week.
      (iii) Auranofin (Ridaura): Oral gold; the starting dose is 6 mg daily or 3 mg two times a day.
      (iv) Effects of gold therapy may take 3–6 months to show signs of improvement.
   b) Hydroxychloroquine (Plaquenil; ACR, 2007, 2009e): Is thought to interfere with communication of cells with the immune system. Dosage is 200–400 mg daily. Symptoms begin to be relieved after 1–2 months of administration of medication.
   c) D-penicillamine (Cuprimine or Depen): 125–100 mg daily
4) Disease-modifying antirheumatic drugs, which are immunosuppressants and decrease swelling and pain in joints, prevent

joint damage and decrease risk of long-term disability. Usually slow-acting drugs that take more than 8 weeks to become effective (Graudal & Jürgens, 2010; Mercier, 2010b; Saag et al., 2008).

- a) Azathioprine (Imuran; ACR, 2009a): 25–150 mg daily
- b) Cyclophosphamide (Cytoxan; ACR, 2009b): 25–150 mg daily (alkylating agent)
- c) Chlorambucil (Leukeran) oral: 0.1–0.2 mg/kg/day
- d) Sulfasalazine (Azulfidine; ACR, 2008): 1,000–1,500 mg BID
- e) Methotrexate (Mexate; PO, IM, IV; ACR, 2009g): 5.0–30 mg per week
- f) Leflunomide (Arava): 10–20 mg daily
- g) Cyclosporine (Sandimmune; ACR, 2009c, 2009f)–Oral: 2.5–5 mg/kg/day

5) Antitumor, necrotizing factor agents (ACR, 2011g; Singh et al., 2009): Tumor necrotizing factor (TNF) is found in the synovial fluid and tissue and has been shown to play a role in the pathology of RA. TNF inhibitors have been shown to inhibit the effects of TNF and prevent inflammation and destruction of joints (Maini, 2004; O'Dell, 2007).

- a) Etanercept (Enbrel): 25–50 mg two times a week subcutaneous
- b) Infliximab (Remicade): 3–10 mg/kg every 4–8 weeks
- c) Adalimumab (Humira): 40 mg every week or every 2 weeks

6) New treatment agents (Mercier, 2010b; Strand & Singh, 2010)

- a) Rituximab (Rituxan; anti-CD20; ACR, 2011d)
- b) Abatacept (Orencia; cytotoxic T-lymphocyte antigen-4 immunoglobulin; ACR, 2011a)
- c) Tocilizumab (Actemra; anti-interleukin-6 receptor; ACR, 2011e; Marti & Scheinberg, 2009; Oldfield, Dhillon, & Plosker, 2009; Oldfield & Plosker, 2009).
- d) Certolizumab pegol (Cimzia)
- e) Golimumab (Simponi)

c. Physical therapy: Encourage participation in an exercise program and use of assistive devices to keep mobile and remain flexible (e.g., hydrotherapy).

1) Rehabilitation therapy is a very important part of the treatment plan.

- a) Goals, early disease
  - (1) Reduce pain and inflammation
  - (2) Prevent muscle atrophy and resulting deformities
  - (3) Improve functional skills
- b) Goals, progressive stage
  - (1) Correct deformities
  - (2) Improve strength and endurance
  - (3) Improve functional skills (Lee & Abramson, 2005)

2) Tai chi (traditional Chinese martial art that combines slow, gentle movements with mental focus) has been shown to improve agility and balance, increase lower-extremity strength and postural balance, and help prevent falls (Arthritis Foundation, 2010d; Uhlig, Fongen, Steen, Christie, & Ødegård, 2010).

d. Occupational therapy: Help make ADLs and IADLs easier by using adaptive aids

e. Splints: Used to give joints rest, correct deformity, and provide physical support to unstable joints

f. Psychological support
1) Antidepressants
2) Support groups

g. Vitamins, minerals, and herbs (e.g., echinacea, ginkgo, St. John's wort)

h. Cartilage matrix enhancers (e.g., glucosamine and chondroitin sulfate)

i. Client education (Mäkeläines, Vehviläinen-Julkenen, & Pietilä, 2009)
1) Choose a treatment regimen.
2) Teach how to incorporate the treatment regimen into life.
3) Manage medication.
4) Teach how to prevent complications.
5) Explain the importance of physical and occupational therapy.
6) Explain how to use assistive devices.
7) Teach joint conservation techniques.
8) Teach energy conservation techniques.
9) Explain what happens if techniques do not work.
10) Teach about coping with disability (Barker & Puckett, 2010).
11) Teach self-management skills (Arthur et al., 2009).

11. Surgical interventions after diagnosis
a. Goals: To relieve pain, stabilize the joint, and correct deformity of the joint
b. Total joint replacement improves joint function

by replacing eroded surfaces with a prosthesis.

    1) Areas include hips, knees, ankles, shoulders, elbows, and phalanges.

    2) Aggressive rehabilitation in acute care, rehabilitation facilities, or subacute care settings is essential to successful outcomes.

    3) For children, joint replacement is delayed as long as possible until bone growth has finished.

c. Osteotomy is performed to correct bone misalignment due to connective tissue defects (Swearingen, 2007a).

d. Arthroscopy may be performed to determine whether joint disease is present and to remove loose bodies and cartilage abrasions.

e. Synovectomy is performed to prevent pannus formation through the removal of synovium that is inflamed.

f. Arthrodesis or fusion of the bony joint is performed to provide stabilization and decrease pain in severely affected joints (Swearingen, 2007a).

g. Laminectomy and spinal fusion for cord compressions

h. Tendon repair (if done within 2 days of rupture)

i. Tenosynovectomies and synovectomies are performed in people with longstanding joint disease with flexion difficulty to decrease pain and to increase hand and finger movement and function.

12. Research topics (Arthritis Foundation, 2010d)

a. Genetic links to RA

b. Long-term effects of biologicals in arthritis

c. Anticyclic citrullinated proteins in RA

d. Use of glucosamine and chondroitin treatment

e. Causes of relapse in JIA

f. Immune cell involvement

g. Treatment parameters that will help the practitioner select the best initial option for each client (O'Dell, 2007)

h. Anakinra use in JIA (ACR, 2011b)

i. Current prevalence and incidence studies

j. Etiology of RA and JIA

k. Causes of and treatment for anemias that accompany chronic inflammatory disease such as JIA in children (NIAMS, 2008)

l. Impact of chronic recurring pain on children and techniques to decrease its impact on their ability to function (NIAMS, 2008)

m. Randomized controlled trials on the long-term effect of medications for arthritis on children (NIAMS, 2008)

D. Osteoarthritis (OA)

1. Definition

a. A progressive, noninflammatory process that affects weight-bearing joints in particular

b. Characterized by degeneration of the articular cartilage at the joint with formation of new bone in the joint space (Meiner & Lueckenotte, 2006)

c. Public health data show that the prevalence, health impact, and economic consequences of OA are expected to increase in the next 2 decades. As a result, the Arthritis Foundation and the CDC joined in 2010 to lead a call to action to develop a national public health agenda for OA, called *A National Public Health Agenda for Osteoarthritis*. This agenda identifies three goals to be accomplished in the next 3–5 years (Arthritis Foundation & CDC, 2010; CDC, 2010).

d. OA involves the following (American Academy of Orthopaedic Surgeons [AAOS], 2007a):

    1) Joints that bear weight (knee, hip, spine)

    2) Joints that are used mainly for work or sports

    3) Joints damaged by fractures or other injuries

2. Etiology

a. Cause remains unknown

b. Contributing risk factors (CDC, 2010; Felson, 2004)

    1) Age

        a) Strongest risk factor but not solely responsible for causing OA

        b) Changes related to aging in cells and tissues may induce development of the disease

    2) Sex: Female

    3) Trauma

        a) Injury to articular cartilage, leaving fragments in the joint, results in degeneration of the cartilage

        b) Recurrent dislocation of the patella

        c) Congenital dislocation of the hip

    4) Obesity: Increases the load on the joints (especially the knee) that causes changes in posture and gait

    5) Lifestyle

        a) Athlete's knee

        b) Dancer's ankle

        c) Tennis elbow

        d) Occupation: Excessive hard labor, mechanical stress, heavy lifting, and repetitive motions such as bending knees

    (1) Men: Often do work such as construction, mechanics, agriculture, blue collar labor, and engineering

    (2) Women: Often do work such as cleaning, agriculture, and small business or retail

6) Intra-articular sepsis

7) Primary diagnoses affecting joints

    a) Hemophilia

    b) Paget's disease

    c) Diabetes mellitus

    d) Charcot-Marie-Tooth disease

8) Menopause

9) Immune response

10) Preexisting joint abnormalities

    a) RA

    b) Legg-Calve-Perthes disease

    c) Avascular necrosis

    d) Structural malalignment, muscle weakness

11) Race: Some Asian populations have a lower risk.

12) Genetic predisposition (Felson, 2004; Meiner & Lueckenotte, 2006; Valdes & Spector, 2009): Approximately 20%–35% of OA of the knee and 50% of OA of the hip and wrist is thought to be genetically determined.

13) Other possible risk factors

    a) Estrogen deficiency: Estrogen replacement therapy may decrease risk of knee and hip OA.

    b) Osteoporosis: Inversely related

    c) Vitamin C, E, and D deficiency

    d) Elevated CRP: Increased risk for OA with higher levels

3. Pathophysiology (Lane & Schnitzer, 2007; Schoen, 2001)

  a. Articular cartilage pits, softens, and frays, losing elasticity and becoming more susceptible to stress damage.

  b. Gradually, full-thickness loss of the articular cartilage occurs, leaving exposed subchondral bone that then goes through a remodeling process.

  c. This bone hypertrophies and forms spurs at the joint margins and at ligaments, tendons, and the joint capsule.

  d. Spurs or osteophytes break off into the joint.

  e. A secondary synovitis occurs later in the process, further affecting the joint's function.

  f. Several cytokines are thought to play a role in the degeneration of cartilage, such as Interleukin-1β, transforming growth factor-β, matrix metalloprotease, and nitric oxide synthesis (Garnero & Delmas, 2003).

  g. With advanced disease, all the cartilage may be destroyed.

4. Incidence (CDC, 2010; National Council on Aging, 2005)

  a. OA is the most common form of arthritis.

  b. The disease may begin when the person is in his or her 20s, but it peaks when the person is in his or her 50s or 60s and levels off at age 80 (Buckwater, Saltzman, & Brown, 2004).

  c. 26.9 million Americans have OA, of whom 13.9% are adults age 25 and older and 33.6% (12.4 million) are adults older than 65 years old (Lawrence et al., 2008).

  d. Each year 632,000 joint replacements are performed as a result of OA (CDC & Arthritis Foundation, 2010).

  e. Incidence rates increase with age but reach a peak at age 80 (Buckwater et al., 2004).

  f. Incidence is higher in Caucasians.

  g. The disease affects women twice as often as men who are older than age 55 (O'Conner, 2007).

    1) The incidence of OA of the knee is 45% lower in men than in women, and the incidence of OA of the hip is 36% lower in men than in women.

    2) The severity of OA of the knee, but not of the hip or hand, is much higher in women than in men (Srinkanth et al., 2005).

  h. Hip, knee, cervical, and lumbosacral joints of the spine and distal and proximal interphalangeal joints are the most frequently involved.

  i. Womens' hands are affected most after menopause.

  j. Lifestyle and occupation may be factors. Job-related OA costs are approximately $3.4–$13.2 billion annually (Buckwater et al., 2004).

  k. Weight gain, lower self-esteem, and loss of sleep may result.

  l. Costs of OA (Maetzel, Li, Pencharz, Tomlinson, & Bombardier, 2004)

    1) $7.9 billion estimated cost in 1997 for hip and knee replacements

    2) The estimated total annual disease cost per person in fiscal year 2000 U.S. dollars was $5,700.

5. Diagnosis (Mercier, 2010a)

  a. History

1) Early stages: Joint stiffness, relieved with activity. The most common symptom is a gradual onset of an aching pain in a joint (Meiner & Lueckenotte, 2006).
2) Later: Pain on movement, relieved with rest
3) Advanced stages
   a) Night pain and pain at rest
   b) Limping
   c) Paresthesias

b. Physical (Altman, Hochberg, Moskowitz, & Schnitzer, 2000; Meiner & Lueckenotte, 2006)
1) Localized symptoms
2) Enlarged joints
3) Decreased ROM
4) Crepitus upon motion (aggravating sound and sensation that can be heard and felt on movement in the affected joints)
5) Joint instability
6) Changes in alignment with flexion deformity
7) Pain on movement
8) Tenderness on palpation
9) Inflammation if present is mild and localized to a specific joint.
10) Degeneration of the structure of the joint may result in
    a) Muscle spasms
    b) Gait changes
    c) Joint disuse
11) Bony enlargements can be seen on the proximal interphalangeal joints, called Bouchard's nodes, and on the distal interphalangeal joints, called Heberden's nodes (Mercier, 2010a).

c. Diagnostic tests
1) Radiologic tests
   a) An X ray of involved joint will not necessarily reflect the severity of clinical symptoms.
   b) Limited in their ability to show non-osseous structures
   c) X rays taken during weight bearing may show deformity.
   d) Radiographs should be performed with the client standing if possible when the knee is involved (Mercier, 2010b).
   e) May show changes such as joint space narrowing, effusions, bone cysts and osteophytes, and subchondral sclerosis (Lane & Schnitzer, 2007)

f) Useful to help exclude other causes of the client's symptoms
2) Other diagnostic studies
   a) Ultrasound and computed tomography: Show more extensive joint detail
   b) Magnetic resonance imaging
      (1) Better visualizes soft tissue and cartilage changes
      (2) More sensitive in identifying soft tissue changes
      (3) Expensive and reserved for evaluating other possible causes of symptoms, such as meniscal tears and tumors (Mercier, 2010a)
3) Laboratory tests
   a) Sedimentation rate: May be minimally elevated
   b) Analysis of synovial fluid after aspiration of the involved joint
   c) CRP (Stumer, Brenner, Koening, & Gunther, 2004).

6. Resulting disabilities (Pollard, Johnston, & Dieppe, 2011)
   a. Pain with rest and movement
   b. Joint contractures
   c. Loss of joint function
   d. Loss of independence
   e. Depression and anxiety

7. Interventions (Altman et al., 2000; Jordan, Arden, & Doherty, 2003)
   a. Goals of treatment (Wilke & Carey, 2009)
      1) Reduce pain.
      2) Protect joints.
      3) Strengthen muscles around affected joints.
      4) Regain joint ROM.
      5) Regain independence with mobility and ADLs.
      6) Lose weight for hip and knee OA if appropriate.
   b. Pharmacological management
      1) Administer early in the morning and before activity.
      2) Acetaminophen (first-line drug for pain management; Michigan Quality Improvement Consortium, 2007)
         a) Recent guidelines to use acetaminophen as initial therapy for OA in addition to nonpharmacological interventions (Zhang et al., 2005)
         b) Effective in OA and associated with fewer adverse reactions than NSAIDs
         c) Treatment must be tailored to the needs of the individual client, taking

into account the severity of symptoms; previous use of acetaminophen; and the client's knowledge, expectations, and preferences.

   d) Caution should be used in clients with hepatic toxicity risk factors (Zhang, Jones, & Doherty, 2004).

  3) NSAIDs: Used for moderate to severe pain both topically and orally. Caution should be taken with the oral form if the client has history of GI bleeding (Lin, Zhang, Jones, & Doherty, 2004; Wegman, Van der Windt, Van Tulder, Stalman, & de Vries, 2004).

  4) COX-2 inhibitors: Celecoxib, Meloxicam (Lane & Schnitzer, 2007; Rosenbaum, O'Mathuna, Chavez, & Shields, 2010)

   a) Specifically inhibits cyclooxygenase-2

   b) Inhibits the inflammatory-mediated production of prostaglandins

   c) More expensive than over-the-counter drugs

   d) Have greater GI safety

   e) Increase risk of cardiovascular events for people with a history of cardiac disease; use with extreme caution in patients with a history of renal and cardiac disease (Maetzel et al., 2004)

  5) Narcotic analgesics: Opioids should be used when nonopioids and nonpharmacologic interventions produce inadequate pain relief (Simon et al., 2002).

  6) Oral corticosteroids

  7) Vitamins and minerals

  8) Oral glucosamine and chondroitin sulfate, 1,500 mg daily (Bruyere & Reginster, 2007; Dahmer & Schiller, 2008; Morris & Smith, 2009)

   a) Appears to relieve pain by an unknown mechanism

   b) Has been demonstrated in several studies to be as effective as acetaminophen and NSAIDs in relieving pain without the side effects

   c) Takes several weeks to take effect but appears to have a sustained effect on pain relief even after discontinuation (Rozendaal et al., 2008; Simon et al., 2002)

 c. Intra-articular (American College of Rheumatology Subcommittee on Osteoarthritis, 2003)

  1) Glucocorticoids: Local intraarticular injection of corticosteroids can produce significant relief of pain and stiffness, with some people reporting long-lasting pain relief (Arroll & Goodyear-Smith, 2004; Godwin & Dawes, 2004).

  2) Viscosupplementation treatments using hyaluronic acid

   a) Used in cases in which OA has not responded to other modalities, but its use is controversial. Routine use is not recommended until further research shows it is definitely beneficial (AAOS, 2009; Lo, LaValley, McAlindon, & Felson, 2003; Wang, Lin, Chang, Lin, & Hou, 2004).

   b) Hyaluronic acid is a naturally occurring substance that is found in the synovial joint fluid. It acts as a lubricant to help the bones move over each other smoothly and is a shock absorber for the joints (AAOS, 2009a).

   c) Approved for use in the United States in 1997

   d) Does not have an immediate pain-relieving effect but does seem to have an anti-inflammatory effect and pain-relieving properties

   e) The injections may also stimulate the body to produce more of its own natural hyaluronic acid.

   f) The long-term effects are not yet known, and more research needs to be continued in this area.

  3) Ultrasound-guided intra-articular viscosupplementation has been shown to be a feasible and safer procedure that provides significant pain relief and functional recovery in younger people with hip osteoarthritis (Migliore et al., 2009; Mulvaney, 2009).

 d. Topical: Aspirin or NSAIDs (ACR Subcommittee on Osteoarthritis, 2003; Mercier, 2010b)

  1) Capsaicin

  2) Methyl salicylate

  3) Alternative to oral medication

  4) Usually reserved for acute flare-ups

  5) Used with more recalcitrant disease

 e. Interdisciplinary approaches (Michigan Quality Improvement Consortium, 2007)

  1) Physical therapy to establish an exercise program

   a) Pool therapy

   b) Home exercise program

c) Assistive devices for ambulation
d) Low-impact, moderate-intensity aerobic physical activity and muscle strengthening exercise (CDC and Arthritis Foundation, 2010)
2) Refer to occupational therapy for devices to assist with maintaining ADLs.
3) Heat and cold applications
4) Splinting or bracing
5) Use of assistive devices
6) Use of transcutaneous electrical nerve stimulation (TENS) for pain reduction
7) Refer to a nutritionist for education and counseling for weight loss if indicated (Simon et al., 2002).
8) Refer to a social worker for social support (Tak, Hong, & Kennedy, 2007).
9) Nontraditional remedies
   a) Meditation
   b) Relaxation exercises
   c) Massage
   d) Biofeedback
f. Surgical interventions
1) Arthroscopy (examination of the interior of a joint with a fiber-optic tube): Performed to remove osteophytes and loose bodies (e.g., particles and fragments of cartilage and bone floating freely in the synovial fluid of the joint; Kirkley et al., 2008)
2) Total joint replacement relieves pain, restores motion, and increases joint stability.
   a) In a total joint replacement, an arthritic or damaged joint is removed and then replaced with an artificial joint, also called a prosthesis (AAOS, 2007b).
   b) Reasons for recommending a total hip replacement include the following (AAOS, 2007b):
      (i) Severe pain that limits everyday activities (walking, climbing stairs, and getting in and out of chairs)
      (ii) Moderate or severe pain in the joint during rest, either day or night
      (iii) Chronic joint inflammation and swelling that does not improve with rest or medications
      (iv) Lack of pain relief from NSAIDs
      (v) Intolerable side effects from pain medications

      (vi) Lack of substantial improvement from other treatments such as cortisone injections, physical therapy, or other surgeries
   b) The joint replacement parts are made of cobalt, chrome, or titanium and smooth, wear-resistant plastic (polyethylene; AAOS, 2007b).
   c) Contraindications to elective surgery
      (i) Acute or chronic infection
      (ii) Major bone loss
      (iii) Poor muscle function
      (iv) History of noncompliance
      (v) Age
      (vi) Malnutrition
      (vii) Bone marrow disease
   d) Postoperative nursing care involves preventing complications, managing pain, and teaching clients how to care for themselves after discharge (Howell, 2007).
   e) Possible complications
      (i) Wound or joint infection with possible prosthesis removal, with extensive intravenous antibiotic therapy and lengthy time before new prosthesis can be used (Anderson & Dale, 1998)
      (ii) Dehiscence of incision line
      (iii) Hematoma
      (iv) DVT or pulmonary embolism
      (v) Neurovascular compromise
      (vi) Dislocation
      (vii) Loosening or fracture of components
      (viii) Wear on components
3) Laminectomy and spinal fusion
4) Arthrodesis: Surgical fusion of the joint
g. Psychological support
8. Trends in total joint replacement
a. Use of critical pathways, which begin 3–4 weeks before surgery and include the following components:
1) Total joint classes to educate the client and coach about what to expect
2) Preoperative therapy session to teach total joint exercises
3) Home evaluation, if necessary, before surgery
4) Preadmission coordination of all equipment and follow-up services
b. Decreased length of stay; on average, 3 days of acute care

c. Discharge with home therapy or outpatient therapy or transfer to a rehabilitation facility or subacute care unit for the remainder of rehabilitation (usually less than 1 week)

9. Client education
   a. What is degenerative joint disease?
   b. How will it affect my body?
   c. Why me?
   d. How is it diagnosed?
   e. What causes it?
   f. How can it be prevented?
   g. Choice of treatment regimen
   h. How to incorporate it into lifestyle
   i. Medication management
   j. Weight reduction
   k. The importance of physical and occupational therapy and assistive devices
   l. Other treatment options
      1) Arthroscopy
      2) Arthroplasty
      3) Arthrodesis
   m. Complications and risks of surgery
   n. Precautions after surgery
   o. Life with an artificial joint
   p. Self-management skills (Arthur et al., 2009)
   q. Ways to prevent disability (Wang, Chern, & Chiou, 2005)

10. Future research
    a. Outcome studies on the use of critical pathways
    b. Improvements in the components used in total joint arthroplasty
    c. Interventions that will better meet the needs of different populations (e.g., ages, ethnic groups)
    d. Measurement of the burden of care for people with arthritis and assessment of ways to improve quality of life
    e. Different strategies to identify other modifiable and nonmodifiable risk factors for the occurrence and progression of the different types of arthritis
    f. Strategies to decrease back pain disability in clients who are socioeconomically vulnerable, including strategies for self-management (CDC, 2010)
    g. Evaluate intervention to reduce the onset and progression of work-related OA.
    h. Evaluate the evidence related to effects of biochemical and mind-body interventions (CDC and Arthritis Foundation, 2010).

E. Metabolic Arthritis (Gout)
   1. Definition: Disturbance in uric acid metabolism in which urate salts are deposited into joints and subcutaneous tissues, associated with hyperuricemia (Choi, Mount, & Reginato, 2005). Historically, gout was thought of as a disease of kings and affluent middle-aged men who ate and drank excessively; however, gout affects all segments of the population (Sunkureddi, Nguyen-Oghalal, & Karnath, 2006).
   2. Etiology
      a. Cause remains unknown
      b. Primary gout results from a genetic defect in purine metabolism and a variation in renal urate transport or upstream regulatory factors, which leads to elevated uric acid production or retention of uric acid (Choi, Atkinson, Karlson, & Curhan, 2005).
      c. Secondary gout
         1) Hydrochlorothiazide and pyrazinamide, which affect urate excretion
         2) Malignant disease, myeloproliferation psoriasis, and sickle-cell anemia may lead to gout because of increased cell turnover, breakdown, or renal dysfunction.
         3) Caused by overindulgence in foods high in protein (e.g., organ meat, shellfish) or alcohol (Choi, Atkinson, Karlson, Willet, & Curhan, 2004b)
   3. Risk factors
      a. Family history in 20% of affected people (O'Dell, 2007)
      b. Overweight or obesity (Choi et al., 2005)
      c. Hypertension
      d. Excessive alcohol intake (beer and spirits more than wine; Choi, Atkinson, Karlson, Willet, & Curhan, 2004a)
      e. Diuretic use (Choi et al., 2004a)
      f. Kidney disease (Baker & Schumacher, 2010)
      g. Intake of fructose in beverages and foods (Bantle, 2009; Choi, Ford, Gao, & Choi, 2008)
   4. Pathophysiology (Teng, Nair, & Saag, 2006; Terkeltaub, 2007)
      a. Four stages of gout (Bieber & Terkeltaub, 2004; Schoen, 2001)
         1) Asymptomatic: Urate levels increase, but no signs or symptoms are present (may last 10–15 years).
         2) Acute attack: First attack is sudden (usually lasts 1–2 weeks).
            a) Involves extreme pain in one or more joints, usually the great toe
            b) Characterized by tissue damage and inflammation
            c) Typically intermittent

3) Intercritical period: Between attacks, symptom free (may last from weeks to years)

4) Chronic gout: Persistent pain and renal dysfunction (this stage usually begins 10 or more years after the first attack)

    a) Tophi: Uric acid crystal lumps found in joints and cartilage (usually the earlobe, fingers, hands, knees, and feet) that lead to the erosion of surrounding tissues, as in RA

    b) Renal tubules: Affected by kidney stone formation

5) Urate crystals directly initiate, amplify, and sustain an acute inflammatory response through their ability to stimulate both synthesis and cellular and humoral inflammatory mediators.

6) Biomarkers such as cytokines, chemokines, proteases, and oxidates are involved in the chronic inflammatory process that leads to effects of chronic gouty synovitis. There is a loss of cartilage and erosion of bone (Choi et al., 2005).

b. Acute inflammation is triggered by an interaction between monosodium urate (MSU) crystals and the local tissue. The cells of the involved tissue react to the deposition of the crystals by phagocytosis, which stimulates a recruitment of inflammatory leucocytes to the site, and their release is the inflammatory mechanism of acute gout (Busso & Alexander, 2010).

5. Incidence

a. Affects approximately 6.1 million Americans (Lawrence et al., 2008)

b. Affects men in 95% of all cases, with the first attack happening after age 30. Prevalence is 2% in men older than 30 years of age, and incidence peaks in the fifth decade of life (Sunkureddi et al., 2006).

c. Affects the foot and great toe in 90% of diagnosed cases

d. Most common form of inflammatory arthritis in men older than age 40 (Baker & Schumacher, 2010)

e. Women may develop gout later in life, and it is more likely to affect the upper extremities. It is rarely seen in premenopausal women (Sunkureddi et al., 2006).

f. Incidence is higher in African-American men than Caucasian men (3.1 vs. 1.8/1,000 person-years; Hochberg et al., 1995)

g. Associated with an increase in healthcare and other economic costs (Wu et al., 2008)

1) The direct burden of care for new cases in the United States is estimated to be $27 million annually (Kim, Schumacher, Hunsche, Wertheimer, & Kong, 2003).

2) People with gout are absent from work more frequently and are less productive (Kleinman & Brook, 2007).

3) Associated with an increase in healthcare utilization and costs in the elderly (Wu et al., 2008)

6. Diagnosis (Teng, Nair, & Saag, 2006)

a. History

1) History of acute rapid development of severe pain and tenderness that develops within 6–12 hours and self-limiting joint pain that is erythematous and swollen (Zhang et al., 2006b)

2) Frequency of attacks and severity and location of symptoms

3) History of podagra (severe pain in the foot, especially that of typical gout in the great toe) and presence of a suspected tophus (a nodular mass of uric acid crystals that are deposited in different soft tissue areas of the body in gout; Baker & Schumacher, 2010)

4) Dietary history (e.g., high protein intake)

5) Assess for history of comorbidities that include features of metabolic syndrome (i.e., obesity, hyperglycemia, hyperlipidemia, and hypertension; Zhang et al., 2006b).

6) In clients diagnosed with gout before the age of 25 years of age and who have a family history of the onset of gout at an early age or have a history or renal stones, a renal uric acid should be tested to assess for overproduction of waste (Baker & Schumacher, 2010).

b. Physical assessment of specific signs and symptoms

1) Red, swollen, deformed, tender, dusky, cyanotic joints, especially in the great toe, ankles, fingers, and wrists

2) Fever and chills

3) Tachycardia, hypertension

4) Headache

5) Joint effusion

6) Severe pain in the joint (during the initial attack the pain is intense, and the joint is sensitive to touch).

7) Decreased ROM

8) Severe back pain

9) Malaise
c. Diagnostic tests
  1) Laboratory tests
     a) Serum uric acid levels: Elevated (Schlesinger, Norquist, & Watson, 2009)
     b) Urinary uric acid levels: Elevated in secondary gout
     c) Urinalysis: Albuminuria
     d) Complete blood count: Leukocytosis
     e) Sedimentation rate: Elevated
     f) MSU crystals to permit definitive diagnosis (Malik, Schumacher, Dinnella, & Clayburne, 2009)
     g) Renal uric acid studies to rule out overproduction of urate in clients with a family history of gout (Baker & Schumacher, 2010)
  2) Radiological examination of the affected joint (useful for a differential diagnosis but not useful to confirm the early or acute diagnosis of gout; Zhang et al., 2006b)
     a) Initially, the joint looks normal.
     b) Later, the joint looks punched out as urate crystals replace bony structures (Crowley, 2004).
     c) Eventually, a narrowing of the joint space is apparent, degenerative arthritic changes occur, and cartilage is destroyed.
  3) Aspiration of synovial fluid: MSU crystals in synovial fluid or tophus aspirate of asymptomatic joints is a definitive diagnosis (Zhang et al., 2006b).
  4) Renal studies determine whether kidneys are affected.
7. Resulting disabilities (Singh & Strand, 2008)
  a. Deformation of the involved joint
  b. Renal dysfunction and calculi
  c. Cardiovascular lesions
  d. Tophus deposits, leading to infection
  e. Thrombosis
  f. Hypertension
  g. Chronic pain
  h. Long-term complications from gout result in a significant decrease in quality of life (Roddy, Zhang, & Doherty, 2007).
8. Interventions (Arthritis Foundation, 2010a; Teng, Nair, & Saag, 2006)
  a. Goals of treatment
     1) Control symptoms.
     2) Terminate acute attacks as promptly as possible.

3) Decrease the frequency of future attacks.
4) Prevent or reverse complications such as obesity, hypertriglyceridemia, hypertension, and alcoholism (Wortmann, 2005).
b. Optimal treatment of gout should include both pharmacological and nonpharmacological therapies (Zhang et al., 2006a).
c. Pharmacological management
  1) Aspirin and acetaminophen for pain management of mild attacks.
  2) NSAIDs: Reduce inflammation caused by deposits of uric acid crystals in the body (Gout & Uric Acid Education Society, 2010; Zhang et al., 2006a)
     a) Indomethacin 50 mg three times daily
     b) Naproxen 500 mg twice daily
     c) Contraindications to be considered
        (1) Renal insufficiency
        (2) Peptic ulcer disease
        (3) GI bleeding
        (4) Severe heart failure
  3) Colchicine 0.6 mg three times daily
     a) Effects are directed against factors responsible for crystal-induced inflammation (Hoskison & Wortmann, 2006).
     b) Prevents or relieves acute attacks
     c) Does not affect uric acid synthesis
     d) Is a prophylactic agent
     e) Is taken at the first sign of an acute attack
     f) Involves side effects
        (1) B_{12} deficiency
        (2) Ongoing diarrhea
        (3) Renal dysfunction (dialysis)
        (4) Abdominal discomfort
     g) Monitor dosage to manage disease process and to decrease number of side effects (Zhang et al., 2006a).
  4) Corticosteroids: Used for inflammation of acute attacks and when NSAIDs and colchicines are contraindicated (Zhang et al., 2006a)
     a) Prednisone 20–60 mg daily
     b) Often preferred for polyarticular gout (Janssens, Janssen, van de Lisdonk, van Riel, & van Weel, 2008)
     c) Shown to be as effective as naproxen 500 mg twice daily
  5) Uricosuric agents: The aim of urate-lowering therapy is to prevent the formation of urate crystals and to promote their dissolution (Zhang et al., 2006a).

a) Probenecid, 250 mg two times a day, to increase kidneys' ability to remove uric acid from the body

b) Sulfinpyrazone, 300–400 mg/day given three or four times a day

c) May be used in clients who are under-excreters of uric acid with otherwise normal renal function

d) Contraindications

   (1) Kidney stones

   (2) Excessive uric acid excretion

   (3) Liver disease

e) Inhibits reabsorption of uric acid

f) Not effective in an acute attack

6) Xanthine oxidase inhibitors

a) Allopurinol: An appropriate long-term urate-lowering drug. Dosage: Start at 100 mg daily and increase by 100 mg every 2–4 weeks if needed to maximum dosage of 800 mg daily. Monitor for renal impairment and allopurinol toxicity.

b) Febuxostat 40–80 mg daily; helps prevent uric acid production by blocking an enzyme that breaks down purines into uric acid

c) Reduces synthesis of uric acid

d) Is not effective in acute attack

e) Increases activity of anticoagulants and hypoglycemics

f) Contraindications

   (1) Previous hypersensitivity

   (2) Abnormal liver function

   (3) Severe renal disease

7) Sodium bicarbonate, citrate solutions: Used to increase urine pH, which increases uric acid excretion by the kidney

d. Dietary guidelines for gout management include the following (Gout & Uric Acid Education Society, 2010):

1) Avoid red meat, shellfish, and alcohol, especially beer; foods that are high in purines (a chemical that can contribute to an elevated uric acid level) can set the stage for an attack of gout that is very painful.

2) Avoid foods with high sugar content that include high-fructose corn syrup, such as soft drinks, fruit juices, and prepackaged baked goods. An increasing amount of evidence associates a diet high in fructose with gout.

3) Eat a healthy, balanced diet including low-fat or nonfat dairy products, nuts, and vegetables.

4) Drink plenty of water (2½–3 L/day to prevent kidney stone formation).

5) Lose weight if overweight.

6) According to Choi, Atkinson, and colleagues (2005), daily consumption of legumes is recommended by the Healthy Eating Pyramid because it provides health benefits and does not increase the risk of gout.

7) Increased vitamin C and coffee intake (more than 4 cups per day) have been shown to moderately increase the excretion of urine uric acid (Choi & Curhan, 2007).

e. Joint protection

f. Pain and symptom management

1) Acute attack

a) Bed rest during episode and until 24 hours after attack

b) Immobilization of affected joint

c) Joint protection

d) Pain management

2) Chronic attack

a) Treat with uricosurics.

b) Increase fluids.

g. Other management techniques

1) Inject corticosteroids into the joint.

2) Intra-articular aspiration of joints: Effective for an acute attack

3) Excise and drain the joint to remove crystals.

4) Use surgery to improve function and decrease deformity.

h. Psychological support

9. Client education

a. Definition of gout

b. Stages of gout

c. Signs and symptoms of gout

d. What to do when you see the signs of gout

e. How to decrease the chances of an attack

f. Medication management: Instruct on importance of lifelong adherence to therapy and how intermittent or discontinued therapy can increase attacks and joint damage.

g. Diet education

1) Importance of weight reduction if client is overweight

2) Diet low in high-purine protein foods

3) Importance of reducing alcohol consumption, especially beer

h. Joint-conservation techniques

10. Future research

a. Additional clinical drug trials to determine the optimal drug dosages and frequency

b. Studies to develop therapeutic approaches to diagnose, treat, and monitor the disease process

c. Optimal drug dosage and duration for prophylactic management of acute attacks

d. Studies to determine the level of serum uric acid that ensures crystal dissolution and cure when administering urate-lowering medications

e. Use of a combination of urate-lowering medications and safety

f. Effectiveness of education programs for lifestyle modifications

g. Management of comorbidities such as hyperlipidemia, hypertension, hyperglycemia, obesity, and smoking (Zhang et al., 2006a)

III. Amputation

A. Overview

1. An amputation is defined as the removal of a limb, a part of the body, or an organ, which is usually a result of a surgical procedure but also can be the result of trauma.

a. The most common reason for amputations in Western countries is a result of peripheral vascular disease (PVD; i.e., lack of blood flow to an extremity) caused by smoking, hypertension, elevated cholesterol levels, inactivity, and uncontrolled diabetes mellitus (Taber, 2005).

b. Other reasons for amputations listed in the literature are crush injuries, electrical shock, severe sepsis, malignant tumors, gangrene, and osteomyelitis.

2. Clients with amputations account for a significant part of the population in most rehabilitation facilities.

3. Loss of a body part is permanent, leaving the person with alterations in mobility and body image and self-care deficits.

4. Rehabilitation interventions are critical for successful adaptation and reintegration into the community.

5. The national health objective for 2010 was to decrease diabetes-related amputations by 40%, from 8.2 per 1,000 people to 4.9 per 1,000 people with diabetes (HHS, 2000). This same objective has been retained in the Healthy People 2020 (2009) proposed objectives. To achieve this goal, regular foot assessments and client education on proper foot care must be stressed long before any problem is noted.

B. Prevention of Amputations

1. Get regular foot assessments by a medical practitioner or podiatrist.

2. Check daily for cracks, sores, and blisters, with prompt medical attention if anything is noted.

3. Cleanse daily with mild soap and water and dry well.

4. Get special care if the person is diabetic.

5. Keep diabetes controlled.

C. Types of Amputation

1. Congenital: Absence of part or all of an extremity at birth

2. Acquired: Loss of part or all of an extremity as a direct result of disease, trauma, or surgery

D. Incidence: In 2007 it was estimated that there were approximately 1.7 million people with limb loss in the United States and that by 2050 this number will double (Amputee Coalition of America [ACA], 2010). The reasons for this estimated prevalence of limb loss by 2050 are the aging of the population, the increased incidence of diabetes mellitus, and the increase in the incidence of PVD (Ziegler-Graham, MacKenzie, Ephraim, Travison, & Brookmeyer, 2008).

1. Age

a. The rate of amputation increases with age.

b. Peak incidence occurs between 41 and 71 years of age; 75% of all amputations occur in people age 65 or older.

2. Sex: The incidence of amputations is higher in men.

3. Race: Among people with diabetes, African Americans have a 1.5:1 to 3.5:1 amputation rate and Hispanic Americans have a 3.6:1 amputation rate compared with Caucasians (Limb Loss Research & Statistics Program, 2006).

4. Type: Lower-extremity amputations usually are related to disease, and upper-extremity amputations usually are related to trauma.

E. Etiology

1. Approximately 185,000 new amputations are performed each year in the United States (ACA, 2008b).

2. Disease-related amputations (American Academy of Physical Medicine and Rehabilitation, 2005)

a. Diabetes mellitus (Refer to Chapter 16 for more information about diabetes.)

1) Diabetes is the leading cause of nontraumatic amputation in the United States, accounting for a majority of all nontraumatic amputations.

2) 50% of these clients are older than age 65 and have vascular, peripheral nerve, cardiac, respiratory, visual, and kidney problems.

b. PVD
   1) Between 1988 and 1996, 80% of clients with amputations had PVD, and 75% had diabetes (Dillingham, Pezzin, & MacKenzie, 2002).
   2) People with diabetes are at higher risk for severe PVD and are five times more likely to have an amputation (Jude, Oyibo, Chalmers, Andrew, & Boulton, 2001).
   3) PVD advances more rapidly in clients with diabetes.
   4) A diabetic client with PVD is unable to form collateral circulation (Spollett, 1998).
   5) Lower-limb amputations account for 97% of all amputations due to PVD (25.8% above knee, 27.6% below knee, and 42.8% at other levels; ACA, 2008b).
   6) At all ages, men and African Americans have the highest risks for an amputation as a result of PVD (Ziegler-Graham et al., 2008).
c. Osteomyelitis
   1) Inflammation of the bone (localized or generalized) caused by a pyrogenic infection
   2) Causes bone destruction, acute pain, and fever
   3) Can be aggravated by diabetes and PVD
d. Gangrene
   1) The death of body tissue, usually associated with a loss of vascular supply and followed by bacterial invasion
   2) Dry gangrene: Common because of the gradual reduction in blood flow to the area
e. Thrombosis: Results from an atherosclerotic event

3. Tumor-related amputations:
   a. Amputations resulting from cancer; 36% of these are of the lower extremity (above or below knee; ACA, 2008a).
   b. There are no notable differences by age or race in the risk for amputations due to cancer (Ziegler-Graham et al., 2008).
   c. Five percent of amputations are caused by sarcomas.
   d. Most common in people 10–20 years of age
   e. No notable differences were found for age or sex (Dillingham et al., 2002)

4. Congenital-related amputations (ACA, 2008a)
   a. Rates among newborn infants with congenital limb anomalies were estimated to be 26/100,000 live births.
   b. Of the newborns with congenital amputation, 58.5% were of the upper limbs (Dillingham et al., 2002).

5. Trauma-related amputations
   a. In a study of trauma-related amputations in the state of Maryland between 1979 and 1993, Dillingham and colleagues (2002) found that the leading causes of amputation were injuries involving the following:
      1) Machinery: 40%
      2) Power tools and appliances: 27.8%
      3) Firearms: 8.5%
      4) Motor vehicle crashes: 8%
   b. They also result from falls, frostbite, electrical shock, explosions, war injuries, burns, and industrial and farm accidents.
   c. They account for 68.8% of upper-extremity amputations and 31% of all amputations (Ziegler-Graham et al., 2008).
   d. Occur more often in men 17–55 years of age
   e. The risk of traumatic amputation for both men and women increases with age and peaks at age 85 (ACA, 2008b).
   f. War-related injuries
      1) Traumatic limb loss involves complex physical and psychological issues.
      2) As of April 2008 it was estimated that there have been more than 900 major limb amputations among U.S. soldiers in Iraq and Afghanistan. This is twice the rate of war-related amputations experienced by military personnel in previous wars (Robbins, Vreeman, Sothmann, Wilson, & Oldridge, 2009).
      3) Predominant causes of war-related injuries are munitions blasts and motor vehicle accidents (ACA, 2008b).
      4) Other war-related injuries include the following (ACA, 2008b):
         a) Open fractures
         b) Damage to soft tissues, arteries, and nerves
         c) Internal bleeding
         d) TBI
         e) Hearing loss
         f) Vision loss
         g) PTSD
      5) Modern munitions have a high kinetic force that can cause extensive injuries to soft tissues and cause complicated wounds that may take a long time to heal.

a) When munitions come into contact with a limb, a complex wound is created, with fragments of the weapon and other debris embedded in the tissue of the wound.

b) The force of the blast may peel away soft tissue and leave the bone exposed, with debris forced into the wound and between the membranes that connect the skin to the muscles (ACA, 2007).

c) As a result of blast injuries, a major complication following amputation is heterotopic ossification (Melcer, Belnap, Walker, Konoske, & Galarneau, 2011; Melcer, Walker, Galarneau, Belnap, & Konoske, 2010). Other complications are phantom pain, mental health problems, and vocational difficulties (Potter, Burns, LaCap, Granville, & Gajewski, 2009).

F. Phases of Amputation Rehabilitation (Meier & Esquenazi, 2004b): From the beginning this process should include not only the surgeon and the prosthetist but also the client and family, the physiatrist, and, when possible, the rehabilitation team. It is important that the client take an integral part in the goal-setting and decision-making process, with the rehabilitation team providing information and recommendations.

1. Preoperative planning for surgery and reconstruction
2. Acute postoperative management
3. Preprosthetic care and management
4. Prescription and fabrication of prosthesis
5. Training in use of prosthesis
6. Reintegration of the client into the community
7. Follow-up management
   a. Physical
   b. Functional
   c. Emotional
   d. Vocational

G. Presurgical Interventions (Department of Veterans Affairs/Department of Defense [VA/DoD], 2008)

1. Obtain a comprehensive baseline assessment of the client's status, including the following:
   a. Medical concerns and comorbidities
   b. Condition of the contralateral limb
   c. Baseline functional abilities
   d. Psychological status
   e. Social environment, home, and community (VA/DoD, 2008)
2. Preamputation treatments
   a. Local treatment of wounds

b. Intravenous antibiotics
c. Debridement procedures
   1) Appropriate dressings
   2) Whirlpool treatment
   3) Surgical debridement
d. Revascularization procedures
e. Hyperbaric oxygen treatments
f. Pain management: Pain must be managed aggressively before the amputation to decrease phantom limb pain after surgery (Beer, 2005).

3. Diagnostic studies (Swearingen, 2007b)
   a. Ankle-arm (ankle-brachial) index (ABI): Used to evaluate PVD. A decrease in the ABI with exercise indicates significant PVD
   b. Doppler ultrasound: Evaluates blood flow to the extremities
   c. Transcutaneous oxygen pressure: Oxygen sensors are placed on the skin, which offers the most accurate assessment of blood supply to the extremities and the best prediction of healing of the residual limb postoperatively.
   d. Angiography: Used to confirm impairment in circulation and to determine the appropriate level for the amputation
   e. Xenon-133: A radioactive isotope is injected intradermally to determine skin clearance, which indicates blood flow to the skin; this is used as another measure to determine the appropriate level for the amputation.

4. Client and family education (Meiner & Lueckenotte, 2006)
   a. What to expect from the preamputation interventions
   b. What happens when conservative treatment fails
   c. What to expect after the amputation
   d. What causes phantom pain
   e. The rehabilitation process
   f. Therapy before surgery (Yetzer, 1996)
      1) Transfer training
      2) Strengthening exercises
      3) Use of assistive devices
   g. The normal grieving process

H. Postoperative Interventions (Pullen, 2010; VA/DoD, 2008)

1. Immediate postoperative nursing care
   a. Assess and monitor vital signs, airway, and breathing.
   b. Check dressing for bleeding at least every 2 hours. Remove dressing every 4–6 hours or according to doctor's orders or policy for the first 2 days and then daily. Assess the surgical site for signs and symptoms of infection, skin

irritation, and skin breakdown. Provide wound care if ordered. Rewrap the residual as directed.

  c. Determine circulation in the residual limb by
    1) Checking color and temperature of skin
    2) Palpating the proximal pulse on the residual limb

  d. Elevate the residual limb to eliminate edema for the first 24–48 hours only, then keep flat and extended.

  e. Turn and position the client every 2 hours side to side to prevent spasms. If ordered and if the client can tolerate it, turn the client prone to help prevent contractures in lower-extremity amputations.

  f. Encourage the client to move the residual limb to prevent stiffness, spasms, contractures, skin breakdown, and thromboembolism.

  g. Adduction exercises of the amputated extremity are recommended after the first 24 hours postoperatively 10 times every 4 hours.

2. Complications after amputation surgery (**Figure 13-3**)

  a. Heterotopic ossification has also been identified as a complication from studies of war-related traumatic amputations, especially as a result of land mine explosions (Melcer et al., 2010).

  b. Other possible postoperative complications (VA/DoD, 2008)
    1) Hemorrhage
    2) Wound dehiscence
    3) Wound infection
    4) Phantom limb pain
    5) Contractures
    6) Abduction deformity
    7) Scar formation

3. Pain management

  a. Acute postoperative pain: Early intervention has been shown to decrease phantom pain the most; the use of epidural analgesia both preoperatively and postoperatively has shown promise (Williams & Deaton, 1997). Immediately postoperatively (24–72 hours), pain medicines should be given on a scheduled basis (Meiner & Lueckenotte, 2006).

  b. Chronic postamputation pain syndromes (Hompland, 2004)
    1) Residual limb pain: A chronic pain localized in the residual limb that occurs after surgical or traumatic amputation
      a) Thought to be caused by the stimulation of peripheral nociceptors and their sensory fibers

Figure 13-3. Potential Complications After Amputation Surgery

Pressure ulcers and skin breakdown (e.g., buttocks, heels)

Nonhealing surgical incisions necessitating revision surgery healing by secondary intention

Infection

Osteomyelitis

Gangrene

Falls without injury

Falls with injuries (e.g., fractures, dehiscence of incision)

Postoperative confusion related to anesthesia, medication, sepsis

Altered mental status, which can worsen dementia, Alzheimer's disease

Depression, anxiety, fear, and adjustment disorders

Embolism (e.g., pulmonary embolism, deep vein thrombosis)

Heart attack or stroke

Diabetic reactions

Flexion contracture

Deconditioning secondary to decreased mobility before surgery

      b) Pain usually resolves during 4–6 weeks postoperatively but it may continue longer.

      c) The primary cause of pain is a prosthesis that does not fit properly, but other causes or types are ischemia of the residual limb, infection, bone spurs, sympathogenic pain, neuromas, and referred pain.

      d) Treatment should be directed toward the mechanism that is causing the pain or symptoms experienced.

      e) Pharmacological therapies
        (1) Nonnarcotic analgesics
        (2) Muscle relaxants
        (3) Antidepressants
        (4) Anticonvulsants
        (5) Local anesthetics
        (6) Hormonal therapy
        (7) Vasodilators
        (8) Beta blockers
        (9) Opioids

      f) Physical therapy
        (1) Heat or cold therapy
        (2) Ultrasound
        (3) TENS
        (4) Massage and desensitization

    2) Phantom sensation: Sensory perceptions that are thought to occur in all people

with amputations (Bang & Jung, 2008)

  a) Thought to fade during the first year after amputation but may last indefinitely or may recur

  b) Some common triggers include residual limb stimulation; feeling happy, cheerful, or frightened; not wearing the prosthesis; and loud noises (Sherman & Sherman, 1985).

  c) It is more likely to occur in the dominant extremity than the nondominant extremity, presumably because of the more intricate neural interconnections of the dominant extremity (Livingston, 1945).

3) Phantom limb pain: Painful sensation that is perceived in a part of the body that is no longer present as the result of a surgical or traumatic removal (Bang & Jung, 2008)

  a) Pain intensity and quality vary between clients from mild to severe.

  b) Pain may completely disrupt the client's ability to function and quality of life.

  c) There is no difference in occurrence related to age or gender of the client or level, side, or etiology of the amputation.

  d) Occurs to some extent in all amputees

  e) Many theories but no known cure

  f) Reported to be related to the following (Bang & Jung, 2008):

    (i) Residual limb pain

    (ii) Physical activity

    (iii) The severity and length of time the person had pain before the amputation

    (iv) Intraoperative stimuli such as pain caused by cutting of tissues

    (v) Pain postoperatively

    (vi) Bilateral extremity amputations

    (vii) Amputation of the lower extremity

  g) Symptoms (Bang & Jung, 2008)

    (i) Worse immediately postoperatively and described as similar to presurgical pain

    (ii) Not static but changes in quality over the years

    (iii) Usually intermittent, but some patients report constant pain

    (iv) Usually localized in the distal parts of the absent limb

    (v) Pain is often described as tingling, throbbing, aching, feeling of pins and needles, knifelike, squeezing, shooting, or cramping.

    (vi) Triggered or worsened by

      (a) Physical stimuli

        1. Change in weather

        2. Use of prosthesis

        3. Bowel and bladder elimination

        4. Muscle tension

      (b) Psychosocial stimuli such as attention

      (c) Emotional stimuli

        1. Stress

        2. Anxiety

  h) Treatment

    (i) Medications

      (a) Anticonvulsants such as carbamazepine, gabapentin, topiramate, and lamotrigine (Harden et al., 2005) were shown to be effective in one study, but in another they did not provide strong pain relief (Smith et al., 2005). Further double-blind studies must be performed (Bone, Critchley, & Buggy, 2002).

      (b) Antidepressants such as amitriptyline have been shown to be effective in some clients (Wilder-Smith, Hill, & Laurent, 2005).

      (c) The use of an analgesic such as tramadol has been shown to be effective (Bang & Jung, 2008).

      (d) A beta blocker (propranolol) can be used to control constant dull ache because it increases serotonin levels and as a result decreases pain transmission to the brain (Swearingen, 2007b).

      (e) Other medications such as topical capsaicin, NSAIDs, and botulinum have been shown to be effective, but additional studies are needed (Jin, Kollewe, Krampfi, Dengler, & Mohammadi, 2008;

Kern, Martin, Scheicher, & Muller, 2004).

(ii) Rehabilitation

    (a) TENS, sensory discrimination, and tactile stimulation have been reported to reduce phantom limb pain.

    (b) Use of myoelectric prosthesis that provides sensory, visual, and motor feedback has been reported to reduce phantom limb pain.

(iii) Desensitization: Believed to decrease pain in the residual limb. It is also thought to help the person with an amputation adjust to a change in body image that includes the loss of a limb (VA/DoD, 2008).

    (a) Tap the distal aspect.

    (b) Rub the distal aspect.

    (c) Stroke the distal aspect.

    (d) Gently massage the proximal residual limb.

(iv) Eye movement desensitization and reprocessing (de Roos et al., 2010; Russell, 2008; Silver, Rogers, & Russell, 2008)

    (a) A psychotherapeutic approach based on the theory that psychopathology often is the result of a traumatic experience of disturbing life events that the person has been unable to integrate within the central nervous system

    (b) Involves activating components of a traumatic experience or disturbing life event and pairing them with alternating bilateral or dual attention stimulation

(v) Psychological: Relaxation techniques, stress management, distraction, and hypnosis have been shown to be helpful.

(vi) Anesthetic: For intractable pain, regional anesthesia, nerve blocks, and sympathetic blocks are helpful.

(vii) Surgical: Generally not recommended except for neuroma resection in selected patents with residual limb pain due to a neuroma (Bang & Jung, 2008)

4. Contracture prevention (VA/DoD, 2008)

  a. Goal: to keep the joint above the site of the amputation in full extension to allow a more functional gait

  b. Lying in prone position

    1) Stretches the hip muscles into full extension

    2) Usually done three or four times a day for 20 minutes each time

    3) Counteracts decreased mobility and increased chair dependency

  c. Knee extension

    1) Prevents contracture of the knee joint and allows a more functional gait

      a) Some surgeons cast the extremity immediately after surgery to decrease the chance of a flexion contracture. A disadvantage of this method is that the surgical incision cannot be examined.

      b) Removable rigid dressing can be used to prevent contractures and can be removed for limb inspection and care.

      c) Some surgeons place a knee immobilizer over the top of the surgical dressing. A benefit of this method is that wound checks can be done.

      d) Exercises to strengthen the quadriceps and gluteal muscles may be ordered.

      e) Encourage the client to perform active ROM if able; if not, assist with passive ROM.

    2) Splints, boards, and wheelchair extensions attempt to keep the limb in extension and allow for wound checks.

  d. Elbow extension: Usually done with a splint made specifically for the client

5. Psychological support (VA/DoD, 2008)

  a. Allow the client to grieve at his or her own pace.

  b. Watch for signs of disturbance. Along with the physical discomfort, psychological distress has been cited as a major reason for nonuse of the prosthesis (Butler, Turkal, & Seidl, 1992).

    1) Refusal to look at or touch residual limb

    2) Unwillingness to discuss predicted limitations or use of prosthesis

    3) Refusal to participate in self-care

    4) Social withdrawal

  c. Make referrals to a psychologist or social worker to help the client adjust to a potential change in lifestyle.

  d. Refer to an amputee support group.

6. Therapy (VA/DoD, 2008)
   a. Transfer training
      1) Standing pivot transfers
      2) Sliding board transfers
   b. Ambulation training
      1) Use of parallel bars, progressing to a walker
      2) Balance training (sitting and standing)
   c. Preprosthetic training
      1) Teach the client to function at the wheelchair level.
      2) Condition the residual limb.
      3) Practice ROM exercises.
      4) Review safety and fall prevention with the client and family.
   d. Deconditioning and strengthening exercises for the entire body
   e. Functional activity training
   f. Prosthetic evaluation and recommendation
7. Wound management
   a. For clients with immediate postoperative casting, monitor for the following:
      1) Signs of increased edema, drainage, and odor
      2) Lack of pulse in the next joint proximally
   b. For clients without casting, monitor for the following:
      1) Dehiscence
      2) Nonhealing
      3) Infection
      4) Progressive gangrene
      5) Lack of pulse in the next joint proximally
   c. For clients with residual limb edema
      1) Decrease pain and prepare the limb for prosthetic fitting.
      2) Use appropriate methods of shrinkage and bandaging (**Figure 13-4**).
         a) Ace wrap: Rewrap the limb every 3–4 hours.
         b) Residual limb (stump) shrinker: Remove every 3–4 hours to assess the incision line. Shrinkers should be washed daily, so two are needed.
         c) Jobst compression boot: Use for 20 minutes three or four times a day along with an ace wrap or shrinker.
         d) Elevation: Do not allow the limb to hang down for extended periods of time.
   d. Open amputation postoperatively
      1) Closure will be staged at a later time
      2) This procedure is performed for wounds that are contaminated with infection and when amputation is related to trauma.
         3) The wound is left open to allow wound drainage and cleansing (VA/DoD, 2008).
I. Prosthetic Management: A prosthesis is a device that artificially replaces a missing body part or extremity such as an artificial extremity (Taber, 2005).
   1. A prosthesis is designed to be functional, cosmetic, or both.
   2. Develop a wearing schedule.
      a. Usually start with 2 hours on, 2 hours off, one or two times a day when sitting
      b. Perform a prewearing and postwearing skin check, looking for areas of redness, irritation, or skin breakdown, which means the adjustment is needed.
      c. If there is an open wound on an amputated limb, the client should not wear the prosthesis until the wound is healed.
   3. Increase wearing times as tolerated.
   4. The client may need to use numerous prostheses over the long term for specific needs related to work, school, home, sports, and leisure activities and growth of a child
   5. Provide prosthetic care before donning the prosthesis.
      a. Check the prosthesis for mechanical stability.
      b. Wipe it off with a damp cloth daily.
      c. Wipe out the socket daily and allow it to dry before donning the prosthesis.
      d. Apply clean, dry socks to the residual limb.
         1) Sock thickness depends on the amount of shrinkage of the limb.
         2) Need several socks of different thicknesses so worn socks can be washed daily
         3) A weight loss or gain of as little as 5 pounds can affect prosthesis fit and function.
   6. Proper foot care of remaining foot to prevent amputation
J. Follow-Up Care After Discharge (Meier & Esquenazi, 2004a): Plan for care on an outpatient basis to plan and assess for
   1. Prosthesis fitting, use, and modifications
   2. Skin care and assessment
   3. Pain status and management
   4. Emotional status
      a. Assess for emotional deterioration. This is often seen after the person is fitted with a prosthesis, training is completed, and the person returns to family and community.
      b. Look for evidence of
         1) Anxiety
         2) Depression
         3) Sleep pattern interruption
         4) Appetite changes

Figure 13-4. Wrapping a Residual Limb

Stump Wrapping

Below-the-Knee Stump

Wrapping the stump with an ace wrap shapes and shrinks the stump to prepare it for the prosthesis. The ace wrap is to be worn at all times, day and night, except during bathing or when wearing the prosthesis.

The ace wrap will need to be reapplied four to five times during waking hours to maintain an even pressure. The pressure should be greater at the end of the stump. Follow the steps as shown.

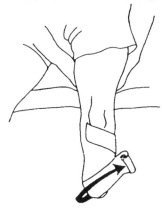

1 To prevent constriction of circulation, all turns must be on the diagonal. Anchor the wrap.

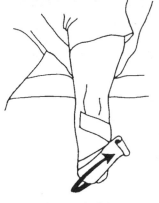

2 Cover the end of the stump at least three times using figure-of-eight turns.

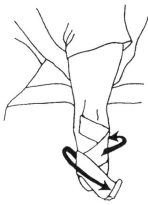

3 Maintain an even tension on the ace wrap. It should be snug, but not tight.

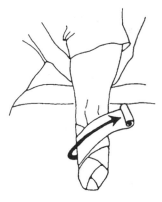

4 Continue up the leg, using figure-of-eight turns. Decrease the tension on the ace wrap as you wrap toward the thigh.

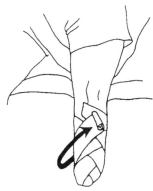

5 Continue wrapping up the leg. The knee can be included in the wrap as a reminder to keep the knee straight.

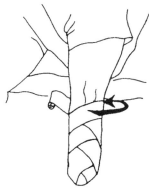

6 If the wrap is extended above the knee, there should be one turn above the knee cap. Do not put excessive pressure on the popliteal area behind the knee as this will decrease the circulation to the leg.

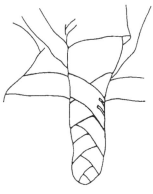

7 Bring the wrap back below the knee, continuing with diagonal turns. Anchor the wrap with tape. Do not use pins as this could injure the skin.

continued

Figure 13-4. Wrapping a Residual Limb *continued*

Stump Wrapping

Above-the-Knee Stump

Wrapping the stump with an ace wrap shapes and shrinks the stump to prepare it for the prosthesis. The ace wrap is to be worn at all times, day and night, except during bathing or when wearing the prosthesis.

The ace wrap will need to be reapplied four to five times during waking hours to maintain an even pressure. The pressure should be greater at the end of the stump. Follow the steps as shown.

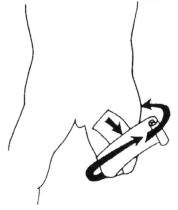

1 To prevent constriction of circulation, all turns must be on the diagonal. Cover the end of the stump well.

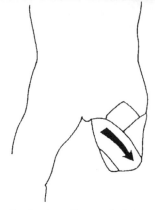

2 Continue figure-of-eight turns to bring the wrap well up into the groin area to prevent adductor muscle from forming roll over bandage.

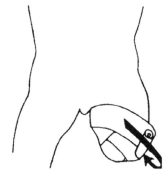

3 Maintain an even tension on the ace wrap. It should be snug, but not tight, on the end of the stump.

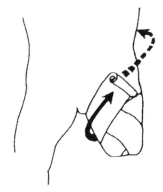

4 The wrap can be finished at this point, or a turn can be taken around the hip to anchor the wrap.

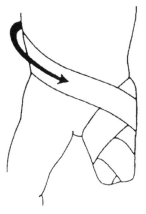

5 Bring the wrap behind the body at the level of the iliac crest. The wrap should not be tight where they cross.

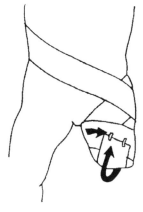

6 Finish the wrap with diagonal turns around the stump. Anchor the wrap with tape. Do not use pins as this could injure the skin.

From "Helping the patient through the experience of an amputation," by E. A. Yetzer, 1996, *Orthapaedic Nursing, 15*(6), pp. 46–47. Copyright 1996 by Lippincott Williams & Wilkins. Reprinted with permission.

K. Results of Disability
   1. Upper-extremity limb loss leaves a client with a complex set of problems. The hand functions in many activities as a sensory organ and a means of communication. Any loss interferes with the client's ability to be productive, feel complete, and interact with environment (Bennett & Alexander, 2004).
   2. Unresolved or chronic pain
   3. Skin breakdown
   4. Unresolved emotional or psychological issues
   5. Contractures
   6. Need for assistance with application and removal of prosthesis or assistive device
   7. Need for vocational training
L. Client Education (VA/DoD, 2008)
   1. Proper foot care
   2. Proper application of external compression devices (e.g., Ace wraps, shrinkers)
   3. Adjustment of prosthetic sock ply for limb volume change as appropriate
   4. Skin care of residual limb
   5. Inspection of the residual limb for signs of pressure or skin irritation
   6. Safe transfers and mobility
   7. Use of assistive devices
   8. Care of prosthetic device
   9. Alternative techniques for pain relief
   10. Donning and doffing techniques
   11. Medication management
   12. Discharge planning
   13. Provide information on resources (McFarlane, Choppa, Betz, Pruden, & Reiber, 2010)
M. Geriatric Considerations
   1. Many amputees are older than age 65, and aging can affect their rehabilitation.
   2. Dual diagnoses and rehabilitation problems are common in this population (Edelstein, 1992).
      a. Cardiopulmonary capacity
      b. Poor neuromuscular coordination
      c. Visual impairments
      d. Weakened musculature
      e. Limited ROM
N. Research Topics
   1. The causes of phantom limb pain and phantom sensations (Davis, 1993)
   2. Preoperative education and pain management's effects on outcomes after surgery (Jahangiri, Jayatunga, Bradley, & Dark, 1994)
   3. Client outcome studies: Inpatient rehabilitation, home care, and outpatient rehabilitation, which helps the client become more functional faster

   4. More double-blind studies to determine the best medication to manage residual limb pain and prosthetic limb pain

IV. **Nursing Diagnoses Associated with Musculoskeletal Disorders**
   A. Overview
      1. Rehabilitation nurses work in many settings: acute care hospitals, rehabilitation hospitals, home care, schools, long-term care facilities, ambulatory care centers, and insurance companies.
      2. Nearly every rehabilitation nurse will someday care for a person with musculoskeletal and orthopedic disorders, no matter what practice setting he or she works in.
      3. As the population ages, nurses will see more clients with these chronic illnesses in everyday practice.
   B. Assessment
      1. Thorough health history
      2. Thorough physical examination
      3. Functional assessment, focusing on the musculoskeletal and neuromuscular systems
      4. Psychological assessment (Bulechek, Butcher, & Dochterman, 2008; Moorehead, Johnson, Maas, & Swanson, 2008).
   C. Nursing Diagnoses and Plans of Care (Ulrich & Canale, 2005)
      1. Impaired physical mobility (**Table 13-5**): Adjust for the client's age, physical ability, and support systems available for assistance.
         a. Related to
            1) Lower-extremity joint stiffness
            2) Contracture or joint or limb deformity
            3) Loss of one or more extremities
            4) Decreased muscle strength or endurance
            5) Altered sense of balance
            6) Pain or discomfort (both acute and chronic)
            7) Activity intolerance or fatigue
            8) Surgical procedure
         b. Outcomes
            1) The client will demonstrate improved ability to move in a designated environment independently or with an assistive device.
            2) The client will demonstrate the safe use of assistive devices or a prosthesis for ambulation.
         c. Interventions
            1) Refer to physical therapy and encourage and facilitate ambulation and other ADLs when possible.
            2) Provide the client with positive support during the activity and allow the client to perform the activity at his or her own rate.

Table 13-5. Nursing Plan of Care: Impaired Physical Mobility

Related to the following:
- Limited movement ability
- Activity restrictions
- Need to use assistive devices
- Need for assistance for ambulation and transfers
- Intolerance to activity
- Pain and discomfort
- Limited strength

Goals	Interventions
Demonstrate optimal independence in mobility skills and activities of daily living (ADLs).	Teach safe use of assistive devices (e.g., walkers, canes).
	Encourage participation in self-care tasks with or without assistive devices.
	Consult a physical therapist (PT) and occupational therapist (OT) for a prescribed exercise program.
	Encourage participation in recreational activities and community outings.
	Teach home safety and fall prevention.
Help the client and family with activity restrictions.	Determine prescribed activity education restrictions and length of the restrictions.
	Educate client and family about why restrictions are needed.
	Teach the client and family how to maintain restrictions in real-life situations.
	Educate the client and family on what to do if restrictions are broken (e.g., notify the physician).
Improve tolerance to activity.	Encourage the use of assistive devices.
	Provide adequate rest periods between activities.
	Teach ways to combine activities.
	Teach the client to pace activities to allow for rest periods.
	Encourage compliance with the exercise program created by PT and OT.
	Educate about the need to adapt the environment to maximize independence.
Manage pain.	Teach about prescribed pain medications and the best times to take them.
	Provide nonpharmacological options for pain management (e.g., heat, ice).
	Provide comfort measures.
	Educate about the need to stay active to avoid further complications of deconditioning.

Expected Outcomes

Maintain a level of independence with mobility and ADLs.

Understand and adhere to activity restrictions as prescribed.

Report improved tolerance to activity.

Report an effective pain-management program.

Maintain safety precautions with all activities.

3) Turn and position the client every 2 hours or as appropriate and maintain body and extremities in proper alignment using pillows, wedges, prefabricated splints, and other supports.
4) Encourage the appropriate use of assistive devices.
5) Teach good body mechanics and encourage the client to maintain.
6) Encourage the client to use a continuous passive motion machine if ordered.

2. Knowledge deficit (**Table 13-6**)
   a. Adjust based on the following factors:
      1) Client's diagnosis
      2) Prior knowledge about the disease
      3) Age of the client
      4) Educational level
   b. Related to
      1) Disease process and management
      2) Pain management
      3) Weight management
      4) Exercise techniques and tolerance
      5) Medications
      6) Identified skills
      7) Surgical procedures and expectations
   c. Outcomes

Table 13-6. Nursing Plan of Care: Knowledge Deficit

Related to the following:
- Chronic illness diagnosis
- Prescribed treatment regimen
- Possible complications

Goals	Interventions
Verbalize an understanding about the diagnosis and prescribed treatment plan.	Teach client and family about the diagnosis.
	• What does the diagnosis mean?
	• How will it affect the body?
	• Why me?
	• How is it diagnosed?
	• What causes the disease?
	• What does the future look like?
	Explain the treatment options presented by the physician.
	Teach the specifics of the treatment plan.
	• Medication management
	• Nutritional management
	• Activity restrictions, use of assistive devices, need for regular exercise
	• Consult physical or occupational therapy regarding an exercise program
	• Encourage proper health maintenance (e.g., eye exams, foot assessments)
	• Community resources available
	• The importance of complying with the treatment plan
	Tailor information to the client's and family's educational level.
	Integrate cultural and religious differences.
	Be creative when presenting information.
	Use age-appropriate education principles.
	Progress from simple to complex topics.
	Repeat information to reinforce learning.
	Provide written information if possible.
Verbalize an understanding of possible complications and what to do about them.	Offer information frequently about complications associated with the diagnosis.
	Teach the client and family what to do if signs and symptoms develop.
	Teach the consequences of complications that are not addressed in a timely manner.
Verbalize an understanding of the disease process and what the future may hold.	Explain the natural progression of the disease.
	Describe treatment changes that may occur as the result of the disease progression (e.g., more aggressive medications, surgical procedures, need for more assistance with mobility and ADLs).
	Describe possible comorbidities that may occur as a result of the disease.

Expected Outcomes

Actively participate in the prescribed treatment plan.

Understand the disease condition and possible complications and comorbidities.

Know what to do if signs and symptoms of complications arise.

---

1) The client verbalizes an understanding of the disease process and management, medications, pain management, weight management, exercise techniques and tolerance, skills, and surgical procedures as appropriate.
2) The client will demonstrate incorporation of appropriate lifestyle changes and diet modifications to decrease effects of the disease process (e.g., weight loss, decreased alcohol intake, and smoking cessation).

d. Interventions
1) Provide information in several forms (e.g., verbal [individual or in classes], written, videos, and apps on iPhones as developed) as appropriate and at numerous times.
2) Provide a quiet, respectful atmosphere without interruption that is conducive to learning.
3) Allow the learner to identify the most important content for him or her to learn.

4) Provide information-seeking opportunities and support for self-directed learning.

5) Allow time for the learner to express feelings and attitudes about changes.

6) Provide the client or learner the opportunity to apply information learned in daily care.

7) Instruct the client about a well-balanced diet related to maintaining proper weight.

8) Teach about the need to supplement diet with calcium and vitamin D as appropriate.

9) Discuss with the client the importance of drinking 2½–4 liters of fluid daily.

10) If appropriate, teach to avoid foods high in purine and provide a list of other protein foods low in purine to use as substitutes.

11) Teach the client about the need to perform adduction and extension exercises 24 hours postamputation and help the client perform exercises.

12) Provide the client and family with information on where and how to purchase needed equipment and supplies.

13) Inform the client about different prosthetic options.

14) Teach the client and family correct technique to perform residual extremity Ace wrapping after amputation.

15) Teach the client and family about phantom pain and sensation and their causes.

16) Teach the client about treatment regimens, including physical and occupational therapy exercises, principles of joint protection, and other modalities.

17) Provide information on medications and supplements including name, dosage, schedule, precautions, and potential side effects (Kleoppel & Henry, 1987).

18) Teach the client about disease process and potential complications and when to seek medical attention.

19) Allow time for the learner to express an understanding of information taught and express feelings about changes.

20) Teach the client about the importance of follow-up appointments, including the following:
    a) Medical appointments
    b) Laboratory follow-up appointments for blood or urine testing needed to monitor effects of medications

21) Provide the client or learner the opportunity to practice information or skills learned.

22) Provide information about community resources.

3. Self-care deficit (impaired ability or inability to perform certain ADLs (e.g., feeding, dressing, bathing, toileting; **Table 13-7**): Tailor to the client's abilities and disabilities, but do not encourage dependency on others.

   a. Related to
      1) Limitations in joint movement
      2) Limitations in strength, weakness
      3) Limitations in limb presence
      4) Impaired ability to perform activity
      5) Decreased endurance, fatigue
      6) Decreased or lack of motivation
      7) Environmental barriers
      8) Pain or discomfort

   b. Outcomes
      1) The client demonstrates an improved ability to safely perform self-care activities to maximum capability.
      2) The client identifies resources to optimize independence in ADLs.
      3) The client demonstrates the use of assistive devices, splints, or prostheses as recommended by therapists.

   c. Interventions
      1) Refer to occupational therapy and encourage and facilitate performance of ADLs when possible.
      2) Encourage independence but provide assistance as needed if the client cannot perform or complete an activity.
      3) Provide the client with positive support during the activity and allow the client to perform the activity at his or her own rate.
      4) Encourage the appropriate use of assistive devices (e.g., plate guards, adapted flatware for eating; long-handled bath sponges, button hooks, zipper pulls; shower chair; safety mats for floor; grab bars for bath or shower).
      5) Provide supervision during an activity until the client is able to perform the skill and is safe in performing the skill independently; reevaluate at intervals to be certain that the client maintains attained skill level and is safe.
      6) Teach the client the proper means of supporting joints to prevent injury.
      7) Teach the client to check skin before and after the application of assistive devices, splints, and prostheses.

Table 13-7. Nursing Plan of Care: Self-Care Deficit

Related to the following:
- Decreased activity tolerance
- Pain and discomfort
- Fear, anxiety, and depression
- Lack of motivation
- Inability to perform or complete bathing
- Inability to perform or complete dressing and grooming self-care activities
- Inability to perform toileting self-care activities

Goals	Interventions
Demonstrate the ability to use adaptive equipment.	Teach or reinforce the use of assistive devices provided by therapy (e.g., plate guards, swivel utensils, universal cuffs, reachers, long-handled sponges, wash mitts, grab bars, tub or shower seats, walkers, crutches, canes). Educate the family about what the client can do and what he or she may need help with.
Perform toileting, bathing, and dressing activities at optimal level of independence.	Set up the environment so the client has easy access to all equipment, hygiene products, and clothing. Allow extra time to complete tasks. Encourage the use of safety measures. Provide privacy based on the client's safety level.
Maintain safe bathing practices.	Teach and reinforce safety measures often (e.g., adequate lighting, no-slip strips on floors and tub or shower floors, electric appliances placed away from water sources, need for rails and grab bars). Provide a means of calling for help as needed (e.g., call bells, panic buttons). Teach how to test water temperature to prevent burns if the client has neurological problems.
Improve tolerance in performing self-care activities.	Teach the client how to pace himself or herself while performing ADLs. Provide rest periods between activities as necessary. Educate the client and family about energy conservation techniques. Provide assistance to the client to prevent exhaustion. Encourage the client to choose loose-fitting clothes that are easy to put on.
Show an interest in hygiene and wear own clothes.	Encourage the client to see himself or herself as becoming healthier. Encourage the client to wear his or her own clothes as much as possible. Adapt clothing for easier application as necessary (e.g., Velcro closures, adjustments to clothing to fit over bulky appliances). Provide assistance with hair, makeup, or shaving as needed. Foster an atmosphere that promotes wellness. Provide psychological counseling as necessary (e.g., for adjustment disorders, depression, anxiety).

Expected Outcomes

Use assistive devices for eating, grooming, dressing, and toileting in a correct, safe, and efficient manner.

Maintain an independent level of functioning for toileting, bathing, grooming, and dressing activities.

Maintain a safe environment.

Demonstrate improved tolerance to performing ADLs.

Demonstrate improved motivation to perform ADLs.

4. Ineffective coping: Denial
   a. Related to
      1) Lack of comprehension of the seriousness of the diagnosis
      2) Denial used as a defense mechanism
      3) Change in or loss of body part
      4) Focusing on past strengths and function
      5) Feelings of helplessness
      6) Changes in lifestyle
   b. Outcomes
      1) The client recognizes his or her inappropriate coping behaviors.
      2) The client seeks out available resources and support systems as appropriate.
      3) The client demonstrates alternative coping strategies.
      4) The client responds positively about the effects of the disease process or disability and resumes personal and employment roles.

c. Interventions
1) Refer for psychosocial counseling for coping strategies.
2) Refer to appropriate support groups.
3) Establish a working relationship with the client by providing care.
4) Provide an opportunity for the client to express feelings and concerns in a safe environment.
5) Encourage the client to identify his or her strengths and abilities.
6) Assist the client in the grieving process related to the loss of body parts or the effects of chronic illness and changes in body function as appropriate.

5. Alterations in comfort level or pain
a. Related to
1) Surgical procedures
2) Joint inflammation, deterioration, and destruction
3) Pathology of the injury or disease
4) Therapy procedures and exercises
5) Medical treatment plan
6) Activity restrictions
7) Paresthesias
8) Phantom pain or sensation
b. Outcomes
1) The client verbalizes relief of pain or the ability to cope with pain that has not been completely relieved.
2) The client verbalizes the tolerance of his or her pain relief level and demonstrates the ability to engage in desired activities.
3) The client exhibits relaxed facial expression.
4) The client sleeps for longer periods at night.
c. Interventions
1) Administer prescribed pain medications.
2) Demonstrate an acceptance of the client's stated pain level.
3) Teach the client about nonpharmacological pain-relieving techniques such as heat and cold applications, TENS, progressive relaxation techniques, music, and diversional activities.
4) Refer to community support groups or other activities such as animal-assisted therapy.
5) Assist the client and family to identify and modify activities that may interfere with pain management.
6) Provide heat and cold therapy as ordered as an adjunct to therapy (e.g., paraffin baths, hot packs, deep ultrasound, and cold applications).

7) Turn and position the client every 2 hours as appropriate and maintain body and extremities in proper alignment using pillows, wedges, and prefabricated splints.
8) Use a firm or pressure-relieving mattress, bed boards, or other devices to provide support and pressure relief to maintain comfort.
9) Handle affected extremities gently, supporting above and below the joint.
10) Explore the client's knowledge and beliefs about pain.
11) Explore with the client factors that improve or worsen pain.
12) Provide optimal pain relief with prescribed medications.
13) Teach diversional techniques to relieve pain (e.g., listening to music; watching TV, videotapes, and DVDs; and using guided imagery and relaxation techniques).
14) Teach about the causes of phantom pain or sensation and techniques to decrease its effect.

6. Alteration in family processes
a. Related to
1) Role changes necessitated by the disability
2) Diagnosis of a chronic illness with disabling features
b. Outcomes
1) The family demonstrates improvement in communication.
2) The family seeks recommended resources for problem solving.
3) The family expresses an understanding of identified problems.
c. Interventions
1) Refer the family for counseling.
2) Provide information on appropriate community support groups.
3) Provide an opportunity for the client and family to express concerns or fears and ask questions.
4) Provide the client and family with information about the client's illness or injury (e.g., pattern of illness, time frames for recovery, and expectations) and how to manage stressful situations.
5) Encourage the client's family to participate with the client in learning care needs and assisting the client with ADLs and ambulation as appropriate.
6) Encourage the family to accompany the client off of the unit to provide social contacts.

THE SPECIALTY PRACTICE OF REHABILITATION NURSING

7. Potential for injury: Falls
    a. Related to
        1) Activity restrictions
        2) Decreased endurance and muscle strength
        3) Loss of limb
        4) Balance changes created by weight-bearing restrictions
        5) Use of assistive devices
        6) Rushing to get things done and not thinking about safety
        7) Unsafe environment
    b. Outcomes
        1) The client will demonstrate taking responsibility to make changes to prevent falls in the home.
        2) The client will report no falls or related injuries.
    c. Interventions
        1) Provide teaching about activity restrictions.
        2) Refer to physical therapy and occupational therapy as appropriate to improve strength and endurance.
        3) Instruct the client to avoid quick movements that could cause falls and fractures.
        4) Provide the client with information about resources to obtain medical supplies and to access medical providers.
        5) Provide the client with a list of emergency phone numbers (e.g., fire department, ambulance, police).
        6) Discuss the importance of maintaining a safe environment and fall prevention.
        7) Instruct about maintaining appropriate lighting.
            a) Place nightlights in hallways, bedrooms, bathrooms, and stairways.
            b) Install light switches at the top and bottom of stairs.
            c) Place a lamp and telephone near the bed.
            d) Maintain uniform lighting in each room and place lighting in dark spaces.
        8) Discuss the need to assess the home to identify any fall risks and make the necessary changes to correct any identified risk factors
            a) Make sure hallways and rooms do not have obstacles that impede safe movement.
            b) Move things such as newspapers, boxes, electrical and phone cords, plants, and furniture out of traffic areas.
            c) Place items such as clothing, bed coverings, and other items used in the house

hold where they can be reached without strain (Administration on Aging, n.d.).
8. Health maintenance behaviors
    a. Related to
        1) Medication regimen
        2) Diet restrictions
        3) Exercise program
        4) Preventive medical care
    b. Outcomes
        1) The client demonstrates positive health maintenance behaviors such as keeping scheduled appointments, following appropriate medication regimens, making diet and exercise changes, improving the home environment, and following other treatment recommendations.
        2) The client seeks out and uses available resources.
    c. Interventions
        1) Involve the family and caregivers in health-planning conferences.
        2) Provide the client and family with a list of medications, dosages, times to be taken, and possible side effects.
        3) Provide the client and family with information on dietary changes.
        4) Provide the client with information on outpatient resources for exercise programs and support groups.
        5) Provide the client and family with a list of scheduled medical appointments and telephone numbers.
9. Alteration in skin integrity
    a. Related to
        1) Surgical procedures (e.g., amputation and joint replacement)
        2) Immobility
        3) Pressure sores
        4) Nutritional deficits
        5) Nodule development in rheumatoid arthritis
        6) Crystal development in gout
        7) Use of splints, casts, braces, orthotic devices, and prosthetics
    b. Outcomes
        1) The client's skin is intact, as evidenced by no discoloration or indurations over bony prominences and no pressure ulcers.
        2) The client's skin is healing or has healed from any surgical procedure performed.
    c. Interventions
        1) If the client is confined to bed, develop an appropriate turning schedule.

2) Assess skin over bony prominences for redness, changes in texture, or any other signs of skin breakdown at frequent intervals.
3) Provide the appropriate pressure-relieving devices.
4) Prevent skin breakdown from excessive moisture.
5) Teach the client and family proper skin-management techniques.
6) Encourage adequate fluids and diet.
7) Instruct the client to follow doctor's orders for the management of surgical wounds and prevent further skin breakdown and infection.
8) Instruct the client to perform regular foot care, including trimming toenails and treating fungal infections as appropriate.
9) Teach surgical site care and signs and symptoms of infection.

10. Social isolation
   a. Related to
      1) Prescribed activity restrictions
      2) Lack of transportation
      3) Lack of social support network
      4) Self-imposed isolation
      5) Self-esteem issues
      6) Lack of motivation
      7) Chronic pain
   b. Outcomes: The client will verbalize participation in social activities and relationships.
   c. Interventions
      1) Discuss with the client the need to identify goals for addressing problematic situations he or she has encountered.
      2) Help the client identify possible activities to improve social relationships.
      3) Provide models and peer support to demonstrate actions and behaviors that are appropriate in different social situations.
      4) Involve significant others and families in social situations with the client in a safe environment.
      5) Provide information on community resources and support groups.
      6) Provide information on public transportation for the disabled.
      7) Refer for counseling if appropriate.

11. Disturbance in body image (a person's subjective perception of his or her body; Meiner & Lueckenotte, 2006)
   a. Related to
      1) Permanent or temporary alteration in appearance, structure, or function of a body part

      2) Amputation
      3) Change in height
   b. Outcomes
      1) The client will demonstrate greater comfort with body image and self-esteem, as evidenced by the ability to look at, touch, talk about, and care for an actual or perceived altered body part or function.
      2) The client will express positive feelings about changes in body image.
   c. Interventions (Thompson, 2002)
      1) Acknowledge the emotional response of the client to an actual or perceived change in body structure or function.
      2) Encourage the client to verbalize both positive and negative feelings related to an actual or perceived change in body image.
      3) Work with the client to identify ways of coping that he or she has used in the past.
      4) Refer the client and caregivers to support groups of people with similar types of problems or body image alterations.
      5) Refer the client for psychosocial counseling as appropriate.
      6) Demonstrate an accepting attitude toward the client and praise him or her for all accomplishments.
      7) Encourage the client to discuss feelings about changes in body image caused by joint deformity, loss of a body part, or the amputation and disease process.
      8) Encourage the client to touch and care for the changed body part.
      9) Encourage the client to discuss coping strengths that he or she has used to deal successfully with other problems in the past.

12. Altered sexuality pattern
   a. Related to
      1) Altered body structure or function
      2) Loss of sexual desire
      3) Pain or discomfort
      4) Changes in body image
      5) Changes in perceived sex role
      6) Changes in desired sexual satisfaction
      7) Knowledge deficits about adaptive positions and assistive techniques
      8) Feelings of rejection due to disability
   b. Outcomes: The client and family will verbalize satisfaction with sexual activity.
   c. Interventions
      1) Provide information on different techniques and positions to improve sexual experience.

THE SPECIALTY PRACTICE OF REHABILITATION NURSING

2) Provide resources for sexual counseling as appropriate.
3) Provide time for the client and significant other to discuss concerns about their ability to have sexual relationships.

13. Fatigue
a. Related to
1) Ineffective sleep pattern
2) Negative body image
3) Discomfort or pain
4) Effects of medications
5) Depression, anxiety, and stress
6) Boring lifestyle
7) Malnutrition
8) Anemia
b. Outcomes: The client will be less fatigued while performing activities.
c. Interventions
1) Assess the client's sleep pattern and suggest strategies to facilitate adequate rest (e.g., warm bath at bedtime, relaxing music).
2) Assess the client's pain and interventions to manage side effects of fatigue and make recommendations.
3) Encourage the client to pace activities and allow for adequate rest periods at intervals during the day.
4) Help the client determine when fatigue begins and explore whether there is a relationship to certain activities; determine which activities aggravate fatigue.
5) Encourage the client to set exercise goals that are realistic and share those goals with healthcare providers and family.
6) Help the client evaluate ADLs and identify ways to decrease fatigue and determine less fatiguing ways of performing activities.
7) Assess the client's diet and make recommendation to include foods for energy.
8) Discuss with the client ways to adapt the environment at work.
9) Monitor and record the client's sleep patterns and amount of time he or she sleeps.
10) Provide interventions to reduce fatigue, including both pharmacological and non-pharmacological.
11) Monitor the client for excess physical and emotional stress.
12) Teach activity organization and time management.
13) Help the client identify tasks and activities that other people (family members and friends) can do for him or her.
14) Encourage alternating periods of activity and rest.

14. Risk for infection
a. Related to
1) Surgical procedure (e.g., amputation, total joint replacement, debridement)
2) Open areas due to pressure
3) Accidental injuries
b. Outcomes: The client will be free of infection, as evidenced by normal temperature, stable vital signs, and no sign of infection at open areas.
c. Interventions
1) Review signs and symptoms of infection with the client.
2) Keep dressings on the surgical site and other open skin areas clean and dry.
3) Administer antibiotics as ordered.
4) Monitor the CBC for signs of infection.
5) Report any signs and symptoms of infection to the physician.

15. Changes in tissue perfusion (Tucker, 2000)
a. Related to
1) Disease process (i.e., diabetes, edema, DVT)
b. Outcomes
1) Distal pulses of affected extremity will be present.
2) Skin on the affected extremity is warm and dry.
c. Interventions
1) Position the client with the affected extremity in the proper position to assist with circulation.
2) Monitor the vascular status of the affected extremity every 2–4 hours as appropriate.
3) Provide ROM exercises.
4) Monitor the temperature and color of the extremity.
5) Check the distal pulses of the affected extremity.
6) Teach the client and family the importance of checking the extremity and noting signs and symptoms to report to the physician.
7) Instruct the client on factors to avoid that interfere with circulation (e.g., smoking, exposure to extreme temperatures, tight clothing, and crossing of the legs).
8) Instruct the client to maintain adequate hydration.

D. Diagnoses Specifically Relevant for Children (Wilson & Hockenberry, 2011).

1. Changes in self-esteem
   a. Related to
      1) Perceived acceptance by peers
      2) Change in appearance and functional ability as a result of disease process
   b. Outcomes
      1) The child or adolescent will verbalize acceptance by peers.
      2) The child or adolescent will participate in activities with peers.
   c. Interventions
      1) Encourage the child to meet with peers and participate in outings.
      2) Assist parents and siblings to explore ways to help the child participate in outings with peers.
      3) Explore with parents and siblings their feelings about the child's inability to perform activities that he or she could do previously.
2. Changes in body image
   a. Related to
      1) Child's or adolescent's expression of having to use assistive devices.
      2) Child's or adolescent's expression of loss of body part or deformed joints.
   b. Outcomes
      1) The child or adolescent will attend therapy as ordered.
      2) The child or adolescent will participate in activities with peers.
   c. Interventions
      1) Determine the client's expectations about body image based on developmental stage.
      2) Determine whether changes in body image are caused by a child's or teenager's perceptions of what society expects.
      3) Determine whether recent physical changes have been incorporated into the client's body image.
      4) Assess the client to determine whether peer groups have influenced the client's body image.
      5) Discuss with the child or adolescent plans to meet with peers and participate in activities.
      6) Encourage the child to meet with peers and participate in outings.
      7) Help parents and siblings explore ways to help the child participate in outings with peers.
      8) Explore with parents and siblings their

feelings regarding the child's loss of extremity or joint deformity and his or her inability to perform activities that he or she could do previously.
3. Changes in growth and development
   a. Related to
      1) Disease process
      2) Change in appearance and functional ability as a result of disease process
   b. Outcomes
      1) Parents will identify children with delayed growth and development.
      2) Parents will verbalize skills that promote their child's growth and development.
      3) Children will demonstrate improved motor skills, language, and personal and adaptive skills.
      4) The child or adolescent will participate in activities appropriate for age and growth and development level.
   c. Interventions
      1) Educate the child and family about normal growth and development.
      2) Educate the parents, child, and school about special accommodations that may need to be made to accommodate changes in the client's growth and development.
      3) Assess the client to determine specific needs and accommodations that may need to be made in relation to the child's changes in growth and development.
      4) Help the client, parents, and siblings explore ways to help the child participate in activities as normally as possible or with adaptations.
      5) Teach the client and family about the changes in the body that occur during normal growth and development.
      6) Instruct children and adolescents about the function of various body parts as appropriate.
4. Ineffective family coping
   a. Related to
      1) Perceived acceptance by peers
      2) Change in appearance and functional ability as a result of disease process
   b. Outcomes
      1) The child or adolescent will verbalize acceptance by peers.
      2) The child or adolescent will participate in activities with peers.
   c. Interventions
      1) Encourage the child to meet with peers

THE SPECIALTY PRACTICE OF REHABILITATION NURSING

and participate in outings.

    2) Help parents and siblings explore ways to help the child participate in outings with peers.

  5. Knowledge deficit related to community resources

    a. Related to lack of knowledge of available community resources

    b. Outcomes

      1) The child and family will verbalize knowledge of different support services and organizations.

      2) The child and family will contact different support services and organizations as appropriate.

    c. Interventions

      1) Provide information on different support services and support organizations for the child and family to access.

      2) Help the child, parents, and siblings explore various community resources.

V. Burns

A. Overview

  1. Burns are injuries to tissues caused by heat, friction, electricity, sunlight, nuclear radiation, or chemicals.

  2. Fires and burns are the seventh leading cause of unintentional injury and death in the United States for people 1–85 years of age (CDC, 2010c).

  3. On average in the United States in 2008, someone was injured by burns every 31 minutes (Karter, 2010).

  4. Death rates from serious burns have declined because of advances in fluid resuscitation, nutritional support, skin replacement, topical antimicrobials to prevent infection, early surgical interventions, and improvement in the management of inhalation injury and hypermetabolism (NIH, 2006).

  5. Rehabilitation of the client with burns requires interdisciplinary teamwork to achieve restoration of function and reintegration into the community.

  6. Rehabilitation nurses must be knowledgeable in wound management and healing and in the pathophysiological and psychological aspects of burn injuries.

B. Skin

  1. The skin is the largest organ of the body.

  2. The skin's major functions are to protect internal organs from infection and trauma, prevent fluid loss, and regulate body temperature.

  3. Exposure to heat above 120 °F will damage the skin, interfere with its primary functions, and cause burn injuries.

C. Epidemiology

  1. More than 1.1 million burn injuries warrant medical assistance in the United States each year, and approximately 50,000 of these warrant hospitalization (CDC, 2006).

  2. Approximately 20,000 of these burns are major burns involving at least 25% of the total body surface.

  3. Children, older adults, and people with disabilities are the high-risk groups for burn injuries. Other high-risk groups include African Americans and Native Americans, those living in rural areas, the poor, and those living in substandard housing (CDC, 2009b).

  4. The most common burn injuries are caused by scalds, building fires, and flammable liquids and gases (National Institute of General Medical Sciences, 2008).

  5. Cooking equipment is the leading cause of home structure fires and fire injuries (Ahrens, 2010).

D. Etiology

  1. Thermal

    a. Flame (e.g., house fire, burning leaves)

    b. Scald (stream of hot liquid [e.g., boiling water])

    c. Flash (e.g., flame burn associated with explosion)

  2. Contact (e.g., hot metal or hot tar)

  3. Chemical: Strong acids or alkalis (e.g., common household cleaning agents) can be ingested or inhaled or come in contact with skin or mucous membranes. The amount of damage depends on the concentration and quantity of the agent, duration of skin contact, and degree of penetration into the tissue (Lewis, Heitkemper, & Dirkson, 2004).

  4. Electrical: The amount of damage caused by exposure to electrical current depends on the type of circuit, voltage and amperage, the pathway of the current through the body, and the duration of contact.

    a. Exposed or faulty wiring

    b. High-voltage power lines

    c. Lightning strikes

  5. Radiation

    a. Sunburn

    b. Therapeutic radiation for cancer treatment

    c. Nuclear radiation accidents

  6. Smoke and inhalation: Directly inhaled smoke, hot air, or flames damage the tissues of the respiratory tract and can also contain chemicals that poison the body's cells, such as carbon monoxide.

E. Pathophysiology

1. Primary injury results from tissue necrosis at the center of the burn from exposure to electricity, chemicals, or heat (Singer, Brebbia, & Soroff, 2007).
2. The extent of a burn depends on the temperature and duration of exposure, skin thickness, and vascular supply (Singer et al., 2007).
3. Burns consist of three zones: necrotic center, ischemic zone (may be reversible), and zone of hyperemia.
4. Burns are classified according to depth and surface area.
   a. Degree (**Figure 13-5**; Singer et al., 2007)
      1) First degree
         a) Epidural layer, pain, erythema
         b) Dry, pink
         c) Usually heals within several days without scarring
      2) Second degree
         a) Entire epidermis and part of underlying dermis
         b) Superficial partial thickness
            (i) Erythema, blisters, weeping
            (ii) Painful
            (iii) Usually heals within 2 weeks with minimal scarring
         c) Deep partial thickness
            (i) Deeper, can convert to third degree
            (ii) Nonelastic white or red layer on top of burn, does not blanch with pressure
            (iii) Up to 3 weeks to heal
            (iv) Potential for scarring
      3) Third degree
         a) Entire epidermis and dermis
         b) White, brown, or tan, leathery
         c) Not sensitive to touch, does not blanch
         d) Warrants excision
   b. Extent of burn
      a) Measured as a percentage of total body surface area (TBSA)
      b) Rule of 9: This is a formula that divides the body into anatomical sections, each representing 9% or a multiple of 9% (head and neck = 9%, arms = 9% each, anterior trunk = 18%, posterior trunk = 18%, legs = 18% each, and perineum = 1%). Calculations are modified for infants and children younger than 10 years because of their larger head and smaller body size.
   c. Level of skin damage (Singer et al., 2007)
      1) Minor

Figure 13-5. Levels of Burn Severity

First Degree (partial thickness)
Does not extend below the epidermis

Is dry and very painful

Heals in a matter of days

Second Degree
Involves the epidermis and part of the dermis

May be superficial (moist, painful, blisters) or deep thickness (less painful); may have a white or red base

Superficial burns heal in 1–2 weeks; deep thickness burns heal in 3 weeks or more

Third Degree (full thickness)
Extends into dermis

Is dry and involves no pain, because sensory nerves are damaged; can be any color (e.g., white, black, yellow, brown)

Autograft is the usual form of treatment

Fourth Degree
Extends beyond fat and into the muscle and bone

Involves no pain and has variable color

Amputation of extremity is often necessary; autografting is the primary method for healing

---

      a) <10% TBSA in adults, <5% TBSA in children or older adults; <2% full-thickness burns
      b) Managed in outpatient setting
   2) Moderate
      a) 10%–20% TBSA in adults, 5%–10% TBSA in children or older adults; 5% full-thickness burns
      b) High-voltage injury, suspected inhalation injury, circumferential burn, co-morbidities that predispose to infection
      c) Treated in hospital
   3) Major
      a) >20% TBSA in adults, >10% TBSA in children or older adults; >5% full-thickness burn
      b) High-voltage burn; inhalation injury; burns to face, eyes, ears, genitalia, joints; significant associated injuries
      c) Treated at burn center
5. Age: Burn victims younger than 2 years and older than 60 years have a higher mortality rate than other age groups with similar burn injuries. In both groups, the skin is thin and more prone to infection.
6. Preexisting conditions that complicate burn recovery: Cardiovascular, respiratory, or renal disease; diabetes; PVD; sickle cell anemia; hepatic disease; obesity; hypertension (American Burn

Association, 2009; Lewis, Heitkemper, & Dirkson, 2004)

7. Clinical manifestations

    a. Local: Capillaries of the injured tissue become leaky; plasma is lost, drawing water with it, resulting in edema of the involved tissue and pain.

    b. Systemic responses: A major burn can affect all body systems and can cause serious complications through excessive fluid loss and tissue damage (**Figure 13-6**).

    c. Complications from burn surface

       1) Pain related to exposed nerve endings in partial-thickness burns and donor sites (American Burn Association, 2009)

       2) Scars

          a) Hypertrophic scars are red, thick, and raised above the level of normal skin but are within the boundaries of the burn wound and result from an imbalance between collagen synthesis and collagen lysis.

          b) Keloid scars are thick, nodular, and ridged scar tissue that grows beyond the site of injury; they can become binding and limit mobility if the keloids are extensive (Burn Survivor Resource Center, n.d.).

          c) Scar tissue affects thermal regulation. Shivering is not possible with a full-thickness scar with extensive grafting.

       3) Contractures: Tightening and shortening of the tendons and muscles, resulting in immobility and decreased ROM. Prevention is the most effective treatment (e.g., splinting, exercising, positioning, using pressure garments). Surgery may be needed depending on the severity and location of contractures.

       4) Heterotopic ossification: Abnormal deposit of new bone in soft tissue surrounding a joint that does not normally ossify. Surgical interventions may be needed if mobility is limited.

       5) Altered sensation: Diminished or absent response to sharp-dull and hot-cold; caution is needed to avoid further injury.

       6) Pruritus or itching as the wound heals (American Burn Association, 2009)

F. Management Options

   1. Prevention (Burn Prevention Network, 2010; CDC, 2009b)

    a. House fires

       1) Use a smoke detector on each floor (one must be outside your bedroom door),

replace batteries at least once a year, and test them monthly.

       2) Keep emergency numbers by your phone.

       3) Have a fire extinguisher in the kitchen.

       4) Use a cooking timer with a loud alarm.

       5) Install a sprinkler system.

       6) Place firefighting decals on the window of children's bedrooms.

Figure 13-6. Systemic Responses to Burn Injury

Vascular Alterations

Vasoconstriction results from exposure to heat and from stress response, resulting in decreased blood flow.

Dilation of adjacent vessels and capillaries and increased capillary permeability occur after the initial vasoconstriction.

Sodium pump is disturbed

Fluid shifts from the vascular space into the extracellular space, resulting in edema. (If edema is not corrected, ischemia in the underlying tissues can occur.)

Cardiac output is decreased as a result of hypovolemia.

Fluid resuscitation must be initiated to prevent cell shock and to maintain cardiac output and renal and tissue perfusion. (Adults with burns of a total body surface area greater than 15% need fluid resuscitation.)

Pulmonary Alterations

Obstruction can occur when damage around the neck area becomes tight or when superheated air, steam, gases, flames, or smoke is inhaled.

Depending on the severity, treatment can range from humidified air to mechanical ventilation.

Hematologic Alterations

Destruction of red blood cells in the burned area results in anemia.

Hematocrit level increases and blood flow decreases as the fluid shifts to the extravascular space, resulting in possible ischemia of underlying tissue and thrombosis.

Immune Response

Immune responses decrease because of damage of the protective skin layer, stress, protein and caloric malnutrition and side effects of immunosuppressant medication and steroids.

The individual is highly susceptible to infection.

Gastrointestinal Alterations

Ileus is due to vasoconstriction.

Parenteral route is used if an ileus is present.

Nutritional Alterations

The metabolic rate increases, resulting in increased caloric need of about two times normal (Wilson, 1996).

The metabolic rate will slowly return to normal when the wound is healed (Wilson, 1996).

Blood glucose rises.

Nutritional support may include oral supplements, tube feeding, intravenous supplements, or total parenteral nutrition.

---

7) Make sure an address is clearly visible on the outside of the house.
8) Keep matches and lighters out of reach of children.
9) Have a fire escape plan, know two ways out of every room, and practice fire drills and meeting at a designated space (a safe distance outside away from the house).
10) Keep fire escape routes free of clutter.

b. Hotels and workplace
1) Become familiar with exits and the posted evacuation plan.
2) Learn the location of building exits.
3) Respond to every alarm as if it were a real fire.
4) Keep a flashlight and room key on the table near the bed for easy access.

c. Hot water
1) Do not exceed 120 °F.
2) Turn handles of pots and pans inward while cooking.
3) Place cold water in the bathtub first, then add hot water to an appropriate temperature.

d. Chemical: Lock all flammable and caustic substances out of reach of children.

e. Electrical
1) Cover outlets with childproof protectors.
2) Do not use appliances with frayed or worn cords.
3) Avoid overloading outlets.
4) Keep electrical appliances and cords away from water.

f. Ultraviolet sun rays
1) Avoid long exposure to sun.
2) Wear hats and sunscreen with a minimum sun protection factor of 15.

g. Static electricity
1) Leave your cell phone inside your vehicle or turn it off during refueling.
2) Do not reenter a vehicle during refueling.
3) If you need to reenter a vehicle during refueling, close the door after getting out and make contact with metal before pulling out the nozzle to discharge static from the body.

h. Precautions for those with disabilities
1) Keep a wheelchair or assistive device close to the bed.
2) Keep a whistle nearby to alert rescuers of your location.
3) Place a sticker on the bedroom window.
4) Do not smoke if using oxygen.

2. Acute phase: Airway management, fluid resuscitation, wound care, pain management, nutritional therapy, and psychosocial care

3. Management of burn surface (Singer et al., 2007)
a. Burn location and severity determine treatment. Wound care should focus on cleaning the wound and removing debris until healthy tissue is present.
b. Wound management includes moist dressing, infection control, debridement of necrotic tissue (i.e., removal of dead tissue), or surgical care.
c. Wound care goals are to reduce pain and contamination, prevent infection, and minimize scarring.
d. Nonsurgical care (Singer et al., 2007)
1) Keep blisters intact if possible.
2) First-degree wounds
a) No specific therapy
b) Superficial partial thickness
c) Topical antimicrobial, synthetic or biological occlusive dressing
d) Specific treatments depend on infection and amount of exudate.
3) Deep-partial-thickness and third-degree burns are managed by a burn specialist.
e. Common topical antimicrobials
1) Silver sulfadiazine, silver nitrate
2) Bacitracin, pupuricin
3) Sulfamylon
f. Burn dressings
1) Acticoat (coated with silver)
2) Duoderm (donor sites)
3) Mepitel (silicone mesh)
4) Biological dressings
a) Integra, TransCyte, Apligraft
b) Surgical debridement needed first
g. Minor burn care (Singer et al., 2007)
1) Treat associated injuries.
2) Cool the burn with cool water.
3) Manage pain.
4) Irrigate with soap and water.
5) Leave blisters intact.
6) Debride as needed.
7) Apply occlusive dressing or topical antimicrobial and absorptive dressing.
8) Update tetanus vaccine.
h. Surgical care (major burns)
1) Change dressings one to three times daily (American Burn Association, 2009).
2) Keep graft and donor sites clean, moist, and covered (American Burn Association, 2009).
3) Surgical excision of damaged tissue (eschar)

THE SPECIALTY PRACTICE OF REHABILITATION NURSING

4) Surgical debridement (American Burn Association, 2009)
5) Escharotomy: Cutting through the burnt tissue until healthy tissue is reached to relieve pressure from circumferential wounds that go around the whole chest, leg, arm, or digits
6) Dermabrasion: Smoothing scar tissue by shaving or scraping off the top layers of the skin to minimize scars, restore function, and correct disfigurement resulting from an injury
7) Grafting to close deep partial-thickness or full-thickness wounds and protect the skin as it heals on its own
   a) Autograft: Use of the client's own skin from another site
      (i) The donor site is the harvested area of the client's own skin.
      (ii) Partial-thickness wounds require an absorbent dressing because of excessive drainage.
   b) Cultured epithelium: Take a small piece of unburned skin from the client and grow skin under special tissue culture conditions until it forms confluent sheets that can be used as skin graft.
   c) Cadaver skin: Obtained through a graft bank
   d) Allograft: From another living or dead person
   e) Xenograft: Usually from pigs because their skin is most similar to human skin
   f) Artificial skin: Synthetic product used to replace burned skin but only as a temporary fix; the use of artificial skins means a thinner skin graft, which allows the donor site and the client to heal faster with fewer surgeries (Shukla, 2008; WHO, 2004a)

4. Management of complications
   a. Begin positioning and splinting immediately on admission to maintain the functional position of joints and prevent contractures. After the graft is stable, the splint should be worn continuously for at least 3 months.
   b. Use pressure garments against the skin to reduce scar formation and deformities for 23 hours per day for 1–2 years until the scar is fully mature, removing for bathing and cleaning of garments only (Burn Survivor Resource Center, n.d.).

   c. Use topical scar treatment gel and massage therapy to limit scar tissue formation.
   d. Manage pain by administering over-the-counter analgesics, NSAIDs, and narcotics and using diversional activities (e.g., music, imagery, relaxation techniques) during dressing changes.
   e. Infection control: Apply topical antimicrobial cream.
   f. Nutritional therapy: Increase protein and increase calories; add vitamin supplements.

5. Nursing process
   a. Assessment
      1) Begin with a history.
      2) Note the cause of the burn and any contributing factors.
      3) Assess pain (e.g., location, quality, duration, intensity).
      4) Assess function, including ROM.
      5) Evaluate diet.
      6) Perform a psychosocial evaluation (e.g., support systems, coping strategies).
      7) Perform a complete physical and functional assessment, including the amount of burn area involved and the depth, severity, and any complications from the injury.
      8) Use a body diagram to document the location and appearance of burns, grafted areas, and donor sites.
   b. Plan of care
      1) Pain management
      2) Nutritional intake to meet caloric needs
      3) Skin and wound care
      4) Interventions to attain and maintain function
      5) Psychological support
   c. Nursing diagnoses
      1) Alteration in comfort related to pain and itching
      2) Self-care deficit related to burn, contracture, wound care, splitting, or pressure garment
      3) Impaired skin integrity related to burn injury
      4) Impaired physical mobility related to burn injury, contracture, wound care, splitting, or pressure garment
      5) Risk of infection related to loss of skin integrity
      6) Inadequate nutrition related to diuresis, metabolic response to burn injury, inactivity, and self-care deficit (inability to self-feed)
      7) Anxiety related to treatment regimen

8) Body image disturbance related to burn injuries, contractures, and scarring
9) Ineffective coping related to burn injury, pain, prognosis, and long-term outcome
10) Knowledge deficit related to burn process, treatment regimen, and signs and symptoms of complications

d. Goals
1) Report pain relief as a result of pain management interventions.
2) Maintain independence or demonstrate progression toward independence in performing ADLs.
3) Show signs of wound healing.
4) Maintain full ROM.
5) Remain free of complications caused by burn injuries such as extensive scarring or contracture.
6) Remain free of signs and symptoms of infection.
7) Maintain present weight and maintain fluid hydration.
8) Verbalize feelings about change in appearance and develop a realistic body image.
9) Develop effective coping strategies to adjust to burn injury.
10) Verbalize understanding about the healing process, treatment options, and signs and symptoms of complications.

e. Interventions
1) Provide pain relief with prescribed analgesics, especially before wound care; elevate legs; and use nonpharmacological methods of pain control (imagery, distraction, relaxation, music).
2) Use therapeutic positioning, splints, and ROM exercises to maintain proper position and prevent contractures.
3) Provide assistive devices for use in performing ADLs.
4) Provide care for the wound and the development of healing tissue.
5) Use a pressure garment to prevent or minimize scarring.
6) Prevent infection by applying topical antimicrobials as ordered, adhering to strict handwashing protocols, maintaining aseptic technique, and monitoring for signs and symptoms of infection.
7) Ensure adequate hydration and nutrition (high protein, high calories, with vitamin supplements for wound healing).
8) Provide psychological support and health education regarding health status, treatments, nutritional needs, prevention of infections, and support groups.
9) Provide education on the healing process, treatment options, pain-relief measures, and complications.

f. Evaluation: Modify care according to the client's response to nursing interventions.

VI. **Blast Injuries**
A. Overview
1. Blast injuries have become more common in rehabilitation settings since the onset of the wars in Iraq and Afghanistan.
2. Blast injuries also occur in industry and in the private sector.
3. Although much is known about blast injury, the long-term effects of blast exposure, particularly repeated blast exposure, are unclear.
4. Common causes of blast injuries in war include bombs and improvised explosive devices.
5. Blast injuries in past wars often called "shell shock"

B. Epidemiology and Incidence
1. Blasts are responsible for about two-thirds of the combat injuries in the Iraq and Afghanistan wars (Kocsis & Tessler, 2009).
2. Forty-seven percent of blast injuries in these wars involve the head, resulting in TBI.
3. Morbidity and mortality are related to proximity to blast, type and strength of the blast device, exposure to repeated blasts, and surroundings (enclosed vs. open space) during explosion.

C. Etiology
1. Primary blast injury results from blast wave–induced changes in atmospheric pressure.
   a. Solids and liquids are converted rapidly into gases; atmospheric pressure changes.
   b. Gases expand rapidly into a pulse of pressure outward (blast overpressure).
   c. Atmospheric pressure then drops, creating a vacuum (blast underpressure).
   d. Pressure causes stress and shear waves that act on the body and organs; the most vulnerable are the lungs, bowel, middle ear, and perhaps brain (Kocsis & Tessler, 2009).
   e. Amputation can result from primary blast injury, although this is an atypical source of amputation injury.
2. Secondary blast injury is caused by objects projected from the blasts into the body. Collision of objects with the body causes injury, including TBI and amputation.

THE SPECIALTY PRACTICE OF REHABILITATION NURSING

3. Tertiary blast injury results from being propelled away from the blast (Kocsis & Tessler, 2009). Collision of the body with solid objects such as buildings or ground causes injury such as fractures and TBI.

4. Quaternary blast injuries encompass all other blast-related injuries such as burns, crush injuries, and toxic inhalations.

D. Risk Factors
1. High-risk environment (e.g., war zone)
2. Industry using large amounts of fuel
   a. Oil and gas wells
   b. Chemical plants
3. Industry using explosives such as TNT
   a. Mining
   b. Rock quarry
   c. Road construction in mountainous areas
   d. Fireworks factory
   e. Military munitions
4. High-risk behaviors
   a. Making methamphetamine
   b. Making bombs
   c. Using fireworks
5. Terrorist attack

E. Pathophysiological Effects of Blast
1. Pulmonary
   a. Pulmonary contusion
   b. Pneumothorax
   c. Inhalation of irritant gases or dusts
   d. Pulmonary edema from myocardial contusion
   e. Adult respiratory distress syndrome
   f. Blast lung: Tearing, hemorrhage, and edema of lung tissue (CDC, 2008)
2. Ears
   a. Tympanic membranes
   b. Rupture
   c. Foreign bodies
3. Musculoskeletal
   a. Amputation
   b. Fracture
4. Abdominal
   a. Liver
   b. Spleen
   c. Hemorrhage
   d. Perforation of bowel (acute or delayed)
5. Neurological
   a. Intracranial hemorrhage
   b. TBI
      1) Mild TBI or concussion
      2) Moderate or severe
6. Skin
   a. Burns

b. Soft-tissue injury
7. Polytrauma
   a. Two or more injuries to physical regions or organ systems, one of which may be life threatening, resulting in physical, cognitive, psychological, or psychosocial impairments and functional disability (VA Polytrauma System of Care, 2010)
   b. Long-term effects
   c. Polytrauma triad: Seen frequently in war-wounded members, the polytrama triad is pain, PTSD, and TBI.
8. Pain
9. PTSD
10. Postconcussive syndrome
   a. May have early or late onset
   b. May last for days, weeks, or months
   c. Severity lessens over time
   d. Symptoms change over time
   e. Possible symptoms include the following:
      1) Dizziness
      2) Headache
      3) Tinnitus, hearing loss
      4) Vision (blurred, double)
      5) Impaired memory, judgment
      6) Sleep disturbance
      7) Poor concentration
      8) Irritability, mood swings
      9) Insomnia
      10) Fatigue
      11) Sensitivity to light or noise
      12) Depression, anxiety
      13) Nausea, vomiting (Lubit, 2008)
11. Management options
   a. Prevention
   b. First-responder training
   c. Intensive care
   d. Rehabilitation
      1) Burns
      2) Amputation
      3) TBI
      4) Soft-tissue injuries
      5) PTSD
      6) Polytrauma
      7) Client and caregiver education
12. Rehabilitation issues
   a. Psychological
      1) PTSD
      2) Depression
      3) Anxiety
      4) Substance abuse potential
      5) Suicide potential
   b. Physiological

1) Wide range of potential injuries
2) Must be alert for hidden or late-onset complications
3) Infection
4) TBI
5) Postconcussive syndrome
6) PTSD
13. Nursing process: Assessment
   a. History
      1) Past medical, surgical, and psychological illnesses and injuries
      2) Current injuries
         a) Characteristics and circumstances of blast
         b) Number, type, and degree of injuries
      3) Medications
      4) Social
         a) Support systems
         b) Family
         c) Friends
         d) Neighbors
         e) Houses of worship
         f) Other
      5) Lifestyle
         a) Drug abuse
         b) Smoking
         c) Alcohol
         d) Activity, exercise
         e) Recreational and diversionary activities
   b. Physical
      1) Neurological
         a) Cognitive function
         b) Memory
         c) Judgment
         d) Behavior
         e) Executive function
         f) Postconcussive syndrome
         g) Sensation
         h) Other
            (i) Cranial nerves
            (ii) Strength, movement of limbs and trunk
            (iii) Hearing
            (iv) Vision
      2) Pulmonary
         a) Lung sounds
         b) Respiratory effort
         c) Perfusion
         d) Pulmonary supports needed
            (1) Oxygen
            (2) Continuous or bilevel airway pressure

3) Cardiovascular
   a) Peripheral circulation
   b) Edema
   c) Chest pain
   d) Heart sounds
4) GI
   a) Bowel sounds
   b) Distention
   c) Tenderness
5) Skin
   a) Burns
   b) Soft-tissue wounds
6) Psychosocial
   a) Support systems
   b) Coping style
   c) Sleep disturbances
   d) PTSD, depression, anxiety
   e) Other stressors
      (i) Family
      (ii) Financial
      (iii) Role
7) Nutritional
   a) Weight over time
   b) Laboratory results
   c) Swallowing function
   d) Appetite
   e) Preferences
8) Sensory
   a) Hearing
   b) Vision
9) Communication
   a) Written
   b) Spoken
   c) Other
10) Functional impairments
   a) ADLs
   b) IADLs
   c) Current level of activity and assistance needed
11) Subjective symptoms
   a) Physical
   b) Psychological
   c) Social
   d) Pain
12) Educational needs
   a) Injury-related
   b) Coping
   c) Community reintegration
13) Secondary complications: Infection
14. Nursing diagnoses (North American Nursing Diagnosis Association [NANDA], 2008)
   a. Activity intolerance
   b. Anxiety

c. Disturbed body image
d. Risk for caregiver role strain
e. Confusion
f. Compromised family coping
g. Ineffective coping
h. Deficient diversional activity
i. Interrupted family processes
j. Fear
k. Grieving
l. Risk for injury
m. Memory impairment
n. Physical mobility impairment
o. Moral distress
p. Acute pain
q. Chronic pain
r. Risk of PTSD
s. Ineffective role performance
t. Self-care deficit
u. Sleep deprivation
v. Social isolation
w. Risk for suicide
x. Disturbed thought processes
y. Impaired tissue integrity
z. Risk for other-directed violence
aa. Impaired walking

15. Plan
a. Demonstrate resolution of cognitive changes.
b. Demonstrate adaptive coping strategies for stress.
c. Demonstrate maximal independence in mobility.
d. Perform ADLs at optimal level of independence with or without adaptive equipment.
e. Demonstrate adequate sleep patterns for rest and rejuvenation.
f. Identify diversional activities to decrease stress.
g. Verbalize an understanding of the treatment of the sequelae of blast injury.

16. Interventions
a. Manage pain.
b. Assess regularly.
c. Guide the client in setting pain goals.
d. Implement nonpharmacological interventions.
   1) Positioning
   2) Massage
   3) Heat and cold
   4) Distraction
e. Allow rest periods.
f. Medicate as indicated.
g. Psychological support
   1) Help the client identify nonadaptive reactions to stress.

2) Assist in identifying coping strategies for stressful situations.
3) Facilitate team and client conferences.
4) Provide socialization opportunities.
5) Refer for psychological services.
6) Educate the client and family on signs, symptoms, and interventions for PTSD.
7) Reduce stress when possible.
8) Share assessments of psychological health with the team.
9) Be alert for threats to staff or client safety (harm to self or others).

h. ADLs and self-care
   1) Ensure privacy and safety.
   2) Allow independence as able.
   3) Include the family with the client's permission.
   4) Allow time for rest between activities.
   5) Support physical and occupational therapists' plan of care.
   6) Contribute to team rounds with assessment of ADL skills.

i. Mobility
   1) Ensure safety.
   2) Use adaptive equipment as indicated.
   3) Maintain a hazard-free environment.
   4) Teach fall-prevention techniques.

j. Client and family education
   1) Assess readiness and motivation for learning.
   2) Provide information at the client's and family's intellectual level.
   3) Use a variety of teaching methods.
   4) Allow privacy and quiet for educational sessions.
   5) Build a knowledge base.

k. Evaluation: Individualize outcome evaluation based on diagnoses and interventions.

VII. Posttraumatic Stress Disorder
A. Overview
1. PTSD is an anxiety disorder that results from the experience or witnessing of a traumatic event (Department of Veterans Affairs, 2010).
2. Posttraumatic stress was recognized as early as the third century BC (Nayback, 2009).
3. References to PTSD occur in Homer's *Iliad* and Shakespeare's *Henry IV* (Nayback, 2009).
4. In 19th-century Great Britain, PTSD was recognized among postal workers and railway workers who witnessed railway crashes.
   a. Symptoms of sleep disorders, nightmares, intolerance to railway travel, chronic pain

b. Called "railway spine" or "accident neurosis" (Nayback, 2009)

5. Also recognized in 19th century by military physicians describing soldiers' responses to combat
   a. Called "soldiers heart," "DeCosta's syndrome," and "effort syndrome"
   b. Attributed to cardiovascular compromise secondary to combat stress (Nayback, 2009)

6. Named "shell shock" by a British psychiatrist in 1915
   a. Symptoms noted included inability to move or speak, unresponsiveness, memory loss, loss of capacity to feel, weeping, and screaming
   b. Symptoms attributed to microtears in the brain secondary to exploding shells (Nayback, 2009)

7. Named "war neurosis" during World War II
   a. 1944: Military focused on prevention and treatment
   b. Front-line psychiatry emerged; soldiers were treated close to the battlefield and returned to combat
   c. Impact of environment and relationships was recognized (Nayback, 2009)

8. PTSD was included in the third edition of the *Diagnostic and Statistical Manual of Mental Disorders (DSM)* as a psychiatric diagnosis in 1980.

9. PTSD is underrecognized by care providers.

B. Epidemiology and Incidence
   1. 50%–90% of all adults and children are exposed to a psychologically traumatic event sometime in their lifetimes (Department of Veterans Affairs, 2010).
   2. Approximately 67% of trauma survivors experience lasting psychological impairment.
      a. PTSD
      b. Panic attacks
      c. Phobias
      d. Anxiety disorders
      e. Depression
      f. Substance abuse (Department of Veterans Affairs, 2010)
   3. Most people experience normal stress reactions after a trauma.
      a. Lasts days to weeks
      b. Emotional reactions: Shock; fear; grief; anger; guilt; shame; helplessness; hopelessness; numbness; emptiness; diminished ability to feel interest, pleasure, or love (Department of Veterans Affairs, 2010)
      c. Cognitive reactions: Confusion, disorientation, worry, shortened attention span, memory loss, self-blame, difficulty concentrating, worry (Department of Veterans Affairs, 2010)

d. Physical reactions: Tension, fatigue, insomnia, nausea, change in appetite and sex drive, elevated startle response, bodily aches and pains (Department of Veterans Affairs, 2010)
e. Interpersonal reactions: Distrust, conflict, withdrawal, irritability, loss of intimacy, feeling rejected or abandoned

4. About one in three trauma survivors has severe stress symptoms that put them at risk for PTSD.
   a. Dissociation (depersonalization, amnesia)
   b. Intrusive reexperiencing (flashbacks, nightmares)
   c. Extreme emotional numbing
   d. Extreme attempts to avoid memories (substance abuse)
   e. Hyperarousal (rage, panic attacks, agitation)
   f. Severe anxiety (compulsions, obsessions, extreme worry)
   g. Severe depression (loss of hope, pleasure, interest; feeling worthless; Department of Veterans Affairs, 2010)

C. Etiology
   1. Traumatic events that might cause PTSD include military combat, natural disasters, terrorist attacks, serious accidents, or physical or sexual assault in adulthood or childhood (Department of Veterans Affairs, 2010).
   2. Certain types of trauma are likely to place the survivor at risk for PTSD.
      a. Life-threatening danger or physical harm
      b. Exposure to gruesome death, bodily injury, or dead or maimed bodies
      c. Extreme environmental or human violence or destruction
      d. Loss of home, valued possessions, neighborhood, or community
      e. Loss of communication with or support from close relations
      f. Intense emotional demands
      g. Extreme fatigue, exposure to weather, hunger, sleep deprivation
      h. Extended exposure to danger, loss, emotional or physical strain
      i. Exposure to toxins (Department of Veterans Affairs, 2010)

D. Risk Factors
   1. Risk of PTSD increases if a person
      a. Was exposed to the traumatic event as a victim or a witness
      b. Was seriously injured during the trauma
      c. Experienced a trauma that was long lasting or very severe

d. Saw themselves or a family member as being in imminent danger

e. Had a severe negative reaction during the event, such as feeling detached from surroundings or having a panic attack

f. Felt helpless during the trauma and was unable to help self or a loved one (Department of Veterans Affairs, 2010)

g. Experienced an interpersonal trauma such as rape or assault

2. Trauma-related risk factors

a. Nature, severity, and duration of the trauma exposure

b. Previous trauma exposure (VA/DoD, 2004)

3. Pretrauma risk factors: Adverse childhood, younger age, female gender, minority race, and low socioeconomic or educational status (VA/DoD, 2004)

4. Posttrauma risk factors: Poor social support and life stress (VA/DoD, 2004)

5. Criteria for diagnosis

a. Exposed to a traumatic event

1) Must involve actual or threatened death or serious injury or a threat to the physical integrity of oneself or others

2) Must involve an intense emotional reaction such as fear, helplessness, or horror

b. The traumatic event is persistently reexperienced (dreams, nightmares, memories, flashbacks).

c. Persistent avoidance of stimuli associated with the trauma and numbing of general responsiveness (avoidance, memory loss)

d. Persistent symptoms of increased arousal

e. Hypervigilance, elevated startle response, loss of sleep, agitation

f. The disturbance lasts more than 1 month.

g. The disturbance causes clinically significant distress or impairment in social, occupational, or other important areas of functioning (Friedman, 2000).

E. Pathophysiology

1. Several key psychobiologic mechanisms that enable humans to cope successfully with stressful situations function abnormally in PTSD clients

a. Fight-or-flight response (sympathetic nervous system [SNS] activation)

b. Abnormal increases in SNS reactivity

c. Hypothalamic-pituitary-adrenocortical mobilization

1) Lower urinary cortisol levels

2) Elevated lymphocyte glucocorticoid receptor levels

3) Dexamethasone supersuppression

d. Exaggerated acoustic startle response

e. Fear conditioning: Neutral cues associated with a traumatic event acquire the capacity to evoke a conditioned emotional (fearful) response in the absence of the aversive stimulus (Pavlovian response; Friedman, 2000).

f. Appraisal: Capacity to evaluate the situation as benign or dangerous is impaired (Friedman, 2000)

2. Physical abnormalities (structure and function)

a. Reduced hippocampal volume

b. Changes in regional cerebral blood flow (rCBF) to limbic and paralimbic areas (Friedman, 2000)

3. Effects of PTSD on health

a. Increased vulnerability to hypertension and atherosclerotic heart disease

b. Abnormalities in thyroid and hormone function

c. Increased susceptibility to infection

d. Problems with pain perception and pain tolerance

4. Behavioral health risks associated with PTSD

a. Smoking

b. Substance abuse

c. Poor nutrition

d. Conflict, violence

e. Anger, hostility

F. Management Options

1. Nonpharmacological

a. Psychotherapy

1) Group

2) Individual

3) Couple and family therapy

4) Cognitive-behavioral therapy (CBT)

a) Consists of cognitive therapy and prolonged exposure to internal and external reminders of the traumatic event

b) Exposure-based, trauma-focused CBT has been shown through research to have better results than other types of therapy early after the event.

c) Used in both acute and chronic PTSD

b. Eye movement desensitization and reprocessing: Technique that combines imaginal exposure to trauma reminders with lateral eye movement (Shalev, 2009)

2. Pharmacological

a. Though found to be helpful in relieving some symptoms, pharmacological treatment of PTSD is not the cure-all.

b. The following medications have had positive results in research studies to date:
   1) Selective serotonin reuptake inhibitors (SSRIs)
      a) First-line pharmacological treatment
      b) Serotonin is important in mood, anxiety, stress modulation, appetite regulation, and sleep.
      c) Reduces symptoms of reexperiencing, hyperarousal, avoidance, and numbing
      d) Paroxetine, fluoxetine, sertraline
   2) Selective serotonin/norepinephrine uptake inhibitor
      a) Similar effects to SSRIs
      b) Venlafaxine
   3) Atypical antipsychotics
      a) Act on dopamine and serotonin systems
      b) May help best if used to augment SSRIs
      c) May elevate glucose and cholesterol levels
      d) Risk of tardive dyskinesia and extrapyramidal side effects
      e) Olanzapine, risperidone, quetiapine
   4) Antiepileptics: Valproate
   5) Beta-adrenergic antagonist
      a) Reduces intrusive recollections, reactivity to traumatic stimuli, hyperreactivity
      b) Small research trials
      c) Propranolol
   6) Antiadrenergic: Prazosin for nightmares and insomnia
   7) Short-term anxiolytics after the event
      a) Include benzodiazepines
      b) Potentially addictive (Shalev, 2009; Department of Veterans Affairs, 2010)
G. Rehabilitation Issues
   1. Screening, recognition, and provision of treatment for PTSD
   2. Family structure and processes
   3. Client and family education
   4. Symptom management
      a. Behavior
         1) Impatience
         2) Anger
         3) Agitation
         4) Violence
         5) Hypervigilance
         6) Elevated startle reflex
      b. Sleep and rest
      c. Lack of concentration
      d. Substance abuse
   5. Safety of self and others
      a. Suicidal ideation

b. Anger, acting out
   6. Inability to join group activities
      a. Trust
      b. Startle
      c. Anger
   7. Comorbidities that either exacerbate or mask symptoms of PTSD
      a. TBI
      b. Depression
      c. Anxiety
H. Nursing Process: Assessment
   1. Presence of PTSD
      a. Recognition of risk
      b. Screening with a validated, reliable instrument: Primary-Care PTSD screen (PC-PTSD; **Figure 13-7**)
      c. Communication with other providers
      d. Knowledge of trauma history: Does it fit with *DSM-IV* criteria listed earlier?
   2. Sleep and rest
      a. Sleep patterns
      b. Nightmares
      c. Recurrent dreams
      d. Difficulty falling and staying asleep
      e. Hypersomnia
   3. Cardiac and pulmonary
      a. Hypertension
      b. Episodes of tachycardia and palpitations
      c. Episodes of tachypnea, breathlessness
      d. Perspiration, hot and cold spells
   4. Psychological
      a. Behaviors
         1) Self-report
         2) Significant-other report
         3) Observation
      b. Concentration
      c. Hypervigilance
      d. Fear
      e. Flashbacks
      f. Anger
      g. Impulse control
      h. Risk of self-harm
         1) Suicidal ideation
         2) Past attempts
      i. Risk of harm to others
      j. Coping measures
         1) Usual
         2) Current
            a) Isolation
            b) Illicit drugs
            c) Alcohol
            d) Cigarettes
   5. Pain

6. Social interactions
   a. Avoidance
   b. Disinterest
7. Medications
8. Therapy received

I. Nursing Diagnoses (NANDA, 2008)
   1. Anxiety
   2. Ineffective coping
   3. Fear
   4. Complicated grieving
   5. Insomnia
   6. Impaired memory
   7. Post-trauma syndrome
   8. Sleep deprivation
   9. Social isolation
   10. Spiritual distress
   11. Overload stress
   12. Risk for suicide
   13. Disturbed thought processes
   14. Risk for other-directed violence
   15. Risk for self-directed violence

J. Plan
   1. Reduce psychological distress and the effects of secondary stressors.

2. Treat specific symptoms when they interfere with normal healing processes.
3. Assist the normal healing process by supporting the client and family.
4. Protect the client from further exposure to stress.
5. Encourage the client to verbalize and express painful emotions as able.
6. Encourage the client to be with others.
7. Educate the client and family on PTSD, interventions, and expected outcomes.
8. Coordinate care with other providers.

K. Interventions
   1. Provide safety for the client and family.
   2. Help the client improve self-esteem and regain a sense of control over feelings and actions.
   3. Encourage the development of assertive, not aggressive, behaviors.
   4. Promote an understanding that the outcome of the present situation can be significantly affected by own actions.
   5. Help the client and family to learn healthy ways to deal with and realistically adapt to changes and events that have occurred.
   6. Provide active listening and support for the client and family.

L. Evaluation
   1. Safety
      a. Client
      b. Significant others
   2. Management of PTSD symptoms
      a. Sleep and rest disturbances
      b. Hypervigilance
      c. Anger, agitation
      d. Fear
   3. Community reintegration

VIII. Advanced Practice
   A. Clinician
      1. Coordination of the multidisciplinary team
         a. Communicate rehabilitation therapy interventions to the bedside nurse.
         b. Coordinate the client's physical and psychological needs with discharge personnel to ensure continuity of care and a safe transition.
      2. Medical and nursing care
         a. Monitor relevant lab values and follow-up interventions related to lab values (e.g., hemoglobin and hematocrit levels after joint replacement).
         b. Monitor and intervene to prevent complications (e.g., DVT prophylaxis, activity).
         c. Troubleshoot care for problem-prone and high-risk clients

d. Create protocols to make care seamless and reduce the chance of error (e.g., develop bowel regimen to prevent constipation in the client taking a lot of pain medication)

B. Educator
1. Nursing personnel
   a. Promote mobility to prevent complications.
   b. Use universal precautions to minimize the spread of infection.
   c. Identify high-risk clients for falls, complications, the development of medical problems, and suicide.
   d. Instruct on pain-management techniques and interventions to prevent oversedation complications.
2. Multidisciplinary personnel
   a. Outline the role of nursing in the multidisciplinary team.
   b. Learn rehabilitation techniques that can be carried over to bedside nursing personnel.
   c. Coordinate new staff orientation to the rehabilitation department and the treatments offered to clients.
3. Community
   a. Promote health.
      1) Early identification of musculoskeletal diseases
      2) Dietary intake needs of preteens and teenagers in osteoporosis prevention
      3) Safety awareness for injury prevention in sports and leisure activities
   b. Prevent illness.
      1) Community methicillin-resistant *Staphylococcus aureus* epidemic
      2) Fall prevention
      3) Circulatory and diabetes care to reduce the need for amputations

C. Leader
1. Facilitate the incorporation of clinical practice guidelines into the care setting.
2. Participate in relevant hospital committees.
   a. Safety committee
   b. Pharmacy and therapeutics
   c. Specialty program development, evaluation, and treatment
   d. Quality-improvement initiatives
3. Interact with relevant community and national organizations to assist in disease prevention and implement evidence-based practice.
   a. National Osteoporosis Foundation
   b. National Institutes of Health
   c. Arthritis Foundation
   d. Society of Vascular Surgery

   e. American Academy of Orthopedic Surgeons
   f. National Association of Orthopedic Nurses
4. Contact local and state representatives regarding health promotion and safety.
   a. Dietary intake in school settings
   b. Helmet and seatbelt laws
   c. Funding for catastrophic care

D. Consultant
1. Identify key areas of care related to a specific diagnosis (e.g., joint replacement: vital signs, lab values, blood loss, activity level, pain management, and incision care).
2. Develop effective mechanisms to communicate this information to the physician and other healthcare providers.
3. Communicate with internal and external financial resources to ensure optimum billing and reimbursement.
4. Product adoption (e.g., assist in medical equipment purchasing to facilitate client recovery and mobility)

E. Researcher
1. Evidence-based practice related to pain management in orthopedic surgery
   a. Pain management is a fundamental component of nursing care in the orthopedic client.
   b. Multiple routes of administration of pain relief are available for use: epidural and intrathecal opioid analgesia, patient-controlled analgesia with systemic opioids, and regional techniques.
   c. Many factors affect how a client experiences pain, such as age, race, gender, and culture.
   d. Pain management continues to be driven by practitioner preference and familiarity of treatment options.
2. Clinical question: Are around-the-clock scheduled pain medications more effective in pain management than patient-controlled analgesia or as-needed pain management practices?
3. Appraisal of evidence
   a. Two national guidelines with good evidence: "Practice Guidelines for Acute Pain Management in the Perioperative Setting: An Updated Report by the American Society of Anesthesiologists Task Force on Acute Pain Management" (2004) and *Acute Pain Management: Operative or Medical Procedures and Trauma. Clinical Practice Guideline* (Agency for Health Care Policy and Research, 1992).
   b. Three level II articles with good evidence (Gimbel, Brugger, Zhao, Verburg, & Geis, 2001; Moizo, Marchetti, Albertin, Muzzolon, & Antonino, 2004; Sinatra et al., 2005)

c. Two level VI articles with good evidence (Herr et al., 2004; Pellino, Willens, Polomano, & Heve, 2003)
4. Recommendations for best rehabilitation nursing practice
    a. There is good support for around-the-clock use of certain analgesic medications such as NSAIDs, COX-2 inhibitors, and acetaminophen.
    b. Clients' perceptions of the staff's ability to care for them influence their satisfaction with pain relief.
    c. Multimodal pain-management treatments can and should be used for effective pain relief.

References

Administration on Aging. (2010). *Fall prevention programs.* Retrieved August 30, 2010, from www.aoa.gov.

Administration on Aging. (n.d.). *Preventing falls at home.* Washington, DC: Author. Retrieved October 22, 2010, from www.eldercare.gov/Eldercare.NET/Public/Resources/Brochures/docs/Preventing_Falls_Brochure_pagebypage.pdf.

Agency for Health Care Policy and Research. (1992). *Acute pain management: Operative or medical procedures and trauma. Clinical practice guideline.* Rockville, MD: Author.

Ahrens, M. (2010). *Home structure fires.* Quincy, MA: National Fire Protection Association. Retrieved August 11, 2010, from www.nfpa.org/assets/files/PDF/OS.Homes.pdf.

Aletaha, D., Neogi, T., Silman, A. J., Funovitis, J., Felson, D. T., Bingham, C.O. III, et al. (2010). 2010 rheumatoid arthritis classification criteria: An American College of Rheumatology/European League Against Rheumatism collaborative initiative. *Arthritis & Rheumatism, 62*(9), 2569–2581.

Alexander, I. M. (2009). Pharmacotherapeutic management of osteoporosis and osteopenia. *The Nurse Practitioner, 34*(6), 30–40.

Altman, R. D., Hochberg, M. C., Moskowitz, R. W., & Schnitzer, T. J. (2000, May 12). Recommendations for the medical management of osteoarthritis of the hip and knee: 2000 update. American College of Rheumatology Subcommittee on Osteoarthritis Guidelines. *Arthritis & Rheumatism, 43*(9), 1905–1915.

American Academy of Orthopaedic Surgeons. (2007a). *Arthritis: An overview.* Retrieved October 22, 2010, from http://orthoinfo.aaos.org/topic.cfm?topic=A00217.

American Academy of Orthopaedic Surgeons. (2007b). *Total joint replacement.* Retrieved October 22, 2010, from http://orthoinfo.aaos.org/topic.cfm?topic=A00233.

American Academy of Orthopaedic Surgeons. (2009a). *Total hip replacement.* Retrieved September 1, 2011, from http://orthoinfo.aaos.org/topic.cfm?topic=A00377.

American Academy of Orthopaedic Surgeons. (2009b). *Viscosupplementation treatment for arthritis.* Retrieved October 22, 2010, from http://orthoinfo.aaos.org/topic.cfm?topic=A002o8.

American Academy of Physical Medicine and Rehabilitation. (2005). *Amputations/prosthetics.* Retrieved October 15, 2005, from www.aapmr.org/condtreat/rehab/amputations.htm.

American Association of Clinical Endocrinologists. (2003). *AACE clinical practice guidelines for the prevention and treatment of postmenopausal osteoporosis.* Retrieved April 20, 2007, from www.aace.com/pub/pdf/guidelines/osteoporosis2001revised.pdf.

American Burn Association. (2009). *White paper: Surgical management of the burn wound and use of skin substitutes.* Retrieved August 11, 2010, from http://ameriburn.org/WhitePaperFinal.pdf?PHPSESSID=238c889e2b37ed68288f844717ba3447.

American College of Rheumatology. (2007). *Information for patients about NSAIDs.* Retrieved September 1, 2011, from www.rheumatology.org/practice/clinical/patients/medications/nsaids.asp.

American College of Rheumatology. (2008). *Sulfasalazine (Azulfidine).* Retrieved September 1, 2011, from www.rheumatology.org/practice/clinical/patients/medications/sulfasalazine.asp.

American College of Rheumatology. (2009a). *Azathioprine (Imuran).* Retrieved September 1, 2011, from www.rheumatology.org/practice/clinical/patients/medications/azathioprine.asp.

American College of Rheumatology. (2009b). *Cyclophosphamide (Cytoxan).* Retrieved September 1, 2011, from www.rheumatology.org/practice/clinical/patients/medications/cyclophosphamide.asp.

American College of Rheumatology. (2009c).*Cyclosporine (Gengraf, Neoral, Sandimmune).* Retrieved September 1, 2011, from ww.rheumatology.org/practice/clinical/patients/medications/cyclosporine.asp.

American College of Rheumatology. (2009d). *Gold preparations (Myochrysine, Ridaura, Solganol).* Retrieved September 1, 2011, from www.rheumatology.org/practice/clinical/patients/medications/gold.asp.

American College of Rheumatology. (2009e). *Hydroxychloroquine (Plaquenil).* Retrieved September 1, 2011, from www.rheumatology.org/practice/clinical/patients/medications/hydroxychloroquine.asp.

American College of Rheumatology. (2009f). *Leflunomide (Arava).* Retrieved September 1, 2011, from www.rheumatology.org/practice/clinical/patients/medications/leflunomide.asp.

American College of Rheumatology. (2009g). *Methotrexate (Rheumatrex, Trexall).* Retrieved September 1, 2011, from www.rheumatology.org/practice/clinical/patients/medications/methotrexate.asp.

American College of Rheumatology. (2010a). *DMARDs, Glucocorticoids, and biologics equally effective for rheumatoid arthritis.* Retrieved September 1, 2011, from www.rheumatology.org/about/newsroom/2010/2010_01_28.asp.

American College of Rheumatology. (2010b). *Denosumab.* Retrieved September 1, 2011, from www.rheumatology.org/publications/hotline/2010_10_18_denosumab.pdf#search="Denosumab".

American College of Rheumatology. (2011a). *Abatacept (Orencio).* Retrieved September 1, 2011, from www.rheumatology.org/practice/clinical/patients/medications/abatacept.pdf#search="abatacept".

American College of Rheumatology. (2011b).*Anakinra.* Retrieved September 1, 2011, from www.rheumatology.org/practice/clinical/patients/medications/anakinra.asp.

American College of Rheumatology. (2011c). *Anti-TNF.* Retrieved September 1, 2011, from www.rheumatology.org/practice/clinical/patients/medications/anti_tnf.asp.

American College of Rheumatology. (2011d). *Rituximab.* Retrieved September 1, 2011, from www.rheumatology.

org/practice/clinical/patients/medications/rituximab. pdf#search="Rituximab".

American College of Rheumatology. (2011e). *Tocilizumab*. Retrieved September 1, 2011, from www.rheumatology. org/publications/hotline/2010_02_03_tocilizumab. pdf#search="Tocilizumab".

American College of Rheumatology Subcommittee on Osteoarthritis. (2003). *Recommendations for the medical management of osteoarthritis of the hip and knee: 2000 update*. Atlanta, GA: Author.

American Medical Association. (2004). *Osteoporosis management: Rehabilitation of the patient with osteoporosis*. Chicago: Author.

American Society of Anesthesiologists Task Force on Acute Pain Management. (2004). Practice guidelines for acute pain management in the perioperative setting. *Anesthesiology, 100*(6), 1573–1581.

Amputee Coalition of America. (2007). Fact sheet. Retrieved July 19, 2007, from www.amputee-coalition.org/easyread/fact_ sheets/dysvascular-ez.html.

Amputee Coalition of America. (2008a). U.S. military builds on rich history of amputee care. *Military-In-Step*. Retrieved August 30, 2010, from www.amputee-coalition.org/military-instep/war-injuries.html.

Amputee Coalition of America. (2008b). The military amputee and the unique characteristics of war injuries. *Military-In-Step*. Retrieved August 30, 2010, from www.amputee-coalition.org/military-instep/rich-history.html.

Amputee Coalition of America. (2010). Limb loss FAQs. National Limb Loss Information Center. Retrieved August 20, 2010, from www.amputee-coalition.org/nllic-faq.html.

Anderson, L. P., & Dale, K. G. (1998). Infections in total joint replacements. *Orthopaedic Nursing, 17*(1), 117–119.

Arroll, B., & Goodyear-Smith, F. (2004). Corticosteroid injections for osteoarthritis of the knee. Meta-analysis. *BMJ, 328*(7444), 869–870.

Arthritis Foundation. (2010a). *Gout: treatment options*. Atlanta, GA: Author.

Arthritis Foundation. (2010b). *Osteoarthritis*. Atlanta, GA: Author.

Arthritis Foundation. (2010c, August). *Research update: Approaches for osteoarthritis*. Atlanta: Author.

Arthritis Foundation. (2010d, August). *Rheumatoid arthritis*. Atlanta, GA: Author.

Arthritis Foundation. (2011). *Rheumatoid arthritis: Who gets rheumatoid arthritis*. Atlanta: Author.

Arthritis Foundation and CDC. (2010). *A national public health agenda for osteoarthritis*. Atlanta: Author.

Arthur, A. B., Kopec, J. A., Klinkhoff, A. V., Carr, S. L., Prince, J. M., Dumont, K. E., et al. (2009). Readiness to manage arthritis: A pilot study using stages-of-change measure for arthritis rehabilitation. *Rehabilitation Nursing, 34*(2), 64-73, 84.

Baker, J. F., & Schumacher, H. R. (2010). Update on gout and hyperuricemia. *International Journal of Clinical Practice, 64*(3), 371–377.

Bang, M. S., & Jung, S. H. (2008). Phantom limb pain. In W. R. Frontera, J. K. Silver, & T. D. Rizzo (Eds.), *Essentials of physical medicine and rehabilitation: Musculoskeletal disorders, pain and rehabilitation* (2nd ed., pp. 575–578). Philadelphia: Saunders/Elsevier.

Bantle, J. P. (2009). Dietary fructose and metabolic syndrome and diabetes. *Journal of Nutrition, 139*(6), 1263S–1268S.

Barker, T. L., & Puckett, T. L. (2010). Rheumatoid arthritis: Coping with disability. *Rehabilitation Nursing, 35*(2), 75–79.

Beer, M. H. (2005). *Merck manual of geriatrics*. Whitehouse Station, NJ: Merck Research Laboratories.

Bennett, J. B., & Alexander, C. B. (2004). Amputation levels and surgical techniques. In R. H. Meier III & D. J. Atkins (Eds.), *Functional restoration of adults with upper extremity amputation* (pp. 9–22). New York: Demos.

Benson, V., & Mariano, M. (1998). Current estimates from the National Health Interview Survey, 1995. *Vital & Health Statistics, 10*(199), 1–428.

Beukelman, T., Patkar, N. M., Saag, K., Tolleson-Rinehart, S., Cron, R. Q., DeWitt, E. M., et al. (2011). 2011 American College of Rheumatology recommendations for the treatment of juvenile idiopathic arthritis: Initiation and safety monitoring of therapeutic agents for the treatment of arthritis and systemic features. *Arthritis Care & Research, 63*(4), 465–482.

Bieber, J. D., & Terkeltaub, R. A. (2004). Gout. On the brink of novel therapeutic options for an ancient disease. *Arthritis & Rheumatism, 50*(8), 2400–2414.

Binkley, N., & Krueger, D. (2005). Current osteoporosis prevention and management. *Topics of Geriatric Rehabilitation, 21*(1), 17–29.

Bischoff-Ferrari, H. A., Dawson-Hughes, B., Stahelin, H. B., Orav, J. E., Stuck, A. E., Theiler, R., et al. (2009). Fall prevention with supplemental and active forms of vitamin D: A meta-analysis of randomized controlled trials. *BMJ, 339*, b3692.

Bischoff-Ferrari, H. A., Dawson-Hughes, B., Willett, W. C., Stoehelin, H. B., Bazemore, M. G., Zee, R. Y., et al. (2004). Effects of vitamin D on falls: A meta-analysis. *JAMA, 291*(16), 1999–2006.

Bischoff-Ferrari, H. A., Rees, J. R., Grau, M. V., Barry, E., Gui, J., & Baron, J. A. (2008). Effects of calcium supplementation on fracture risk: A double-blind randomized controlled trial. *American Journal of Clinical Nutrition, 87*(6), 1945–1951.

Bischoff-Ferrari, H. A., Willett, W. C., Wong, J. B., Giovannucci, E., Dietrich, T., & Dawson-Hughes, B. (2005). Fracture prevention with vitamin D supplementation: A meta-analysis of randomized controlled trials. *JAMA, 293*(18), 2257–2264.

Blick, S. K. A., Dhillon, S. & Keam, S. J. (2008). Teriparatide: A review of its use in osteoporosis. *Drugs, 68*(18), 2709–2737.

Bock, O., & Felsenberg, D. (2008). Bisphosphonates in the management of postmenopausal osteoporosis—optimizing efficacy in clinical practice. *Clinical Interventions in Aging, 3*(2), 279–297.

Bone, M., Critchley, P., & Buggy, D. J. (2002). Gabapentin in post amputation phantom limb pain: A randomized double-blind placebo-controlled cross-over study. *Regional Anesthesia and Pain Medicine, 27*(5), 481–486.

Bonner, F. J., Sinaki, M., Grabois, M., Shiipp, K. M., Lane, J. M., Lindsay, R., et al. (2003). Health professional's guide to rehabilitation of the patient with osteoporosis. *Osteoporosis International, 14*(Suppl. 2), S1–S22.

Boonen, S., Bischoff-Ferrari, H. A., Cooper, C., Lips, P., Ljunggren, O., Meunier, J., et al. (2006). Addressing the musculoskeletal components of fracture risk with calcium and vitamin D: A review of the evidence. *Calcified Tissue International, 78*(5), 257–270.

Brandes, V. A., Stulberg, D. S., & Chang, R. W. (1994). Rehabilitation following hip and knee arthroplasty. *Physical Medicine and Rehabilitation Clinics of North America, 5*, 815–836.

Bren, L. (2004). Joint replacement. An inside look. *FDA Consumer, 38*(2), 12–19.

Bruyere, O., & Reginster, J. Y. (2007). Glucosamine and chondroitin sulfate as therapeutic agents for knee and hip osteoarthritis. *Drugs & Aging, 24*(7), 537–580.

Buchbinder, R., Osborne, R. H., Ebeling, P. R., Wark, J. D., Mitchell, P., Wriedt, C., et al. (2009). A randomized trial of vertebroplasty for painful osteoporotic vertebral fractures. *New England Journal of Medicine, 31*(6), 557–568.

Buckwater, J. A., Saltzman, C., & Brown, T. (2004). The impact of osteoarthritis: Implications for research. *Clinical Orthopaedics and Related Research, 427S*, S6–S15.

Bulechek, G. M., Butcher, H., & Dochterman, J. M. (2008). *Nursing interventions classification (NIC)* (5th ed.). St. Louis: Mosby.

Burn Prevention Network. (2010). *Resources.* Retrieved August 11, 2010, from www.burnprevention.org/site/resources/.

Burn Survivor Resource Center. (n.d.). *Medical care guide: Types of scars.* Retrieved August 10, 2010, from www.burnsurvivor.com/scar_types.html.

Busso, N., & Alexander, S. (2010). Mechanisms of inflammation in gout. *Arthritis Research & Therapy, 12*(206). Retrieved February 3, 2011, from http://arthritis-research.com/content/12/2/206.

Butler, D., Turkal, N., & Seidl, J. (1992). Amputation: Preoperative psychological preparation. *Journal of American Board of Family Practice, 5*(1), 69–73.

Carda, S., Cisari, C., Invernizzi, M., & Bevilacqua, M. (2009). Osteoporosis after stroke: A review of the causes and potential treatments. *Cerebrovascular Disease, 28,* 191–200.

Cassidy, J. T., Petty, R. E., Lindsley, C. B., & Laxer, R. N. (Eds.). (2005). *Textbook of pediatric rheumatology* (5th ed.). Philadelphia: Saunders.

Centers for Disease Control and Prevention. (2006). *Mass casualties: Burns.* Retrieved August 10, 2010, from www.bt.cdc.gov/masscasualties/burns.asp.

Centers for Disease Control and Prevention. (2008). *Blast injuries essential facts.* Retrieved July 29, 2010, from http://emergency.cdc.gov/masscasualties/blastessentials.asp.

Centers for Disease Control and Prevention. (2009a, October 28). *Arthritis basics.* Retrieved August 13, 2010, from www.cdc.gov/chronicdisease/resources/publications/aag/arthritis.html.

Centers for Disease Control and Prevention. (2009b). *Fire deaths and injuries.* Retrieved August 10, 2010, from www.cdc.gov/homeandrecreationalsafety/Fire-prevention/fires-factsheet.html.

Centers for Disease Control and Prevention. (2010). *Arthritis: Meeting the challenge.* Retrieved August 13, 2010, from www.cdc.gov/chronicdisease/resources/publications/aag/arthritis.html.

Centers for Disease Control and Prevention. (2010c). *WISQARS leading causes of death.* Retrieved August 10, 2010, from http://webappa.cdc.gov/sasweb/ncipc/leadcaus10.html.

Centers for Disease Control and Prevention & The Arthritis Foundation. (2010). *CDC and the Arthritis Foundation launch the 1st national agenda for osteoarthritis to help millions.* Retrieved February 13, 2011, from www.cdc.gov/arthritis/osteoarthritis.html.

Chan, K. M., Anderson, M., & Lau, E. M. C. (2003). Exercise interventions: Defusing the world's osteoporosis time bomb. *Bulletin of the World Health Organization, 81*(11), 827–839.

Chen, C. M., Chen, L., Gu, Y., Xu, Y., Liu, Y., Bai, X. L., et al. (2010). Kyphoplasty for chronic painful osteoporotic vertebral compression fractures via unipedicular approach-ment: A comparative study in early stage. *Injury: International Journal of the Care of the Injured, 41*(4), 356–359.

Cheng, Y. J., Hootman, J. M., Murphy, L. B., Langmaid, G. A., & Helmick, C. G. (2010). Prevalence of doctor-diagnosed arthritis and arthritis-attributable activity limitation: United States, 2007–2009. *MMWR, 59*(39), 1261–1265.

Chesnut, C. A., Silverman, S., Andriano, K., Genant, H., Gimona, A., Harris, S., et al. (2000). A randomized trial of nasal spray salmon calcitonin in post-menopausal women with established osteoporosis: The Prevent Recurrence of Osteoporotic Fracture study: PROOF Study Group. *American Journal of Medicine, 109*(4), 267–276.

Chesnut, C. A., Skay, A., Christiansen, C., Recker, R., Stakkestad, J. A., Hoiseth, A., et al. (2004). Effects of oral ibandronate administered daily or intermittently on fracture risk in postmenopausal osteoporosis. *Journal of Bone and Mineral Research, 19*(8), 1241–1249.

Choi, H. K., Atkinson, K., Karlson, E. W., & Curhan, G. (2005). Obesity, weight change, hypertension, diuretic use and risk of gout in men. *Archives of Internal Medicine, 165*(7), 742–749.

Choi, H. K., Atkinson, K., Karlson, E. W., Willet, W., & Curhan, G. (2004a). Alcohol intake and risk of incident gout in men: A prospective study. *Lancet, 363*(9417), 1277–1281.

Choi, H. K., Atkinson, K., Karlson, E. W., Willet, W., & Curhan, G. (2004b). Purine-rich foods, dairy and protein intake, and the risk of gout in men. *New England Journal of Medicine, 350*(11), 1093–1103.

Choi, H. K., & Curhan, G. (2007). Coffee, tea and caffeine consumption and serum uric acid level: The Third National Health and Nutrition Examination survey. *Arthritis & Rheumatism, 57*(5), 816–821.

Choi, H. K., Mount, D. B., & Reginato, A. N. (2005). Pathogenesis of gout. *Annals of Internal Medicine, 143*(7), 499–516.

Choi, J. W. J., Ford, E. S., Gao, X., & Choi, H. K. (2008). Sugar sweetened soft drinks, and serum uric acid level: The Third National Health and Nutrition Examination Survey. *Arthritis & Rheumatism, 59*(1), 109–116.

Coupaud, S., McLean, A. N., & Allan, D. B. (2009). Role of peripheral quantitative computed tomography in identifying disease osteoporosis in paraplegia. *Skeletal Radiology.* Retrieved August 30, 2010, from http://eprints.gla.ac.uk/5106.pdf.

Cranney, A., Tugwell, P., Zytarak, N., Robinson, V., Weaver, B., Shea, B., et al. (2002). Meta-analysis of calcitonin for the treatment of postmenopausal osteoporosis. *Endocrine Review, 23*(4), 540–541.

Crowley, L. V. (2004). *An introduction to human disease: Pathology and pathophysiology correlations.* Sudbury, MA: Jones & Bartlett.

Cumming, R., & Nevitt, M. C. (1997). Calcium for osteoporotic fractures in postmenopausal women. *Journal of Bone and Mineral Research, 12,* 1321–1329.

Cummings, S. R., San Martin, J., McClung, M. R., Siris, E. S., Eastell, R., Reid, I. R., et al. (2009). Denosumab for prevention of fractures in postmenopausal women with osteoporosis. *New England Journal of Medicine, 361*(8), 756–765.

Dahmer, S., & Schiller, R. M. (2008). Glucosamine. *American Family Physician, 78*(4), 471–476, 481.

Davis, R. W. (1993). Phantom sensation, phantom pain, and stump pain. *Archives of Physical Medicine and Rehabilitation, 74,* 243–256.

Dawson-Hughes, B., Mithal, A., Bonjour, J. P., Boonen, S., Burck-hardt, P., Fulcihan, G. E. H., et al. (2010). IOF position statement: Vitamin D recommendations for older adults. *Osteoporosis International, 21*(7), 1151–1154.

Delmas, P. D., Recker, R. R., Chesnut, C. H. III, Skag, A., Stakkestad, J. A., Emkey, R., et al. (2004). Daily and intermittent oral ibandronate normalize bone turnover and provide significant reduction in vertebral fracture risk: Results from the BONE study. *Osteoporosis International, 15*(10), 792–798.

Department of Veterans Affairs. (2010). National Center for PTSD. Retrieved August 10, 2010, from www.ptsd.va.gov/professional/index.asp.

Department of Veterans Affairs/Department of Defense. (2004). *Clinical practice guideline for the management of post-traumatic stress.* Retrieved August 10, 2010, from www.healthquality.va.gov/ptsd/ptsd_full.pdf.

Department of Veterans Affairs/Department of Defense. (2008). *Clinical practice guideline for rehabilitation of lower limb amputation.* Washington, DC: Author.

de Roos, C., Veenstra, V. C., de Jongh, A., den Hollander-Gijisman, V., van der Wee, N. J., Zitman, F.G., et al. (2010). Treatment of chronic phantom limb pain using a trauma-focused psychological approach. *Pain Research & Management: The Journal of the Canadian Pain Society, 15*(2), 65–71.

Dheerendra, S., Khan, W., Saeed, M. Z., & Goddard, N. (2010). Recent developments in total hip replacements. Cementation, articulation, minimal-invasion and navigation. *Journal of Perioperative Practice, 20*(4), 133–137.

Diaz-Borjon, A. (2009). Guidelines for the use of conventional and newer disease-modifying antirheumatic drugs in elderly patients with rheumatoid arthritis. *Drugs & Aging, 26*(4), 273–293.

Dillingham, T. R., Pezzin, L. E., & MacKenzie, E. J. (2002). Limb amputation and limb deficiency: Epidemiology and recent trends in the United States. *Southern Medical Journal, 95*(8), 875–883.

Dudley-Javoroski, S. S., & Shields, R. K. (2008). Muscle and bone plasticity after spinal cord injury: Review of adaptations to disuse and to electrical muscle stimulation. *Journal of Rehabilitation Research & Development, 45*(2), 283–296.

Edelstein, J. (1992). Preprosthetic and nonprosthetic management of older patients. *Topics in Geriatric Rehabilitation, 8*(1), 22–29.

Eli Lilly. (2007). *Evista (raloxifene hydrochloride).* Indianapolis, IN: Author. Retrieved August 10, 2010, from www.fda.gov/downloads/Drugs/DrugSafety/ucm088593.pdf.

Eli Lilly. (2008). *Forteo (teriparatide [rDNA origin] injection).* Indianapolis, IN: Author. Retrieved August 10, 2010, from www.accessdata.fda.gov/drugsatfda_docs/label/2008/021318s015lbl.pdf.

Engelke, K., Adams, J. E., Armbrecht, G., Augat, P., Bogado, C. E., Bouxsein, M. L., et al. (2008). Clinical use of quantitative computed tomography and peripheral quantitative computed tomography in the management of osteoporosis in adults: The 2007 ISCD official positions. *Journal of Clinical Densitometry: Assessment of Skeletal Health, 11*(1), 123–162

Felson, D. T. (2004). Risk factors for osteoarthritis. *Clinical Orthopaedics and Related Research, 427S,* S16–S21.

Finckh, A., Bansback, N., Marra, C. A., Anis, A. H., Michaud, K., Lubin, S., et al. (2009). Treatment of very early rheumatoid arthritis with symptomatic therapy, disease-modifying antirheumatic drugs, or biologic agents: A cost-effectiveness analysis. *Annals of Internal Medicine, 151*(9), 61–621

Friedman, M. A. (2000). *Posttraumatic stress disorder.* Retrieved August 10, 2010, from www.acnp.org/g4/GN401000111/CH109.html.

Gabriel, S. E., Crowson, C. S., Campion, M. E., & O'Fallon, W. M. (1997a). Direct medical costs unique to people with arthritis. *Journal of Rheumatology, 24*(4), 719–725.

Gabriel, S. E., Crowson, C. S., Campion, M. E., & O'Fallon, W. M. (1997b). Indirect and nonmedical costs among people with rheumatoid arthritis and osteoarthritis compared with non-arthritic controls. *Journal of Rheumatology, 24*(1), 43–48.

Gafeo, A., Saag, K. G., & Curtis, J. R. (2006). Treatment of Rheumatoid arthritis. *American Journal of Health-System Pharmacy, 63,* 2451–2465.

Gan, M., Yang, H., Zhou, F., Zou, J., Wang, G., Mei, X., et al. (2010). Kyphoplasty for the treatment of painful osteoporotic thoracolumbar burst fractures. *Orthopedics, 33*(2), 88–92.

Garnero, P., & Delmas, P. D. (2003). Biomarkers in osteoarthritis. *Bulletin of the World Health Organization, 15*(5), 641–646.

Gass, M., & Dawson-Hughes, B. (2006). Preventing osteoporosis-related fractures: An overview. *American Journal of Medicine, 119*(4 Suppl. 1), S3–S11.

Gennari, L., Merlotti, D., Valleggi, F., Martini, G., & Nuti, R. (2007). Selective estrogen receptor modulators for postmenopausal osteoporosis: Current state of development. *Drugs & Aging, 24*(5), 361–379.

Gimbel, J., Brugger, A., Zhao, W., Verburg, K., & Geis, G. (2001). Efficacy and tolerability of celecoxib versus hydrocodone/acetaminophen in the treatment of pain after ambulatory orthopedic surgery in adults. *Clinical Therapeutics, 23*(2), 228–241.

Godwin, M., & Dawes, M. (2004). Intra-articular steroid injections for painful knees: Systematic review with meta-analysis. *Canadian Family Physician, 50,* 241–248.

Gout & Uric Acid Education Society. (2010, May). *Gout & Uric Acid Education Society survey reveals Americans underestimate serious health implications of gout.* Retrieved August 25, 2010, from www.Gout&UricAcidEducationSociety.com.

Graudal, N., & Jürgens, G. (2010). Similar effects of disease-modifying antirheumatic drugs, glucocorticoids, and biologic agents on radiographic progression in rheumatoid arthritis: meta-analysis of 70 randomized placebo-controlled or drug-controlled studies, including 112 comparisons. *Arthritis & Rheumatism, 62*(10), 2852–2863.

Grossman, J. M., Gordon, R., Ranganath, V. K., Deal, C., Caplan, L., Chen, W., et al. (2010). American College of Rheumatology 2010 recommendations for the prevention and treatment of glucocorticoid-induced osteoporosis. *Arthritis Care & Research, 62*(11), 1515–1526.

Harden, R. N., Houle, T. T., Remble, T. A., Lin, W., Wang, K., & Saltz, S. (2005). Topiramate for phantom limb pain: A time series analysis. *Pain Medicine, 6*(5), 375–378.

Harris, N. T., Watts, N. B., Genant, H. K., McKeever, C. D., Hangartner, T., Keller, M., et al. (1999). Effects of risedronate treatment on vertebral and non-vertebral fractures in women with postmenopausal osteoporosis: A randomized controlled trial: Vertebral Efficacy with Risendronate Therapy (VERT) Study Group. *JAMA, 282*(14), 1344–1352.

Healthy People 2020. (2009, October 30). *Developing Healthy People 2020: Healthy People 2020 public meetings—2009 draft objectives.* Retrieved August 10, 2010, from www.healthypeople.gov/HP2020.

Heaney, R. P. (1998). Recommended calcium intakes revisited: Round table. In P. Burckhardt, B. Dawson-Hughes, & R. P. Heaney (Eds.), *Nutritional aspects of osteoporosis* (pp. 317–325). New York: Springer-Verlag.

Heaney, R. P., & Weaver, C. M. (2003). Calcium and vitamin D. *Endocrinology and Metabolism Clinics of North America, 32,* 181–194.

Helmick, C., Felson, D., Lawrence, R., Gabriel, S., Hirsch, R., Kwoh, C.K., et al. (2008). Estimates of the prevalence of arthritis and other rheumatic conditions in the United States. *Arthritis & Rheumatism, 58*(1), 15–25.

Herr, K., Titler, M. G., Schilling, M. L., Marsh, J. L., Xie, X., Ardery, G. et al. (2004). Evidence-based assessment of acute pain in older adults: Current nursing practices and perceived barriers. *Clinical Journal of Pain, 20*(5), 331–340.

Hochberg, M. C., Thomas, J., Thomas, D. J., Mead, L., Levine, D. M., & Klag, M. J. (1995). Racial differences in the incidence of gout. The role of hypertension. *Arthritis & Rheumatism, 38*(5), 628–632.

Holick, M. F. (2009). Vitamin D deficiency. *New England Journal of Medicine, 357*(3), 266–281.

Hompland, S. (2004). Pain management for upper extremity amputation. In R. H. Meier III & D. J. Atkins (Eds.), *Functional restoration of adults with upper extremity amputation* (pp. 89–111). New York: Demos.

Hootman, J. M., Bolen, J., Helmick, C., & Langmaid, G. (2006). Prevalence of doctor-diagnosed arthritis and arthritis attributed activity limitation: United States, 2003–2005. *MMWR, 55*(40), 1089–1092.

Hootman, J. M., & Helmick, C. (2006). Projections of U.S. prevalence of arthritis and associated activity limitations. *Arthritis & Rheumatism, 54*(1), 226–229.

Hoskison, T. K., & Wortmann, R. L. (2006). Advances in the management of gout and hyperuricaemia. *Scandinavian Journal of Rheumatology, 35*(4), 251–260.

Howell, B. (2007). Joint surgery: Paving the way to a smooth recovery. *RN, 70*(1), 32–38.

Iesaka, K., Kubiak, E. N., Bong, M. R., Su, E. T., & DiCesare, R. E. (2006). Orthopedic surgical management of hip and knee involvement in patients with juvenile arthritis. *American Journal of Orthopedics, 35*(2), 67–73.

Institute for Clinical Systems Improvement. (2008). *Health care guideline: Diagnosis and treatment of osteoporosis* (6th ed.). Retrieved August 10, 2010, from www.ICSI.org.

Institute of Medicine. (2010). *Dietary reference intakes for calcium and vitamin D.* Retrieved February 12, 2011, from www.iom.edu/Reports/.Calcium-and-Vitamin-D/DRI-Values.aspx.

International Osteoporosis Foundation. (2009a). *Basic bone biology.* Retrieved August 10, 2010, from www.iof.com/health-professionals/aboutosteoporosis/basic-bone-biology.html.

International Osteoporosis Foundation. (2009b). *Bisphosphonates.* Retrieved August 10, 2010, from www.iof.com/health-professionals/about-osteoporosis/treatment/biphosphonates.html.

International Osteoporosis Foundation. (2009c). *Calcitonin.* Retrieved August 10, 2010, from www.iof.com/health-professionals/about-osteoporosis/treatment/calcitonin.html.

International Osteoporosis Foundation. (2009d). *Calcium.* Retrieved August 10, 2010, from www.iof.com/patients-public/about-osteoporosis/prevention/nutrition/calcium.html.

International Osteoporosis Foundation. (2009e). *Calcium and vitamin D.* Retrieved August 21, 2010, from www.iofbone health.org/health-professionals/about-osteoporosis/treatment/calcium-vitamin-D.html.

International Osteoporosis Foundation. (2009f). Diagnosis and follow-up. Retrieved August 21, 2010, from www.iofbone health.org/health-professionals/about-osteoporosis/diagnosis.html.

International Osteoporosis Foundation. (2009g). *Epidemiology.* Retrieved August 21, 2010, ffrom www.iof.com/epidemiology.html.

International Osteoporosis Foundation. (2009h). *Facts and statistics about osteoporosis and its impact.* Retrieved August 10, 2010, from www.iofbonehealth.org/facts-and-statistics.html.

International Osteoporosis Foundation. (2009i). *FRAX®: Information and resources.* Retrieved August 21, 2010, ffrom www.iofbonehealth.org/health-professionals/frax.html.

International Osteoporosis Foundation. (2009j). *Risk factors.* Retrieved August 21, 2010, f] from www.iofbonehealth.com/risk-factors.html.

International Osteoporosis Foundation. (2009k). *Vertebroplasty and kyphoplasty.* Retrieved August 21, 2010, f from www.iofbonehealth.org.

International Osteoporosis Foundation. (2009l). *Vitamin D.* Retrieved August 10, 2010, from www.iofbonehealth.com/patients-public/about-osteoporosis/prevention/nutrition/vitamin-D.html.

International Osteoporosis Foundation. (2009m). *Vitamin D deficiency and insufficiency.* Retrieved August 10, 2010, from www.iof.com/health-professionals/about-osteoporosis/treatment/Vitamin-d-Ideficiency.html.

International Osteoporosis Foundation. (2010a). *Anabolic agents; PTH and teriparatide.* Retrieved August 10, 2010, from www.iof.com/health-professionals/about-osteoporosis/treatment/pth.html.

International Osteoporosis Foundation. (2010b). *Hormone replacement therapy.* Retrieved August 10, 2010, from www.iof.com/health-professionals/about-osteoporosis/treatment/hrt.html.

International Osteoporosis Foundation. (2010c). *Selective estrogen receptor modulators (SERM).* Retrieved August 10, 2010, from www.iof.com/health-professionals/about-osteoporosis/treatment/serms.html.

International Osteoporosis Foundation. (2010d). *Treatment of osteoporosis.* Retrieved August 10, 2010, from www.iof.com/health-professionals/about-osteoporosis/treatment.html.

International Osteoporosis Foundation. (2010e). *Vitamin D can prevent falls and fractures in older adults.* Retrieved August 10, 2010, from www.news-medical.net/news/20100511/IOf-vitamin-d-can-prevent-falls-and-fractures.html.

Jahangiri, M., Jayatunga, A. P., Bradley, J. W., & Dark, C. H. (1994). Prevention of phantom pain after major lower limb amputation by epidural infusion of diamorphine, clonidine and bupivacaine. *Annals of the Royal College of Surgeons of England, 76,* 324–326.

Janssens, H. J. E., Janssen, M., van de Lisdonk, E. H., van Riel, P. L. C. M., & van Weel, C. (2008). Use of oral prednisolone or naproxen for the treatment of gout arthritis: A double-blind, randomized equivalence trial. *Lancet, 371*(9627), 1854–1860.

Jiang, S. D., Dai, L. Y., & Jiang, L. S. (2006). Osteoporosis after spinal cord injury. *Osteoporosis International, 17,* 180–192.

Jin, L., Kollewe, K., Krampfi, K., Dengler, R., & Mohammadi, B. (2008). Treatment of phantom limb pain with botulinum toxin type A. *American Academy of Pain Medicine, 10*(2), 300–303.

Joint Commission & National Pharmaceutical Council. (2008). *Improving and measuring osteoporosis management.* Reston, VA: Author.

Jones, K. B., & Higgins, G.C. (2009). Juvenile rheumatoid arthritis. In P. J. Allen (Ed.), *Primary care of the child with a chronic condition* (5th ed., pp. 587–606). St. Louis: Mosby. .

Jordan, K. M., Arden, N. K., & Doherty, M. (2003). EULAR recommendations 2003: An evidence based approach to the management of knee osteoarthritis: Report of a task force of the Standing Committee for International Clinical Studies Including Therapeutic Trails (ESCISIT). *Annals of Rheumatic Disease, 62,* 1145–1155.

Jordan, A., & McDonagh, J. E. (2006). Juvenile idiopathic arthritis: The paediatric patient. *Pediatric Radiology, 36,* 734–742.

Jude, E. B., Oyibo, S. O., Chalmers, N., Andrew, J. M., & Boulton, A. J. M. (2001). Peripheral arterial disease in diabetic and non-diabetic patients: A comparison of severity and outcome. *Diabetes Care, 24,* 1433–1437.

Kalyani, R. R., Stein, B., Valiyil, R., Manno, R., Maynard, J. W., & Crews, D. C. (2010). Vitamin D treatment for the prevention of falls in older adults: Systematic review and meta-analysis. *Journal of the Geriatrics Society, 58*(7), 1299–1310.

Kanis, J. A. (1999). The use of calcium in the management of osteoporosis. *Bone, 24,* 279–290.

Kanis, J. A., Johansson, H., Johnell, O., Odén, A., de Laet, C., Eisman, J., et al. (2005). Alcohol intake as a risk factor for fracture. *Osteoporosis International, 16,* 737–742.

Kanis, J. A., Johnell, O., De Laet, C., Johansson, H., Oden, A., Delmas, P., et al. (2004). A meta-analysis of previous fracture and subsequent fracture risk. *Bone, 35*(2), 375–382.

Kanis, J. A., Johnell, O., Odén, A., Johansson, H., de Laet, C., Eisman, J. A., et al. (2005). Smoking and fracture risk: A meta-analysis. *Osteoporosis International, 16*(2), 155–162.

Karter, M. J., Jr. (2010). *Fire loss in the United States 2008.* Retrieved August 10, 2010, from www.nfpa.org/assets/files/PDF/OS.fireloss.pdf.

Kebicz, R. B. (2007). Nursing care of patients with musculoskeletal and connective tissue disorders. In L. S. Williams & P. D. Hopper (Eds.), *Understanding medical/surgical nursing* (3rd ed., pp. 991–1033). Philadelphia: F. A. Davis.

Kern, U., Martin, C., Scheicher, S., & Muller, H. (2004). Does botulinum toxin A make prosthesis use easier for amputees? *Journal of Rehabilitation Medicine, 36,* 238–239.

Kessenich, C. R. (1997). The pathophysiology of osteoporotic vertebral fractures. *Rehabilitation Nursing, 22*(4), 192–195.

Kim, K. Y., Schumacher, H. R., Hunsche, E., Wertheimer, A. I., & Kong, S. X. (2003). A literature review of the epidemiology and treatment of acute gout. *Clinical Therapeutics, 25*(6), 1593–1617.

Kimball, S., Fuleihan, G. E. H., & Vieth, R. (2008). Vitamin D: A growing perspective. *Critical Review in Clinical Laboratory Sciences, 45*(4), 339–414.

Kirkley, A., Birmingham, T. B., Litchfield, R. B., Giffin, J. R., Willits, K. R., Wong, C. J., et al. (2008). A randomized trial of arthroscopic surgery for osteoarthritis of the knee. *New England Journal of Medicine, 359*(11), 1097–1107.

Kleinman, N. L., & Brook, R. A. (2007). The impact of gout on work absence and productivity. *Value Health, 10,* 231–237.

Kleoppel, J. W., & Henry, D. W. (1987). Teaching patients, families and communities about their medications. In C. E. Smith (Ed.), *Patient education. Nurses in partnership with other health professions* (pp. 271–296). Philadelphia: W. B. Saunders.

Kocsis, J. D., & Tessler, A. (2009). Pathology of blast-related brain-injury. *Journal of Rehabilitation Research and Development, 46*(6), 667–672.

Lane, N. E., & Schnitzer, T. J. (2007). Osteoarthritis. In L. Goldman & D. Ausiello (Eds.), *Cecil medicine* (23rd ed., pp. 1993–1997). Philadelphia: Saunders.

Larsen, E. R., Mosekilde, L., & Foldspang, A. (2004). Vitamin D and calcium supplementation prevents osteoporotic fractures in elderly community dwelling residents: A pragmatic population-based 3-year intervention study. *Journal of Bone and Mineral Research, 19*(3), 370–378.

Law, M. R., & Hackshaw, A. K. (1997). A meta-analysis of cigarette smoking, bone mineral density and risk of hip fracture: Recognition of a major effect. *British Medical Journal, 315*(7112), 841–846.

Lawrence, R. C., Felson, D. T., Helmick, C. G., Arnold, L. M., Choi, H., Deyo, R.A., et al. (2008). Estimates of the prevalence of arthritis and other rheumatic conditions in the United States, Part II. *Arthritis & Rheumatism, 58*(1), 26–35.

Lee, S. H., & Abramson, S. B. (2005). Rheumatic diseases. In H. H. Zaretsky, E. F. Richter III, & M. G. Eisenberg (Eds.), *Medical aspects of disability: A handbook for the rehabilitation professional* (3rd ed.). New York: Springer.

Lemke, D. M. (2005). Vertebroplasty and kyphoplasty for treatment of painful osteoporotic compression fractures. *Journal of the American Academy of Nurse Practitioners, 17*(7), 268–276.

Lewis, S. M., Heitkemper, M. M., & Dirkson, S. R. (2004). *Medical-surgical nursing: Assessment and management of clinical problems* (6th ed.). St. Louis: Mosby.

Limb Loss Research & Statistics Program. (2006). *People with amputations speak out.* Retrieved September 4, 2010, from www.amputee-coalition.org/people-speak-out/background.html.

Lin, J., Zhang, W., Jones, A., & Doherty, M. (2004). Efficacy of topical non-steroidal anti-inflammatory drugs in the treatment of osteoarthritis: Meta-analysis of randomized controlled trials. *BMJ, 329*(7461), 324.

Livingston, K. E. (1945). The phantom limb syndrome: A discussion of the role of major peripheral nerve neuromas. *Journal of Neurosurgery, 2*(3), 251–255.

Lo, H. G., LaValley, M., McAlindon, T., & Felson, D. T. (2003). Intra-articular hyaluronic acid in treatment of knee osteoarthritis. *JAMA, 290*(230), 3115–3121.

Lubit, R. (2008). *Postconcussive syndrome.* Retrieved July 29, 2010, from http://emedicine.medscape.com/article/292326-overview.

Maetzel, A., Li, L. C., Pencharz, J., Tomlinson, F., & Bombardier, C. (2004). The economic burden associated with osteoarthritis. Rheumatoid arthritis and hypertension: A comparative study. *Annals of Rheumatologic Diseases, 63*(4), 395–401.

Maini, R. N. (2004). Review: Current and new antitumor necrosis factor agents in perspective. *Arthritis Research & Therapy, 8*(Suppl. 2), S1–S2.

Mäkeläines, P., Vehviläinen-Julkenen, K., & Pietilä, A.M. (2009). Rheumatoid arthritis patient education: RA patient's expressions. *Journal of Clinical Nursing, 18*(14), 2058–2065.

Malik, A., Schumacher, H. R., Dinnella, J. E., & Clayburne, G. M. (2009). Clinical diagnostic criteria for gout: Comparison with the gold standard of synovial fluid crystal analysis. *Journal of Clinical Rheumatology, 15*(1), 22–24.

Marti, L., & Scheinberg, M. (2009). Anti-interleukin 6: First line in rheumatoid arthritis? *Clinical Rheumatology, 28*, 877–879.

Mauck, K. F., & Clarke, B. L. (2006). Diagnosis, screening, prevention, and treatment of osteoporosis. *Mayo Clinic Proceedings, 81*(5), 662–672.

Mauk, K. L. (2006). Medications to treat arthritis. *ARN Network, 23*(5), 7–8.

Maunier, P. J. (1999). Calcium, vitamin D and vitamin K in the prevention of fractures due to osteoporosis. *Osteoporosis International, 9*(Suppl. 2), S48–S52.

Mayes, S. L. (2007). Review of postmenopausal osteoporosis pharmacotherapy. *Nutrition in Clinical Practice, 22*(3), 276–285.

McClung, B. L. (1999). Using osteoporosis management to reduce fractures in elderly women. *The Nurse Practitioner, 24*(3), 26–42.

McClung, M. R. (2003). Bisphosphonates. *Endocrinology and Metabolism Clinics of North America, 32*, 253–271.

McFarlane, L. V., Choppa, A. J., Betz, K., Pruden, J. D., & Reiber, G.E. (2010). Resources for wounded warriors with major traumatic limb loss. *Journal of Rehabilitation Research & Development, 47*(4), 1–13.

Meier, R. H., & Esquenazi, A. (2004a). Follow-up, outcomes and long-term experiences in adults with upper extremity amputation. In R. H. Meier III & D. J. Atkins (Eds.), *Functional restoration of adults with upper extremity amputation* (pp. 327–337). New York: Demos.

Meier, R. H., & Esquenazi, A. (2004b). Rehabilitation planning for the upper extremity amputee. In R. H. Meier III & D. J. Atkins (Eds.), *Functional restoration of adults with upper extremity amputation* (pp. 56–61). New York: Demos.

Meiner, S. E., & Lueckenotte, A. G. (2006). Musculoskeletal function. In S. E. Meiner & A. G. Lueckenotte (Eds.), *Gerontologic nursing* (3rd ed., chapter 27). St. Louis: Mosby/Elsevier.

Melcer, T., Belnap, B., Walker, G. J., Konoske, P., & Galarneau, M. (2011). Heterotopic ossification in combat amputees from Afghanistan and Iraq wars: Five case histories and results from a small series of patients. *Journal of Rehabilitation, Research & Development, 48*(1), 1–12.

Melcer, T., Walker, G. J., Galarneau, M., Belnap, B., & Konoske, P. (2010). Midterm health and personnel outcomes of recent combat amputees. *Military Medicine, 175*(3), 147–154.

Mercier, L. R. (2010a). Osteoarthritis: Basic information. In F. F. Ferri (Ed.), *Ferri's clinical advisor 2011*. St. Louis: Mosby.

Mercier, L. R. (2010b). Rheumatoid arthritis: Basic information. In F. F. Ferri (Ed.), *Ferri's clinical advisor 2011*. St. Louis: Mosby.

Michigan Quality Improvement Consortium. (2007). *Medical management of adults with osteoarthritis*. Southfield, MI: Author.

Michigan Quality Improvement Consortium. (2010). *Management and prevention of osteoporosis*. Southfield, MI: Author.

Migliore, A., Bizzi, E., Massafra, U., Vacca, F., Alimohti, A., Iannessi, F., et al. (2009). Viscosupplementation: A suitable option for hip osteoarthritis in young adults. *European Review for Medical and Pharmacological Sciences, 13*(6), 465–472.

MMWR. (2006). Prevalence of doctor-diagnosed arthritis and arthritis-attributable activity limitation, United States, 2003–2005. *MMWR, 55*(40), 1089–1092. Retrieved August 20, 2010, from www.cdc.gov/mmwr/preview/mmwrhtml/mm5540a2.htm?s_cid=mm5540a2_e.

Moizo, E., Marchetti, C., Albertin, A., Muzzolon, F., & Antonino, S. (2004). Acute pain service and multimodal therapy for postsurgical pain control: Evaluation of protocol efficacy. *Minerva Anesthesiology, 70*(11), 779–787.

Moorehead, S., Johnson, M., Maas, M., & Swanson, E. (2008). *Nursing outcomes classification (NOC)* (94th ed.). St. Louis: Mosby/Elsevier.

Morris, J. D., & Smith, K. M. (2009). Chondroitin sulfate in osteoarthritis therapy. *Orthopedics, 32*(4), 268–272.

Mosby Great Performance. (1995). *Helping at home, preventing falls* [Pamphlet]. Available from 14964 NW Greenbrier Parkway, Beaverton, OR 97006.

Mudano, A. S., Bian, J., Cope, J. U., Curtis, J. R., Gross, T. P., Allison, J. J., et al. (2009). Vertebroplasty and kyphoplasty are associated with an increased risk of secondary vertebral compression fractures: A population-based study. *Osteoporosis International, 20*, 819–826.

Mulvaney, S. W. (2009). A review of viscosupplementation for osteoarthritis for the hip and a description of an ultrasound: Guided hip injection technique. *Current Sports Medicine Reports, 8*(6), 291–294.

Nakamura, H., Masuko, K., Yudoh, K., Kato, T., Kamada, T., & Kawahara, T. (2007). Effects of glucosamine administration on patients with rheumatoid arthritis. *Rheumatology International, 27*(3), 213–218.

National Center for PTSD. (2010). *What is PTSD?* Retrieved August 20, 2010, from www.ptsd.va.gov/public/pages/what-is-ptsd.asp.

National Council on Aging. (2005). *New survey uncovers impact of osteoarthritis on sufferer's everyday lives*. Retrieved July 19, 2007, from www.redhotmamas.org/component/content/article/44-volume14/330-new-survey-uncovers-significant-impact-of-osteoarthritis-on-sufferers-lives.

National Institute of Arthritis and Musculoskeletal and Skin Diseases. (2008). *Juvenile arthritis*. Retrieved August 27, 2010, from www.niams.nih.gov/Health-Info/Juv-Arthritis.asp.

National Institute of General Medical Sciences. (2008). *Burn basics*. Retrieved August 10, 2010, from www.nigms.nih.gov/Publications/Factsheet_burns.htm.

National Institutes of Health. (2006, September). *Fact sheet: Burns and traumatic injury*. Retrieved August 10, 2010, from www.nih.gov/about/researchresultsforthepublic/BurnsandTraumaticInjury.pdf.

National Institutes of Health. (2011a). *Calcium*. Retrieved February 10, 2011, from http://ods.od.nih.gov/factsheets/calcium-HealthProfessional.html.

National Institutes of Health. (2011b). *Vitamin D*. Retrieved February 10, 2011, from http://ods.od.nih.gov/factsheets/VitaminD-HealthProfessional.

National Institutes of Health Consensus Development Panel. (2004). National Institute of Health Consensus Development Panel on optimal calcium intake. *Journal of the American Medical Association, 272*(13), 1942–1948.

National Limb Loss Information Center. (2008). *Recent trends in the United States*. Retrieved August 20, 2010, from www.amputee-coalition.org/fact_sheets/amp_stats_cause.html.

National Osteoporosis Foundation. (2008). BMD testing. Retrieved July 28, 2010, from www.nof.org/osteoporosis/bmdtest.htm.

National Osteoporosis Foundation. (2010a). Clinician's guide to prevention and treatment of osteoporosis. Washington, DC: Author. Retrieved July 28, 2010, from www.nof.org.

National Osteoporosis Foundation. (2010b). *Diagnosing osteoporosis: Understanding osteoporosis*. Retrieved August 10, 2010, from www.nof.org.

National Osteoporosis Foundation. (2010c). *Fast facts on osteoporosis*. Retrieved August 10, 2010, from www.nof.org/osteoporosis/disease facts.htm.

Nayback, A.M. (2009). Posttraumatic stress: A concept analysis. *Archives of Psychiatric Nursing, 23*(3), 210–219.

Neal-Boylan, L. (2009). Update on rheumatology, Part 1. *Home Healthcare Nurse, 27,* 286–296.

Nelson, H. D., Haney, E. M., Dana, T., Bougatsos, C., & Chou, R. (2010). Screening for osteoporosis: An update for the U.S. Preventive Services Task Force. *Annals of Internal Medicine, 153*(2), 1–13, W-5–W-11.

The North American Menopause Society. (2010). Management of osteoporosis in postmenopausal women: 2010 position statement of the North American Menopause Society. *Menopause: The Journal of the North American Menopause Society, 17*(1), 25–54.

North American Nursing Diagnosis Association. (2008). *Approved nursing diagnoses 2007–2008*. Retrieved July 29, 2010, from www.scribd.com/doc/8465961/NANDA-Nursing-Diagnosis-2008.

NYU Hospital for Joint Diseases Spine Center. (2005). *Types of osteoporosis*. Retrieved September 1, 2011, from http://hjd.med.nyu.edu/spine/patient-education/spine-problems/osteoporosis/types-osteoporosis.

Oaseem, A., Snow, V., Shekelle, P., Hopkins, R. Jr., Forciea, M. A., & Owens, D. K. (2008). Pharmacologic treatment of low bone density or osteoporosis to prevent fractures: A clinical practice guideline from the American College of Physicians. *Annals of Internal Medicine, 149*(6), 404–415.

O'Conner, M. I. (2007). Sex differences in osteoarthritis of the hip and knee. *Journal of the American Academy of Orthopedic Surgery, 15*(Suppl. 1), S22–S25.

O'Dell, J. R. (2007). Rheumatoid arthritis. In L. Goldman & D. Ausiello (Eds.), *Cecil medicine* (23rd ed., chapter 285). Philadelphia: Saunders.

Oldfield, V., Dhillon, S., & Plosker, G. L. (2009). Tocilizumab: A review of its use in the management of rheumatoid arthritis. *Drugs, 69*(5), 609–632.

Oldfield, V. ,& Plosker, G. L. (2009).Golimumab: In the treatment of rheumatoid arthritis, psoriatic arthritis and ankylosing spondylitis. *BioDrugs, 23*(2), 125–135.

Olubumma, C. A. (2009). Rheumatoid arthritis: A chronic inflammation. *Nursing Made Incredibly Easy*. Retrieved September 2, 2010, from www.NursingMadeincrediblyEasy.com.

Oshima, M., Matsuzaki, M., Tokuhashi, Y., & Okawa, A. (2010). Evaluation of biomechanical and histological features of vertebrae following vertebroplasty using hydroxyapatite blocks. *Orthopedics, 33*(2), 89–93.

Pang, M. Y. C., Ashe, M. C., & Eng, J. J. (2007). Muscle weakness, spasticity and disuse contribute to demineralization and geometric changes in the radius following stroke. *Osteoporosis International, 18,* 1243–1252.

Pellino, T., Willens, J., Polomano, R., & Heve, R. (2003). The American Society of Pain Management Nurses role-delineation study. National Association of Orthopaedic Nurses respondents. *Orthopedic Nursing, 22*(4), 289–297.

Pitocco, D., Ruotolo, V., Caputo, S., Mancini, L., Collina, C. M., Manto, A., et al. (2005). Six months treatment with alendronate in acute Charcot neuropathy. *Diabetes Care, 28*(5), 1214–1215.

Pollard, B., Johnston, M., & Dieppe, P. (2011). Exploring the relationships between International Classification of Functioning, Disability and Health (ICF) constructs of Impairment, Activity Limitation and Participation Restriction in people with osteoarthritis prior to joint replacement. *BMC Musculoskeletal Disorders, 12,* 97.

Post, T. M., Cremers, S. C. L. M., Kerbusch, T., & Danhof, M. (2010). Bone physiology, disease and treatment: Towards disease system analysis in osteoporosis. *Clinical Pharmacokinetics, 49*(2), 89–118.

Potter, B. K., Burns, T. C., LaCap, A. P., Granville, R. R., & Gajewski, D. A. (2007). Heterotopic ossification following traumatic and combat-related amputations: Prevalence, risk factors, and preliminary results of excision. *Journal of Bone & Joint Surgery, 89*(3), 496–486.

Pratelli, E., Cinotti, I., & Pasquetti, P. (2010). Rehabilitation in osteoporotic vertebral fractures. *Clinical Cases in Mineral and Bone Mineralism, 7*(1), 45–47.

Pullen, R. L. Jr. (2010). Caring for a patient after amputation. *Nursing, 40*(1), 15.

Ragnarsson, K. T. (2008). Functional electrical stimulation after spinal cord injury: Current use, therapeutic effects and future directions. *Spinal Cord, 46,* 255–274.

Rahmani, P., & Morin, S. (2009). Prevention of osteoporosis-related fractures among postmenopausal women and older men. *Canadian Medical Association Journal, 181*(11), 815–820.

Rawlins, S. (2009). Approaches to osteoporosis: Screening and implementing treatment in clinical practice. *Journal of Family Practice, 58*(7), S39–S44.

Reginster, J. Y., & Burlet, N. (2006). Osteoporosis: A still increasing prevalence. *Bone, 38*(2), 1573–1581.

Reid, I. R., Ames, R. W., Evans, M. C., Gamble, G. D., & Sharpe, S. J. (1995). Long-term effects of calcium supplementation on bone loss and fractures in postmenopausal women: A randomized controlled trial. *American Journal of Medicine, 98*(4), 31–35.

Richter, E. F. III, & Deporto, R. (2005). Orthopedic impairments. In H. H. Zaretsky, E. F. Richter III, & M.G. Eisenberg (Eds.), *Medical aspects of disability: A handbook for the rehabilitation professional* (3rd ed.). New York: Springer.

Robbins, C. B., Vreeman, D. J., Sothmann, M. S., Wilson, S. L., & Oldridge, N. B. (2009). A review of the long-term health outcomes associated with war-related amputation. *Military Medicine, 4*(6), 588–592.

Roddy, E., Zhang, W., & Doherty, M. (2007). Is gout associated with reduced quality of life? A case-control study. *Rheumatology (Oxford), 48*(9), 1441–1444.

Rosen, C. (2007). Osteoporosis. In L. Goldman & D. Ausiello (Eds.), *Cecil medicine* (23rd ed., pp. 1879–1888). Philadelphia: Saunders.

Rosenbaum, C. C., O'Mathuna, D. P., Chavez, M., & Shields, K. (2010). Antioxidants and antiinflammatory dietary supplements for osteoarthritis and rheumatoid arthritis. *Alternative Therapies in Health and Medicine, 16*(2), 32–40.

Rossouw, J. E., Anderson, G., Prentice, R. L., LaCroix, A. Z., Kooperberg, C., Stefanick, M. L., et al. (2002). Risk and benefits of estrogen plus progestin in healthy postmenopausal women: Principal results from the Women's Health Initiative randomized control trial. *JAMA, 288*(3), 321–333.

Rozendaal, R. M., Koes, B. W., Van Osch, G. J. V. M., Uitterlinden, E. J., Garling, E. H., Willemsen, S. P., et al. (2008). Effect of glucosamine sulfate on hip osteoarthritis. *Annals of Internal Medicine, 146*, 580.

Russell, M. C. (2008). Treating traumatic amputation-related phantom limb pain: A case study utilizing eye movement desensitization and reprocessing within the armed forces. *Clinical Case Studies, 7*(1), 136–153.

Saag, K. G., & Geusens, P. (2009). Progress in osteoporosis and fracture prevention: Focus on post menopausal women. *Arthritis Research & Therapy, 11*(5), 251.

Saag, K. G., Teng, G. G., Patkar, N. M., Anuntiyo, J., Finney, C., Curtis, J. R., et al. (2008). American College of Rheumatology 2008 recommendations for the use of nonbiologic and biologic disease-modifying anti-rheumatic drugs in rheumatoid arthritis. *Arthritis & Rheumatism, 59*(6), 762–784.

Sacks, J. J., Helmick, C. G., Luo, Y. H., Ilowik, N. T., & Bowyers, S. (2007). Prevalence of annual ambulatory health care visits for pediatric arthritis and other rheumatologic conditions in the United States in 2001–2004. *Arthritis Care & Research, 57*(8), 1439–1445.

Sambrook, P., & Cooper, C. (2006). Osteoporosis. *Lancet, 367*(9527), 2010–2018.

Schlesinger, N., Norquist, J. M., & Watson, J. D. (2009). Serum urate during acute gout. *Journal of Rheumatology, 36*, 1287–1289.

Schoen, D. C. (2001). *NAON core curriculum for orthopaedic nursing* (4th ed.). Pitman, NJ: Anthony J. Jannetti.

Schongerb, M. A., Marcantonio, E. R., & Hamel, M. B. (2009). Perceptions of physician recommendations for joint replacement surgery in older patients with severe hip or knee osteoarthritis. *Journal of American Geriatric Society, 57*(1), 82–88.

Shalev, A. Y. (2009). Posttraumatic stress disorder and stress-related disorders. *Psychiatric Clinics of North America, 32*, 687–704.

Shea, B., Wells, G., Cranney, A., Ztaruk, N., Robinson, V., Griffith, L., et al. (2002). Meta-analysis of calcium supplementation for the prevention of post menopausal osteoporosis. *Endocrine Reviews, 23*(4), 552–559.

Sherman, R. A., & Sherman, C. J. (1985). A comparison of phantom sensations among amputees whose amputations were of civilian and military origins. *Pain, 21*(1), 91–97.

Shin, J. J., Chin, D. K., & Yoon, Y. S. (2009). Percutaneous vertebroplasty for the treatment of osteoporotic burst fractures. *Acta Neurochirurgica, 151*, 141–148.

Shukla, P. C. (2008). *Initial evaluation and management of the burn patient.* Retrieved August 10, 2010, from http://emedicine.medscape.com/article/435402-overview

Sierakowska, M., Krajewska-Kulak, E., Lewko, J., Przeorska-Najgebauer, T., Jankowiak, B., Rolka, H., et al. (2005). The education of patients with rheumatoid arthritis: The knowledge and expectations of patients: The opinions of rheumatology nurses. *Roczniki Akademii Medycznej w Bialymstoku (Annales Academiae Medicae Bialostocensis), 50*(Suppl. 1), 107–110.

Silver, S. M., Rogers, S., & Russell, M. (2008). Eye movement desensitization and reprocessing (EMDR) in the treatment of war veterans. *Journal of Clinical Psychology: In Session, 64*(8), 947–957.

Silverman, S. L. (2003). Calcitonin. *Endocrinology and Metabolism Clinics of North America, 32*, 273–284.

Silverman, S. L., Minshall, M. E., Shen, W., Harper, K. D., & Xie, S.; Health-Related Quality of Life Subgroup of the Multiple Outcomes of Raloxifene Evaluation Study. (2001). The relationship of health-related quality of life to prevalent and incident vertebral fractures in postmenopausal women with osteoporosis: Results from the Multiple Outcomes of Raloxifene Evaluation Study. *Arthritis & Rheumatism, 44*(11), 2611–2619.

Siminoski, K., O'Keeffe, M., Levesque, J., Henley, P., & Brown, P. (2011). Canadian Association of Radiologists technical standards: Bone mineral densitometry reporting. *Canadian Association of Radiologists Journal, 62*(3), 166–175.

Simon, L. S., Lipman, A. G., Caudill-Slosberg, M., Gill, L. H., Keele, F. J., Kerr, K. L., et al.(2002). *Pain in osteoarthritis, rheumatoid arthritis and juvenile chronic arthritis* (2nd ed.). Glenview, IL: American Pain Society.

Sinatra, R., Jahr, J., Reynolds, L., Viscusi, E., Groudine, S., & Paen-Champenois, C. (2005). Efficacy and safety of single and repeated administration of 1 gram intravenous acetaminophen injection (paracetamol) for pain management after major orthopedic surgery. *Anesthesiology, 102*(4), 822–831.

Singer, A. J., Brebbia, J., & Soroff, H. H. (2007). Management of local burn wounds in the ED. *American Journal of Emergency Medicine, 25*, 666–671.

Singh, J.A., Christensen, R., Wells, G. A., Suarez-Almazor, M. E., Buchbinder, R., Lopez-Olivo, M. A., et al. (2009). A network meta-analysis of randomized controlled trials of biologics for rheumatoid arthritis: A Cochrane overview. *CMAJ, 181*(11), 787–796.

Singh, J. A., & Strand, V. (2008). Gout is associated with more comorbidities, poorer health-related quality of life and higher healthcare obligation in US veterans. *Annals of the Rheumatic Diseases, 67*(9), 1310–1316.

Smith, D. G., Ehde, D. M., Hanley, M. A., Campbell, K. M., Jensen, M. P., Hoffman, A. J., et al. (2005). Efficacy of gabapentin in treating chronic phantom limb and residual limb pain. *Journal of Rehabilitation, Research & Development, 42*(5), 645–654.

Solomon, J. (1998). Osteoporosis: When supports weaken. *RN, 61*(5), 37–40.

Sommers, M. S., Johnson, S. A., & Beery, T. A. (2007). Rheumatoid arthritis. In M. S. Sommers, S. A. Johnson, & T. A. Beery (Eds.), *Diseases and disorders: A nursing therapeutic manual* (3rd ed.). Philadelphia: F. A. Davis.

Song, B. K., Eun, Y. M., & Oh, Y. M. (2009). Clinical and radiological comparison of unipedicular versus bipedicular balloon kyphoplasty for the treatment of vertebral compression fractures. *Osteoporosis International, 20*, 1717–1723.

Southwood, T. (2008). Juvenile idiopathic arthritis: Clinically relevant imaging in diagnosis and monitoring. *Pediatric Radiology, 38*(Suppl. 3), S305–S402.

Spollett, G. R. (1998). Preventing amputations in the diabetic population. *Nursing Clinics of North America, 33*(4), 629–637.

Spratto, G. R., & Woods, A. L. (1998). *PDR nurses' handbook* (3rd ed.). Montvale, NJ: Medical Economics.

Srikanth, V. K., Fryer, J. L., Zhai, G., Winzenberg, T. M., Hosmer, D., & Jones, G. (2005). A meta-analysis of sex difference prevalence, incidence and severity of osteoporosis. *Osteoporosis Cartilage, 13*(9), 769–781.

Strand, V., & Singh, J. A. (2010). Newer biological agents in rheumatoid arthritis. *Drugs, 70,* 121–145.

Stumer, T., Brenner, H., Koening, W., & Gunther, K. P. (2004). Severity and extent of osteoarthritis and low grade systemic inflammation as assessed by high sensitivity C-reactive protein. *Annals of Rheumatologic Disease, 63,* 200–205.

Sunkureddi, P., Nguyen-Oghalal, T. U., & Karnath, B. M. (2006). Clinical signs of gout. *Hospital Physician, 47,* 39–42.

Supervía, A., Nogués, X., Enjuanes, A., Vila, J., Mellibovsky, L., Serrano, S., et al. (2006). Effect of smoking and smoking cessation on bone mass, bone remodeling, vitamin D, PTH and sex hormones. *Journal of Musculoskeletal & Neuronal Interactions, 6*(3), 234–241.

Swearingen, P. L. (2007a). Osteoarthritis. In P. L. Swearingen (Ed.), *Manual of medical-surgical nursing care* (6th ed., pp. 553–557). St. Louis: Mosby Elsevier.

Swearingen, P. L. (2007b). Amputation. In P. L. Swearingen (Ed.), *Manual of medical–surgical nursing care* (6th ed., pp. 602–605). St. Louis: Mosby Elsevier.

Sweet, M. G., Sweet, J. M., Jeremiah, M. P., & Galazka, S. S. (2009). Diagnosis and treatment of osteoporosis. *American Family Physician, 79*(3), 193–200.

Taber, V. D. (2005). *Taber's cyclopedic medical dictionary* (20th ed.). Philadelphia: F. A. Davis.

Tak, S. H., Hong, S. H., & Kennedy, R. (2007). Daily stress in elders with arthritis. *Nursing Health Science, 9*(1), 29–33.

Tang, B. M., Eslick, G. D., & Nowson, C. (2007). Use of calcium or calcium in combination with vitamin D supplementation to prevent fractures and bone loss in people aged 50 years and older: A meta-analysis. *Lancet, 370*(9588), 657–666.

Tanner, S. (2003–2004). Back pain, vertebroplasty, and kyphoplasty: Treatment of osteoporotic vertebral compression fractures. *Bulletin on the Rheumatic Diseases, 52*(2), 1–7.

Teng, G. G., Nair, R., & Saag, K. G. (2006). Pathophysiology, clinical presentation and treatment of gout. *Drugs, 66*(12), 1547–1563.

Terkeltaub, R. (2007). Crystal deposition diseases. In L. Goldman & D. Ausiello (Eds.), Cecil medicine (23rd ed., pp. 2069–2077). Philadelphia: Saunders Elsevier.

Thalgott, J., LaRocca, H., & Gardner, V. O. (1993). Arthritis affecting the spinal column. In S. H. Hochschuler, H. B. Cotler, & R. D. Guyer (Eds.), *Rehabilitation of the spine.* St. Louis: Mosby.

Thompson, J. M. (2002). Amputation: Collaborative interventions and related nursing care. In J. M. Thompson, G. K. McFarland, J. E. Hirsch, & S. M. Tucker (Eds.), *Mosby's clinical nursing* (5th ed.). St. Louis: Mosby.

Traon, A. P. L., Heer, M., Narici, M. V., Rutweger, J., & Vernikos, J. (2007). From space to Earth: Advances in human physiology from 20 years of bedrest studies (1986–2006). *European Journal of Applied Physiology, 101,* 143–194.

Tucci, J. R. (2006). Importance of early diagnosis and treatment of osteoporosis to prevent fractures. *American Journal of Managed Care, 12*(Suppl. 7), S181–S190.

Tucker, K. L., Jugdaohsingh, R., Powell, J. J., Qiao, N., Hannan, M. T., Sripanyakorn, S., et al. (2009). Effects of beer, wine and liquor intake on bone mineral density in older men and women. *American Journal of Clinical Nutrition, 89*(4), 1188–1196.

Tucker, S. M. (2000). Amputation of leg: Above or below knee. In S. M. Tucker, M. M. Cannobbio, E. V. Paquetto, & M. F. Wells (Eds.), *Patient Care Standards: Collaborative Planning and Nursing Interventions* (7th ed.). St. Louis: Mosby.

Uhlig, T., Fongen, C., Steen, E., Christie, A., & Ødegård, S. (2010). Exploring tai chi in rheumatoid arthritis: A quantitative and qualitative study. *BMC Musculoskeletal Disorders, 11*(43).

Ulrich, S. P., & Canale, S. W. (2005). *Nursing care planning guide* (6th ed.). St. Louis: Elsevier/Saunders.

University of Minnesota Research. (2006). *Osteoporosis research.* Retrieved April 11, 2007, from www.epi.umn.edu/research/osteop.shtm.

U.S. Army Wounded Warrior Program (AW2). (n.d.). Loss of a limb. Alexandria, VA: Author. Retrieved from www.AW2.army.mil.

U.S. Department of Health and Human Services. (2000, August 14). Diabetes-related amputations of lower extremities in the Medicare population: Minnesota, 1993–1995. *Morbidity and Mortality Weekly Report (MMWR), 47*(31), 649–652.

U.S. Department of Health and Human Services. (2004). *Bone health and osteoporosis: A report of the surgeon general.* Retrieved August 25, 2010, from www.surgeongeneral.gov.library/bone-health/content.html.

U.S. Department of Health and Human Services. (2006). *Progress review: Arthritis, osteoporosis and chronic back conditions.* Retrieved August 31, 2011, from www.healthypeople.gov/Data/midcourse/pdf/fa02.pdf.

Valdes, A. M., & Spector, T. D. (2009). The contribution of genes to osteoarthritis. *Medical Clinics of North America, 93*(1), 45–66.

Veteran's Administration Polytrauma System of Care. (2010). *Definition of polytrauma.* Retrieved July 29, 2010, from www.polytrauma.va.gov/definitions.asp#polytrauma.

Villa-Blanco, J. I., & Calvo-Alen, J. (2009). Elderly onset rheumatoid arthritis: Differential diagnosis and choice of first-line and subsequent therapy. *Drugs & Aging, 26*(9), 739–750.

Walsh, N. C., Crotti, T. N., Goldring, S. R., & Gravallese, E. M. (2005). Rheumatic disease: The effects of inflammation on bone. *Immunological Reviews, 208*(1), 228–251.

Wang, C., Lin, J., Chang, C. J., Lin, Y. T., & Hou, S. M. (2004). Therapeutic effects of hyaluronic acid in osteoarthritis of the knee. *Journal of Bone & Joint Surgery, 86-A*(3), 538–545.

Wang, T. J., Chern, H. L., & Chiou, Y. E. (2005). A theoretical model for preventing osteoarthritis-related disability. *Rehabilitation Nursing, 30*(2), 62–67.

Watts, N. B. (1997, September). Osteoporosis: Prevention, detection and treatment. *Journal of the Medical Association of Georgia,* 224–226.

Watts, N. B. (2010). Postmenopausal osteoporosis: What's new and What's next? *SRM (Sexuality, Reproduction and Menopause), 8*(2), 17–22.

Wegman, A., Van der Windt, D., Van Tulder, M., Stalman, W., & de Vries, T. (2004). Nonsteroidal anti-inflammatory drugs or acetaminophen for osteoarthritis of the hip or knee? A systematic review of evidence and guidelines. *Journal of Rheumatology, 31*(2), 344–354.

Weiss, J. F., & Ilowite, N. T. (2005). Juvenile idiopathic arthritis. *Rheumatic Diseases Clinics of North America, 33*(3), 441–470.

Wells, G. A., Cranney, A., Peterson, J., Boucher, M., Shea, B,, Robinson, V., et al. (2008a). Alendronate for the primary and secondary prevention of osteoporotic fractures in postmenopausal women. *Cochrane Database of Systematic Reviews, 4,* CD001155.

Wells, G. A., Cranney, A., Peterson, J., Boucher, M., Shea, B., Robinson, V., et al. (2008b). Risedronate for the primary and secondary prevention of osteoporotic fractures in postmenopausal women. *Cochrane Database of Systematic Reviews, 4,* CD004523.

Wilder-Smith, C. H., Hill, L. T., & Laurent, S. (2005). Postamputation pain and sensory changes in treatment-naïve patients: Characteristics and responses to treatment with tramadol, amitriptyline and placebo. *Anesthesiology, 103*(3), 619–628.

Wilke, W. S., & Carey, J. (2009). *Osteoarthritis.* Retrieved August 17, 2010, from www.clevelandclinicmeded.com/medical-pubs/diseasemanagement/rheumatology.

Williams, A. M., & Deaton, S. B. (1997). Phantom limb pain: Elusive, yet real. *Rehabilitation Nursing, 22*(2), 73–77.

Wilson, R. E. (1996). Care of the burn patient. *Ostomy/Wound Management, 42*(8), 16–34.

Wilson, D., & Hockenberry, M. J. (2011). The process of nursing infants and children: Nursing diagnoses and the nursing process. In D. Wilson & M. J. Hockenberry (Eds.), *Wong's Clinical Manual of Pediatric Nursing* (8th ed.). St. Louis: Mosby.

Woodhead, G. A., & Moss, M. M. (1998). Osteoporosis: Diagnosis and prevention. *The Nurse Practitioner, 23*(11), 18–35.

World Health Organization. (1994). *Assessment of fracture risk and its implication to screening for postmenopausal osteoporosis.* Technical report series 843. Geneva, Switzerland: Author.

World Health Organization. (2003). *Prevention and management of osteoporosis.* WHO Technical Report Series #921. Geneva, Switzerland: Author.

World Health Organization. (2004a). *Management of burns.* Retrieved August 10, 2010, from www.who.int/surgery/publications/Burns_management.pdf.

World Health Organization. (2004b, May). *WHO Scientific Group on the Assessment of Osteoporosis at Primary Health Care Level: Summary meeting report.* Brussels, Belgium: Author.

World Orthopedic Osteoporotic Organization. (2002). *Recommendations to care for the osteoporotic patient to reduce the risk of future fracture.* Retrieved August 1, 2010, from www.iofbonehealth.org.

Wortmann, R. L. (2005). Recent advances in the management of gout and hyperuricemia. *Current Opinion in Rheumatology, 17*(3), 319–324.

Wu, E. Q., Patel, P. A., Yu, A. P., Mody, R. R., Cahill, K. E., Tang, J., et al. (2008). Disease-related and all-cause healthcare costs of elderly patients with gout. *Journal of Managed Care Pharmacy, 14*(2), 164–173.

Yelin, E., Murphy, L., Cisternos, M., Foreman, A., Pasta, D., & Helmick, C. (2007). Medical care expenditures and earning losses among persons with arthritis and other rheumatic conditions in 2003 and comparisons to 1997. *Arthritis and Rheumatism, 56*(5), 1397–1407.

Yetzer, E. A. (1996). Helping the patient through the experience of an amputation. *Orthopaedic Nursing, 15*(6), 45–49.

Youngblood, N. M., & Edwards, P. A. (1999). Autoimmune and endocrine conditions. In P. A. Edwards, D. L. Hertzberg, S. R. Hays, & N. M. Youngblood (Eds.), *Pediatric rehabilitation nursing* (pp. 412–419). Philadelphia: W. B. Saunders.

Yurkow, J., & Yudin, J. (2002). Musculoskeletal problems. In V. T. Cotter & N. E. Strumpf (Eds.), *Advanced practice nursing with older adults: Clinical guidelines* (pp. 229–242). New York: McGraw-Hill.

Zhang, W., Doherty, M., Arden, N., Bannwarth, B., Bijlsma, J., Gunther, K., et al. (2005). EULAR evidence based recommendations for the management of hip osteoarthritis: Report of a task force of the EULAR Standing Committee for International Clinical Studies Including Therapeutics (ESCISIT). *Annals of the Rheumatic Diseases, 64*(5), 669–685.

Zhang, W., Doherty, M., Bardin, T., Pascual, E., Barskova, V., Conaghan, P., et al. (2006a). EULAR evidence based recommendations for gout. Part II: Management. Report of a task force of the EULAR Standing Committee for International Clinical Studies Including Therapeutics (ESCOSOT). *Annals of Rheumatic Disease, 65*(10), 1312–1324.

Zhang, W., Doherty, M., Pascual, E., Bardin, T., Barskova, V., Conaghan, P., et al. (2006b). EULAR evidence based recommendation for gout. Part I: Diagnosis. Report of a task force of the Standing Committee for International Clinical Studies Including Therapeutics (ESCISIT). *Annals of Rheumatic Disease, 65*(10), 1301–1311.

Zhang, W., Jones, A., & Doherty, M. (2004). Does paracetamol (acetaminophen) reduce the pain of osteoarthritis? A meta-analysis of randomized control trials. *Annals of Rheumatic Disease, 63*(8), 901–907.

Zhu, K., Austin, N., Devine, A., Bruce, D., & Prince, R. L. (2010). A randomized controlled trial of the effects of vitamin D on muscle strength and mobility in older women with vitamin D II sufficiency. *Journal of the American Geriatrics Society, 58*(11), 2063–2068.

Ziegler-Graham, K., MacKenzie, E. J., Ephraim, P. L., Travison, T. G., & Brookmeyer, R. (2008). Estimating the prevalence of limb loss in the United States: 2005 to 2050. *Archives of Physical Medicine and Rehabilitation, 89*(3), 422–427.

Suggested Resources

American Burn Association: http://ameriburn.org
The Amputation Surgery Education Center: http://ampsurg.org
Amputee Coalition of America: www.amputee-coalition.org
The Arthritis Foundation: www.arthritis.org
Arthritis Today: www.arthritistoday.org
MedlinePlus: Burns: www.nlm.nih.gov/medlineplus/ency/article/000030.htm
MedlinePlus: Gout: www.nlm.nih.gov/medlineplus/gout.html
National Amputation Foundation: www.nationalamputation.org
National Center for PTSD: www.ptsd.va.gov
National Osteoporosis Foundation: www.nof.org

Suggested Resources: Blast

Blast- and explosion-induced illness pocket card available at www.healthquality.va.gov/Biological_Radiation_Chemical_or_Blast_Induced_Illnesses.asp
Blast injury fact sheets for professionals available at http://emergency.cdc.gov/masscasualties/blastinjuryfacts.asp
CDC blast training modules available at www.bt.cdc.gov/masscasualties/bombings_injurycare.asp
Clinical practice guideline: Management of Concussion-Mild Traumatic Brain Injury, available at www.healthquality.va.gov/management_of_concussion_mtbi.asp

Suggested Resources: PTSD

Gateway to PTSD Information: www.ptsdinfo.org
National Institutes of Mental Health: www.nimh.nih.gov/
health/topics/post-traumatic-stress-disorder-ptsd/index.shtml
VA/DoD Clinical Practice Guideline: Posttraumatic stress
disorder: www.healthquality.va.gov/ptsd/ptsd_full.pdf
VA PTSD screening guidelines for PTSD: www.ptsd.va.gov/
professional/pages/screening-and-referral.asp

Suggested Resources: Burns

Joint Theater Trauma System Clinical Practice Guideline:
www.usaisr.amedd.army.mil/cpgs/Burn_CPG_20_Dec_10.pdf

CHAPTER 14
Cardiac and Pulmonary Rehabilitation: Acute and Long-Term Management

Holly Evans Madison, PhD RN

As treatments for cardiovascular disease (CVD) and pulmonary disease improve, more people in the United States are living with these diseases; therefore, rehabilitation nurses must be knowledgeable about these diseases and treatments so they can support these clients and their families through rehabilitation and beyond. It is estimated that 81.1 million Americans have CVD (American Heart Association [AHA], 2010), and 35 million Americans experience some form of chronic lung disease (American Lung Association [ALA], 2010). CVD is the leading cause of death, and chronic obstructive lung disease is the fourth leading cause of death in the United States (AHA, 2010; ALA, 2010). The estimated direct and indirect cost of CVD in 2010 for the United States was $503.2 billion.

Cardiac and pulmonary rehabilitation programs provide a way for people to increase strength and functional ability in a supervised setting. In addition, the educational component teaches people how to manage their disease. These interdisciplinary programs have been shown to yield positive outcomes including increased quality of life, increased functional ability, and adoption of health-promoting behaviors. In this chapter, select cardiovascular disease processes will be presented, followed by information on cardiac rehabilitation. In the second half of the chapter, pulmonary diseases and rehabilitation will be presented.

I. Types of Cardiovascular Disease

A. Coronary heart disease (CHD) or coronary artery disease: A disorder of the coronary arteries that leads to disruption of the blood flow that supplies oxygen and nutrients to the myocardium (AHA, 2010; **Figure 14-1**)

1. Epidemiology: A progressive atherosclerotic disease of the coronary arteries that results in a narrowing of the vessel lumen (AHA, 2010)

2. Etiology: Progressive disease related to risk factors (AHA, 2010; **Figure 14-2**)

3. Pathophysiology: Arteriosclerosis (thickening, reduced elasticity, and calcification of the coronary arteries) and atherosclerosis (plaque buildup) in the coronary arteries (AHA, 2010; Osborn, Wraa, & Watson, 2010)

4. Risk factors for CHD: Factors have been identified that increase a person's likelihood of developing CHD. Some of these factors cannot be changed, such as age and family history. However, other factors can be changed; these are called modifiable risk factors. Making changes that

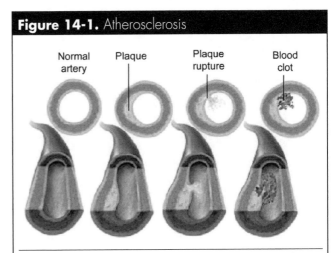

Figure 14-1. Atherosclerosis

Normal artery · Plaque · Plaque rupture · Blood clot

From "Atherosclerosis," by Medmovie.com, 2007, Lexington, KY: Medmovie.com. Copyright 2007 by Medmovie.com. Reprinted with permission.

reduce risk can help stop the progression of heart disease. The at-risk criteria have been included.

a. Tobacco smoke
b. High cholesterol level
   1) Total cholesterol higher than 200 mg/dL
   2) HDL: Men, lower than 40 mg/dL; women, lower than 50 mg/dL
   3) LDL higher than 100 mg/dL
   4) Triglycerides higher than 150 mg/dL
c. Hypertension: Blood pressure 140/90 mm Hg or higher
d. Physical inactivity
e. Overweight and obesity
f. Diabetes mellitus
g. Stress
h. Alcohol consumption
   1) More than two drinks a day for men
   2) More than one drink a day for women
i. Diet and nutrition (AHA, 2010)

5. Complications (AHA, 2010; Osborn, Wraa, & Watson, 2010)

a. Angina: 10.2 million people experience angina, or transient chest pain due to myocardial ischemia, per year.
   1) Stable: Triggered by a predictable degree of exertion, its duration, and frequency
   2) Unstable: Transitory syndrome in which a thrombus forms but is lysed and there are no residual deficits

Factors have been identified that increase a person's likelihood of developing coronary heart disease. Some of these factors cannot be changed, such as age and family history. However, other factors can be changed or modified. These are called modifiable risk factors. Making changes that reduce risk can help stop the progression of heart disease. Review this list with your practitioner so the two of you can develop a plan to reduce your risk. The criterion that puts you at risk has been included.

Tobacco smoke

High cholesterol level

- Total cholesterol: more than 200 mg/dL
- High-density lipoprotein (HDL)
- Men, less than 40 mg/dL
- Women, less than 50 mg/dL
- Low-density lipoprotein (LDL): more than 100 mg/dL
- Triglycerides: more than 150 mg/dL

High blood pressure

- Blood pressure ^{3}140/90

Physical inactivity

Overweight and obesity

Diabetes mellitus, diagnosed through blood glucose

Other factors that may affect the development of heart disease:

Stress

Alcohol

- More than 2 drinks a day for men
- More than 1 drink a day for women

Diet and nutrition

3) Variant, Prinzmetal, or vasospastic angina, caused by vasospasms

b. Myocardial infarction (MI): 8.5 million people per year experience an MI, or death of myocardial tissue from inadequate coronary perfusion, when blood supply to a portion of the heart is severely reduced or stopped. MI may occur at rest or with exertion. Pain may last longer than 30 minutes, is continuous, and is unrelieved by rest, position change, or nitroglycerin tablets.

6. Symptoms

    a. Chest pain characterized as crushing, squeezing, stabbing, or heavy pressure

    b. May radiate down the left arm and to neck, jaws, teeth, epigastric area, and back

    c. Extreme fatigue

    d. Diaphoresis

    e. Syncope

    f. Dyspnea, orthopnea

    g. Nausea, vomiting

    h. Dysrhythmias: Include premature atrial and ventricular contractions, conduction abnormalities, and tachycardia and bradycardia

7. Treatment (AHA, 2010; Osborn, Wraa, & Watson, 2010; Aschenbrenner & Venable, 2006)

    a. Invasive interventions (AHA, 2010)

        1) Percutaneous transluminal coronary angioplasty is an invasive nonsurgical procedure performed via a catheter introduced into the coronary artery. Patency is restored to the coronary artery by inflating and deflating a balloon at the distal end of the catheter to compress plaques in the arteries.

        2) Stent placement: After angioplasty, a small metal stent is inserted to maintain patency of the arterial lumen.

        3) Ablation: This is a laser procedure that focuses on an area of the heart causing a dysrhythmia; the area is lysed to stop the cycle.

    b. Surgical procedures

        1) Coronary artery bypass graft: Conduits for blood are created from arteries or veins, bypassing areas of stenosis.

        2) Pacemaker or automatic implantable cardioverter-defibrillator placement (for dysrhythmias)

    c. Medications, which can be used alone or in combination, depending on the CHD and the severity of symptoms (Aschenbrenner & Venable, 2006)

        1) Vasodilators

        2) Beta-adrenergic blocking agents

        3) Angiotensin-converting enzyme inhibitors

        4) Anticoagulation and antiplatelet medications

        5) Antiarrhythmics

        6) Calcium antagonists

        7) Antihyperlipidemic agents

        8) Cardiac glycosides

        9) Diuretics

       10) Nitrates

       11) Calcium channel blockers

       12) Angiotensin II receptor blockers

       13) Alpha-2 agonists

       14) Thrombolytics

       15) Oxygen

       16) Morphine (for acute pain)

8. Management measures (AHA, 2010): Risk factor modification for CHD
   a. Stop smoking.
   b. Control blood pressure.
   c. Control cholesterol: AHA-recommended cholesterol levels
      1) Lower LDLs to <100 mg/dL.
      2) Raise HDLs to >50 mg/dL (women) or >40 mg/dL (men).
      3) Maintain total cholesterol level of <200 mg/dL.
      4) Lower fasting triglyceride level to <150 mg/dL.
   d. Ways to lower elevated cholesterol levels
      1) Diet (**Figure 14-3**)
      2) Exercise
      3) Weight control
      4) Medications
      5) Smoking cessation
      6) Diabetes management
   e. Perform physical activity (**Figure 14-4**).
      1) Consult with a physician before beginning an exercise program.
      2) Exercise
         a) Aerobic exercise most days a week
         b) Strength training three times a week
         c) Flexibility three times a week
      3) Monitor response and target heart rate.
   f. Manage stress (**Figures 14-5** and **14-6**).
      1) Identify stressors.
      2) Use relaxation techniques.
      3) Seek social support.
      4) Exercise.
      5) Explore spiritual resources.
      6) Seek counseling.
   g. Resuming sexual activity
      1) Be well rested.
      2) Wait until at least 30 minutes after a meal.
      3) Cease activity if angina or other symptoms occur and call a cardiologist.
   h. Teach cardiopulmonary resuscitation (CPR) to family members.
B. Congestive Heart Failure (CHF) or Heart Failure: A complex syndrome that results from the heart's inability to increase cardiac output sufficiently to meet the body's metabolic demands. Currently, 5.8 million Americans have CHF (AHA, 2010; Osborn, Wraa, & Watson, 2010).
   1. Epidemiology: The rising prevalence is related to the aging population and increased survival rates among people with CHD and hypertension (AHA, 2010; Osborn, Wraa, & Watson, 2010).

Figure 14-3. Diet to Promote Cardiac Health

Whether you want to lose a few pounds or consume a more heart-healthy diet, there are certain strategies that you can use to increase your health through your diet.

Know what you're eating.

Keep a food diary for a couple of weekdays and a weekend to assess your consumption. Look at the number of calories a day you consume and the amount of fiber and fat in the foods you eat. Read the nutrition labels of food.

Eat a variety of foods. Variety includes eating foods of different colors.

Eat food as close to their natural state as possible.

Eat fresh fruits and vegetables and whole grains as often as possible.

If you drink, do so in moderation. Moderation means no more than one drink per day for women, two drinks a day for men.

Eat small, frequent meals.

American Dietetic Association. (2010). www.eatright.org/.
Madison, H. E. (2010). *What women want to know: Assessing the value, relevance, and efficacy of a self-management intervention for rural women with coronary heart disease.* Unpublished doctoral dissertation, University of Massachusetts, Amherst.

---

2. Etiology: The leading causes of CHF include CHD, hypertension, and cardiomyopathy. Risk factors for CHF include all the risk factors for CHD and valvular abnormalities (AHA, 2010; Osborn, Wraa, & Watson, 2010).
3. Pathophysiology: Loss or dysfunction of the cardiac muscle or an inability of the ventricle to fill or pump blood (AHA, 2010; Osborn, Wraa, & Watson, 2010)
4. Complications: New York Heart Association Classification (AHA, 2010; Osborn, Wraa, & Watson, 2010)
   a. Class I: No symptoms
   b. Class II: Symptoms with ordinary exertion
   c. Class III: Symptoms with less than ordinary exertion
   d. Class IV: Symptoms at rest
5. Treatment (AHA, 2010; Osborn, Wraa, & Watson, 2010; Aschenbrenner & Venable, 2006)
   a. Device therapy: Pacemakers (including cardiac resynchronization therapy), implantable cardiac defibrillators, and mechanical assist devices
   b. Cardiac transplantation
   c. Medications
      1) Angiotensin-converting enzyme inhibitors
      2) Angiotensin II receptor blockers
      3) Beta-adrenergic blockers
      4) Diuretics
      5) Cardiac glycosides

Figure 14-4. Fitness

Exercise has many benefits. Some of these include increased feelings of well-being, lower blood pressure, weight control, increased levels of HDLs (the "good" cholesterol), increased immunity, increased muscle and bone strength, and restful sleep. There are three types of physical activity: aerobic, strengthening, and flexibility exercises. A balanced exercise program contains all three.

Aerobic exercise: Aerobic exercise is designed to strengthen your heart. When you engage in aerobic exercises you will experience an increase in your heart rate. Using large muscles, such as your legs when walking, is the most effective way to do this. You should aim to engage in aerobic activity 30 minutes at least 3 times a week.

Strengthening: Strengthening or resistance training will increase muscle strength. There are several benefits of this type of exercise. It increases muscle mass, which helps when performing activities of daily living. Also, the increased muscle mass burns calories effectively, helping with weight management. Strengthening exercises should be performed three times a week, allowing at least a day between sessions so the muscles can recover.

Flexibility: Flexibility protects you from injury, assists with balance, and is relaxing. Flexibility exercises can be performed before and after aerobic activities or as a separate exercise program, such as yoga or tai chi.

Beginning an exercise program is as easy as 1, 2, 3.

1. Consult with your practitioner.

Before you begin an exercise program, you should consult with your practitioner. There may be types of exercise that you should avoid. When you visit your practitioner, find out your target heart range. This is the range where you get the most benefits from aerobic exercise. It also gives you the upper limit of heart rate, the rate you do not want to exceed. The target heart range can be determined by several methods, but for someone with heart disease, a stress test is the most effective way to gauge your target heart range.

2. Obtain baseline data.

Take your pulse either manually or with a heart rate monitor. Monitor your normal activity for several days by keeping a journal. One way is to do this is to use a pedometer to keep track of the number of steps you take in a day. Compare it with the guidelines for activity and make decisions about what types of exercise you will adopt to increase your activity level. Set daily and weekly goals for yourself.

3. Begin.

Continue your journal. Review it on a weekly basis and compare it with your goals. Celebrate your success!

American Association of Cardiovascular and Pulmonary Rehabilitation. (2010). *Fast facts for cardiac rehabilitation.* Retrieved August 20, 2010, from www.aacvpr.org/Resources/CardiacPulmonaryRehabFundamentals/tabid/256/Default.aspx.

American Heart Association. (2010). *Heart disease and stroke statistics.* Retrieved February 10, 2010, from www.americanheart.org?presenter.jtml?identifier=4977.

Madison, H. E. (2010). *What women want to know: Assessing the value, relevance, and efficacy of a self-management intervention for rural women with coronary heart disease.* Unpublished doctoral dissertation, University of Massachusetts, Amherst.

6) Aldosterone antagonists
7) Antiarrhythmic or dysrhythmic agents
8) Anticoagulant and antiplatelet agents
9) Inotropic, vasopressor, and vasodilator therapeutic agents

6. Management measures (AHA, 2010; Osborn, Wraa, & Watson, 2010) to maintain functionality
  a. Self-monitor pulse and blood pressure.
  b. Weigh daily.
  c. Advance activity as tolerated.
  d. Monitor diet, especially sodium consumption.
  e. Monitor respiratory function.
  f. Monitor for complications.

C. Cardiomyopathy: Diseases that affect the myocardium, resulting in enlargement or restriction, leading to cardiac dysfunction. Types include dilated (accounts for 87% of all cardiomyopathies), nonobstructive, obstructive, and restrictive cardiomyopathies. This section describes dilated cardiomyopathy. With dilated cardiomyopathy, the myocardium is dilated and there is impaired contraction of the ventricles.

1. Epidemiology: Found in all ages, but the majority is in older adults (Osborn, Wraa, & Watson, 2010)
2. Etiology: CHD is the most common cause of dilated cardiomyopathy, accounting for more than half of the cases.
3. Pathophysiology: Some people have a genetic predisposition, whereas for others it is idiopathic. Tissue remolding occurs when myocardial fibers disintegrate and become necrotic and fibrotic tissue forms.
4. Complications: CHF and dysrhythmias.
5. Treatment
  a. Medications: Treat symptoms (e.g., heart failure)
  b. Surgical: Heart transplantation
6. Management measures are the same as those for CHF.

D. Congenital Heart Defects: Structural or functional abnormalities of the heart or great vessels existing from birth that obstruct blood flow in and to the heart and cause the blood to flow abnormally

Figure 14-5. Stress

"Don't compromise yourself. You're all you've got."

—Janis Joplin

Stress has been shown to put people at risk for coronary heart disease. Are you one of them? Do you feel stressed? There are things you can do to manage your stress.

Exercise
Besides all the other benefits of exercise, endorphins are released in the brain, and that improves mood. Regular exercise has been shown to increase immunity, assist in weight control, and build bone and muscle mass that help to achieve the activities of daily living. When you look at it, there is no reason not to exercise.

Sleep
It is important to get enough sleep. Most people need a minimum of 7 hours of sleep a night. If you have trouble falling asleep or staying asleep, it is important to have proper sleep hygiene. Some tips for restful sleep include going to sleep and getting up at the same time every day, sleeping in a dark room, and not keeping a computer or a TV in the room because the light from these screens can disturb sleep.

Laugh
Laughter links the logical left brain function with the creative right brain function. Laughter is almost like exercise: It increases heart rate and respiration, triggers the release of endorphins, and diminishes anxiety.

Share
Connect with others. We are social beings, and being with others can decrease stress. Get out with friends. And if you can include any of the other things on this list (exercise, laughter), that makes it even better.

Eat
It is always important to eat a balanced diet, but it is especially important when you are feeling stressed. Examine your diet and make sure that you are consuming adequate amounts of protein, fruits, and vegetables, things that people often do not eat enough of when they are stressed. Do not eat too many "comfort foods" that are high in fat, calories, and sugar or stimulants such as caffeine because all these things can actually cause "discomfort" as they pile on pounds, cause gastrointestinal upsets, and cause your blood sugar and energy levels peak and then drop.

Pray
Just as it is important to connect with other people, it is important to see how you connect with the rest of the universe. Prayer or meditation can help you with that. Throughout history, people have recognized a connection between spiritual practices and health and healing. Prayer is a spiritual ritual that takes many different forms; it includes solitary meditation or singing in a group. Find the type of prayer that works best for you.

Relax
Practice relaxation techniques. There are a variety of relaxation techniques that you can use. Relaxation techniques can be as simple as taking a few deep breaths, doing progressive relaxation exercises, or meditating. To perform progressive relaxation exercises, you need to sit or lie down in a comfortable position. Starting with your toes and moving up your body to your head, you consciously relax the muscles in each part of your body. Whatever relaxation technique you adopt, you need to practice it regularly for it to be effective.

Condon, M. C. (2004). *Women's health: An integrated approach to wellness and illness.* Upper Saddle River, NJ: Prentice Hall. Eliopoulos, C. (2004). *Invitation to holistic health: A guide to living a balanced life.* Boston: Jones & Bartlett. Leddy, S. K. (2003). *Integrative health promotion: Conceptual bases for nursing practice.* Thorofare, NJ: Slack Incorporated. Madison, H. E. (2010). *What women want to know: Assessing the value, relevance, and efficacy of a self-management intervention for rural women with coronary heart disease.* Unpublished doctoral dissertation, University of Massachusetts, Amherst.

---

through the heart. There is a range of severity from life-threatening to undetected (AHA, 2010). The following are the most common types of congenital heart defects and their prevalence in the population:

- Tetralogy of Fallot (9%–14%)
- Transposition of the great arteries (10%–11%)
- Coarctation of the aorta (8%–11%)
- Atrioventricular septal defect (4%–10%)
- Hypoplastic left heart syndrome (4%–10%)
- Ventricular septal defect (14%–16%)
    1. Epidemiology: Congenital heart defects occur in approximately 0.9% of live births (AHA, 2010).

2. Etiology: Congenital heart defects occur during heart development, which occurs soon after conception. In most cases the cause is not known, although sometimes medications, maternal infections, and genetics may be responsible (AHA, 2010).
3. Pathophysiology: This depends on the particular defect.
4. Complications (AHA, 2010): These defects can result in a number of medical conditions.
    a. CHF
    b. Pulmonary hypertension

Figure 14-6. Sleep and Rest

Sleep is the time when your body renews itself. Getting enough sleep affects how we feel and the quality of our lives. Our daily pattern of sleep and wakefulness is one of our circadian rhythms. Although sleep patterns vary between individuals, most people need between 7 and 8 hours of sleep a night. It has been found that as people age, changes occur in the circadian rhythm, resulting in feelings of drowsiness in the afternoon or evening. Whether we are getting enough sleep to satisfy our needs is not found in the number of hours of sleep but in how we feel and carry out our activities of daily living. A person who has had enough sleep awakens refreshed and able to perform at his or her best.

Difficultly falling asleep or staying asleep is called insomnia. Some of the causes of insomnia are short term in nature, such as stress or excitement. Others can last a longer period of time and include depression, general anxiety, or chronic illness. Some medications or things such as caffeine can contribute to insomnia.

Proper sleep is important for your health. Here are some tips that may be help you get the rest you need.

Sleep Tips

Do	Do Not
Try to go to sleep and get up at the same time every day. As boring as that may sound, your body will respond to the regularity of your schedule.	Consume caffeine in the evening.
Exercise regularly.	Exercise vigorously right before you are planning to go to sleep.
Sleep in quiet surroundings.	Consume alcohol in excess.
Sleep in a restful, darkened room.	Use sleep medications without the knowledge of your physician.
Keep the room a comfortable temperature.	Use your bed for stress-producing things, such as paying bills.
Make your room a peaceful spot and use relaxing fragrances such as lavender to scent the room or your pillow.	Eat a large meal within 3 hours of going to sleep.
Use "white noise" if helpful.	Consume sugar in the evening.
Do relaxation exercises such as deep breathing, progressive relaxation exercises, or meditation at bedtime.	Keep the lights on.
If you experience difficulty breathing when lying flat, elevate the head of your bed. This can be accomplished by adding pillows or elevating the bed with blocks.	Ignore it when you wake up in the night short of breath; consult your physician.
Take a warm bath before bedtime.	Take a brisk shower.

If you continue to have problems sleeping, you may want to maintain a sleep diary, a record of your sleeping and waking events. The diary may help you see patterns and assist in identifying the underlying problem. Contact your practitioner if you have explored other alternatives and have not been successful getting adequate sleep.

Madison, H. E. (2010). *What women want to know: Assessing the value, relevance, and efficacy of a self-management intervention for rural women with coronary heart disease.* Unpublished doctoral dissertation, University of Massachusetts, Amherst. National Sleep Foundation. (2010). www.sleepfoundation.org/.

c. Dysrhythmias
5. Treatment (AHA, 2010)
    a. Medication: Treats symptoms
    b. Surgery: Used for repair of defects
6. Management measures are the same as for CHF.
E. Cardiac Valve Disease: Classified according to the valve involved and the functional alterations (AHA, 2010; Osborn, Wraa, & Watson, 2010)
    1. Epidemiology, etiology, and pathophysiology depend on the valve involved. For example, the most common cause of mitral regurgitation is rheumatic heart disease.
    2. Complications include such things as CHF and dysrhythmias.
    3. Treatment
        a. Invasive treatments: Surgery

b. Annuloplasty: Corrects regurgitation by repairing the enlarged annulus
c. Valvuloplasty: Repair of the valve leaflet
d. Prosthetic heart valves: Replacement of valves with a mechanical or biological valve
4. Management measures (AHA, 2010; Osborn, Wraa, & Watson, 2010)
    a. Monitor vital signs.
    b. Monitor coagulation.
    c. Check for bleeding.
    d. Progress activity as tolerated.

II. **Cardiac Rehabilitation**
Cardiac rehabilitation programs serve people with congenital or acquired heart disease.
A. Benefits of Cardiac Rehabilitation
    1. Clients attending cardiac rehabilitation programs have been shown to have

a. Reduced symptoms (angina, dyspnea, fatigue)

b. Mortality benefit (approximately 20%–25%)

c. Reduction in nonfatal recurrent MI over median follow-up of 12 months

d. Increased exercise performance

e. Improved lipid panel (total cholesterol, HDL [good cholesterol], LDL [bad cholesterol], and triglycerides)

f. Increased knowledge about cardiac disease and its management

g. Enhanced ability to perform activities of daily living (ADLs)

h. Improved health-related quality of life

i. Improved psychosocial symptoms (reversal of anxiety and depression, increased self-efficacy)

j. Reduced hospitalizations and use of medical resources

k. Increased ability to return to work or leisure activities (American Association of Cardiovascular and Pulmonary Rehabilitation [AACVPR], 2010)

2. Although cardiac rehabilitation enhances recovery and secondary prevention measures prevent further complications from the disease, fewer than one-third of eligible people access rehabilitation programs. That number is even lower for women, older adults, and people who reside in rural areas (Beckie, 2006; Grace et al., 2009).

3. Researchers have found differences between sexes with regard to development of the disease, prodromal symptoms and diagnosis, treatment, and short- and long-term outcomes (Espnes & Byrne, 2008; Gleeson & Crabbe, 2009; Godfrey & Manson, 2008; Madison, 2010; Pollin et al., 2008; Shaw et al., 2008; Yang, Kuper, & Weiderpass, 2008).

B. Phases of Cardiac Rehabilitation: There are four phases of cardiac rehabilitation programs (AACVPR, 2010)

1. Phase I: Inpatient

a. First 1–4 days after cardiac event

b. Usually in cardiac care unit

c. Goal: Minimize damage from event

d. Insurance coverage

1) Medicare

2) Private insurance

2. Phase II: Restoration

a. In hospital care, Day 1–discharge

b. Goals

1) Assessment of hemodynamic response to activity

2) Determination of medication effectiveness

3) Gathering baseline data

4) Behavior modification

5) Risk factor reduction

6) Family education

7) Progressive activities

8) Bed rest

9) Bed rest with minimal activities

10) Sitting up as long as comfortable

11) Beginning ambulation

12) Progressing activity as able

c. Insurance coverage

1) Medicare

2) Private insurance

3. Phase III: Outpatient supervised program

a. Duration: 2–12 weeks

b. Goals

1) Increase activity capacity and endurance in a safe, progressive manner.

2) Continue exercise program in home environment.

3) Assess cardiovascular response to increased workloads.

4) Teach self-monitoring.

5) Relieve anxiety and depression.

6) Increase client knowledge of risk factors.

c. Education

1) Cardiovascular anatomy and physiology

2) Personal risk factors

3) Controlling risk factors

4) Resuming sexual activity

5) Benefits of exercise

6) Diet and stress

7) Healthy living

d. Exercise program is individualized and based on principles of frequency, intensity, and duration.

e. Insurance coverage

1) Medicare

2) Private insurance (some)

4. Phase IV: Maintenance of physical activity and lifestyle changes

a. Duration: Lifelong

b. Goals

1) Maintain improved endurance and fitness

2) Reduce risk factors

c. Insurance coverage

1) No Medicare

2) Some private insurance

3) Private insurance may have health club benefit

5. In cardiac rehabilitation, the modification of risk factors is achieved through a supervised exercise program and education. The exercise component

consists of aerobic exercise, strength training, and flexibility exercises. Aerobic exercises contribute to cardiovascular health by increasing the strength of the heart, reduce risk factors, and increase feelings of well-being. Strength training promotes the ability to manage ADLs and bone health. Flexibility training protects clients from injury.

C. Nursing Process
1. Assessment (AHA, 2010; Osborn, Wraa, & Watson, 2010)
   a. Subjective elements
      1) Palpitations, dizziness, lightheadedness, syncope, shortness of breath, fatigue, poor appetite, insomnia, restlessness, anxiety and fear, nausea, jaw pain, indigestion
      2) Chest discomfort: Quality, location, precipitating factors, duration, alleviating factors
   b. Objective elements
      1) Skin: Pallor, diaphoresis
      2) Cardiac output: Tachycardia, bradycardia, irregular heart rhythm, heart murmur, hypotension, hypertension, confusion, decreased urine output, peripheral edema, sacral or genital edema, weight gain, abdominal distention, electrocardiogram changes, elevated cardiac serum enzymes (creatine kinase myocardial band) and muscle proteins
      3) Pulmonary status: Crackles; wheezes; dyspnea; labored breathing; frothy, blood-tinged sputum; cyanosis
      4) Nutritional: Anorexia, decreased skin turgor and integrity
   c. History
      1) Health habits
      2) Medical
      3) Surgical
      4) Social support
      5) Previous independence level
      6) Medications
2. Diagnoses (Doenges, Moorhouse, & Murr, 2010)
   a. Activity intolerance
   b. Anxiety
   c. Cardiac output, decreased
   d. Shock, risk for
   e. Coping, ineffective
   f. Electrolyte imbalance, risk for
   g. Fatigue
   h. Fear
   i. Fluid volume, imbalanced, risk for
   j. Health maintenance, ineffective
   k. Health-seeking behaviors
   l. Knowledge deficit
   m. Mobility, impaired
   n. Self-care deficits (e.g., feeding, bathing, grooming, dressing, toileting)
   o. Nutrition, readiness for enhanced
   p. Pain
   q. Perfusion, risk for decreased
   r. Powerlessness, risk for
   s. Skin integrity, risk for impaired
   t. Sleep pattern, disturbed
   u. Spiritual distress, risk for
   v. Therapeutic regimen management, infective
   w. Tissue integrity, impaired
   x. Tissue perfusion, ineffective
   y. Gas exchange, impaired
3. Plan: Goals for client and family (ALA, 2010; Osborn, Wraa, & Watson, 2010)
   a. Demonstrate understanding of exercise plan and verbalize understanding of activity intolerance by modifying activity and rest to prevent fatigue, palpitations, shortness of breath, and diaphoresis.
   b. Verbalize pain relief after measures are taken and reduce symptoms of angina, dyspnea, and fatigue.
   c. Demonstrate understanding of and participation in self-management, including ADLs, exercise programs, dietary management, and lifestyle changes.
   d. Maintain adequate nutritional status to lower risk of progression of cardiac disease and promote healing.
   e. Maintain adequate mentation, heart rate, rhythm, and urine output.
   f. Demonstrate decreased anxiety and verbalize understanding of disease, procedures, and expected outcomes.
   g. Identify stressors and develop strategies to decrease stress.
   h. Verbalize an understanding of the importance of taking medications as prescribed, actions of medications, how to administer medications, and potential side effects.
   i. Maintain skin integrity.
   j. Verbalize and demonstrate an understanding of the importance of following therapeutic and medical treatment recommendations.
   k. Verbalize improved health-related quality of life.
   l. Reduce hospitalizations and use of medical resources (AACVPR, 2010).
4. Implementation (AHA, 2010; Osborn, Wraa, & Watson, 2010)

a. Activity intolerance; mobility impaired; self-care deficits, fatigue
   1) Monitor activities that aggravate the condition (e.g., type of activity, intensity, frequency of symptoms).
   2) Monitor blood pressure, heart rate, and respiratory rate before, during, and after exercise, staying within target heart rate parameters.
   3) Increase activities gradually.
b. Cardiac pain management
   1) Administer medications for chest pain and symptoms.
   2) Administer oxygen therapy as ordered to increase oxygen to myocardium.
   3) Monitor vital signs.
   4) Assess effectiveness of interventions.
c. Nutrition; readiness for enhanced
   1) Consult with a dietitian for special dietary instructions and meal planning.
   2) Monitor weight daily.
   3) Offer caloric supplements (if needed).
   4) Offer measures to improve appetite (e.g., appropriate environment; good oral care; small, frequent meals).
   5) Administer antiemetics before meals (if necessary).
   6) Administer medications so they do not interfere with meals.
d. Tissue perfusion, impaired or ineffective; cardiac output, decreased; fluid volume, imbalanced, risk for; perfusion, risk for decreased; shock, risk for; skin integrity, risk for
   1) Monitor level of consciousness, signs and symptoms of hypoxemia.
   2) Monitor laboratory values of blood urea nitrogen, creatinine, and electrolytes.
   3) Monitor vital signs for changes.
   4) Monitor electrocardiogram.
   5) Document changes in the client's condition.
e. Anxiety; coping, ineffective; fear; powerless, risk for; spiritual distress, risk for; sleep pattern, disturbed
   1) Explain procedures, disease process, and expected outcomes.
   2) Allow the client to express feelings.
   3) Involve the family, significant other, and spiritual counselor.
   4) Encourage participation in the decision-making process and lifestyle changes.
   5) Provide information about support groups, social services, and vocational counseling.
f. Fluid volume excess; electrolyte imbalance, risk for
   1) Administer diuretics as ordered and monitor their effectiveness (e.g., increased urine output, decreased edema, clear lung sounds).
   2) Monitor weight daily and report weight gain of 2 pounds in 24 hours.
   3) Restrict sodium and fluid intake.
g. Knowledge deficit; health-seeking behaviors; health maintenance, ineffective
   1) Instruct about disease process and expected outcomes.
   2) Instruct about medications: Purpose, dosage, how to administer, potential side effects, take only as prescribed, and the importance of follow-up with physician.
   3) Practice energy-conservation techniques, teaching signs and symptoms of overexertion.
   4) Instruct on dietary restrictions and infection prevention.
   5) Offer counseling for employment, genetics, marriage, childbearing, contraceptive use, resuming sexual relations, and learning CPR.
   6) Instruct about oxygen safety.
   7) Instruct about proper protection of sternum (and grafts) if the client has had surgery.
   8) Instruct on modification of risk factors.
   9) Include significant other and family members in all instructions.
h. Gas exchange
   1) Monitor chest X ray.
   2) Elevate the head of the bed.
   3) Monitor breath sounds and respiratory function.
   4) Encourage coughing and deep breathing.
i. Therapeutic regimen, ineffective
   1) Promote performance of ADLs.
   2) Promote therapeutic regimen.
   3) Teach proper incision care for surgical patients.
   4) Assess the client's and family members' readiness to learn and follow the therapeutic regimen.
   5) Stress the importance of administering medications as prescribed, reporting untoward reactions or responses to medications, and difficulties obtaining recommended medications (e.g., expenses, accessibility).

6) Assess understanding of the treatment regimen.
5. Evaluation
    a. Assess the efficacy of the treatment regimen.
    b. If goals are not met as originally designed, then reassessment should be done and revisions to the plan of care developed.

III. Pulmonary Disease

More than 400,000 Americans die annually from obstructive pulmonary diseases (ALA, 2010; Osborn, Wraa, & Watson, 2010). The estimated direct cost of pulmonary disease in the United States for 2010 was $69 billion, and the indirect cost was $186 billion (National Institutes of Health, 2011).

A. Chronic Obstructive Pulmonary Disease (COPD): Persistent airway obstruction that decreases lungs' capacity to take in and excrete oxygen. It is estimated that 12 million people have chronic bronchitis or emphysema.
   1. Chronic bronchitis: Excessive secretion of bronchial mucus, obstructing air flow and causing chronic coughing and scarring of the bronchial tissue
   2. Emphysema: Abnormal alterations of the air spaces distal to the terminal bronchiole; damaged alveoli are less able to transfer oxygen to the blood, causing shortness of breath; lung tissue loses flexibility, making it difficult to exhale (ALA, 2010).
   3. Epidemiology (ALA, 2010): COPD is the fourth-leading cause of death in the United States, with 120,970 deaths in 2006. Women in the United States have surpassed the death rate of men. It is estimated that 80%–90% of deaths from COPD are caused by smoking.
   4. Etiology (ALA, 2010; Osborn, Wraa, & Watson, 2010)
      a. Chronic bronchitis: The causes of chronic bronchitis include smoking, recurrent infections, and environmental irritants such as coal mines, industrial pollutants, grain handlers, metal molders, and dust.
      b. Emphysema: The causes of emphysema include smoking, recurrent infections, and environmental irritants. In addition, alpha 1-antitrypsin (a1AT) deficiency is an inherited form of emphysema.
   5. Pathophysiology (ALA, 2010; Osborn, Wraa, & Watson, 2010)
      a. Chronic bronchitis
         1) Acute: Not associated with fever
         2) Chronic: Mucus-producing cough most days of the month for 3 months out of a year for 2 successive years without underlying disease

3) Hypertrophy and hypersecretion of goblet and mucous gland cells in bronchioles extend into terminal bronchioles.
4) Increased secretions cause bronchial congestion and narrowing of the bronchioles and small bronchi.
5) The lower respiratory tract becomes colonized by bacteria and stimulates secretions by leukocytes.
6) Leukocytes cause swelling and tissue destruction of the bronchial walls so that they become granulated and fibrotic, leading to stenosis and obstruction that impair the exchange of oxygen to and from the lungs.
      b. Emphysema
         1) Recurrent infections, history of smoking, and exposure to environmental irritants cause deficiency in the protease inhibitor a1AT.
         2) Elastase, a neutral protease that is produced by leukocytes and alveolar macrophages, proliferates and destroys lung elastin as it becomes uninhibited because of the deficiency of a1AT.
         3) Alveoli are destroyed, creating permanent holes in the lower lung tissues.
         4) Oxygen-carbon dioxide transfer in the blood is inhibited.
         5) Lungs lose their elasticity and bronchial tubes collapse, trapping air in the lungs.
   6. Complications (ALA, 2010; Osborn, Wraa, & Watson, 2010) include shortness of breath, coughing, change in chest circumference (increased anteroposterior diameter), sputum production, and weight loss (with emphysema) and obesity (with chronic bronchitis).
   7. Treatments
      a. Medications (Aschenbrenner & Venable, 2010)
         1) Beta agonists (sympathomimetics)
         2) Anticholinergic agents
         3) Xanthine derivatives
         4) Mucolytic drugs
         5) Inhaled glucocorticoid steroids
         6) Leukotriene receptor antagonists
         7) Oxygen therapy
      b. Management measures: To stop the progression of the disease; maximize breathing; reduce airway secretions, inflammation, and bronchospasm; and prevent complications
         1) Maximize breathing (**Figure 14-7**).
         2) Maintain or improve functional status.
         3) Enhance coping skills, identify stressors, and modify behavior (see Figure 14-5).

4) Maintain or improve nutritional status.

5) Educate about the disease process and prognosis.

6) Use mechanical ventilation as needed.

7) Identify irritants.

8) Identify and manage precipitating factors.

9) Encourage smoking cessation.

10) Encourage prevention and early treatment of airway infections and vaccinations (influenza and pneumococcal disease).

11) Encourage use of chest physiotherapy techniques (**Figure 14-8**).

12) Administer medications, including oxygen, as needed.

13) Provide pulmonary rehabilitation for stable clients.

B. Asthma: Inflammation of the trachea and bronchi lining in response to various stimuli, causing narrowing of the airway passages, tightening of the muscles, and increased mucus secretions in the airways (ALA, 2010). Management for asthma is based on Global Initiatives for Asthma guidelines (2010).

1. Medical management incorporates four treatment components.

a. Objective measures of lung function

b. Avoidance of risk factors and environmental control factors

c. Comprehensive pharmacological management

d. Client education

2. Epidemiology (ALA, 2010): More than 36 million Americans have asthma that has been diagnosed. After a steady increase in deaths related to asthma, the number of deaths has declined.

3. Etiology (ALA, 2010): Asthma is caused by an interaction between genetics and the environment that is not fully understood.

4. Pathophysiology (ALA, 2010; Osborn, Wraa, & Watson, 2010)

a. Irritants stimulate bronchoconstriction of the smooth muscles that line the bronchial tubes, causing fluid to leak from blood vessels and stimulating inflammation.

b. The inflammation narrows the airways and mucus becomes so thick the cilia are unable to remove it from the airways effectively.

c. This impairs oxygen delivery to the blood and lungs, trapping carbon monoxide.

5. Complications (ALA, 2010): May be fatal; complications include COPD

6. Treatment

a. Medications (Aschenbrenner & Venable, 2006)

1) Beta agonists

2) Anticholinergic agents

Figure 14-7. Breathing Techniques

Certain exercises can be used to improve your breathing. They include pursed-lip breathing and abdominal breathing.

Pursed-Lip Breathing

Pursed-lip breathing decreases how often you take breaths and keeps your airways open longer. This allows more air to flow in and out of your lungs so you can be more physically active.

To do pursed-lip breathing, you breathe in through your nostrils. Then you slowly breathe out through slightly pursed lips, as if you're blowing out a candle. You exhale two to three times longer than you inhale. Some people find it helpful to count to two while inhaling and to four or six while exhaling.

Illustrations are available at www.nhlbi.nih.gov/health/dci/Diseases/pulreh/pulreh_during.html

The illustration shows the pursed-lip breathing technique. The "inhale" illustration shows how to inhale correctly using this technique. The "exhale" illustration shows how to exhale correctly. Click your mouse on the "inhale" and "exhale" tabs at the top of the illustration to view each step of the technique.

Abdominal Breathing

Abdominal breathing is the process of contracting the diaphragm, the muscle that separates the lungs from the stomach and liver. It enables the lungs to expand more fully and expel carbon dioxide more effectively.

1. Adjust your posture so that your lungs, chest, and abdomen can expand fully (standing, sitting or lying down).

2. Place your hand on your abdomen to assess the effectiveness of your breathing.

3. Breathe in through the nose slowly, feeling your abdomen expand.

4. Rest for a moment.

5. Slowly exhale through your mouth.

6. Repeat the process for several minutes or as tolerated.

From *Pursed-lip breathing*, by the National Heart and Blood Institute, 2010. Retrieved August 3, 2011, from www.nhlbi.nih.gov/health/dci/Diseases/pulreh/pulreh_summary.html. Copyright 2010 by the National Heart and Blood Institute. Reprinted with permission.

Figure 14-8. Airway Clearance Techniques

If a client has a condition that is causing a buildup of mucus in his or her airways such as cystic fibrosis, he or she will be taught how to loosen and expel the mucus. These are called airway clearance techniques (ACTs). The following is a brief overview of ACTs. The ACTs a client uses will be based on his or her needs and his or her disease.

Coughing

Coughing is the most basic and effective of ACTs. Mucus is cleared from the lung by the speed of the airflow. However, coughing a lot can make a client feel short of breath. One type of coughing is called huffing. The technique involves taking a breath in and actively exhaling. To huff, imagine breathing onto a mirror and steam it up. Although huffing is not as forceful as a cough, it can be very effective and is not as tiring.

Chest Physical Therapy (CPT or Chest PT) or Postural Drainage & Percussion (PD&P)

CPT or chest PT or PD&P is an ACT that includes postural drainage and chest percussion. Postural drainage involves the client getting into certain positions (postures) that drain mucus from different parts of the lung. It works by using gravity to it drain from airways where it can be coughed. Chest percussion involves clapping and using vibration to dislodge and move mucus.

Oscillating Positive Expiratory Pressure (Oscillating PEP)

Oscillating PEP is an ACT in which the client exhales many times through a device. Breathing with these devices vibrates the large and small airways and dislodges mucus so it can be expelled. After blowing through the device many times, the client coughs or huffs to expel the mucus. This entire process is repeated many times.

High-Frequency Chest Wall Oscillation

High-frequency chest wall oscillation is done with an inflatable vest attached to a machine that vibrates it at high frequency. The vest vibrates the chest to loosen the mucus so it can be expelled. Every 5 minutes the client turns off the machine and coughs or huffs to expel the mucus.

PEP Therapy

PEP therapy moves air into the lungs and behind the mucus using extra (collateral) airways. PEP keeps the airways open. A PEP system includes a mask or mouthpiece attached to a resistor. During this treatment, the client breathes in normally and breathes out a little harder against the resistance.

Active Cycle of Breathing Technique (ACBT)

ACBT involves breathing techniques. It can be changed to meet each person's needs. It moves mucus through air pressure and decreases airway spasm. ACBT includes the following:

- Breathing control: This is normal, gentle breathing of the lower chest while relaxing the upper chest and shoulders.

- Thoracic expansion exercises: During thoracic expansion exercises, the client inhales deeply. Some people hold their breath for 3 seconds to increase its effectiveness. This may be combined with chest clapping or vibrating, followed by breathing control.

- Forced expiration technique: huffs of varied lengths with breathing control.

Autogenic Drainage (AD)

AD is self-drainage. It uses varied airflows to move mucus from small to large airways. AD has three parts

- Dislodging mucus

- Collecting mucus

- Clearing mucus

The client inhales at different levels and then adjusts exhalation to increase airflow and move mucus. AD takes practice to be successful, and it is most effectively used with people older than 8 years.

From *Airway clearance techniques*, by Cystic Fibrosis Foundation, 2010. Retrieved August 3, 2011, from www.cff.org/treatments/Therapies/Respiratory/ AirwayClearance/#Airway_clearance_techniques. Copyright 2010 by Cystic Fibrosis Foundation. Reprinted with permission.

3) Combination inhalers
4) Xanthine derivatives
5) Anti-inflammatory agents
6) Mast cell stabilizers
7) Leukotriene receptor antagonists
8) Inhaled steroids
b. Management measures (ALA, 2010; Osborn, Wraa, & Watson, 2010): Maximize breathing; reduce airway secretions, inflammation, and bronchospasm; and prevent complications.

1) Maximize breathing (see Figure 14-7).
2) Maintain or improve functional status.
3) Enhance coping skills, identify stressors, and modify behavior (see Figure 14-5).
4) Maintain or improve nutritional status.
5) Educate about the disease process and prognosis.
6) Use mechanical ventilation as needed.
7) Identify irritants.
8) Identify and manage precipitating factors,

including environmental and emotional triggers.

9) Encourage smoking cessation.

10) Encourage prevention and early treatment of airway infections and vaccinations against influenza and pneumococcal disease.

11) Use a peak flow meter, a handheld device that measures air flow from the lungs. Benefits include better asthma management through indication of worsening or improvement of symptoms, allowing titration of medication.

C. Cystic Fibrosis (CF): Genetic disorder of the exocrine glands, causing secretion of abnormally thick mucus that obstructs glands and ducts of various organs, most commonly the respiratory, pancreatic, and sweat glands, causing respiratory infections and malabsorption (ALA, 2010)

1. Epidemiology (ALA, 2010): CF is the second most common life-threatening inherited pulmonary disease of children, with the incidence higher in white children than in other races. About 30,000 people in the United States have CF, with about 1,000 new cases each year. More than 10 million Americans are symptomless carriers of the CF gene. More than 80% of cases are diagnosed by the age of 3.

2. Etiology (ALA, 2010; Osborn, Wraa, & Watson, 2010): CF is caused by a defective gene, the CF trans-membrane conductive regulator. This gene controls the production of a protein that regulates how sodium is carried across the membrane that separates cells.

3. Pathophysiology (ALA, 2010; Osborn, Wraa, & Watson, 2010): The gene disturbance leads to production of thick mucus that blocks bodily passages, particularly in the digestive and respiratory systems. The disorder affects all exocrine glands. People with only one copy of the gene carry it but have no symptoms.

4. Complications (ALA, 2010; Osborn, Wraa, & Watson, 2010)

a. Bronchial obstruction: Causes infections, respiratory disease, cor pulmonale, coughing, wheezing, and shortness of breath

b. Pancreatic duct obstruction: Inability of pancreatic enzymes to be released, causing malabsorption, nutritional deficiencies, and diabetes mellitus

c. Intestinal obstruction and gastrointestinal malabsorption (excessive appetite with poor weight gain and greasy, bulky stools)

d. Bile duct obstruction: Causes portal hypertension and liver failure

e. Blocked sweat glands: Decreases absorption of sodium and chloride, leading to dehydration, salty-tasting skin

f. Reproductive tract: Causes sterility by obstructing the vas deferens in men and producing thick cervical secretions in women, blocking sperm from entering the uterus (ALA, 2010)

5. Treatment is directed toward slowing of organ dysfunction and pancreatic insufficiency.

a. Medications (Aschenbrenner & Venable, 2006)
1) Pancreatic enzymes
2) Mucolytics
3) Antibiotics (as needed)
4) Bronchodilators
5) Hypertonic saline
6) Anti-inflammatory medicines (as needed)
7) Oxygen therapy (as needed)

b. Physical therapy: Chest physical therapy with postural drainage

c. Nutritional therapy
1) Balanced, high-calorie diet
2) Fat-soluble vitamins (A, D, E, and K) must be supplemented.

d. Surgery: Lung transplant for end-stage disease

6. Management measures: Early diagnosis and comprehensive interdisciplinary therapy are important in lengthening survival time and alleviating symptoms (ALA, 2010; Osborn, Wraa, & Watson, 2010).

a. Maximize breathing (see Figure 14-7).

b. Maintain or improve functional status.

c. Enhance coping skills, identify stressors, and modify behavior (see Figure 14-5).

d. Maintain or improve nutritional status.

e. Educate about the disease process and prognosis.

f. Use mechanical ventilation as needed.

g. Identify irritants.

h. Psychological and genetic counseling

i. Administer chest physiotherapy (see Figure 14-8).

j. Administer medications as needed, including oxygen.

k. Encourage prevention and early treatment of airway infections and vaccinations against influenza and pneumococcal disease.

D. Restrictive Pulmonary Diseases (ALA, 2010; Osborn, Wraa, & Watson, 2010)

1. Interstitial lung disease: A group of about 130 disorders that share the following characteristics:

a. The lung is damaged in some known or unknown way.

b. The walls of the air sacs are inflamed.

c. The lung stiffens from scaring of the tissue between the air sacs.

2. Examples: Interstitial pulmonary fibrosis (IPF), occupational lung disease, sarcoidosis.

3. Epidemiology, etiology, and pathophysiology: Currently about 200,000 Americans have IPF, one form of interstitial lung disease. The severity of symptoms varies from disease to disease and person to person. Scientists are looking for a genetic cause and other possible causes of these diseases.

4. Complications: These conditions can lead to respiratory failure.

5. Treatment: Current treatment is focused on treatment of inflammation.

6. Medication

a. Medications used to treat symptoms

b. Oxygen therapy

7. Management measures (ALA, 2010; Osborn, Wraa, & Watson, 2010). Goal: prevent inflammation and relieve symptoms.

a. Maximize breathing (see Figure 14-7).

b. Maintain or improve functional status.

c. Enhance coping skills, identify stressors, and modify behavior (see Figure 14-5).

d. Maintain or improve nutritional status.

e. Educate about the disease process and prognosis.

f. Use mechanical ventilation as needed.

g. Identify irritants.

h. Encourage prevention and early treatment of airway infections and vaccinations against influenza and pneumococcal disease.

E. Neuromuscular and Neurologic Conditions: Parkinson's disease, postpolio syndrome, amyotrophic lateral sclerosis, multiple sclerosis, Guillain-Barré syndrome, myasthenia gravis, Duchenne's muscular dystrophy, spinal cord injury, diaphragm dysfunction

1. Epidemiology, etiology, and pathophysiology: These conditions affect the neurological and neuromuscular control of the lungs.

2. Complications: These conditions can lead to respiratory distress or failure.

3. Treatment

a. Oxygen (if needed)

b. Mechanical ventilator support (if needed)

c. Chest physical therapy

4. Management measures

a. Maximize breathing.

b. Maintain or improve functional status.

c. Enhance coping skills, identify stressors, and modify behavior.

d. Maintain or improve nutritional status.

e. Educate about the disease process and prognosis.

f. Use mechanical ventilation as needed.

g. Identify irritants.

h. Encourage prevention and early treatment of airway infections and vaccinations against influenza and pneumococcal disease.

F. Other Conditions

1. Lung cancer (ALA, 2010): Lung cancer is the second most commonly diagnosed type of cancer in both men and women.

2. Epidemiology and etiology (ALA, 2010; Osborn, Wraa, & Watson, 2010): Smoking accounts for 87% of all lung cancer deaths. Repeated exposure to carcinogens such as radon and asbestos is also a factor. There are two major types of lung cancer.

a. Small-cell lung cancer (SCLC).

b. Non-small-cell lung cancer (NSCLC), including squamous cell carcinoma, adenocarcinoma, and large-cell carcinoma. These types of cancer make up 80% of cases of lung cancer.

3. Pathophysiology

a. SCLC is likely to spread and is widely distributed by the time of diagnosis, making treatment difficult.

b. NSCLC

1) Squamous cell: A slow-growing mass typically originates in the proximal bronchi.

2) Adenocarcinoma: This is the most common type of lung cancer in nonsmokers; cells are found in the periphery of the lungs. Progression is slow, although the cells can be found in the lymph and blood.

3) Large cell: Cells are found in the periphery of the lungs, spreading to bronchi and larger airways.

4. Complications (ALA, 2010; Osborn, Wraa, & Watson, 2010): Cancer cells can metastasize to other areas of the body (most commonly the liver, bone, adrenal glands, and brain) or be fatal. Treatment can cause other health problems.

a. Surgical treatment: Weakened arm and chest muscles; fluid may build up in space left after resection

b. Radiation therapy: Loss of appetite related to nausea, vomiting, loss of taste, oral and throat sores affecting swallow; weight loss; pulmonary fibrosis; and dry, itching, tender skin

c. Chemotherapy: Immunosuppression, decreased clotting time, fatigue, alopecia, nausea, vomiting, and oral sores affecting appetite

5. Treatment (ALA, 2010; Osborn, Wraa, & Watson, 2010): Staging and type of cancer affect the treatment plan.
   a. Surgery involves removal of tumor and the diseased portion of the lung. For small tumors that have not spread outside the lung, surgery offers a cure rate higher than 50%. Lobectomy, pneumonectomy, and segmental resection are performed.
   b. Radiation targets the tumor. Radiation may be used to shrink the tumor before surgery or after surgery to kill any remaining cells.
   c. Chemotherapy: Medications may be used systemically to kill any cancer cells. It may be used after surgery to kill any remaining cancer or in advanced stages to eliminate symptoms.
6. Management measures (ALA, 2010; Osborn, Wraa, & Watson, 2010)
   a. Maximize breathing (see Figure 14-7).
   b. Maintain or improve functional status.
   c. Enhance coping skills, identify stressors, and modify behavior (see Figure 14-5).
   d. Maintain or improve nutritional status.
   e. Educate about the disease process and prognosis.
   f. Use mechanical ventilation as needed.
   g. Encourage prevention and early treatment of airway infections and vaccinations against influenza and pneumococcal disease.
G. Pulmonary Rehabilitation: Pulmonary rehabilitation is a multidisciplinary and comprehensive intervention to treat clients with chronic respiratory diseases or to prepare for or recover from lung surgery. Pulmonary rehabilitation is designed to reduce symptoms and optimize functional status. The goal is to stabilize or reverse the manifestations of the disease. The components of pulmonary rehabilitation include the following:
   1. Physician-prescribed exercise: Includes exercise conditioning through strength training and aerobic exercises
   2. Education or training: Includes self-management of the disease and nutritional counseling
   3. Psychosocial assessment: Evaluation of the client's mental and emotional status
   4. Outcome assessment: Evaluation of progress as it relates to the client's goals and program (AACVPR, 2010; National Heart, Lung, and Blood Institute, 2010)
H. Nursing Process
   1. Assessment (Osborn, Wraa, & Watson, 2010)
      a. Medical and family history

1) Medical history
2) Surgical history
3) Use of supplemental oxygen, medical devices, and knowledge of appropriate use
4) Medications: Including allergies and drug intolerance
5) Triggers in work and home environments
6) Lifestyle
   a) Smoking history
   b) Work and home activities
7) Recent illnesses: Complete blood cell count to monitor white blood cells for signs of infection and hematocrit to follow anemia, bleeding, cirrhosis, and dehydration
8) Self-care skills
9) Knowledge and use of medications
10) Test results: Pulmonary function, blood tests, electrocardiogram, chest radiography
      b. Physical
         1) Activity
            a) Physical limitations (e.g., strength, functional ability, orthopedic limitations)
            b) Exercise tolerance, need for supplemental oxygen, cardiac function
         2) Neurological: Cognition changes, lethargy, restlessness
         3) Pulmonary: Dyspnea, tachypnea, wheezes, crackles, rhonchi, decreased breath sounds, cough, hoarseness, clubbed fingers, chest retractions, barrel chest, decreased chest wall movement, productive thick sputum that may be odorous, hemoptysis, postnasal drainage
         4) Cardiovascular: Tachycardia, dysrhythmia, fatigue, chest pain, edema
         5) Gastrointestinal
            a) General: Weight loss or gain, appetite, oral sores, constipation, dehydration, reflux
            b) Special gastrointestinal considerations for clients with CF: Bulky, foul-smelling, pale, or watery stool; intestinal obstruction, fecal impaction, and tarry stools if bleeding; jaundice; ascites; abnormal liver function laboratory results
         6) Skin: Decreased skin turgor with dehydration, diaphoresis
            a) Color
            b) Temperature

7) Nutritional: Weight loss, lack of appetite, loss of taste, swallowing difficulties, constipation, hydration, serum albumin

8) Psychosocial
   a) Support systems
   b) Individual and family coping
   c) Psychosocial: Fear of suffocation, sleep disturbance, depression, anxiety
   d) Willingness to participate in program, health-changing behavior
   e) Symptoms of depression
   f) Knowledge of disease process, description and interpretation of medical tests

2. Diagnoses (Doenges et al., 2010)
   a. Airway clearance, ineffective
   b. Anxiety
   c. Coping, ineffective
   d. Activity intolerance
   e. Constipation, risk for
   f. Electrolyte imbalance, risk for
   g. Fatigue
   h. Fluid balance, risk for imbalance
   i. Gas exchange, impaired
   j. Infection, risk for
   k. Knowledge deficit
   l. Mobility, impaired
   m. Nutrition, imbalanced, less or more than body needs
   n. Powerlessness, risk for
   o. Self-care deficit (bathing and hygiene, dressing and grooming, feeding, toileting)
   p. Sexual dysfunction
   q. Skin integrity, risk for impaired
   r. Spiritual distress, risk for
   s. Stress, overload
   t. Therapeutic regimen management, readiness for enhanced
   u. Tissue perfusion, ineffective

3. Plan: Goals for client and family (ALA, 2010; Osborn, Wraa, & Watson, 2010)
   a. Demonstrate effective breathing patterns without fatigue and use energy conservation measures.
   b. Demonstrate improved airway clearance through use of postural drainage when appropriate, coughing, deep breathing, and taking medications as directed.
   c. Demonstrate resolution of cognitive changes if they have not become permanent; resolve cyanosis.
   d. Demonstrate ability to perform ADLs using compensation measures when necessary to

prevent dyspnea or fatigue; for children, demonstrate ability to participate in normal activities using preactivity medications.

   e. Demonstrate stable weight for age and size, take adequate caloric intake daily, and have a normal albumin level.
   f. Have regular bowel movements without constipation or dehydration and take in adequate amounts of fluid daily.
   g. Remain free of infection and prevent influenza and pneumonia.
   h. Demonstrate adequate sleep patterns for rest and rejuvenation.
   i. Verbalize decreased spiritual distress, increasing sense of integrity while living with chronic disease.
   j. Demonstrate support for the person with the disability and verbalize resources available for family support.
   k. Acknowledge fear and anxiety and demonstrate ways to decrease anxiety (e.g., hobbies, social activities, relaxation techniques).
   l. Verbalize understanding of compensation measures while engaging in sexual activity.
   m. Verbalize knowledge of the disease process, precipitating factors of respiratory difficulties and how to avoid or minimize effects, how to administer medication and oxygen therapy properly, and when to call the physician.
   n. Verbalize and demonstrate understanding of the therapeutic regimen and the importance of self-monitoring and compliance with therapeutic recommendations.

4. Interventions (ALA, 2010; Osborn, Wraa, & Watson, 2010)
   a. Observe respiration depth and rate, dyspnea, nasal flaring.
   b. Inspect thorax or symmetry of respiratory movement, chest muscle retractions, changes in skin color and capillary refill, changes in mentation or behavior.
   c. Auscultate lungs for adventitious sounds.
   d. Administer oxygen, bronchodilators, antibiotics, corticosteroids, and other medications as directed.
   e. Teach breathing techniques and exercises to conserve energy (see Figure 14-8).
   f. Identify ways to conserve energy in daily activities.
   g. Adapt ways to increase endurance and conserve energy.
   h. Slowly increase activity as tolerance allows, promoting as much independence as possible.

THE SPECIALTY PRACTICE OF REHABILITATION NURSING

i. Encourage a regular exercise program with planned rest periods between activities.

j. Teach clients receiving intermittent, continuous, or nocturnal ventilator support to do the following:

1) Strengthen skeletal muscles that have atrophied from illness and bedrest.

2) Strengthen skeletal muscles by beginning exercises during periods while the client is receiving ventilator support, adjusting ventilator settings as needed, and including strengthening techniques (e.g., free weights, gravity, manual resistance, elastic bands).

3) Improve nutritional support through supplements, considering the possibility of using a feeding tube to increase muscle strength and endurance. Clients with a tracheotomy have limited speech and are at risk of aspiration.

4) Assist with communication by exploring different modalities.

5) Prevent aspiration by teaching compensatory swallowing techniques.

6) Provide uninterrupted periods of rest.

k. Identify triggers.

1) Air particles (indoor and outdoor)

2) Cold air or sudden temperature change

3) Tobacco or smoke from burning wood or leaves

4) Perfume, paint, hairspray

5) Allergens (e.g., dust mites, pollen, pollution, animal dander)

6) Common cold, flu, or respiratory illness

7) Vigorous exercise

8) Stress or excitement

9) Certain foods

l. Control measures (ALA, 2010)

1) Do skin testing to identify allergens.

2) Keep an asthma diary to identify triggers.

3) Use pillow and mattress covers.

4) Remove carpets.

5) Use air-filtering devices or air conditioning.

6) Keep pets out of bedrooms.

7) Ensure early detection of respiratory infections.

8) Stop smoking.

9) Monitor the pollution index and adjust outdoor activities accordingly.

10) Avoid exposure to colds and flu and encourage vaccinations against influenza and pneumonia.

m. Promote caloric intake to support adequate growth.

1) Provide frequent small meals to lessen fatigue.

2) Provide appropriate food consistency to enhance energy conservation during meals.

3) Maintain good oral care.

4) Monitor for swallowing difficulties and risk for aspiration.

5) Monitor for nutritional risk

a) Weigh daily and monitor for dehydration (keep records of intake and output and skin turgor).

b) Monitor intake.

c) Monitor albumin levels and offer protein supplements as needed for healing and weight maintenance.

d) Administer vitamins and pancreatic enzymes for clients with CF as ordered.

6) Monitor stools.

a) Encourage fluids, fiber, stool softeners, or laxatives.

b) Encourage ambulation.

c) Note color, amount, consistency, frequency, and presence of blood.

7) Teach about medications.

a) Explain usage and symptoms of effectiveness, ineffectiveness, and toxicity.

b) Monitor theophylline levels (if prescribed).

c) Maintain inhalation equipment.

8) Teach about safe oxygen use in the home.

a) Explain that oxygen is combustible and must be kept away from open flames and heat, including a running gas stove or gas or kerosene space heater.

b) Prevent leakage.

(1) Keep the tank upright.

(2) Turn off the system when not in use.

(3) Do not place anything over the tubing.

(4) Keep an all-purpose fire extinguisher available.

(5) In case of fire, turn off the oxygen and leave the home.

(6) Notify the fire department that there is oxygen in the home. Many fire departments offer free safety inspections.

c) Monitor for symptoms of not enough or too much oxygen.

(1) Difficult, irregular, or slow breathing

(2) Restlessness or anxiousness

(3) Tiredness or drowsiness

(4) Difficulty waking up

(5) Persistent headache

(6) Confusion, difficulty concentrating, or slurred speech

(7) Cyanotic fingertips or lips

d) Teach the client to notify the practitioner if any of these symptoms occur and to never change the flow rate without guidance from the physician.

e) Teach about diagnostic tests, disease processes, prognoses, and therapies.

f) Assist the client and family with coping and stress reduction.

(1) Develop trust with the client and family, encourage family members to express feelings, assist in problem solving, identify support systems, and offer support network as needed.

(2) Promote normal growth and development.

(3) Encourage personal control.

(4) Teach relaxation and stress-reduction techniques.

g) Consult with the chaplain or the client's spiritual guide to offer spiritual support.

h) Offer education on sexual and other physical activity.

5. Evaluation

a. Client follow-up is crucial.

b. Evaluate the client's understanding of instructions and how the interventions are affecting them, positively or negatively.

c. Revise goals and interventions with the client and the physician as needed.

Acknowledgment

We would like to thank Lynn Carbone, RN CRRN, for her contributions to the 5th edition of the *Core Curriculum*.

References

American Association of Cardiovascular and Pulmonary Rehabilitation. (2010). *Cardiac and pulmonary rehabilitation fundamentals.* Retrieved August 20, 2010, from www.aacvpr.org/Resources/CardiacPulmonaryRehabFundamentals/tabid/256/Default.aspx.

American Heart Association. (2010). *Heart disease and stroke statistics.* Retrieved February 14, 2011, from www.americanheart.org?presenter.jtml?identifier=4977.

American Lung Association. (2010). Retrieved August 6, 2010, from www.lungusa.org/.

Aschenbrenner, D. S., & Venable, S. J. (2008). *Drug therapy in nursing.* Philadelphia: Lippincott, Williams & Wilkins.

Beckie, T. M. (2006). A behavior change intervention for women in cardiac rehabilitation. *Journal of Cardiovascular Nursing, 21*(2), 146–153.

Condon, M. C. (2004). *Women's health: An integrated approach to wellness and illness.* Upper Saddle River, NJ: Prentice Hall.

Doenges, M. E., Moorhouse, M. F., & Murr, A. C. (2010). *Nursing diagnosis manual: Planning, individualizing & documenting client care.* Philadelphia: F. A. Davis.

Eliopoulos, C. (2004). *Invitation to holistic health: A guide to living a balanced life.* Boston: Jones & Bartlett.

Espnes, G. A., & Byrne, D. (2008). Gender differences in psychological risk factors for development of heart disease. *Stress and Health, 24,* 188–195.

Gleeson, D., & Crabbe, D. L. (2009). Emerging concepts in cardiovascular disease risk assessment: Where do women fit in? *Journal of the American Academy of Nurse Practitioners, 21,* 480–487.

Global Initiatives for Asthma. (2010). *GINA report, global strategy for asthma management and prevention.* Retrieved August 23, 2011, from ww.ginasthma.org/guidelines-gina-report-global-strategy-for-asthma.html.

Godfrey, J. R., & Manson, J. E. (2008). Toward optimal health: Strategies for prevention of heart disease in women. *Journal of Women's Health, 17*(8), 1271–1276.

Grace, S. L., Gravely-Witte, S., Kayaniyil, S., Brual, J., Suskin, N., & Stewart, D. E. (2009). A multisite examination of sex differences in cardiac rehabilitation barriers by participant status. *Journal of Women's Health, 18*(2), 209–216.

Leddy, S. K. (2003). *Integrative health promotion: Conceptual bases for nursing practice.* Thorofare, NJ: Slack Incorporated.

Madison, H. E. (2010). *What women want to know: Assessing the value, relevance, and efficacy of a self-management intervention for rural women with coronary heart disease.* Unpublished doctoral dissertation, University of Massachusetts, Amherst.

National Heart, Lung, and Blood Institute. (2010). Pulmonary rehabilitation: Key points. Retrieved August 5, 2011, from www.nhlbi.nih.gov/health/dci/Diseases/pulreh/pulreh_summary.html.

National Institutes of Health. (2011). *2010 factbook.* Retrieved February 14, 2011, from www.nhlbi.nih.gov/about/factbook/chapter4.htm.

Osborn, K. S., Wraa, C. E., & Watson, A. (2010). *Medical surgical nursing: Preparation for practice.* Boston: Prentice Hall.

Pollin, I. S., Kral, B. G., Shattuck, T., Sadler, M. D., Boyle, J. R., McKillop, L., et al. (2008). High prevalence of cardiometabolic risk factors in women considered low risk by traditional risk assessment. *Journal of Women's Health, 17*(6), 947–953.

Shaw, L. J., Merz, C. N. B., Bittner, V., Kip, K., Johnson, B. D., Reis, S. E., et al. (2008). Importance of socioeconomic status as a predictor of cardiovascular outcome and costs of care in women with suspected myocardial ischemia. Results from the National Institute of Health, National Heart, Lung, and Blood Institute-sponsored women's ischemia syndrome evaluation (WISE). *Journal of Women's Health, 17*(7), 1081–1092.

Yang, L., Kuper, H., & Weiderpassa, E. (2008). Anthropometric characteristics as predictors of coronary heart disease in women. *Journal of Internal Medicine, 264,* 39–49.

CHAPTER 15
Acute and Chronic Pain

Diane B. Monsivais, PhD CRRN

Pain is defined as an "unpleasant sensory and emotional experience associated with actual or potential tissue damage, or described in terms of such damage" (International Association for the Study of Pain [IASP], 2011b). In addition, the classic definition by Margo McCaffery should always be kept in mind: "Pain is whatever the experiencing person says it is, existing whenever he (or she) says it does" (McCaffery, 1979, p. 11).

Although these two definitions of pain seem straightforward, effective pain management is one of the most complicated challenges in health care. Successful management relies on continuous holistic care from a multidisciplinary team, not always an easy feat in today's healthcare system. Rehabilitation nurses must evaluate the client's pain in its entirety, including the effects on the client's personal, family, and community roles. It is only through a holistic interdisciplinary team approach that successful pain management outcomes can be achieved.

The Association of Rehabilitation Nurses (n.d.) supports the following definition of the pain management rehabilitation nurse: "The pain management rehabilitation nurse promotes and advances the professional rehabilitation nursing practice of caring for people with pain. Excellence in this specialized practice area is achieved through education, advocacy, research, and networking."

Extent of the Pain Problem

The societal and economic extent of the pain problem is striking. With 116 million Americans affected by pain and costs for health care and lost productivity estimated at $560–$635 billion annually, the Institute of Medicine (IOM) has declared pain to be a major public health problem (2011).

I. **Pain Classifications**

There are many ways to categorize pain, including duration, source, mode of transmission, or etiology (Taylor, Lillis, Lemone, & Lynn, 2006).

A. Duration

1. Acute pain stems from tissue damage and is rapid in onset and protective in nature, and it varies from mild to severe. When the underlying cause resolves, pain should resolve. Burns, fractures, muscle injury, childbirth, and surgery are examples of conditions that cause acute pain. Commonly injured tissues are skin, muscle, bone, ligaments, tendons, and visceral organs (IASP,

2011a). Fewer than 50% of postoperative clients receive adequate pain relief (Apfelbaum, Chen, Mehta, & Gan, 2003).

2. Chronic pain occurs when acute pain persists beyond the expected healing period, or it may be present without noticeable past injury.

   a. Chronic pain is associated with the following disease conditions: osteoarthritis, rheumatoid arthritis, headache, backache, cancer pain, neuralgias, chronic renal failure, chronic pancreatitis, and phantom pain.

   b. Persistent pain often becomes debilitating and causes severe disruptions in work, family, and social roles. Clients are often questioned as to the legitimacy of the pain (Craig, 2006).

B. Source

1. Cutaneous pain involves skin or subcutaneous tissue.

2. Somatic: Diffuse and originates in tendons, ligaments, bones, blood vessels, or nerves

3. Visceral: Poorly localized and originates within organs in the thorax, cranium, and abdomen when organs are stretched abnormally. Stretching may create distention, ischemia, or inflammation, which initiates pain (Taylor et al., 2006).

C. Neuropathic Pain

1. Central pain is pain initiated or caused by a primary lesion or dysfunction in the central nervous system (IASP, 2011b). Rehabilitation examples include cerebrovascular lesions, multiple sclerosis, and traumatic spinal cord injuries correlated with sensory abnormalities (primarily to temperature and pain) and hyperesthesia (Boivie, 2006).

2. Peripheral neuropathic pain is pain initiated or caused by a primary lesion or dysfunction in the peripheral nervous system (IASP, 2011b).

   a. Rehabilitation examples include diabetes, polyarteritis, alcoholic nutritional deficiency states, entrapment neuropathies, and amputation stump pain.

   b. Usually localized to affected area

   c. Mechanisms underlying pain in neuropathies remain obscure (Scadding & Koltzenburg, 2006).

II. Pain Pathways and Processes (Transduction, Transmission, Modulation, Response; Figure 15-1)

The concept of pain processing and the definitions of terms are the combined work of many scientists. There is not one definitive source on the topic, so summaries from textbooks reflect multiple authors' contributions to the literature.

A. Transduction (Activating Nociceptors): Nociceptors are specialized nerve endings found at the ends of small, unmyelinated and myelinated afferent neurons that are preferentially sensitive to a stimulus, such as heat, pressure, or other tissue damage (Meyer, Ringkamp, Campbell, & Raja, 2006). Nociceptors may be polymodal, responding to many different types of stimulus such as heat, chemical, or mechanical, or they may be more specialized and may share both afferent and efferent functions (Meyer et al.). The IASP defines a nociceptor as a receptor that is preferentially sensitive to a noxious stimulus or to a stimulus that would become noxious if prolonged.

1. Transduction starts with nociceptors being activated by various stimuli.
   a. Chemical or electrical changes (ischemia or substances from injured tissue)
   b. Mechanical (stretching or pressure on organs)
   c. Thermal (temperature changes of heat or cold)
2. Damaged tissue cells release chemicals (e.g., prostaglandins, histamine, bradykinin, serotonin, substance P) that stimulate the pain process (Taylor et al., 2006).

B. Transmission: Pain sensations are transmitted to the spinal cord and higher centers.

1. Acute: Localized pain along fast-conducting A-delta fibers
2. Visceral (diffuse) pain (burning, aching) through slow-conducting C-fibers (Taylor et al., 2006)
3. The transmission of impulses in primary afferent nerves is facilitated by neurotransmitters, particularly glutamate. Other neurotransmitters include aspartate, neuropeptides such as substance P, and calcitonin gene-related peptide (Julius & McKleskey, 2006).
4. Ascending pain impulses are then transmitted contralaterally to pathways in the dorsal horn of the spinal cord (Bradley & McKendree-Smith, 2002).
5. Most afferent impulses ascend via the lateral spinothalamic tract and spinoreticular tract (Bradley & McKendree-Smith, 2002).
6. The impulses then ascend to the thalamus and reticular formation in the brain and on to the cortex (Bradley & McKendree-Smith, 2002).

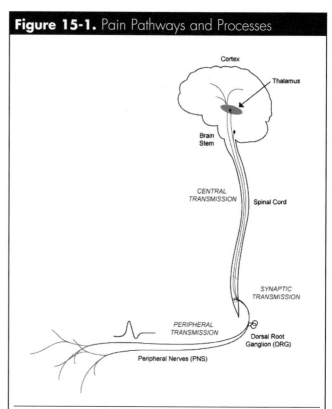

Figure 15-1. Pain Pathways and Processes

From *Pain pathway*, by University of Wisconsin School of Medicine and Public Health, 2010. Retrieved August 8, 2011, from http://projects.hsl.wisc.edu/GME/PainManagement/session2.2.html. Copyright 2010 by University of Wisconsin School of Medicine and Public Health. Reprinted with permission.

7. Mode of Transmission: Referred pain is transmitted to a cutaneous site different from its original site. For example, pain associated with myocardial infarction is referred to the neck, shoulder, and arm (Taylor et al., 2006).

C. Modulation: Neuromodulators (endorphins and enkephalins) are endogenous opioid substances in the brain and spinal cord that alter pain perception.

1. Endorphins are produced at neural synapses in the central nervous system pathway and have powerful analgesic effects and produce euphoria.
2. Enkephalins are less potent than endorphins and hypothesized to reduce pain by inhibiting release of substance P from terminals of afferent neurons (Taylor et al., 2006).

D. Perception of Pain: Perception of pain is formed in the primary and secondary somatosensory cortex, the insular cortex, and other parts of the limbic forebrain (Bradley & McKendree-Smith, 2002). The somatosensory cortex formulates the "affective expression of pain (how . . . pain looks to an observer)" (Huether & DeFriez, 2006, p. 450).

1. The threat presented by acute and especially chronic pain is based in part on the effect on

daily activities, ability to cope with the pain, and potential long-term consequences of the pain or its cause (Bond, 2006).

2. Personality, environmental factors (e.g., presence or absence of social support), and affective disorders (e.g., depression or anxiety) or other psychiatric conditions also affect the person's expression of pain and behaviors surrounding the pain experience (Bond, 2006).

E. Common Responses to Pain (Taylor et al., 2006)

1. Physiologic (involuntary) responses
   a. Sympathetic responses to superficial and moderate pain
      1) Increased blood pressure
      2) Increased pulse and respirations
      3) Pupil dilation
      4) Muscle tension and rigidity
      5) Pallor
      6) Increased adrenalin output
      7) Increased blood glucose
   b. Parasympathetic responses to deep and severe pain
      1) Nausea and vomiting
      2) Fainting
      3) Decreased blood pressure
      4) Decreased pulse rate
      5) Rapid and irregular breathing
   c. Intermittent pain imitates acute pain
      1) Persistent pain allows physiological adaptation, resulting in lack of the typical pain symptoms without pain relief (Huether & DeFriez, 2006). Therefore, the nurse may not have typical signs and symptoms to assess, making McCafferey's definition very important: "Pain is whatever the experiencing person says it is, existing whenever he (or she) says it does" (McCaffery, 1979, p. 11).
      2) Suspected nervous system alterations may cause "misinterpretation of nociceptive input" (Huether & DeFriez, 2006, p. 458). Physiological factors that may contribute to chronic pain include the following:
         a) Decreased level of endorphins
         b) Alterations in the neuronal sensitivity
         c) Spontaneous impulses arising from regenerating nerves
         d) Changes in dorsal root ganglia
         e) Reduced pain inhibition in the spinal cord (Huether & DeFriez, 2006)

2. Behavioral (voluntary responses)
   a. Moving away from painful stimuli
   b. Grimacing, moaning, crying
   c. Restlessness
   d. Protecting the area and refusing to move

3. Psychological responses
   a. Weeping and restlessness
   b. Withdrawal
   c. Stoicism
   d. Anxiety
   e. Depression
   f. Fear
   g. Anger
   h. Anorexia
   i. Fatigue
   j. Hopelessness
   k. Powerlessness

III. **Pain Theories**

A. Gate Control Theory (Melzack & Wall, 1965): This is the most widely accepted theory of pain, but it remains controversial.

1. The theory postulates a gating mechanism in the spinal cord.
2. Nociceptor impulses are transmitted from specific skin sites via large A-delta and small C-fibers to the spinal cord, terminating in the substantia gelatinosa.
3. The cells of the substantia gelatinosa function as the gate. The large, fast-conducting fibers close the gate, and the small, slower cells open the gate.
4. The closed gate results in a decrease in the stimulation of trigger cells, a decrease in pain impulses, and a decrease in pain perception. If persistent stimulation of the large fibers occurs, it results in adaptation.
5. The opposite occurs with an open gate. Stimulation of trigger fibers, transmission of impulses, and pain perception increase when the substantia gelatinosa opens the gate.

B. Neuromatrix Theory: This theory proposes an explanation for pain that does not correlate with actual injury or with a specific cause.

1. This theory suggests that the central nervous system contains a built-in body-self neuromatrix, which is capable of generating nerve impulses that represent the multidimensional somatosensory experience (Huether & DeFriez, 2006).
2. These nerve impulses, called the neurosignature patterns, may be activated by peripheral sensory stimulation or by brain processes to produce persistent pain.
3. Phantom limb pain is an example of this activation; there is no real body part to feel pain, yet the brain perceives that the limb is both present and painful (Huether & DeFriez, 2006; Melzack, 1999).

Table 15-1. Nursing Process Expanded with Cultural Negotiation Model

Nursing Process	Cultural Negotiation (Engebretson & Littleton, 2001)
Assess	Exchange of expert knowledge between client and provider
Diagnose • Chronic pain related to neuropathic pain • Anxiety related to potential lifestyle and job changes • Deficient knowledge related to individual pain control needs • Misinformation about use of pain medication	Analysis and interpretation of information about communication of pain symptoms and beliefs about pain medication
Plan (Nursing Outcomes Classification) • Pain control • Quality of life	Joint decision making • Increased family role in housework • Most effective way to inform coworkers about pain • Discussion of beliefs about pain medications
Implement (Nursing Intervention Classification) • Analgesic administration • Pain management • Medication management • Standardized templates often used to create the plan	Mutually derived plans • Desired outcomes for home setting • Desired outcomes for work setting • Desired outcomes for pain control
Evaluate	Outcome appraisal

4. The neuromatrix provides an explanation for chronic pain, which may exist with no discernible cause or stimulus (Huether & DeFriez, 2006; Melzack, 1999).

IV. **Middle-Range Nursing Theories Applicable to Pain Management**
   A. Theory of Symptom Management examples applied to pain experiences (Humphreys et al., 2008)
      1. Symptom experience. Example: Clients with chronic pain develop distrust because they feel they are not believed and are delegitimized.
      2. Symptom management strategies. Example: Clients may keep silent or withhold information from providers. They may not take medications because of misconceptions about taking pain medications.
      3. Symptom status outcomes. Example: Pain is not under control, and the client becomes angry and frustrated.
   B. Cultural Negotiation Model (Engebretson & Littleton, 2001). The cultural negotiation model is an interactive process that enhances the traditional nursing process (**Table 15-1**).

   The negotiation model views the client as providing expert knowledge of his or her own condition. McCafferey's definition of pain (1979) is a good fit for the model because the client expressing pain brings his or her own ideas about what pain is and beliefs about how it should be treated. Often, clients perceive barriers to taking pain medication related to misinformation or deeply held beliefs.

V. **Assessment and Management of Pain**
   The guidelines included in the grey section are excerpted from the Registered Nurses Association of Ontario's (RNAO's) *Assessment and Management of Pain* (2002, 2007) with permission.
   A. Assessment
      1. Screen all clients at risk for pain at least once a day, asking the client or caregiver about the presence of pain, ache, or discomfort. If the client is nonverbal, use behavioral indicators to identify the presence of pain.
      2. Self-report is the primary source of assessment for verbal, cognitively intact people. Family or caregiver reports of pain are included for children and adults unable to give self-report.
      3. A systematic, validated pain assessment tool is selected to assess the following basic parameters of pain:
         a. Location of pain
         b. Effect of pain on function and activities of daily living (ADLs; e.g., work, interference with usual activities)
         c. Level of pain at rest and during activity
         d. Medication use and adverse effects
         e. Provoking or precipitating factors
         f. Quality of pain (words the person uses to describe pain, such as *aching* or *throbbing*)
         g. Radiation of pain (Does the pain extend from the site?)
         h. Severity of pain (intensity, 0–10 scale), pain-related symptoms, and timing (occasional, intermittent, constant)

4. A standardized tool with established validity is used to assess the intensity of pain.
    a. Visual Analog Scale (VAS)
    b. Numeric Rating Scale (NRS)
    c. Verbal Scale
    d. Faces Scale
    e. Behavioral Scale
5. Pain assessment in clients who are unable to give self-report (noncommunicative) may include behavioral indicators using standardized measures and physiological indicators where appropriate.
6. The following parameters are part of a comprehensive pain assessment:
    a. Physical examination, relevant laboratory and diagnostic data
    b. Effect and understanding of current illness
    c. History of pain
    d. Meaning of pain and distress caused by the pain (current and previous)
    e. Coping responses to stress and pain
    f. Effects on ADLs
    g. Psychosocial and spiritual effects
    h. Psychological and social variables (anxiety, depression)
    i. Situational factors: culture, language, ethnic factors, economic effects of pain and treatment
    j. Person's preferences, expectations, beliefs, and myths about pain management methods
    k. Person's preferences and response to receiving information related to his or her condition and pain
7. Pain is reassessed on a regular basis according to the type and intensity of pain and the treatment plan.
    a. Pain intensity and function (impact on activities) are reassessed at each new report of pain and new procedure, when intensity increases, and when pain is not relieved by previously effective strategies.
    b. The effectiveness of an intervention (both pharmacological and nonpharmacological) is reassessed after the intervention has reached peak effect (e.g., 15–30 minutes after parenteral opioid therapy, 1 hour after immediate-release analgesic).
    c. Acute postoperative pain should be regularly assessed as determined by the operation and severity of pain, with each new report of pain or instance of unexpected pain, and after each analgesic, according to peak effect time.

    d. The following parameters should be monitored continuously in persistent pain situations:
        1) Current pain intensity, quality, and location
        2) Intensity of pain at its worst in past 24 hours, at rest, and on movement
        3) Extent of pain relief achieved, response (reduction on pain intensity scale)
        4) Barriers to implementing the treatment plan
        5) Effects of pain on ADLs, sleep, and mood
        6) Adverse effects of medications for pain treatment (e.g., nausea, constipation)
        7) Level of sedation
        8) Strategies used to relieve pain, both pharmacological and nonpharmacological
8. Unexpected intense pain, particularly if sudden or associated with altered vital signs such as hypotension, tachycardia, or fever, should be evaluated immediately.
9. Document on a standardized form that captures the person's pain experience specific to the population and setting of care. Documentation tools will include the following:
    a. Initial assessment, comprehensive assessment, and reassessment
    b. Monitoring tools that track efficacy of intervention (0–10 scale)
10. Document pain assessment regularly and routinely on standardized forms that are accessible to all clinicians involved in care.
11. Teach clients and families (as proxy recorders) to document pain assessment on the appropriate tools when care is provided. This will facilitate their contributions to the treatment plan and will promote continuity of effective pain management across all settings.
12. Validate with clients and caregivers that the findings of the pain assessment (healthcare provider's and client's or caregiver's) reflect the client's experience of pain.
13. Communicate to members of the interdisciplinary team pain assessment findings by describing parameters of pain obtained through the use of a structured assessment tool, the relief or lack of relief obtained from treatment methods and related adverse effects, the client's goals for pain treatment, and the effect of pain on the client.
14. Advocate on behalf of the client for changes to the treatment plan if pain is not being relieved. The nurse will engage in discussion with the interdisciplinary healthcare team regarding identified need for changes in the treatment plan. The

nurse supports his or her recommendations with appropriate evidence, providing a clear rationale for the needs for change, including the following:

   a. Intensity of pain using a validated scale
   b. Change in severity pain scores in past 24 hours
   c. Change in severity and quality of pain after administration of analgesics and length of time the analgesic is effective
   d. Amount of regular and breakthrough pain medication taken in past 24 hours
   e. Client's goals for pain relief
   f. Effect of unrelieved pain on the client
   g. Absence or presence of adverse effects or toxicity
   h. Suggestions for specific changes to the treatment plan that are supported by evidence

15. Provide instruction to the client and caregiver on the following:

   a. The use of a pain log or diary (provide a tool)
   b. Communicating unrelieved pain to the appropriate clinician and advocating on behalf of the client

16. Report situations of unrelieved pain as an ethical responsibility using all appropriate channels of communication in the organization, including client and caregiver documentation.

17. Refer clients whose pain is not relieved after following standard principles of pain management to the following:

   a. A clinical team member skilled in dealing with the particular type of pain
   b. A multidisciplinary team to address the complex emotional, psychosocial, spiritual, and concomitant medical factors involved

B. Management

1. Establishing a plan for pain management

   a. Establish a plan for management in collaboration with interdisciplinary team members that is consistent with client and family goals for pain relief, taking into consideration the following factors:

      1) Assessment findings
      2) Baseline characteristics of pain
      3) Physical, psychological, and sociocultural factors shaping the experience of pain
      4) Etiology
      5) Most effective pharmacological and nonpharmacological strategies
      6) Management interventions
      7) Current and future primary treatment plans

   b. Provide clients, families, and other caregivers with a written copy of the treatment plan to promote their decision making and active involvement in the management of pain. The plan will be adjusted according to the results of assessment and reassessment. Changes to the treatment plan will be documented and communicated to everyone involved in the implementation of the plan.

2. Pharmacological management of pain: Selecting appropriate analgesics

   a. Ensure the selection of analgesics is individualized to the client, taking into account

      1) The type of pain (acute, persistent, nociceptive, or neuropathic)
      2) Intensity of pain
      3) Potential for analgesic toxicity (age, renal impairment, peptic ulcer disease, thrombocytopenia)
      4) General condition of the client
      5) Concurrent medical conditions
      6) Response to prior or present medications
      7) Cost to the client and family
      8) Care setting

   b. Advocate for use of the most effective analgesic dosage schedules and least invasive pain management modalities.

      1) Tailor the route to the client's pain control needs and the care setting.
      2) The oral route is the preferred route for persistent pain and for acute pain as healing occurs.
      3) Intravenous administration is the parenteral route of choice after major surgery, usually via bolus and continuous infusion.
      4) Consider using a butterfly injection system to administer intermittent subcutaneous analgesics.
      5) Regional analgesia provides site-specific relief and is an effective pain-management modality in certain populations and should be considered.
      6) The intramuscular route is not recommended because it is painful and not reliable.
      7) Epidural patient-controlled analgesia (PCA) is more effective than intravenous PCA in certain surgical procedures and should be considered for eligible clients.

   c. Use a stepwise approach in making recommendations for the selection of analgesics for pharmacological management to match the intensity of pain unless contraindicated because of age, renal impairment, or other issues related to the drug.

1) Mild to moderate pain should be treated with acetaminophen or nonsteroidal anti-inflammatory drugs (NSAIDs) unless the client has a history of ulcers or a bleeding disorder.

2) Moderate to severe pain should be treated initially with an opioid analgesic, taking into consideration previous opioid use and adverse effects.

d. Recognize that a multimodal analgesic approach is most effective for pain treatment and includes the use of adjuvant medications as part of treatment for mild pain and for specific types of pain, unless contraindicated.

1) Adjuvant medications such as anticonvulsants, NSAIDs, and antidepressants are important adjuncts because they provide independent analgesia for specific types of pain, such as neuropathic pain.

2) Caution is needed in administering adjuvant medications to older adults, who may experience significant anticholinergic and sedative adverse effects.

e. Consider the following pharmacological principles in the use of opioids for the treatment of severe pain:

1) Mixed agonist-antagonists (e.g., pentazocine) are not administered with opioids because the combination may precipitate a withdrawal syndrome and increase pain.

2) Older adults generally receive greater peak and longer duration of action from analgesics than younger adults, so dosing should be initiated at lower dosages and increased more slowly (careful titration).

3) Special precautions are needed in the use of opioids for neonates and infants younger than the age of 6 months. Drug dosages, including those for local anesthetics, should be calculated carefully based on the current or most appropriate weight of the neonate. Initial dosages should not exceed maximum recommended amounts.

f. Recognize that meperidine is not recommended for the treatment of pain.

1) Meperidine is contraindicated for persistent pain because buildup of the toxic metabolite normeperidine can cause seizures and dysphoria. Meperidine toxicity is not reversible by naloxone.

2) Meperidine has limited use in acute pain because of a lack of drug efficacy and a buildup of toxic metabolites, which can occur within 72 hours.

g. Advocate for consultation with a pain management expert for complex pain situations, including the following:

1) Pain unresponsive to standard treatment

2) Multiple sources of pain

3) Mix of neuropathic and nociceptive pain

4) History of substance abuse

3. Pharmacological management of pain: Optimizing pain relief with opioids

a. Ensure the timing of analgesics is appropriate according to personal characteristics of the client, pharmacology (i.e., duration of action, peak effect, half life), and route of the drug.

b. Recognize that opioids should be administered on a regular time schedule according to the duration of action and depending on the expectation regarding the duration of severe pain.

1) If severe pain is expected for 48 hours postoperatively, routine administration may be needed for that period of time. Late in the postoperative course, analgesics may be effective given as needed.

2) In persistent cancer pain, opioids are administered on an around-the-clock basis, according to their duration of action.

3) Long-acting opioids are more appropriate when dosing needs are stable.

c. Use principles of dose titration specific to the type of pain to reach the analgesic dosage that relieves pain with minimal adverse effects, according to the following:

1) Cause of the pain

2) Client's response to therapy

3) Clinical condition

4) Concomitant drug use

5) Onset and peak effect

6) Duration of the analgesic effect

7) Age

8) Known pharmacokinetics and pharmacodynamics of the drugs administered. Dosages are usually increased every 24 hours for clients with persistent pain on immediate-release preparations and every 48 hours for clients on controlled-release

opioids. The exception to this is transdermal fentanyl, which can be adjusted every 3 days.

d. Promptly treat pain that occurs between regular doses of analgesic (breakthrough pain) using the following principles:

1) Breakthrough doses of analgesic in the postoperative situation depend on the routine dosage of analgesic, the client's respiratory rate, and the type of surgery and are usually administered as bolus medications through PCA pumps or the epidural route.

2) Breakthrough doses of analgesics should be administered as needed according to the peak effect of the drug (oral or rectal, hourly; subcutaneous, every 30 minutes; intravenous, every 10–15 minutes).

3) It is most effective to use the same opioid for breakthrough pain that is being given for around-the-clock dosing.

4) Clients with persistent pain should have

a) An immediate-release opioid available for pain (breakthrough pain) that occurs between the regular administration times of the around-the-clock medication.

b) Breakthrough doses of analgesic for continuous cancer pain should be calculated as 10%–15% of the total 24-hour dose of the routine around-the-clock analgesic.

c) Breakthrough analgesic dosages should be adjusted when the regular around-the-clock medication is increased.

d) Adjustment to the around-the-clock dosage is necessary if more than two or three doses of breakthrough analgesic are needed in a 24-hour period and pain is not controlled.

e. Use an equianalgesic table to ensure equivalency when switching analgesics. Recognize that the safest method when switching from one analgesic to another is to reduce the dosage of the new analgesic by 25%–50% in a stable pain situation.

f. Ensure that alternative routes of administration are prescribed when medications cannot be taken orally or if refractory nausea and vomiting occur, taking into consideration the most efficacious and least invasive route, individual preferences, care setting, cost, and resources.

1) Transdermal preparations for clients with persistent pain

2) Continuous subcutaneous opioid infusions for persistent cancer pain

g. Recognize the difference between drug addiction, tolerance, and dependency to prevent these from becoming barriers to optimal pain relief.

4. Monitoring for safety and efficacy: Monitor clients taking opioids, recognizing that opioids used for people not in pain, or in dosages larger than necessary to control the pain, or when they have not been titrated appropriately, can slow or stop breathing.

a. Monitor clients taking opioids for potential toxicity when the client exhibits the following:

1) Unacceptable adverse effects such as myoclonus, confusion, or delirium refractory to prophylactic treatment

2) In the presence of inadequate pain relief after appropriate dosage titration

b. Advocate for a change in the treatment plan, as needed.

c. Evaluate the efficacy of pain relief with analgesics at regular intervals and after a change in dosage, route, or timing of administration. Recommend changes in analgesics when inadequate pain relief is observed.

d. Refer to a pain specialist for clients who need increasing dosages of opioids that are ineffective in controlling pain. Evaluation should include assessment for residual pathology and other pain causes, such as neuropathic pain.

5. Anticipating and preventing common adverse effects of opioids

a. Anticipate and monitor clients taking opioids for common adverse effects such as nausea, vomiting, constipation, and drowsiness, and institute prophylactic treatment as appropriate.

b. Counsel clients that adverse effects to opioids can be controlled to ensure adherence with the medication regimen.

c. Recognize and treat all potential causes of adverse effects, taking into consideration medications that potentiate opioid adverse effects.

1) Sedation: Sedatives, tranquilizers, antiemetics

2) Postural hypotension: Antihypertensives, tricyclics
3) Confusion: Phenothiazines, tricyclics, antihistamines, and other anticholinergics

6. Anticipating and preventing common adverse effects of opioids: Nausea and vomiting
   a. Assess all clients taking opioids for the presence of nausea and vomiting, paying particular attention to the relationship of the symptom to the timing of analgesic administration. Ensure these clients are prescribed an antiemetic for use as needed, with routine administration if nausea or vomiting persists.
   b. Recognize that antiemetics have different mechanisms of action, and selection of the right antiemetic is based on this understanding and etiology of the symptom.
   c. Assess the effect of the antiemetic on a regular basis to determine relief of nausea or vomiting and advocate for further evaluation if the symptom persists despite adequate treatment.
   d. Consult with the prescribing clinician regarding switching to a different antiemetic if nausea or vomiting is determined to be related to the opioid and does not improve with adequate dosages of antiemetic.

7. Anticipating and preventing common adverse effects of opioids: Constipation
   a. Institute prophylactic measures for the treatment of constipation unless contraindicated and monitor constantly for this adverse effect.
      1) Laxatives should be prescribed and increased as needed to achieve the desired effect as a preventive measure for clients receiving a routine administration of opioids.
      2) Osmotic laxatives soften stool and promote peristalsis and may be an effective alternative for clients who find it difficult to manage an increasing volume of pills.
      3) Stimulant laxatives may be contraindicated if there is stool impaction. Enemas and suppositories may be needed to clear the impaction before oral stimulants are resumed.
      4) Bulk-forming agents should be avoided when bowel motility is compromised, for example, with opioids.
   b. Counsel clients on dietary adjustments that increase bowel peristalsis, recognizing personal circumstances (seriously ill clients may not tolerate such changes) and preferences.

   c. Urgently refer clients with refractory constipation accompanied by abdominal pain or vomiting to the appropriate clinician.
   d. Recognize that transitory sedation is common and counsel the client and caregiver that drowsiness is common upon initiation of opioid analgesics and with subsequent dosage increases.

8. Anticipating and preventing common adverse effects of opioids: Drowsiness and sedation. Notify the appropriate clinician of confusion or hallucinations to evaluate drowsiness that continues beyond 72 hours and to determine the underlying cause.

9. Anticipating and preventing procedural pain
   a. Anticipate pain that may occur during procedures (e.g., medical tests, dressing changes, chest tube removal, line insertion or removal).
      1) Combine pharmacologic (e.g., topical anesthetic) with nonpharmacologic options for prevention.
      2) Anticipate and prevent pain when performing procedures on infants to prevent sensitization for pain in the future.
   b. Recognize that analgesics and local anesthetics are the foundation for pharmacological management of painful procedures. Anxiolytics and sedatives are specifically used for the reduction of associated anxiety. If used alone, anxiolytics and sedatives blunt behavioral responses without relieving pain.
   c. Ensure that skilled supervision and appropriate monitoring procedures are instituted when moderate sedation is used.

10. Educating the client and family
    a. Provide the client and family with information about their pain and the measures used to treat it. Use an individualized approach, with particular attention focused on strategies for preventing and treating adverse effects, and address myths.
    b. Ensure that clients understand the importance of promptly reporting unrelieved pain, changes in their pain, new sources or types of pain, and adverse effects from analgesics.
    c. Clarify the differences between addiction, tolerance, and physical dependence to correct misbeliefs that can prevent optimal use of pharmacological methods for pain management.
       1) Addiction is a psychological dependence and is rare with clients taking opioids for persistent pain.

2) Clients using opioids on a long-term basis for pain control may be on the same dosage for years but may need upward adjustments with signs of tolerance. Tolerance is usually not a problem, and clients can be on the same dosage for years.

3) Clients who no longer need an opioid after long-term use need to reduce their dosage slowly over several weeks to prevent withdrawal symptoms because of physical dependence.

11. Maintaining effective documentation

a. Document all pharmacological interventions on a systematic pain record that clearly identifies the effect of analgesic on pain relief. Use this record to communicate with interdisciplinary colleagues regarding the titration of analgesic. The date, time, severity, location, and type of pain should all be documented.

b. Provide the client and family in the home setting with a simple strategy for documenting the effect of analgesics.

12. Managing pain nonpharmacologically

a. Combine pharmacological methods with nonpharmacological methods to achieve effective pain management.

1) Nonpharmacological treatment methods should not be substitutes for adequate pharmacological management.

2) Any potential contraindications to nonpharmacological methods should be considered before application.

3) Selection of nonpharmacological methods should be based on individual preference and may include strategies such as the following:

a) Superficial heat and cold
b) Massage
c) Relaxation
d) Imagery
e) Pressure or vibration
f) Music

b. Implement educational and psychosocial interventions that facilitate coping for the client and family early in the course of treatment.

c. Institute educational and psychoeducational interventions as part of the overall treatment plan.

d. Recognize that cognitive-behavioral strategies combined with other approaches, including multidisciplinary rehabilitation, can be helpful for treatment of persistent nonmalignant pain.

13. Assessing and managing pain in at-risk populations: The RNAO pain management guidelines are used as a starting point, but at-risk populations may have special problems not addressed in the general guidelines. This section provides more detailed information about at-risk populations rehabilitation nurses may encounter, including older adults, clients who are nonverbal, clients with dementia, and poststroke clients.

a. Older adults

1) Pain assessment is critical to creating a useful treatment plan. Pain assessment in older adults is often more challenging because of comorbidities, sensory and cognitive impairments, and misinformation about pain in aging. Establishing an institutionally appropriate procedure for evaluating pain and response to treatment, and then regular reassessment using the same methods, is key to effective management (Herr, 2011). The American Geriatrics Society Panel on Persistent Pain in Older Persons (2002) provides the following examples of common pain behaviors in cognitively impaired older adults:

a) Facial expressions (frowns, grimaces, closed eyes)

b) Vocalizations (sighing, groaning, grunting, calling out, asking for help)

c) Body movements (rigid, tense; guarding, fidgeting, pacing rocking; mobility changes)

d) Changes in interactions with others (aggressive, resisting care, disruptive, withdrawn)

e) Changes in activity patterns (refusing to eat, changing sleep patterns, suddenly stopping common routines)

f) Mental status changes (crying or tears, increased confusion, irritability)

2) Pain behavior tools useful in cognitively impaired older adults

a) The City of Hope website includes English-language tools available for assessing pain in nonverbal older adults (http://prc.coh.org/PAIN-NOA.htm).

b) Pain Assessment in Advanced Dementia (PAINAD) and Pain Assessment Checklist for Seniors with Limited Ability to Communicate (PACSLAC) are supported by consensus recommendations from expert groups for use in assessing pain in nonverbal residents in nursing homes (Herr, Bursch, Ersek, Miller, & Swafford, 2010).

3) Several factors may impede appropriate pain management in older adults.

a) Clients may fear addiction to or side effects of pain medications.

b) Clients may believe pain is the inevitable consequence of aging or that reporting pain may indicate something more serious is wrong (e.g., if the healthcare provider does not ask about the pain, the older client may perceive that it should not exist).

c) Clients may believe that if they admit to pain, family or caregivers will label them as "bad patients" (Hanks-Bell, Halvey, & Paice, 2004).

d) Healthcare providers may not manage an older adult's pain properly because of the inaccurate perception that older adults experience less pain.

e) Healthcare providers may believe that if the client does not report pain, he or she is not experiencing it.

f) Older adults' sensitivity to the side effects of pain medications, especially narcotics, may indicate that these medications should be avoided. Older adults experience diminishing renal and liver function, which affects metabolism of medications commonly used for pain and its sequelae, such as opiates, benzodiazepines, and anticholinergics.

g) Nurses may lack the ability to evaluate pain in people with cognitive impairment (Hanks-Bell et al., 2004).

b. Pain assessment in the nonverbal client

1) See Herr and colleagues (2006) for the American Society for Pain Management Nursing position statement and clinical practice recommendations.

2) Hierarchy of Pain Assessment Technique

a) Self-report remains the gold standard even in clients with severe cognitive impairment.

b) Search for potential causes by reviewing acute and chronic conditions and procedures that may affect the client.

c) Assess pain-related behaviors.

d) Include surrogate reporting by caregivers, family members, or anyone who knows the client well.

e) Attempt an analgesic trial to see if behavior changes.

c. Cancer pain

1) Cancer survival rates have increased, but treatments that allow longer survival may lead to chronic pain syndromes (Paice, 2011).

a) Chemotherapy-induced painful peripheral neuropathies: Rehabilitation is essential for maintaining and improving function, gait training, muscle strengthening, use of assistive devices, and fall risk assessment and intervention (Stubblefield et al., 2009).

b) Graft versus host disease: Multiple systems are affected, but treatment has not been well studied (Paice, 2011).

c) Radiation therapy: Chest pain, cystitis, enteritis, myelopathy, osteoporosis, pelvic fractures, pelvic nerve entrapment, plexopathies, and secondary malignancies may occur (Paice, 2011)

d) Hormonal therapies and arthralgias

i. Aromatase inhibitors are associated with significant joint pain.

ii. Treatments have not undergone trials (Paice, 2011).

2) Numerous barriers to cancer pain management remain. Some examples include fear of addiction, fear of becoming tolerant to the medication, the idea that pain is inevitable with cancer, the idea that medication will weaken the immune system, and the idea that good clients do not complain (Gunnarsdottir, Donovan, Serlin, Voge, & Ward, 2002).

3) The representational approach to client education (RidCancerPain) is one of the more fully developed educational interventions in cancer pain management (Donovan & Ward, 2001; Donovan et al., 2007). During this counseling intervention, the client is helped to develop an individualized cancer pain management plan.

VI. Cultural Diversity

A. Strategies for Culturally Appropriate Assessment and Management of Pain (Davidhizar & Giger, 2004, pp. 47–55).

1. Use assessment tools to assist with measuring pain.

2. Appreciate variations in affective response to pain.

3. Be sensitive to variations in communication styles.

4. Recognize that the communication of pain may not be acceptable within a culture.

5. Appreciate that the meaning of pain varies between cultures.

6. Use knowledge of biological variations.

7. Develop personal awareness of values and beliefs that may affect responses to pain.

B. The Clinically Relevant Continuum Model of Cultural Competence (Engebretson, Mahoney, & Carlson, 2008) provides a useful framework that links the cultural competency continuum (Cross, Bazron, Dennis, & Isaacs, 1989) and evidence-based practice (**Figure 15-2**). Examples of how the model can be used in client-centered pain care are provided here.

1. "Standardization" would equate to clinical practice guidelines, which provide current best practices based on the highest level of evidence available (such as the RNAO pain management guidelines).

2. "Outcomes focused" includes measures such as functioning, mood, and depression.

3. The evidence-based practice triangle includes client values and circumstances, provider expertise, and evidence. Provider expertise includes specific knowledge of client populations to help provide anticipatory guidance. For example, clients often do not take their pain medications because they do not want to associate themselves with the alleged type of person who takes pain medication or because of fear of addiction or loss of control. For the provider, this means some clients must be encouraged to take medication (Monsivais, 2011; Monsivais & McNeill, 2007).

4. Cultural subgroups are created by people who share a chronic illness. Among people with chronic pain, there are many shared pain-related behaviors. According to a review of the literature, somatizing, overdramatizing, withholding information from the provider, and leaving the healthcare system when they felt ignored were common pain-related behaviors (Monsivais & Engebretson, 2011). Knowledge of such behaviors becomes both research evidence and part of the provider's expertise in recognizing them.

Case Study

Mrs. K. is a 45-year-old office worker with a 10-year history of a pain who is the main wage earner in her family. Her husband is disabled and unemployed and she has two teenage children. Medication alleviated her pain for a brief period of time when it first started. She works frequently at a computer, and she states that the computer work makes it worse, especially at the elbow. She says she takes pain medicines only when she really needs them to get through work or so she can sleep. She admits to being afraid of addiction and the long-term medication side effects on her body.

When she comes home from work she takes care of some of the housework, although her husband does contribute to cleaning, shopping, and cooking on a regular basis. Mrs. K. says she has been putting in more hours at work, and that is when symptoms increase. Her coworkers are helpful when she asks for assistance lifting, but she is worried about asking for too much help, fearing such requests could jeopardize her job. She tries to work through her breaks because the agency is short of staff, but she realizes this habit may be increasing her pain levels.

Discussion Questions

- What assessment tools will you use to get a comprehensive pain assessment for Mrs. K?
- How will you use the results of your assessment to create a client-centered plan that meets best practices? (See Section IV, "Middle-Range Nursing Theories Applicable to Pain Management," for application to the Cultural Negotiation Model.)
- How would you evaluate the outcomes of pain-management strategies?

References

American Geriatrics Society Panel on Persistent Pain in Older Persons. (2002). The management of persistent pain in older persons. *Journal of the American Geriatrics Society, 50,* S204–S224.

American Pain Society. (2010). *Media resources: About the American Pain Society* [APS press room media backgrounder]. Retrieved August 8, 2011, from www.ampainsoc.org/press/backgrounder.htm.

Apfelbaum, J. L., Chen, C., Mehta, S. S., & Gan, T. J. (2003). Postoperative pain experience: Results from a national survey suggest postoperative pain continues to be undermanaged. *Anesthesia and Analgesia, 97,* 534–540.

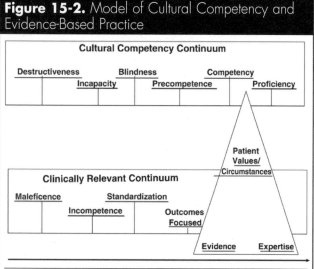

Figure 15-2. Model of Cultural Competency and Evidence-Based Practice

From "Cultural competency in the era of evidence-based practice," by J. Engebretson, J. Mahoney, & E. Carlson, 2008, *Journal of Professional Nursing, 24*(3), pp. 172–178. Copyright 2008 by the American Association of Colleges of Nursing. Reprinted with permission.

Association of Rehabilitation Nurses. (n.d.). *Role descriptions: The pain management rehabilitation nurse.* Retrieved June 14, 2011, from www.rehabnurse.org/pubs/role/painmgmt.html.

Boivie, J. (2006). Central pain. In S. McMahon & M. Koltzenburg (Eds.), *Wall and Melzack's textbook of pain* (5th ed., pp. 1057–1074). Philadelphia: Elsevier.

Bond, M. R. (2006). Psychiatric disorders and pain. In A. B. McMahon & M. Koltzenburg (Eds.), *Wall and Melzack's textbook of pain* (5th ed., pp. 259–266). Philadelphia: Elsevier.

Bradley, L. A., & McKendree-Smith, N. (2002). Central nervous system mechanisms of pain in fibromyalgia and other musculoskeletal disorders: Behavioral and psychologic treatment approaches. *Current Opinion in Rheumatology, 14*(1), 45–51.

Craig, K. D. (2006). Emotions and psychobiology. In S. McMahon & M. Koltzenburg (Eds.), *Wall and Melzack's textbook of pain* (5th ed., pp. 231–239). Philadelphia: Elsevier.

Cross, T., Bazron, B., Dennis, K., & Issacs, M. (1989). *Towards a culturally competent system of care: Vol. 1. Child and Adolescent Service System Program Technical Assistance Center.* Washington, DC: Georgetown University Child Development Center.

Davidhizar, R., & Giger, J. N. (2004). A review of the literature on care of clients in pain who are culturally diverse. *International Nursing Review, 51,* 47–55.

Donovan, H. S., & Ward, S. (2001). A representational approach to patient education. *Journal of Nursing Scholarship, 33*(3), 211–216.

Donovan, H. S., Ward, S. E., Song, M. K., Heidrich, S. M., Gunnarsdottir, S., & Phillips, C. M. (2007). An update on the representational approach to patient education. *Journal of Nursing Scholarship, 39*(3), 259–265.

Engebretson, J., & Littleton, L. (2001). Cultural negotiation: A constructivist-based model for nursing practice. *Nursing Outlook, 49*(5), 223–230.

Engebretson, J., Mahoney, J., & Carlson, E. (2008). Cultural competency in the era of evidence-based practice. *Journal of Professional Nursing, 24*(3), 172–178.

Gunnarsdottir, S., Donovan, H. S., Serlin, R. C., Voge, C., & Ward, S. (2002). Patient-related barriers to pain management: The Barriers Questionnaire II (BQ-II). *Pain, 99*(3), 385–396.

Hanks-Bell, M., Halvey, K., & Paice, J. A. (2004). Pain assessment and management in aging. *Online Journal of Issues in Nursing, 9*(3), 65–82.

Herr, K. (2011). Pain assessment strategies in older adults. *Journal of Pain, 12*(3, Suppl. 1), 53.

Herr, K., Bursch, H., Ersek, M., Miller, L., & Swafford, K. (2010). Use of pain-behavioral assessment tools in the nursing home: Expert consensus recommendations for practice. *Journal of Gerontological Nursing, 36,* 18–29.

Herr, K., Coyne, P. J., Key, T., Manworren, R., McCaffery, M., Merkel, S., et al. (2006). Pain assessment in the nonverbal patient: Position statement with clinical practice recommendations. *Pain Management Nursing, 7*(2), 44–52.

Huether, S. E., & DeFriez, C. B. (2006). Pain, temperature regulation, sleep, and sensory function. In K. L. McCance & S. E. Huether (Eds.), *Pathophysiology: The biologic basis for disease in adults and children* (5th ed., pp. 447–490). Philadelphia: Elsevier Mosby.

Humphreys, J., Lee, K.A., Carrieri-Kohlman, V., Puntillo, K., Faucett, J., Janson, S., et al. (2008). Theory of symptom management. In M. J. Smith & P. R. Liehr (Eds.), *Middle range theory for nursing* (2nd ed., pp. 145–158). New York: Springer.

Institute of Medicine. (2011). *Relieving pain in America: A blueprint for transforming prevention, care, education, and research.* Washington, DC: National Academies Press.

International Association for the Study of Pain. (2011a). *Mechanisms of acute pain* [Fact sheet]. Retrieved March 15, 2011, from www.iasp-pain.org/Content/NavigationMenu/GlobalYearAgainstPain/GlobalYearAgainstAcutePain/FactSheets/default.htm.

International Association for the Study of Pain. (2011b). "Resources" to "IASP Taxonomy" to "Pain Terms." Retrieved May 1, 2011, from www.iasp-pain.org.

Julius, D., & McKleskey, E. W. (2006). Cellular and molecular properties of primary afferent neurons. In A. B. McMahon & M. Koltzenburg (Eds.), *Wall and Melzack's textbook of pain* (5th ed., pp. 35–48). Philadelphia: Elsevier.

McCaffery, M. (1979). *Nursing management of the patient with pain* (2nd ed.). Philadelphia: J. B. Lippincott.

Melzack, R. (1999). From the gate to the neuromatrix. *Pain, Suppl. 6,* S121–S126.

Melzack, R., & Wall, P. D. (1965). Pain mechanisms: A new theory. *Science, 150*(699), 971–979.

Meyer, R. A., Ringkamp, M., Campbell, J. N., & Raja, S. N. (2006). Peripheral mechanisms of cutaneous nociception. In A. B. McMahon & M. Koltzenburg (Eds.), *Wall and Melzack's textbook of pain* (5th ed., pp. 3–34). Philadelphia: Elsevier.

Monsivais, D. (2011). Promoting culturally competent chronic pain management using the clinically relevant continuum model. *Nursing Clinics of North America, 46*(2), 163–169.

Monsivais, D., & Engebretson, J. (2011). Cultural cues: Review of qualitative evidence of patient-centered care in patients with nonmalignant chronic pain. *Rehabilitation Nursing, 36*(4), 166–171.

Monsivais D., & McNeill, J. (2007). Multicultural influences on pain medication attitudes and beliefs in patients with nonmalignant chronic pain syndromes. *Pain Management Nursing, 8*(2), 64–71.

Paice, J. A. (2011). Chronic treatment-related pain in cancer survivors. *Pain, 152*(Suppl.), 84–89.

Registered Nurses Association of Ontario. (2002). *Assessment and management of pain.* Toronto, ON. Canada: Author.

Registered Nurses Association of Ontario. (2007). *Assessment and management of pain: Supplement.* Toronto, ON, Canada: Author.

Scadding, J. W., & Koltzenburg, M. (2006). Painful peripheral neuropathies. In S. McMahon & M. Koltzenburg (Eds.), *Wall and Melzack's textbook of pain* (5th ed., 973–999). Philadelphia: Elsevier.

Stubblefield, M. D., Burstein, H. J., Burton, A. W., Custodio, C. M., Deng, G. E., Ho, M., et al. (2009). MCCM task force report: Management of neuropathy in cancer. *Journal of the National Comprehensive Cancer Network, 7*(Suppl. 5), S1–S26.

Taylor, C. R., Lillis, C., Lemone, P., & Lynn, P. (2006). *Fundamentals of nursing: The art and science of nursing care* (6th ed.). Philadelphia: Lippincott Williams & Wilkins.

Suggested Resources

The IASP Task Force site (www.iasp-pain.org/AM/Template.
cfm?Section=Home&Template=/CM/HTMLDisplay.
cfm&ContentID=3011) provides definitions and clear guidelines for desirable characteristics of different types of pain facilities, such as

- Pain treatment facilities
- Multidisciplinary pain centers
- Multidisciplinary pain clinics
- Pain clinics
- Modality-oriented clinics

Resources for clinicians are available through the American Pain
Society website at www.ampainsoc.org/resources/clinician1.
htm.

Resources for people in pain are available through the American
Pain Foundation website at www.painfoundation.org.

CHAPTER 16

Specific Disease Processes Requiring Rehabilitation Interventions

Joan K. McMahon, MSA BSN CRRN

Rehabilitation nurses play an important role in caring for people with a wide variety of chronic illnesses and disabilities. This chapter covers the following specific disease processes that warrant rehabilitation interventions:

- Diabetes mellitus
- Human immunodeficiency virsu (HIV) and acquired immune deficiency syndrome (AIDS)
- Cancer
- Obesity

Coping with a chronic condition is very stressful, and rehabilitation nurses are the ideal practitioners to provide and coordinate client and family education and interventions to help clients integrate illness into daily life and become as independent as possible. It is important for rehabilitation nurses to have current knowledge and the requisite skills to prevent complications and modify the effects of chronic conditions regardless of practice setting.

I. Diabetes Mellitus (DM)

A. Overview

1. Diabetes consists of a group of diseases marked by high fasting, preprandial, or postprandial blood glucose levels resulting from defects in insulin production, insulin action, or both. It requires a partnership between the client and health professional for medical care and self-management. Diabetes care is complex and entails addressing many issues beyond glycemic control. A large body of evidence supports a range of interventions to control the disease and lower the risk of complications.

2. Substantial progress has been made in the treatment and management of diabetes during the past 30 years, and many new options for treatment are being researched and marketed. New products and new medications are becoming available.

3. Involves an increasing number of people who need rehabilitation nursing care

   a. DM is a comorbid condition commonly treated in rehabilitation (along with stroke, heart disease, amputation, and renal failure) and is a major management issue.

   b. Optimal recovery from any of these conditions relies primarily on the control of acute and chronic hyperglycemia.

4. Rehabilitation nurses can make a difference in client outcomes by using current standards of care in diabetes management and effective client teaching to empower behavior changes (e.g., lifestyle changes in diet, exercise, stress management, and self-administration of medications).

B. Types (Centers for Disease Control and Prevention [CDC], 2007)

1. Type 1

   a. Previously known as insulin-dependent DM or juvenile-onset diabetes

   b. Affects 5%–10% of the total number of people with diabetes

   c. Results from B-cell destruction, usually leading to absolute insulin deficiency

2. Type 2

   a. Previously known as noninsulin-dependent DM or adult-onset diabetes

   b. Affects 90%–95% of the total number of people with diabetes

   c. Results from a progressive insulin secretory defect on the background of insulin resistance

3. Gestational diabetes (American Diabetes Association [ADA], 2010b; CDC, 2007b)

   a. Hyperglycemia that first appears in pregnancy, usually around 28 weeks or later, and usually resolves at birth

   b. An estimated 200,000 American women (approximately 5% of total pregnancies) are diagnosed with gestational diabetes annually.

   c. Five to ten percent of those with gestational diabetes are found to have diabetes, and 40%–60% may develop diabetes in the next 5–10 years.

4. Other types

   a. Result from specific genetic conditions (e.g., maturity-onset diabetes of youth), surgery, drugs, malnutrition, infections, and other illnesses

   b. Account for 1%–5% of all diagnosed cases (CDC, 2007b)

5. Prediabetes

   a. Affected 57 million adults in the United States in 2007 and raises the risk of developing type 2 diabetes, heart disease, and stroke

b. People with prediabetes have blood glucose levels higher than normal but not high enough to be classified as diabetes.

C. Epidemiology and Incidence (CDC, 2007b)

1. Diabetes is a global epidemic and burden, with more than 285 million people worldwide having diabetes in 2010, and this number is estimated to increase to 438 million by 2030 (Unwin, Whiting, Gan, Jacqmain, & Ghyoot, 2009).

2. In the United States 23.6 million people (7.8% of the population) have diabetes: 17.9 million with diagnosed diabetes and 5.7 million with undiagnosed diabetes.

3. The CDC predicts the prevalence of diabetes in the United States will double by 2050 and affect more than 48 million people (or 12% of the population).

4. Ethnic minorities (Hispanic and Latino Americans, American Indians, some Asian Americans, and Native Hawaiians) and older adults are expected to be disproportionately affected by the increase, with the number of Hispanics with diabetes predicted to rise almost sixfold.

5. People 65 years or older account for almost 40% of the population with diabetes.

6. Diabetes was the seventh most common cause of death in the United States in 2006 and is the leading cause of adult blindness, chronic renal failure, and nontraumatic lower-extremity amputations.

7. People with diabetes have a risk of death about twice that of people without diabetes of the same age.

8. People with diabetes have two to four times the risk of atherosclerosis and are three times more likely to have a heart attack or stroke than those who do not have diabetes.

9. The direct and indirect costs of diabetes are staggering, totaling more than $174 billion a year in 2007. However, the full burden of diabetes is hard to measure because death records often fail to reflect the role of diabetes, and the costs related to undiagnosed diabetes are unknown.

10. Diabetes is the fourth most common comorbid condition among hospital discharges.

11. Martz and colleagues (2006) reported a 31% rate of known diabetes in hospitalized people with stroke and an additional 16% of people with unrecognized diabetes and hospital-related hyperglycemia.

D. Etiology (ADA, 2010b)

1. Type 1 diabetes is an autoimmune disorder involving B-cell destruction by islet cell antibodies leading to absolute insulin deficiency.

2. Type 2 diabetes results from a progressive defect in the secretion of insulin on the background of insulin resistance.

3. Gestational diabetes is a form of glucose intolerance diagnosed during pregnancy that, if uncontrolled, puts both mother and baby at risk for complications during the pregnancy; the mother has a 20%–50% chance of developing diabetes in the next 5–10 years.

4. Other types of diabetes result from specific genetic defects in B-cell function, genetic defects in insulin action, diseases of the exocrine pancreas (e.g., cystic fibrosis), and drug- or chemical-induced diabetes (e.g., in the treatment of AIDS or after organ transplantation).

5. Prediabetes (CDC, 2007b), now classified as Categories of Increased Risk (ADA, 2010b)

   a. Prediabetes is an elevated risk of developing diabetes, as indicated by an impaired fasting glucose (IFG), impaired glucose tolerance (IGT), or higher than average hemoglobin A1c (HbA1c).

   b. IFG is a condition in which the fasting blood sugar level is elevated (100–125 mg/dL) after an overnight fast but is not high enough to be classified as diabetes.

   c. IGT is a condition in which the blood sugar level is elevated (140–199 mg/dL) after a 2-hour oral glucose tolerance test but is not high enough to be classified as diabetes.

   d. An HbA1c between 5.7 and 6.4 is at the borderline of diagnosis but not high enough to be classified as diabetes.

   e. Progression to diabetes among those at elevated risk is not inevitable because weight loss and increased physical activity may prevent or delay diabetes and may return blood glucose levels to normal.

   f. People in this category are already at elevated risk for other adverse health outcomes such as heart disease and stroke.

   g. The CDC (2007) reported that at least 57 million American adults had prediabetes in 2007. The number has undoubtedly increased since then.

E. Risk Factors for Diabetes

1. Type 1
   a. Family history of diabetes
   b. Age: Usually associated with children and young adults, although disease onset can occur at any age
   c. Environmental factors

2. Type 2

a. Obesity: Body fat of more than 25% for men and more than 30% for women
b. Physical inactivity
c. Environmental factors
d. Family history of diabetes or history of gestational diabetes
e. Race or ethnicity: African Americans, Hispanic and Latino Americans, American Indians, and some Asian Americans and Native Hawaiians or other Pacific Islanders are at particularly high risk for type 2 diabetes and its complications.
f. Age: Usually associated with older adults, but type 2 diabetes in children and adolescents is being diagnosed more frequently, particularly in the non-White populations listed earlier.
g. Previous IGT or IFG
h. Polycystic ovary disease (in women)
i. Hypertension (≥140/90 or on therapy for hypertension)
j. HDL cholesterol level <35 mg/dL or triglyceride level >250
k. History of cardiovascular disease

F. Pathophysiology
1. Impaired release of insulin from the pancreas
   a. Normal
      1) Phase 1: Stored insulin from beta cells is released within the first 5 minutes after glucose ingestion.
      2) Phase 2: More insulin is released and newly synthesized by beta cells.
   b. In diabetes
      1) Type 1: Endogenous insulin release is deficient.
      2) Type 2: Endogenous insulin release may be normal, inefficient, or deficient.
2. Insulin resistance (need for the beta cells of the pancreas to make more insulin to accommodate, or secondary hyperinsulinemia)
   a. The condition in which normal amounts of insulin are inadequate to produce a normal insulin response from fat, muscle, and liver cells
   b. Insulin resistance in fat cells results in hydrolysis of stored triglycerides, which elevates free fatty acids in the blood plasma.
   c. Insulin resistance in muscle reduces glucose uptake, whereas insulin resistance in liver reduces glucose storage, with both effects elevating blood glucose.
   d. High plasma levels of insulin and glucose caused by insulin resistance often lead to the metabolic syndrome and type 2 diabetes.
   e. Leads to insulin deficiency as the pancreas

works harder to meet the increasing need to overcome the resistance
3. Insulin deficiency
   a. Primary problem in type 1 diabetes
   b. Common in thin people with type 2 diabetes
   c. Increases in type 2 diabetes with longevity of the disease
4. Clinical manifestations (**Table 16-1**)

G. Diagnostic Criteria (ADA, 2010b; **Table 16-2**): Diagnosis for type 1 or type 2 is confirmed by one of the following tests, plus symptoms of diabetes (e.g., polyuria, polydipsia, polyphagia, unexplained weight loss, blurry vision, slow healing, weight loss, numbness or tingling in the hands and feet). The diagnosis of diabetes has been based on glucose levels for many years. In 2010 an international expert committee recommended the use of the HbA1c test to diagnose diabetes with a threshold of ≥6.5%, and the ADA confirmed that decision.
1. HbA1c (glycosylated hemoglobin test, also called the A1c test)
   a. Measurement of average glycemic levels on a time scale of 6–9 weeks, which reflects the lifespan of red blood cells (Leahy, Clark, & Cefalu, 2000)
   b. Use of point-of-care testing for HbA1c (A1c) allows timely therapy decisions.
   c. The A1c goal for people in general is less than 7% (ADA, 2010b).
   d. The A1c goal for the individual client is an A1c as close to normal (less than 6%) as possible without significant hypoglycemia (ADA, 2010b).
   e. Two studies, the Diabetes Control and Complications Trial and the United Kingdom Prospective Diabetes Study, found that lowering HbA1c levels dramatically reduces the risks of complications in people with type 1 and 2 diabetes (Genuth, 2006).
2. Blood glucose testing
   a. Casual nonfasting plasma glucose (any time of day without consideration of last meal) at least 200 mg/dL
   b. Fasting plasma glucose (no food for at least 8 hours) higher than 126 mg/dL
   c. Two-hour oral glucose tolerance test, 75-g glucose load test at least 200 mg/dL (not routinely used because of inconvenience and cost)

H. Management Options (ADA, 2010b)
1. Glycemic control
   a. Two primary techniques
      1) Client self-monitoring of blood glucose

Table 16-1. Symptomatic Manifestations of Diabetes Mellitus

Primary Symptoms	Secondary Symptoms	Tertiary Symptoms
Poor wound healing	Infection, chronic ulceration, limb amputation	Dysfunctional denial
Skin and feet	Dryness and cracking, callus formation, ulceration, deformities (e.g., Charcot's foot)	Dysfunctional grief
		Body image crisis
		Social isolation
Peripheral neuropathy (e.g., numbness, tingling, pain, decreased sensation in extremities)	Cold intolerance, rest and sleep disturbance, inadequate hand and finger movement (e.g., carpal tunnel syndrome)	Ineffective coping with anxiety, reactive depression, anger
		Marital conflict or divorce
Gastroparesis (e.g., bowel, bladder, sexual dysfunction)	Constipation, urinary retention, urinary tract infections, gastroparesis, vaginal dryness, decreased libido and orgasmic ability	Loss of job, financial stability, self-esteem, and self-worth
		Loss of ability to provide adequate self-care, causing loss of independence and control over life, living situation, location (i.e., often needing nursing home placement if unable to do self-insulin management)
Blurred vision, cataracts, blindness, retinopathy	Errors with insulin drawing and mixing, declining ability to visually inspect skin and feet	Falls, accidents
Hypoglycemia	Mild symptoms (sweating, trembling, impaired concentration, dizziness), severe symptoms (mental confusion, lethargy, unconsciousness)	End-stage renal disease
		Microvascular disease
		Macrovascular disease
Hyperglycemia	Specific symptoms (polyuria, polydipsia, blurred vision, polyphagia, weight loss), nonspecific symptoms (weakness, malaise, lethargy, headaches), gastrointestinal symptoms (nausea, vomiting, abdominal pain), respiratory symptoms (Kussmaul's, ketonuria, metabolic acidosis, hyperventilation, coma)	
Weight changes (i.e., more or less than ideal body weight)	Obesity (body fat more than 25% in men and 30% in women), central adipose tissue accumulation, inadequate nutrition	
Chronic systemic dysfunction	Orthostatic hypertension, cardiac denervation, hypoglycemia unaware, proteinuria	

Table 16-2. Criteria for the Diagnosis of Diabetes

1. A1c ≥6.5%. The test should be performed in a laboratory using a method that is NGSP certified and standardized to the DCCT assay.*

or

2. FPG ≥126 mg/dL (7.0 mmol/L). Fasting is defined as no caloric intake for at least 8 h.*

or

3. 2-h plasma glucose ≥200 mg/dL (11.1 mmol/L) during an OGTT. The test should be performed as described by the World Health Organization, using a glucose load containing the equivalent of 75 g anhydrous glucose dissolved in water.*

or

4. In a patient with classic symptoms of hyperglycemia or hyperglycemic crisis, a random plasma glucose ≥200 mg/dL (11.1 mmol/L).

*In the absence of unequivocal hyperglycemia, criteria 1–3 should be confirmed by repeat testing.
From "Diagnosis and classification of diabetes mellitus," by American Diabetes Association, 2010, *Diabetes Care, 33*(Suppl. 1), S62–S69. Copyright 2010 by the American Diabetes Association. Reprinted with permission.

2) Interstitial glucose and A1c
  b. Glucose monitoring
  c. A1c
  d. Glycemic goals in adults
2. Medical nutritional therapy (ADA, 2010b)
  a. Focus on serving size and total carbohydrates.
  b. Shift to individualized meal plans based on the client's needs and preferences.
  c. Have a registered dietitian individualize meal plans with specific amounts of carbohydrates, fats, and protein according to height, weight, eating habits, food preferences, lipid profile, blood protein, and other medical conditions (e.g., end-stage renal disease).
  d. Emphasize that both the amount (grams) of carbohydrate and the type of carbohydrate in a food influence blood glucose level.
  e. Monitoring total grams of carbohydrate, whether by use of exchanges or carbohydrate counting, remains a key strategy in achieving glycemic control.
  f. The use of the glycemic index or glycemic load may provide an additional benefit over that observed when total carbohydrate is considered alone.
  g. Low-carbohydrate (restricting total carbohydrate to less than 130 g/day) and low-fat, calorie-restricted diets may be helpful for a limited amount of time (up to 1 year).
  h. To reduce the risk of neuropathy, protein intake should be limited to the recommended dietary allowance (0.8 g/kg) in those with any degree of chronic kidney disease.
  i. Saturated fat intake should be less than 7% of total calories.
  j. The intake of trans fat should be minimized.
  k. Weight loss is recommended for all overweight (body mass index [BMI] 25.0–29.9 kg/m^2) or obese (BMI greater than 30.0 kg/m^2) adults who have or are at risk for developing type 2 diabetes.
  l. The primary approach for achieving weight loss is therapeutic lifestyle change that includes regular physical activity (150 minutes per week) and a diet low in fat and calories for a moderate weight loss (7% of body weight).
  m. Nonnutritive sweeteners and sugar alcohols are safe when consumed within the acceptable daily intake levels established by the U.S. Food and Drug Administration (FDA).
  n. Alcohol use should be limited to a moderate amount (one drink per day or less for adult women and two or fewer drinks per day for adult men); one drink is defined as 12 ounces of beer, 5 ounces of wine, or 1.5 ounces of distilled spirits.
  o. Routine supplementation with antioxidants, such as vitamins E and C and beta-carotene, is not advised because of lack of evidence of efficacy and concern over long-term safety.
  p. The benefit of chromium supplementation in people with diabetes or obesity has not been conclusively demonstrated and is not recommended.
  q. Individualized meal planning should include optimization of food choices to meet recommended dietary allowances for all micronutrients.
3. Physical activity
  a. Initial physical activity recommendations should be modest and based on the client's willingness and ability, gradually increasing the duration and frequency to 30–45 minutes of moderate aerobic activity 3–5 days per week. The goal is at least 150 minutes/week of moderate-intensity aerobic physical activity (50%–70% maximum heart rate).
  b. In the absence of contraindications, people with Type 2 diabetes should be encouraged to perform resistance training three times per week.
  c. Activity levels of at least 1 hour a day of moderate (e.g., walking) or 30 minutes a day of vigorous (e.g., jogging) activity may be needed to achieve successful long-term weight loss.
  d. Exercise options and strategies for self-directed exercise can be identified by a physical therapist.
  e. Benefits, effects, risks, and precautions vary depending on
    1) Age and type of diabetes
    2) Physical conditioning and presence of other chronic diseases
    3) Presence of ketonuria
  f. Providers should assess clients for comorbidities that might predispose clients to injury (e.g., hypertension, diabetic neuropathy, unstable proliferative retinopathy).
4. Bariatric surgery
  a. Should be considered for adults with a BMI greater than 35 kg/m^2 and type 2 diabetes, especially if the client is unable to control diabetes with lifestyle and pharmacologic therapy. (There is not enough evidence to

recommend surgery in clients with a BMI less than 35.)

   b. People who have had bariatric surgery will need lifelong lifestyle support and medical monitoring.

5. Medication therapy (Chitre & Burke, 2006; Diabetes Mall, 2010)

   a. Oral agents

     1) Classifications of oral antidiabetic agents include the following:

       a) Sulfonylureas stimulate the pancreas to make more insulin. The second- and third-generation agents are the best (tolazamide, glyburide, glipizide, glimepiride).

       b) Biguanides shut off the liver's excess glucose production (metformin).

       c) Meglitinides or nonsulfonylurea secretagogues stimulate the pancreas to make more insulin (repaglinide, nateglinide).

       d) Alpha-glucosidase inhibitors slow absorption of carbohydrates in the intestine (acarbose, miglitol).

       e) Thiazolidinediones increase the body's sensitivity to insulin (pioglitazone, rosiglitazone).

       f) Dipeptidyl peptidase-4 inhibitors (e.g., sitagliptin) slow the inactivation of incretin hormones and improve pancreatic beta cell insulin synthesis and release, lower pancreatic alpha cell glucagon secretion, and reduce hepatic glucose production.

     2) Each class of drugs differs in its modes and sites of action, advantages, and disadvantages, and the choice of agent for each person should be made with consideration of the person's overall health status.

     3) Medication regimens can be simple or complex, with options for monotherapy or polytherapy.

     4) Complexity of the regimen is increased by addition of insulin therapy to oral therapy (e.g., bedtime insulin and daytime orals) when oral therapy alone is no longer effective.

     5) Evidence supports the combination of biguanides with insulin to improve weight management and glycemic control and reduce congestive heart disease risk.

   b. Injectable agents other than insulin (Odegard, Setter, & Iltz, 2006)

     1) Exenatide (Amylin Pharmaceuticals, Inc., Byetta, 2010), an incretin mimetic for the treatment of type 2 DM in people experiencing inadequate glycemic control with oral DM medications, is not approved to be used with insulin. It reduces fasting and postprandial glucose concentrations though glucose-dependent insulin secretion, restores first-phase insulin response, regulates glucagon secretion, delays gastric emptying, reduces appetite, and helps to lower weight (McKennon & Campbell, 2007; Odegard et al., 2006).

     2) Pramlintide, a synthetic analog of the hormone amylin found to be deficient in type 1 DM, is used as an adjunct therapy with mealtime insulin, slows gastric emptying, curbs appetite, suppresses postprandial plasma glucagon and hepatic glucose output, and helps mediate satiety centrally, resulting in decreased caloric intake and promoting weight loss; approved for people with type 1 DM and type 2 DM taking insulin. It should not be put into the same syringe as insulin (Odegard et al., 2006).

   c. Insulin types usually address basal insulin (e.g., fasting) and bolus (e.g., preprandial glucose level and postprandial excursion; LaSalle, 2006; **Table 16-3**)

   d. Insulin regimens are numerous, ranging from simple to complex, and will challenge the rehabilitation nurse; the following is limited to the basic regimens because the ideal is an individualized program suited to the person's needs, lifestyle, and resources (Diabetes Health, 2006).

   e. Combination regimens

     1) Daily routine doses of long-lasting insulin (basal; e.g., neutral protamine Hagedorn [NPH], glargine, or detemir) may be combined with a secretagogue with or without additional oral sensitizer.

     2) Premixtures (e.g., NPH 50/regular 50, NPH 70/regular 30, Humulin R 70/30 or Novolin R 70/30, NPH 75/lispro 25, Humalog mix 75/25, NPH 70/aspart 30, Novolog mix 70/30) twice daily with or without oral sensitizers are normally used for convenience and to improve compliance.

   f. Intensive conventional therapy (LaSalle, 2006)

     1) Multiple daily injections of 0.2–0.6 initial units per kilogram with or without oral sensitizers, 50% bolus (rapid-acting

Table 16-3. Overview of Insulin Types and Characteristics

Type of Insulin	Brand Name/Generic Name	Onset	Peak	Duration
Rapid acting	NovoLog/aspart	15 min	30–90 min	3–5 hr
	Apidra/glulisine	15 min	30–90 min	3–5 hr
	Humalog/lispro	15 min	30–90 min	3–5 hr
Short acting	Humulin/regular	30–60 min	2–4 hr	5–8 hr
	Novolin/regular	30–60 min	2–4 hr	5–8 hr
Intermediate acting	Humulin/NPH	1–3 hr	8 hr	12–16 hr
	Novolin	1–3 hr	8 hr	12–16 hr
Long acting	Levemir/detemir	1 hr	None	20–26 hr
	Lantus/glargine	1 hr	None	20–26 hr
Premixed neutral protamine Hagedorn (NPH)	Humulin 70/30 70% NPH and 30% regular	30–60 min	Varies	10–16 hr
	Novolin 70/30 70% NPH and 30% regular	30–60 min	Varies	10–16 hr
	Humulin 50/50 50% NPH and 50% regular	30–60 min	Varies	10–16 hr
Premixed insulin lispro protamine suspension and rapid-acting lispro	Humalog mix 50/50 50% insulin lispro protamine and 50% insulin lispro	10–15 min	Varies	10–16 hr
Premixed insulin aspart protamine suspension and rapid-acting insulin aspart	Novolog mix 70/30 70% insulin aspart protamine and 30% insulin aspart	5–15 min	Varies	10–16 hr

insulin) at meals, and 50% basal insulin (i.e., NPH, glargine, or detemir) once or twice a day

2) Daily routine doses of basal insulin (i.e., NPH, glargine, or detemir) once or twice daily with fast-acting insulin boluses using carbohydrate/insulin ratios calculated according to future carbohydrate consumption

3) Provides flexibility (e.g., a meal can be delayed and less consumed because the bolus amount is determined by the amount of food eaten rather than having to take the right amount of food at the right time to match the action of the traditional insulin, such as NPH)

g. Correction dose (previously called sliding scale): Bolus dose of rapid- or fast-acting insulin calculated on actual blood glucose level

h. Injection therapy (LaSalle, 2006)
1) Absorption rates differ between sites and types of insulins: The abdomen is the fastest, followed by the arms, thighs, and buttocks. Absorption is less variable with analog insulins.

2) Lipohypertrophy usually slows absorption; this is less of a problem with analog insulins.

3) Exercise increases the rate of absorption by providing increased blood flow to the injection site; this is less of a problem with analog insulins.

i. Inhaled insulin therapy (Lifeclinic, 2010)
1) Inhaled powder form of recombinant human insulin that is administered into the mouth through an inhaler device

2) Rapid-acting insulin only, causing the continued need for injections of a basal (long-acting) insulin

3) Exubera, the first inhaled insulin, was FDA approved in 2006 but then removed from the market in 2007 because of disappointing sales.

4) Recent research involving a new inhaled insulin (Afreszza) shows promise, but it is not yet FDA approved (Bailey & Barnett, 2010).

5) Trials with inhaled insulin demonstrated few episodes of hypoglycemia in those using the inhaler.

j. Insulin pump therapy (Lifeclinic, 2010)
   1) Insulin pumps are devices used for administering insulin, consisting of controls, a processing module, batteries, an insulin reservoir, and a catheter to carry the insulin into the subcutaneous tissue.
   2) Insulin pumps make it possible to deliver continuous small amounts of fast-acting (basal) and a mealtime bolus dose, providing tighter control over blood sugar and reducing the chance of long-term complications (i.e., blindness, amputation, renal disease).
   3) Costs can run into the thousands of dollars for initial setup and continued maintenance, including the costs of insulin, batteries, and infusion catheter sets.
   4) Insurance and Medicare may pay up to 80% of the costs of pump therapy.
   5) Numbers of insulin pump users continue to rise, and pump features continue to advance.
   6) People using their pumps often rebel against forced removal.
   7) Rehabilitation nurses must be prepared to deal with the client who continues to use the pump during an inpatient stay.
   8) Pump use may be helpful in achieving glycemic control by matching the typical insulin pattern of a person without diabetes.
   9) Transitioning on and off a pump can entail a complex series of insulin management plans and orders from the physician and coordination of pharmacy and nursing staff.
   10) A comprehensive plan should be in place for the safe use of an insulin pump using the Joint Commission standards regarding a facility's responsibility for the cleanliness and maintenance of any home medical equipment and the competency of staff responsible for overseeing the equipment.
   11) Implantable insulin pumps are in the development stage. When surgically implanted, they will be able to deliver a basal dose continuously and a bolus dose as needed.
I. Hospital Inpatient Diabetes and Glycemic Control (ADA, 2010b)
   1. Poorly controlled blood glucose levels are associated with increased morbidity and mortality and higher healthcare costs caused by increased length of stay, complications, and readmissions.
   2. Both undertreatment and overtreatment of hyperglycemia are safety issues in hospitalized clients and are considered errors of omission because hyperglycemia can negatviely affect the treatment of illness and diabetes.
   3. All people with diabetes admitted to the hospital should have an order for blood glucose monitoring, with results available to the healthcare team.
   4. Critically ill clients: Insulin therapy to treat persistent hyperglycemia should start at a threshold no greater than 180 mg/dL. Once insulin therapy is started, a glucose range of 140–180 mg/dL should be maintained. (An intravenous insulin protocol has demonstrated efficacy and safety in achieving this range without increasing risk for hypoglycemia).
   5. New glucose guidelines for hospitalized clients established by the American Association of Clinical Endocrinologists and the ADA: 80–110 mg/dL for intensive care units and less than 140 mg/dL fasting and less than 180 random blood sugar on other units with or without a diagnosis of diabetes; modify for unstable cardiac disease, hypoglycemia unawareness, or recurrent hypoglycemia (ADA, 2010b).
   6. ADA targets for most adults with diabetes: Premeal 70–130 mg/dL and postmeal (1–2 hours after eating) less than 180 mg/dL
   7. Lower or higher targets may be recommended for certain people who are at lower or higher risk for hypoglycemia, especially clients going to physical therapy as part of their rehabilitation program.
   8. Protocols or algorithms and order sets guide the management of hyperglycemia and hypoglycemia.
J. Acute Problems Associated with Diabetes
   1. Hypoglycemia
      a. Eating too little; too much insulin or oral diabetes medication; excessive exercise; alcohol; certain cancers; critical illnesses such as kidney, liver, or heart failure; hormonal deficiencies
      b. Symptoms
         1) Mild: Sweating, trembling, difficulty concentrating, lightheadedness, blurred vision
         2) Specific: Inability to self-treat, mental confusion, lethargy, unconsciousness
         3) Hypoglycemia unawareness may be present due to autonomic neuropathy, with loss of warning neuroglycopenic symptoms resulting from deficient sympathetic neuronal (norepinephrine) and adrenomedullary (epinephrine) responses to falling glucose levels.

4) Some medications may mask symptoms (e.g., beta blockers).
c. Treatment options (ADA, 2010b)
   1) Begin with administration of 15–20 g (5–10 g for children) of fast-acting carbohydrate (e.g., three glucose tablets or one small tube of glucose gel, 2 tablespoons raisins, 8 ounces of lowfat milk, half a can of regular soda).
   2) Retest the blood glucose level after 15 minutes.
   3) Give an additional 15 g carbohydrate if blood glucose is still less than 70 mg/dL.
   4) Consider preference, allergies, and food intolerance when making treatment choices (e.g., glucose gel for clients with dysphagia).
   5) People taking glucosidase inhibitors (acarbose or nateglinide) must use glucose (dextrose) tablets or, if unavailable, milk or honey (Meriter Health Services, 2010).
   6) Be careful not to overtreat and cause rebound hyperglycemia.
   7) Using a food with added fat (e.g., chocolate bar) is not recommended because fat may slow down the body's absorption of the carbohydrate.
   8) The use of protein to keep blood glucose up after a low is not necessary and may add calories and promote weight gain.
   9) Follow the treatment with a snack or scheduled meal if it is 2 hours before the next meal.
   10) Severe hypoglycemia may be treated with glucagon injection or intravenous glucose.
   11) Prevention of low blood glucose is the best treatment (e.g., not skipping meals, eating six small meals a day instead of three large ones, taking the fast-acting bolus insulin after a meal instead of before, reducing the amount of insulin or oral diabetes medications before exercise, frequent monitoring of blood glucose before and after exercise, and taking a snack if indicated before exercising; Feigenbaum, 2006).

2. Hyperglycemia
a. Causes: Eating too much food; not enough insulin or oral diabetes medication; physical stress such as a cold, infection, or the flu; emotional stress such as family conflict; problems with the insulin; or other medications (e.g., corticosteroids, phenytoin)

b. Symptoms
   1) Specific: Polyuria, polydipsia, blurred vision, dysphagia, weight loss
   2) Nonspecific: Weakness, malaise, lethargy, headache
   3) Gastrointestinal: Nausea, vomiting, abdominal pain
   4) Respiratory: Kussmaul's breathing, metabolic acidosis, hyperventilation
c. Treatment: Insulin and fluids
d. Prevention of hyperglycemia: Eating the correct number and portion sizes of carbohydrates established per individual needs, taking medications on time, limiting snacking, treating infections and illness, controlling stress, increasing exercise, limiting fats

3. Other complications associated with diabetes
a. Cardiovascular disease is the major cause of mortality for people with diabetes (ADA, 2010b).
b. Diabetes is an independent risk factor for macrovascular disease and its common coexisting conditions (e.g., hypertension and dyslipidemia).
c. Consider aspirin therapy as a primary prevention strategy in people with diabetes at elevated cardiovascular risk (ADA, 2010b).
d. Other complications include Charcot's foot, amputations, neuropathy, gastroparesis, depression, retinopathy, nephropathy, and autonomic nerve disease, which affects nerves that control heartbeat, digestion, and other automatic functions.

4. Self-blood glucose testing and diabetes medication administration
a. The rehabilitation nurse often is responsible for initiating self-monitoring of blood glucose and self-medication administration (e.g., self-administering of insulin) for newly diagnosed clients and ensuring that those with previous skills are competent, knowledgeable, and safe.
b. Facilities that follow Joint Commission standards and allow clients to use their own glucose monitors and provide new monitors for education purposes should review the home medical equipment standards from the Joint Commission.
c. The rehabilitation nurse may find it helpful to refer the client learning diabetes self-management skills to a certified diabetes educator on staff or in the community.
d. Adding the specialty practice of diabetes education is a possibility for every rehabilitation nurse; information about this

additional specialty can be obtained from the American Association of Diabetes Educators (www.diabeteseducator.org).

e. Facilities need written policies and procedures and medical staff approval to ensure the safety and legality of self-monitoring and self-medication administration programs.

K. Nursing Process

1. Assessment

a. Gather objective data: Determine the type of diabetes and classification. People with hyperglycemia can be classified into one of three categories: previously diagnosed DM, unrecognized DM, or hyperglycemia related to hospitalization (ADA, 2010b).

b. Gather subjective data: Determine the client's self-perceived compliance with medical and nutritional prescriptions for medication administration, blood glucose monitoring, meal planning, exercise, foot and skin care, sick day management, and treatment and preventive methods for high and low glucose levels.

c. Determine the client's acceptance of the disease, the effect on his or her lifestyle, and perceived social and economic barriers to compliance.

d. Observe the client's functional ability and physical and psychological barriers (e.g., verbal and nonverbal communication, mobility, vision, cognition).

e. Observe the client's ability in self-glucose testing, self-insulin drawing and administration, and foot and skin care.

f. Identify the family support system.

2. Plan of care

a. Nursing diagnoses

1) Ineffective individual coping related to denial and depression

2) Knowledge deficit related to disease cause, progression, and treatments

3) Self-care deficits related to the following:

a) Physical, social, economic, and psychological barriers and limitations (e.g., medication administration, self-glucose testing)

b) Neuropathy, limited mobility, and poor vision (e.g., foot and skin care)

c) Lack of knowledge of target blood glucose levels

d) Lack of financial and social support systems

e) Lack of knowledge of follow-up needs and prevention of further complications related to the disease process

4) Altered nutritional intake (more or less than the body needs) related to lack of awareness about serving sizes, limited self-discipline, and noncompliance with dietary guidelines

5) Sensory-perceptual alterations related to neuropathy

6) Sexual dysfunction related to microvascular and macrovascular impairment

b. Goals

1) State barriers to and develop methods of effective coping with diabetes.

2) Increase level of independent self-administration of medication and glucose testing.

3) Perform or direct daily foot checks and skin care.

4) Identify adequate nutritional intake according to ADA guidelines.

5) Practice selecting proper serving sizes of favorite foods.

6) Identify ways to compensate for altered sensory-perceptual sensations.

7) Identify individual concerns with and compensate for sexual dysfunction.

8) Learn normal and target blood glucose levels.

9) Identify variances of blood glucose levels, corrective actions, and when to call for help.

10) State sick day care.

11) Identify and obtain needed adaptive equipment (e.g., talking meters, insulin bottle holders, dose-dialing insulin syringes, premixed syringes, magnifying guides).

12) Identify and obtain insurance and Medicare and Medicaid benefits for diabetes education and equipment (e.g., meters, strips, lancets, therapeutic shoes).

13) Maintain appropriate weight loss as needed.

14) Identify proper use and disposal of needles and syringes.

15) Involve family or a significant other in management of diabetes as needed.

16) Learn preventive measures and identification and treatment of acute and chronic complications.

3. Interventions
    a. Teach coping strategies (e.g., stress management, humor, breathing exercises).
    b. Provide opportunities for assisted practice with a self-medication program (e.g., storing, drawing, mixing, and injecting insulin).
    c. Direct daily self-foot checks and skin care (e.g., using skin cream).
    d. Promote identification and selection of the proper number and size of carbohydrate servings for individualized meal programs (e.g., four carbohydrate servings would total 60 g carbohydrate, or 15 g carbohydrate times four food choices).
    e. Suggest ways to compensate for altered sensory-perceptual sensations (e.g., wear diabetic socks at night to increase warmth, circulation, and comfort).
    f. Teach compensation for sexual dysfunction (e.g., cream for vaginal dryness, enhancer medications and pumps for men).
    g. Teach problem-solving skills to treat and prevent blood glucose variances and to know when and how to get help.
    h. Teach use of adaptive equipment (e.g., talking meters, insulin bottle holders).
    i. Teach survival skills and suggest follow-up education and self-management support as needed after dismissal from the hospital.
    j. Discuss insurance and Medicare and Medicaid benefits for education, equipment, and continued assistance (e.g., nursing home or assisted living placement, support groups).
    k. Discuss follow-up care (e.g., annual eye exam, HbA1c test, kidney function test).
    l. Teach sick day management (e.g., increase frequency of blood glucose testing, when to call the doctor).
    m. Encourage the client to perform at least 150 minutes per week of moderate-intensity aerobic activity and, if no contraindications, encourage him or her to perform resistance training three times per week after discharge to home.
    n. Teach proper disposal of needles and syringes.
    o. Involve family or a significant other in management of diabetes.
    p. Discuss acute and chronic complications that can occur with diabetes and management of complications.
L. Rehabilitation

1. The need for rehabilitation usually results from the complications of diabetes rather than the disease itself.
2. Stroke, heart disease, peripheral neuropathy, and amputation are the consequences of diabetes that rehabilitation nurses treat.
3. Key rehabilitation nursing strategies
    a. Incorporate all interventions identified in the nursing process assessment into the daily care of the client.
    b. Observe for neuropathy, lack of proprioception, and instability as you treat the client.
4. The rehabilitation team should include the following in addition to the basic team:
    a. Nutritional counselor or dietitian
    b. Diabetic educator, if available
    c. Pain management specialist
    d. Endocrinologist or primary care physician who is managing the diabetes

II. **HIV and AIDS**
    A. Overview (Fan, Conner, & Villarreal, 2011)
        1. AIDS was first recognized in 1981 as a serious life-threatening illness and has since become a worldwide epidemic.
        2. In 1985 the causative agent HIV was identified, and AIDS was determined to be the end stage of the HIV infection.
        3. Although significant breakthroughs in prevention, treatment, and diagnosis have increased survival times, the long-term prognosis for people with HIV and AIDS remains poor.
        4. Drug therapy to treat the infection became available in 1987 and has since expanded, but despite research and new developments, no cure or vaccine is available, and the HIV epidemic is far from over (Lewis, Heitkemper, & Dirksen, 2004).
        5. An estimated 1.2 million people in the United States were living with HIV or AIDS at the end of 2009.
        6. It is estimated that 25 million people worldwide have died of AIDS since the start of the epidemic, including 583,298 Americans.
        7. Avoiding behaviors that put a person at risk of infection is the only way to prevent the infection.
        8. Nurses play a vital role in caring for people with HIV and AIDS and are challenged to stay up to date on the most current research because information in this area is constantly developing.
    B. Types
        1. AIDS is the most advanced stage of a progressive immune function disorder caused by the retrovirus HIV.
        2. HIV

a. Attacks the immune system and leaves the body defenseless to numerous infections and health problems

b. Includes two strains that cause AIDS but have differing geographic distributions

   1) HIV-1 accounts for the majority of infections worldwide (Avert.org., 2010).

      a) Classified into four groups: The "major" group M, the "outlier" group O, and two new groups, N and P. These four groups may represent four separate introductions of simian immunodeficiency virus into humans. Group O appears to be restricted to west-central Africa, and group N, a strain discovered in 1998 in Cameroon, is extremely rare.

      b) More than 90% of HIV-1 infections belong to group M.

   2) HIV-2 appears to be prevalent in West African countries but has only limited distribution in other areas.

C. Epidemiology (CDC, 2009)

1. In 2008, 33 million people in the world were living with HIV or AIDS.

2. The *09 AIDS Epidemic Update* (Joint United Nations Programme on HIV/AIDS, 2009) reported that 2.7 million people were newly infected with HIV in 2008, and approximately 2 million people died from the virus.

3. Blacks/African Americans accounted for 51% of the HIV/AIDS diagnoses made in 2007 in the United States, followed by Whites (29%) and Hispanics and Latinos (18%).

4. Advances in treatment slowed the progression of HIV infection to AIDS, leading to dramatic decreases in AIDS deaths. The number of AIDS diagnoses has remained relatively stable.

D. Etiology

1. The origin of HIV is unknown.

2. The causative agent of HIV infection is HIV, a retrovirus.

3. A person with HIV may be asymptomatic for many years and not even know that he or she is infected; however, as the immune system weakens, the person will become ill more often.

4. Differentiate between exposure, infection, and disease: When an HIV-infected person has intimate contact with an uninfected person (exposure), this does not always result in transmission of HIV to the uninfected person. Likewise, not all people who become infected with the virus (infection) will develop physical symptoms.

5. HIV is one continuous disease process that ranges from asymptomatic to AIDS, which is characterized by potentially life-threatening opportunistic infections (OIs; CDC, 2009).

a. Primary infection or early chronic infection: Period from infection with HIV to the development of HIV-specific antibodies, which results in viremia (large amounts of virus in the blood)

   1) Onset is 0–12 weeks from initial infection.

   2) Virus infects white blood cells called CD4+ T-lymphocytes (T-helper cells), which are the master coordinators of the immune system.

   3) Immune system clears virus to lymphatic organs.

   4) The CD4+ T-cell count declines and is greater than or equal to 500 cells/mm^3.

   5) Physical characteristics are similar to those of flu or mononucleosis (e.g., fever, fatigue, headache, arthralgia, myalgia, generalized lymphadenopathy, pharyngitis, anorexia, weight loss, and night sweats). Symptoms usually disappear after a week to a month.

b. Chronic asymptomatic infection

   1) Onset is 12 weeks–12 years or more from initial infection.

   2) Anti-HIV antibodies have been produced at about 12 weeks and can be detected by antibody screening.

   3) The virus is present primarily in lymphatic tissue and slowly spreads throughout the body.

   4) Clinical symptoms usually are absent or mild. Vague symptoms include fatigue, headache, lymphadenopathy, and night sweats.

   5) As the viral load increases, the CD4+ T-cell count gradually declines (200–499 cells/mm^3).

c. AIDS

   1) As the immune system fails, symptoms increase, and the illnesses that occur become more severe.

   2) Signs and symptoms progress from mild to moderate (e.g., chills, frequent fever, night sweats, dry productive cough, dyspnea, lethargy, confusion, stiff neck, seizures, headaches, malaise, oral lesions, generalized lymphadenopathy, skin rashes, abdominal discomfort, chronic diarrhea, weight loss, fatigue, short-term memory loss, tuberculosis, oral hairy

leukoplakia, shingles, thrombocytopenia, pelvic inflammatory disease in women that does not respond to treatment, developmental delays and failure to thrive in children) to life-threatening OIs.

3) CD4+ T-cell counts continue to decline to less than 200 cells/mm^3.

4) One or more OIs or diseases (AIDS indicator conditions) develop (**Figure 16-1**). Children may get the same OI or disease as do adults, but they also have severe forms of common childhood bacterial infections such as conjunctivitis, ear infections, and tonsillitis (Health-Disease.org, 2011).

5) Clinical manifestations involve the loss of lean body mass and wasting syndrome.

6) Without treatment, death occurs in 3–5 years and usually results from infection, cancer, or wasting syndrome.

E. Pathophysiology
1. Overview (Fan et al., 2011)
  a. HIV is a retrovirus that consists of RNA virus that contains a special viral enzyme called reverse transcriptase, which allows the virus to replicate backward, going from RNA to DNA, and then integrate and take over a cell's own genetic material.
  b. HIV cannot replicate unless it is inside a living cell.
  c. HIV interacts with human cells that have CD4 receptors on their surface membrane, which include lymphocytes, monocytes, macrophages, astrocytes, and oligodendrocytes (white blood cells that fight infections); once attached, HIV virus enters the cell.
  d. After the virus enters the cell, viral RNA is transcribed into DNA with the assistance of the enzyme reverse transcriptase, becoming a permanent part of the cell's genetic structure and replicated during normal cell processes.
  e. It uses the cell to make copies of itself, produces new HIV retroviruses, and kills primarily CD4+ T lymphocytes because they have more CD4+ receptor-bearing cells.
  f. Viral load increases (the number of circulating HIV retroviruses in the person's serum).
  g. Antibodies are produced and detectable between 6 weeks and 6 months after infection; however, these antibodies are not able to fight the infection.
  h. Millions of CD4+ T cells are destroyed every day, but the bone marrow and thymus are

---

Figure 16-1. Opportunistic Infections (OIs) Associated with AIDS

Viral: Cytomegalovirus disease, herpes simplex, pneumonitis or esophagitis

Bacterial: *Mycobacterium* tuberculosis, recurrent pneumonia, recurrent *Salmonella* septicemia

Protozoal: *Pneumocystis carinii* pneumonia (PCP), toxoplasmosis of the brain

Fungal: Candidiasis of bronchi, trachea, lungs, or esophagus

Neurological: Dementia, headaches

Neoplastic processes: Lymphoma, Kaposi's sarcoma (KS), cervical carcinoma

Wasting syndrome: Chronic diarrhea, weakness, weight loss, constant or intermittent fever for at least 30 days

---

able to produce enough CD4+ T cells to replace the destroyed cells for many years.

i. Once the ability of HIV to destroy CD4+ T cells exceeds the body's ability to make them, they will not be able to regulate immune responses, resulting in the most serious stage of HIV infection, AIDS, with OIs.

j. Immune problems start to occur when the CD4+ T cell count drops to 200–499 cells/mm^3; severe problems develop with fewer than 200 CD4+ T cells/mm^3.

2. Transmission
  a. HIV is transmitted from human to human through exposure to infected body fluid (e.g., blood, semen, vaginal secretions, breast milk).
  b. No evidence has been found that HIV is transmitted through tears, sweat, saliva, vomit, urine, or feces.
  c. Common modes of transmission:
    1) Sexual contact (e.g., oral, vaginal, anal)
    2) Sharing a needle or syringe (e.g., intravenous drug use, tattooing, body piercing)
    3) Blood transfusion (risk extremely small because of blood screening and heat treatment)
    4) Tissue or organ donation
    5) Prenatal contact from mother to infant before or during birth or during breastfeeding
    6) Occupational exposure (e.g., needlestick)
  d. HIV is not spread through casual contact (e.g., touching; hugging; shaking hands; sharing eating utensils; eating food prepared by a person with HIV; coughing; sneezing; using restrooms; touching animals or insects; or living, working, or attending school with an HIV-infected person).

3. Clinical manifestations

a. Common signs and symptoms of HIV infection include chills, fever, flulike symptoms, rash, fatigue, malaise, arthralgias, headache, loss of appetite, weight loss, myalgias, nausea, vomiting, pharyngitis, oral ulcers, dry productive cough, sore throat, rash, night sweats, shortness of breath, stiff neck, yeast infection, lymphadenopathy, gastrointestinal distress, diarrhea, pain, dementia, confusion, infected gums, sores on anus and genitals, and photophobia (Zingman, 2010).

b. People with AIDS are susceptible to OIs, which are life-threatening illnesses caused by organisms that normally do not cause problems in healthy people (Fan et al., 2011).

   1) OIs can affect every organ and body system.
   2) Diagnosis and treatment of OIs are essential to increase longevity.
   3) Pneumocystis pneumonia caused by a fungus microbe is a common OI in adults.
   4) Children are susceptible to OIs, conjunctivitis, ear infections, and tonsillitis.

4. Diagnosis

   a. Early testing and routine voluntary testing for HIV will alert the HIV-infected person to avoid high-risk behavior, reducing HIV transmission and enabling appropriate treatment, resulting in improved health, extended life, and prevention of OIs (CDC, 2006).

   b. Recommendations for HIV testing (CDC, 2006)

      1) Routine HIV screening for people 13–64 years of age in all healthcare settings after the client is notified that the testing will be performed unless he or she declines (opt-out screening)
      2) HIV testing at least once per year for people at high risk unless the client declines (opt-out screening)
      3) HIV screening included in a panel of prenatal screening tests for all pregnant women and repeat screening in the third trimester in certain areas with elevated HIV infection rates unless the client declines (opt-out screening)

   c. Written consent is not recommended and HIV screening should be incorporated into the general consent for medical care (CDC, 2007a).

   d. Prevention and pretest counseling are encouraged but not required for diagnostic testing as part of routine screening programs in healthcare settings (CDC, 2007a).

      1) Pretest counseling
         a) Review test procedures.
         b) Explain the meaning of positive and negative test results.
         c) Provide information on HIV and AIDS.
         d) Set a plan for risk reduction.
         e) Describe the importance of follow-up care.
         f) Prepare the client for potential psychological and emotional reactions to a positive test result.
      2) Posttest counseling
         a) If the test is negative, provide advice on retesting (if the person engages in high-risk behavior) and preventing the spread of HIV.
         b) If the test is positive, evaluate the person's potential for suicide; provide crisis intervention if needed and information on symptoms of HIV and AIDS; teach health maintenance; refer for medical follow-up and tuberculosis screening, support groups, clinical trials, or experimental protocols; and discuss potential discrimination.

   e. Confidentiality with HIV testing is very important because disclosure may result in discrimination.

   f. Diagnostic tests available (CDC, 2007a; Fan et al., 2011)

      1) Antibody testing (rapid test [20 minutes], enzyme-linked immunosorbent assay [ELISA], Western blot)
         a) Detects the presence of antibodies to HIV
         b) Involves a delay (window period) of 3 weeks to 6 months before a detectable antibody is produced
         c) A positive test should be repeated and then confirmed by an alternative method, usually Western blot.
         d) Most widely used
      2) Antigen testing
         a) Detects the virus (HIV RNA) in the blood
         b) Is detectable 1 week earlier than antibody testing but is labor intensive and costly
         c) May be performed if an antibody test is negative and the person is highly likely to test positive

3) Viral load: Measures plasma HIV RNA levels in a sample of blood, indicating the amount of virus in the person's serum, how well the immune system is controlling the virus, or whether the medication regimen is working
   a) No antiretroviral medication: Viral load every 3–4 months
   b) With antiretroviral medication: Viral load 2–8 weeks after initiation of treatment and then every 3–4 months to make sure the drug is still working
4) CD4 cell count: Used to measure the extent of immune damage that has occurred, to stage HIV infection and prognosis, and to determine whether the medication regimen is working
5) Drug resistance testing: Determines whether a person's HIV strain is resistant to any anti-HIV medication

F. Management Options (Panel on Antiretroviral Guidelines for Adults and Adolescents, 2009)
1. Early intervention allows the person to survive longer. Research has focused on antiretroviral agents to inhibit disease progression, prophylactic therapy to prevent OIs, therapy to restore the damaged immune system, and vaccine development (Monahan, Sands, Neighbors, Marek, & Green, 2007).
2. The primary goals driving the decision to initiate antiretroviral therapy (ART) include the following:
   a. Maximally and durably suppress plasma HIV viral load
   b. Reduce HIV-associated morbidity and prolong survival
   c. Improve quality of life
   d. Restore and preserve immunologic function
   e. Prevent HIV transmission
3. HIV suppression with ART may also decrease inflammation and immune activation, which are thought to increase rates of cardiovascular and other comorbidities.
4. The FDA has approved a number of drugs for treating HIV infection (Fan et al., 2011).
   a. Nucleoside analog reverse transcriptase inhibitors (NRTIs)
      1) Target the viral enzyme reverse transcriptase. These drugs specifically block the virus from replicating while having little effect on the host.
      2) Include azidothymidine (AZT), zalcitabine (ddC), didanosine (ddI), stavudine (d4T),

lamivudine (3TC), abacavir (Ziagen), tenofovir (Viread), and emtricitabine (Emtriva)
   b. Nonnucleoside reverse transcriptase inhibitors (NNRTIs)
      1) Bind to the reverse transcriptase enzyme and prevent it from functioning
      2) Include delavirdine (Rescriptor), nevirapine (Viramune), and efavirenz (Sustiva)
      3) In 2010 a single dose of nevirapine was found to be effective in substantially reducing HIV transmission from pregnant women to their children.
   c. Protease inhibitors
      1) Prevent the virus from making long protein molecules necessary to create a new virus, thus halting replication
      2) Include ritonavir (Norvir), saquinavir (Invirase), indinavir (Crixivan), nelfinavir (Viracept), lopinavir (Kaletra), atazanavir (Reyataz), amprenavir (Agenerase), darunavir (Prezista), lopinavir (Kaletra), tipranavir (Aptivus), and fosamprenavir (Lexiva)
   d. Integrase inhibitors
      1) The most recently developed antiviral drug that targets the viral integrase, which is the enzyme responsible for integration of viral DNA into the host cell.
      2) Raltegravir (Isentress) was approved for use in 2007 and when used with other anti-HIV drugs is effective in controlling viral loads.
   e. Fusion inhibitors
      1) Interfere with HIV-1's ability to enter cells by blocking the merging of the virus with the cell membrane
      2) Include enfuvirtide (T-20, Fuzeon)
5. The most effective treatment strategy is combination drug therapy, which can attack viral replication in several different ways, attack different stages of the HIV life cycle, produce a more sustained antiviral effect in a person with HIV, and decrease the likelihood of drug resistance.
   a. Current recommendations are to monitor a client with HIV and to initiate ART after the CD4T counts drop below 200 cells/mm^3. ART initiation is also recommended for people with CD4 counts below 350 and an AIDS-defining illness (Fan et al., 2011).
   b. The current guidelines recommend achieving the maximum suppression of symptoms for as long as possible. This used to be called highly

active antiretroviral therapy (HAART) but now is referred to as ART (Fan et al., 2011).

   c. In addition, because quality of life is important, the overall goal of AIDS treatment is to find the strongest possible regimen that is also simple and has the fewest side effects.

     1) With effective ART therapies, HIV-infected people experience a drop in viral loads to below the level of detectability for several years.

     2) ART is not a cure but reduces the amount of virus circulating in the bloodstream.

     3) Drops in viral loads are accompanied by recoveries of T-cell counts, increases in immune function, and the disappearance of AIDS symptoms.

6. A number of treatments are available for some opportunistic diseases (e.g., radiation and chemotherapy for Kaposi's sarcoma and other forms of cancer, ganciclovir to treat cytomegalovirus eye infections, fluconazole to treat yeast and other fungal infections, and pentamidine or trimethoprim/sulfamethoxazole to treat *Pneumocystis carinii* pneumonia).

7. The influenza vaccine is recommended; people with advanced AIDS may have a poor response to immunization and should be given antiviral medications if they are likely to be exposed to other people with influenza.

8. Alternative and complementary therapies include therapeutic touch, massage therapy, meditation, imagery, tai chi, and herbal medicine.

9. Health promotion and disease prevention can be effective in preventing the spread of infection.

   a. Promote a lifestyle that prevents or decreases the risk of HIV infection.

     1) Abstain from sexual activity or use a condom for all insertive sexual practices with a partner who has or may have HIV.

     2) Stop using intravenous drugs, stop sharing needles and equipment, use a clean needle and syringe or disinfect them after each use, decrease the number of injections, and avoid engaging in risky sexual activity.

     3) Early testing and routine screening for all clients 13–64 years of age

     4) Screen all potential blood donors for high-risk behaviors and signs and symptoms of AIDS and test all human tissue for transplantation for HIV antibodies.

     5) Adhere to safety guidelines to prevent occupational exposure.

   b. Promote a healthy lifestyle in people who are already infected.

     1) Decrease high-risk behavior.

     2) Attend regular medical and psychiatric evaluations and follow-ups.

     3) Maintain proper nutrition and diet (high calorie, high protein to prevent weight loss), which improve immune function.

     4) Maintain food safety by keeping food at the proper temperature, cooking food thoroughly, avoiding foods that may be contaminated or harbor bacteria, and washing fruits and vegetables before eating (because people with HIV infection are vulnerable to foodborne illness).

     5) Remove fresh flowers and plants from the room.

     6) Avoid cleaning the litter box.

     7) Ask visitors to wear a mask if they have a cold.

     8) Maintain proper hand washing.

     9) Reduce and control stress.

     10) Avoid or limit cigarettes, alcohol, and drugs.

     11) Exercise regularly.

G. Nursing Process

  1. Assessment

   a. Obtain a complete history of current high-risk behaviors that could put other people at risk and signs and symptoms that may indicate the progression of HIV and the presence of OIs.

   b. Perform a neurological evaluation.

   c. Perform a psychosocial evaluation (e.g., support systems, financial state, coping strategies).

   d. Observe the client's overall health and appearance and conduct a complete physical and functional assessment because any body system can be affected.

   e. Investigate nutritional status, energy level, and preventive strategies to protect others and self from further infectious insult.

   f. Assess for weight loss, fever, skin lesions, short-term memory loss, and cold symptoms.

   g. Assess compliance with treatment, effectiveness of the treatment regimen, and side effects.

  2. Plan of care

   a. Nursing diagnoses

     1) Hopelessness related to terminal disease process

     2) Fear related to possible death

3) Anticipatory grieving related to terminal diagnosis
4) Ineffective individual coping or compromised family coping related to diagnosis
5) Inadequate nutrition related to the disease process, wasting syndrome, and side effects of the treatment regimen
6) Pain related to the disease process
7) Fatigue related to poor nutrition, the disease process, and muscle weakness
8) Activity intolerance related to weakness, poor nutrition
9) Risk for infection related to deficient immune system
10) Knowledge deficit related to diagnosis, prognosis, and long-term care

b. Goals (Lewis et al., 2004)
1) For the asymptomatic stage
   a) Demonstrate a healthy lifestyle.
   b) Verbalize an understanding of measures to prevent further HIV transmission.
   c) Identify and use effective strategies for coping with stressful situations and adjustment to illness.
   d) Verbalize an understanding of the disease process, significant implications, and treatment options.
2) For the symptomatic stage
   a) Verbalize an understanding of the prevention and treatment of OIs.
   b) Verbalize an understanding of and appropriately manage problems caused by HIV infection.
   c) Maintain a maximal level of function.
   d) Verbalize understanding of and adhere to the drug regimen to keep the viral load as low as possible for as long as possible.
3) For the terminal stage
   a) Maintain a desired level of comfort.
   b) Verbalize wishes and declare preferences regarding treatment options.
   c) Experience a dignified and comfortable death.

3. Interventions
   a. Asymptomatic stage
   1) Provide education about the diagnosis of HIV, prevention of the spread of HIV, disease progression, and treatment options.
   2) Use strategies to prevent infection.
   3) Provide education for HIV-negative people who are at risk for contracting HIV

and prevent the HIV-infected person from transmitting the virus to others.
4) Empower the client to take control of preventive measures.
5) Encourage the client to maintain social and community activities.
6) Monitor for signs and symptoms of infection, which may indicate disease progression.
7) Provide emotional support, include significant others in the plan of care, and help identify additional sources of financial and emotional support.
8) Assess the psychological response to situations.

b. Symptomatic stage
1) Provide education about medications and adverse effects.
2) Assess effectiveness of the treatment regimen (viral load, CD4+ T-cell count), adverse reactions, and compliance with medication regimens.
3) Educate about changing treatment options and encourage continued adherence.
4) Monitor weight and provide a high-calorie, high-protein diet and nutritional supplements as necessary.
5) Manage and treat HIV-related symptoms with antibiotics, antifungals, or antiviral medication for infection; antiemetics for nausea; analgesics for pain; and antidiarrheal medication for diarrhea.
6) Balance energy with rest to maintain a normal or nearly normal activity level and use assistive devices (wheelchair, cane) to conserve energy.
7) Encourage verbalization of fears and concerns.

c. Terminal stage
1) Assist with end-of-life comfort measures in a suitable care setting and appropriate services (e.g., hospice).
2) Administer pain medication to relieve pain and discomfort.
3) Administer antianxiety medication for anxiety and restlessness.
4) Promote a calm environment.
5) Provide emotional and spiritual support to the client and significant others.
6) Maintain the client's dignity and wishes throughout the dying process.
7) Instruct significant others on the dying process.

8) Provide bereavement counseling for significant others.

4. Evaluation: Modify care according to the stage of HIV and the client's response to nursing interventions.

H. Rehabilitation

1. Rehabilitation needs are determined by the stage of HIV and the client's response to nursing interventions.

2. HIV and AIDS rehabilitation should include the following:

   a. Client and family education and counseling

   b. Functional activities with introduction of assistive devices as needed

   c. Nutritional counseling

   d. An exercise program to help build strength, endurance, and mobility

3. In addition to the basic rehabilitation team, the team should include the following:

   a. Primary care physician or physician handling the HIV or AIDS

   b. Counselor

   c. Representative of hospice or palliative care

III. Cancer

A. Overview

1. Cancer encompasses a group of diseases characterized by the growth and spread of abnormal cells that result in death if not controlled.

2. Cancer is the second most common cause of death in the United States, exceeded only by heart disease, and smoking alone causes one-third of all cancer deaths (American Cancer Society [ACS], 2010).

3. Adult cigarette smoking prevalence in the United States has been slowly declining since 1991. The prevalence among adolescents has declined since the late 1990s, but one in five adults and adolescents is a smoker (NCI, 2010e).

4. Prostate, breast, lung, and colorectal cancers are the most common cancers in the United States (NCI, 2011).

5. The cancer incidence rate has declined since the early 2000s. However, incidence rates for some cancers (e.g., melanoma of the skin; non-Hodgkin's lymphoma; childhood cancers; leukemia; and cancers of the kidney, renal pelvis, thyroid, pancreas, liver, testis, and esophagus) are rising (NCI, 2010e).

6. Categories of cancer (NCI, 2009)

   a. Carcinoma: Cancer that begins in the skin or internal and external linings of the body (e.g., skin, lungs, breast, pancreas, and other organs and glands)

   b. Sarcoma: Cancer that begins in bone, cartilage, fat, or other connective tissue (e.g., bone, skeletal muscle, fibrous tissue, or cartilage)

   c. Myeloma: Cancer of plasma cells of bone marrow

   d. Lymphoma: Cancer of cells in the glands or nodes of the lymphatic system

   e. Leukemia: Cancer that affects the blood-forming elements of the bone marrow

   f. Central nervous system (CNS) cancers: Cancers that begin in the tissues of the brain and spinal cord

   g. Mixed type: Cancer of multiple tissue types

7. Not all tumors are cancerous.

   a. Benign tumors are not cancerous. They can be removed and in most cases do not return.

   b. Malignant tumors are cancerous. Cells in these tumors can invade nearby tissues and spread to other parts of the body (metastasis).

8. Early detection and treatment improve the chances of a cure.

B. Epidemiology and Incidence (ACS, 2011)

1. Approximately 1,596,670 new cancer cases are expected to be diagnosed in 2011 in the United States.

2. Approximately 571,950 Americans are expected to die of cancer in 2011.

3. One out of every two American men and one out of every three American women will develop cancer during their lifetime.

4. Seventy-eight percent of all cancers are diagnosed in people 55 years and older.

5. The 5-year survival rate for all cancers diagnosed between 1999 and 2005 was 68%, up from 50% in 1975.

C. Etiology and Risk Factors

1. The exact cause of cancer remains a mystery.

2. Development of cancer is a multistep process that is influenced by many independent variables causing damage to DNA, resulting in mutation within the genes of cells.

3. These mutations can be caused by chemicals or physical agents, called carcinogens, or they may occur spontaneously and may be passed down from one generation to the next.

4. Risk factors (CDC, 2010d)

   a. Age: The risk of nearly all cancers increases with age.

   b. Genetic factors: Some cancers are inherited and create a significant predisposition to cancer. About 5% of cancers are strongly hereditary (an inherited genetic alteration confers a very high risk of developing one or more specific types of cancer).

c. Hormonal factor: Evidence suggests that hormones may be connected with the development of certain cancers.

d. Exposure to environmental factors: 75%–80% of cancer in the United States is attributed to environmental factors.

1) Tobacco smoke is the most lethal known carcinogen (responsible for 30% of cancer deaths in the United States).

2) Radiation: Ionizing and ultraviolet radiation (sunlight) can cause cancer.

3) Nutrition, obesity, and inactivity are responsible for 35% of cancer deaths in the United States. Research shows that approximately one-third of all cancer deaths are related to an unhealthy diet and lack of physical activity in adulthood (ACS, 2010).

    a) Some research indicates that grilled meats may cause cancer. The apparent culprit is meat that is charred (About. com: Cancer, 2007).

    b) People who have diets high in saturated fats have a higher cancer risk than those with lower-fat diets.

    c) Inactivity has been linked to a higher risk of colon cancer.

4) Certain viruses: A number of cancers have been linked to viruses (sexually transmitted disease organisms) that suppress the immune system.

5) Occupational exposure (responsible for 4% of cancer deaths in the United States): Exposure to carcinogens (e.g., drugs, chemicals, radiation) increases the risk of cancer.

6) Alcohol: Drinking alcohol has been linked with an elevated risk of cancer of the esophagus, oral cavity, pharynx, and larynx (ACS, 2010).

e. Precancerous lesions: Benign lesions and tumors (polyps of the colon and rectum, certain pigmented moles) tend to progress to cancer.

f. Psychosocial factors: Extreme stress activates the body's endocrine (hormone) system, which in turn can cause changes in the immune system. There is no research directly linking cancer with stress.

D. Pathophysiology

1. Overview: Cancer develops when a number of mechanisms, either alone or in combination, cause abnormalities in cell growth and multiplication.

2. Cancer cells

a. Characteristics

1) Variable size and shape

2) Loss of capacity for specialized function

3) Continued growth after division

    a) Normal cells usually die after 50–60 divisions; however, cancer cells continue in an uncontrolled growth pattern.

    b) Cancer cells continue to grow despite a diminished concentration of growth hormones.

b. Tumor growth

1) Cancer cells accumulate and form a mass of abnormal cells (or tumors) that may compress, invade, and destroy normal tissues.

2) Most cancers form tumors, but not all tumors are cancerous.

    a) Benign: Noncancerous tumors that stop growing and do not spread to other parts of the body

    b) Malignant: Cancerous tumors

c. Carcinogenesis

1) The process through which cancer develops and abnormal cells grow and proliferate out of control

2) Change or mutation in the nucleus of a cell: Millions of cells in the human body die and are replaced every second. The body's immune system typically recognizes mutant cells and destroys them before they multiply, but some mutant cells survive and cause cancer.

3) Carcinogenesis may occur after exposure to carcinogens, which are substances that start or promote the process (e.g., various chemicals, gases, and other substances found in the air, water, foods, pesticides, and industrial settings; tobacco smoke; cleaning products; paints; certain viruses [HIV, hepatitis B, Epstein–Barr]).

4) Two models of carcinogenesis (NCI, 2010d)

    a) Vogelstein and Kinzler emphasized that cancer is ultimately a disease of damaged DNA, comprised of a sequence of genetic mutations that can turn normal cells into cancerous cells.

    b) Hanahan and Weinberg focused on the hallmark events at the cellular level that lead to a tumor.

d. Metastasis

1) Abnormal cells multiply out of control.

2) A tumor spreads from the original site to another site via the lymphatic system or blood vessels.

3) This uncontrolled growth and spread of cancer cells can eventually interfere with vital organs or functions, resulting in a variety of other tissue changes in the body such as pain, cachexia, lowered immunity, anemia, leukopenia, and thrombocytopenia, and if not controlled can result in death.

4) The primary sites of cancer metastasis are the bone, lymph nodes, liver, lungs, and brain.

5) Cancer is classified by the body part where it started.

3. Symptoms that may signal the presence of cancer (ACS, 2010)

a. A change in the size, color, shape, or thickness of a wart, mole, or mouth sore

b. A sore that resists healing

c. Persistent cough, hoarseness, or sore throat

d. Thickening or lumps in the breasts, testicles, or elsewhere

e. A change in bowel or bladder habits

f. Any unusual bleeding or discharge

g. Chronic indigestion or difficulty swallowing

h. Persistent headaches

i. Unexplained loss of weight or appetite

j. Persistent fatigue, nausea, or vomiting

k. Persistent low-grade fever, either constant or intermittent

l. Repeated instances of infection

4. Diagnosis

a. Diagnostic testing: Laboratory testing (e.g., CBC, chemistry profile, liver function test, tumor markers [i.e., substances measurable in the blood that are not produced or are produced in a lesser amount in healthy people]).

b. Noninvasive: Radiological studies, computed tomography (CT), magnetic resonance imaging (MRI), ultrasonography, nuclear medicine studies

c. Invasive procedures: Biopsy (ranges from needle biopsy to surgical procedure), endoscopy

d. Staging

1) Staging is the process used to describe the extent of the disease or the spread of cancer from the original site.

2) The tumor-node-metastasis staging system is a uniform system used worldwide that assesses tumors in three ways to determine a stage, ranging from I to IV (Monahan et al., 2007).

a) T: Extent of the primary tumor. TX means the primary tumor cannot be evaluated. T0 means there is no evidence of a primary tumor. Carcinoma in situ (CIS) means abnormal cells are present but have not spread to neighboring tissue. Although not cancer, CIS may become cancer and is sometimes called preinvasive cancer. T1 to T4 describe the size or level of invasion into nearby structures (the higher the T number, the larger the tumor).

b) N: Absence or presence of regional lymph node involvement. NX means regional lymph nodes cannot be evaluated. N0 means no regional lymph node involvement. N1 to N3 describe the size, location, or number of lymph nodes involved. The higher the N number, the more involved the lymph nodes are.

c) M: Absence or presence of metastases. MX means distant metastases cannot be evaluated. M0 means there are no known distant metastases, and M1 means that distant metastases are present.

e. Pap smear: Cells found in body secretions are spread, stained, and examined for tissue classification.

f. Tumor marker blood test: Measures for the presence of tumor markers or proteins associated with specific cancers (e.g., CA-125 for ovarian cancer, prostate-specific antigen for prostate cancer)

g. Screening examinations by healthcare professionals can help detect cancer of the breast, colon, rectum, cervix, prostate, testis, oral cavity, and skin.

h. Self-examination for breast and skin cancer may result in early detection of tumors.

E. Management Options

1. Prevention measures (Fayed, 2009)

a. Do not smoke or chew tobacco. Avoid exposure to smoke. Tobacco is believed to play a role in 90% of all lung cancer deaths (ACS, 2010).

b. Limit alcohol intake. Alcohol increases the risk of cancers of the mouth, pharynx, larynx, esophagus, liver, and breast and probably of the colon and rectum (ACS, 2010).

c. Eat a well-balanced diet.
1) Studies suggest that people who eat more fruits and vegetables, which are rich sources of antioxidants, may have a lower risk for some types of cancer (ACS, 2010).
2) Reduce the intake of fat.
3) Limit red meat and animal fat.
4) Avoid processed, smoked, cured, fried, or barbecued foods.
5) Balance caloric intake with physical activity.
6) Maintain a healthy weight and avoid excessive weight gain throughout life.
d. Practice sun safety and recognize when skin changes occur.
1) Stay out of the sun between 10 am and 3 pm.
2) Use sunscreen with an SPF of 15 or higher outdoors. Wear a hat and shirt when in the sun.
3) Wear ultraviolet light–filtering sunglasses.
4) Avoid tanning booths.
e. Exercise regularly. Exercise reduces the risk of several types of cancer (e.g., breast, colon, endometrium, prostate) and reduces the risk of other health problems (e.g., heart disease, high blood pressure, diabetes, osteoporosis).
f. Follow occupational hazard guidelines if exposed to carcinogens.
1) Limit exposure to carcinogens at home.
2) Avoid using aerosol cleaning products.
3) Wear gloves when using carcinogenic chemicals.
4) Follow safety warnings when using paint, solvents, pesticides, household cleaners, and other carcinogenic chemicals.
g. Remove precancerous adenomatous polyps to prevent colon cancer.
h. Practice safe sex.
1) Human papilloma virus is a known cause for cervical cancer and a risk factor for other cancers.
2) HIV and AIDS are associated with some types of cancers.
i. Get screened for cancer regularly. Screening tests such as colonoscopy, mammogram, and pap smear can detect abnormal changes before they turn cancerous.
2. Cancer treatment modalities are used to cure, control, or provide palliation; options depend on the stage of the tumor and the level of metastasis.
a. Surgery: The oldest form of treatment offers the greatest chance for cure for many types of cancer.
1) Biopsy: Obtain specimens of suspected tissue.
2) Curative resection: Resect lesions.
3) Palliation: Relieve symptoms to improve quality of life.
b. Radiation: A stream of high-energy particles or waves is used to destroy or damage cancer cells in a specific area.
1) Used before surgery to shrink a tumor so it can be removed more easily
2) Used after surgery to stop the growth of cancer cells that remain
3) Side effects: Irritation to the overlying skin, nausea, vomiting, anorexia, bone marrow depression, anemia, thrombocytopenia, leukopenia
c. Chemotherapy is the use of drugs to treat cancer by interfering with the stages of the dividing cell cycle and is used to treat cancer cells that have metastasized.
1) Anticancer drugs are more powerful when used in combination. More than 50 anticancer drugs are currently in use.
a) Drugs of different actions can work together to kill more cancer cells.
b) The use of multiple drugs can reduce the chance of developing a resistance to one particular drug.
c) Drugs can be administered by mouth, intravenously, intramuscularly, or topically.
2) Side effects vary with the drug and the client. They may include nausea, vomiting, fatigue, temporary hair loss, mouth sores or dryness, difficulty swallowing, diarrhea, and increased vulnerability to infection.
d. Bone marrow transplantation (BMT) and peripheral blood stem cell transplantation (PBSCT) are procedures that restore stem cells that have been destroyed by high doses of chemotherapy or radiation therapy (NCI, 2008b).
1) Autologous BMT: The client's own bone marrow is used.
2) Allogenic BMT: The client receives a donor's bone marrow.
a) Syngenic: Donor is an identical twin
b) Related: Donor is a relative
c) Unrelated: Donor is not a relative
3) The stem cells used in BMT come from the liquid center of the bone, called the marrow. The stem cells used in PBSCT come from the bloodstream.

e. Hormone therapy consists of drug treatment that interferes with hormone production or action to kill or slow the growth of cancer cells.

f. Biologic therapies (immunotherapy or biologic response modifier therapy) manipulate the immune system through the use of naturally occurring biologic substances or genetically engineered agents that promote or support the immune system's response to cancer.

g. Gene therapy manipulates genetic material inside cancerous cells to make them easier to destroy or prevent their growth and in some approaches targets healthy cells to increase their ability to fight cancer (NCI, 2006).

h. Alternative and complementary therapy are unconventional therapies that have not been scientifically tested but may complement conventional care, may help relieve certain symptoms and side effects, and may include vitamins, herbs, dietary supplements, or procedures such as acupuncture.

  1) Body work promotes relaxation and reduces cancer-related fatigue (e.g., massage, reflexology).

  2) Exercise controls fatigue, muscle tension, and anxiety.

  3) Mind-body medicine improves quality of life through behavior modification (e.g., guided imagery, hypnotherapy, biofeedback, art or music therapy).

  4) Acupuncture has been found to be effective in the management of chemotherapy-associated nausea and vomiting and in controlling pain associated with surgery (NCI, 2010a)

i. Nutrition and diet can play a role in cancer prevention, but no diet can cure cancer. A proper diet with vitamins, minerals, and other nutrients may inhibit the development of cancer by neutralizing carcinogens, ensuring proper immune function, and preventing tissue and cell damage.

3. Treatment of side effects

a. Pain: The goal of pain management is to relieve suffering and control pain.

  1) Medication

    a) For mild to moderate pain: Nonopioids, including aspirin, acetaminophen, and nonsteroidal anti-inflammatory drugs such as ibuprofen and naproxen

    b) For moderate to severe pain

      i. Opioids, including morphine, hydromorphone, oxycodone, hydrocodone, codeine, fentanyl, and methadone. A prescription is needed for these medicines. Nonopioids may also be used along with opioids for moderate to severe pain.

      ii. Adjunct medications

    c) For tingling and burning pain: Antidepressants, including amitriptyline, imipramine, doxepin, and trazodone; antiepileptics, including gabapentin and pregabalin

    d) For pain caused by swelling: Steroids, including prednisone and dexamethasone

  2) Other methods: Relaxation techniques, imagery, distraction, music, humor, biofeedback, hypnosis

  3) Invasive techniques: Surgery, nerve block, acupuncture

b. Nausea: Provide small, light meals throughout the day rather than heavy meals.

  1) Avoid gas-forming foods.

  2) Eat small, frequent meals to keep the stomach from feeling too full.

  3) Ginger candy, tea, or capsules

  4) Bland foods such as rice, applesauce, crackers, toast

  5) Cold or room-temperature foods

  6) Relaxation, imagery, and distraction techniques

  7) Antiemetics: Dronabinol (Marinol), ondansetron (Zofran)

  8) Antiulcer medications: Ranitidine (Zantac), sucralfate (Carafate), metoclopramide (Reglan)

  9) Lorazepam (Ativan) may produce adjunct antiemetic therapy.

c. Increased risk for infection

  1) Arises from underlying disease, side effects of treatment (e.g., neutropenia, immune suppression), disruption of mucous membranes or skin, presence of a long-term venous access device, impaired nutrition, and prolonged hospitalization

  2) Can be managed via prevention; prompt recognition of suspected infection; treatment of skin complications; administration of antibiotics, antifungals, or antiviral agents; fever management; or platelet or blood transfusion for bleeding

d. Fatigue
  1) Minimize symptoms that interfere with sleep.
  2) Avoid stimulants.
  3) Pace activities to save energy.
  4) Exercise.
e. Weight loss
  1) Can be caused by treatment side effects that impair nutritional status, uncontrolled pain that impairs appetite, or fatigue that affects the ability to obtain and eat food
  2) Can be treated according to the cause of the weight loss and the overall goals
  3) Can be treated with oral or parenteral nutritional supplementation
f. Pruritus
  1) Systemic histamine
  2) Topical corticosteroid cream may reduce localized urticaria; antifungal cream can be used for fungal infections.
  3) Tepid bath with aloe vera or oatmeal
  4) Creams containing aloe vera or lanolin for radiation dermatitis
  5) Stop medications suspected of causing pruritus.
g. Arm care precautions for women after breast or axillary surgery
  1) Perform range-of-motion exercises.
    a) Ensures full use and flexibility of the arm to help alleviate damage to the nerves and muscles that accompanies breast cancer surgery
    b) Reduces the risk and severity of lymphedema (i.e., the accumulation of lymph fluid in the tissues of the upper extremity after breast cancer surgery), which occurs most commonly in women with breast cancer who had axillary node dissection followed by radiation
  2) Avoid sunburn and burns while cooking, baking, or smoking.
  3) Wear protective gloves while gardening.
  4) Wear loose-fitting watches, jewelry, and clothing.
  5) Treat cuts immediately and monitor for signs of infection.
  6) Use the unaffected arm for intravenous access, blood draws, and blood pressure; avoid getting chemotherapy in the affected arm.

  7) Avoid carrying heavy objects with the affected arm.
h. Monitor for oncologic emergencies: Hypercalcemia, disseminated intravascular coagulation, alterations in blood-clotting mechanisms, septic shock, pleural effusion, spinal cord compression, neoplastic cardiac tamponade, superior vena cava syndrome, elevated intracranial pressure, airway obstruction, urinary obstruction., massive hemoptysis (Monahan et al., 2007).

F. Clinical Management of Cancers Necessitating Rehabilitation
  1. Brain tumors (NCI, 2010b)
    a. Brain cancer is the second leading cause of cancer death in people younger than 20 years old and accounts for 2% of all malignancies and 2.5% of all cancer deaths (Vogel, Wilson, & Melvin, 2004).
    b. Each year 35,000 people in the United States are diagnosed with a primary brain tumor.
    c. Metastasis to the brain is more common, with an incidence 10 times that of primary brain cancer (Vogel et al., 2004).
    d. Exposure to chemicals, such as pesticides, herbicides, fertilizers, petrochemicals, and viruses; bioelectromagnetic fields and cellular telephones have been studied as potential contributors to brain cancer (Muscat et al., 2000; Vogel et al., 2004).
    e. Anaplastic astrocytoma and glioblastoma account for approximately 38% of primary brain tumors; meningiomas and other mesenchymal tumors account for approximately 27% of these tumors.
    f. Brain tumors result in better outcomes in children than in adults.
    g. Clinical manifestations vary according to the location and size of the tumor but may include headache; seizures; nausea and vomiting; memory deficit; and changes in speech, motor skills, and vision.
    h. Diagnosis: Neurologic assessment, CT, MRI, biopsy
    i. Treatment: Surgery, radiation therapy, chemotherapy
      1) Chemotherapy may prolong survival in people with some tumor types and has been reported to lengthen disease-free survival in people with gliomas, medulloblastoma, and some germ-cell tumors.
      2) Complications of CNS surgery include intracranial bleeding, cerebral edema,

infection, neuromotor deficits, thrombosis, and hydrocephalus.

2. Spinal cord tumors (Mayo Clinic, 2010)
   a. The spine is the third most common site for metastatic cancer, after the lungs and liver. Most tumors that affect the vertebrae have spread to the spine from another site in the body.
   b. Cancerous tumors that originate in the bones of the spine are far less common and include osteosarcomas (osteogenic sarcomas), the most common type of bone cancer in children, and Ewing's sarcoma, a particularly aggressive tumor that affects young adults.
   c. Spinal cord lymphomas are more common in people whose immune systems are compromised by medications or disease.
   d. Many cases of spinal cord tumors run in families. Examples of these hereditary tumors are neurofibromatosis 2 and Von Hippel-Lindau disease.
   e. Intradural-extramedullary tumors develop in the spinal cord's arachnoid membrane (meningiomas), in the nerve roots that extend out from the spinal cord (schwannomas and neurofibromas), or at the spinal cord base (filum terminale ependymomas).
   f. Intramedullary tumors begin in the supporting cells in the spinal cord. Most are either astrocytomas, which affect mainly children and adolescents, or ependymomas, the most common type of spinal cord tumor in adults.
   g. Clinical manifestations are related to the site and size of tumor and may include pain, weakness, sensory loss (numbness, decreased skin sensitivity to temperature), muscle spasms, and loss of bowel and bladder control. If left untreated, symptoms may progress to include muscle wasting and paralysis.
   h. Diagnosis: Neurologic assessment, CT, MRI, biopsy
   i. Treatment: Surgery, radiation therapy, chemotherapy

3. Bone cancer (NCI, 2008a)
   a. Cancer that originates in the bone (primary bone cancer) is rare; cancer that spreads to the bones (metastatic cancer) from other parts of the body is more common.
      1) Primary bone cancer generally attacks young people and is more likely to occur in bones that have been fractured or infected in the past.
      2) The likelihood of a cure for primary bone cancer depends on how early it is detected and how rapidly it spreads.
      3) Primary bone cancers make up a small percentage of all cancers.
      4) For 2010 there were an estimated 2,650 new cases of cancer of the bones and joints and 1,460 deaths from it in the United States (NCI, 2010c).
   b. Symptoms: A hard lump felt on the surface of the bone, pain (especially at night), swelling in bones and joint, spontaneous bone fracture, fever, weight loss, fatigue, and impaired mobility (Monahan et al., 2007)
   c. Diagnosis: X rays, other imaging tests, biopsy
   d. Treatment
      1) Surgical removal when possible. If the cancer is in the arm or leg, amputation usually is avoided and the bone is reconstructed with a metal prosthesis.
      2) Radiation and chemotherapy
         a) May be given before surgery to reduce the size of the tumor
         b) May be used after surgery to kill remaining cells
         c) Used to treat inoperable bone cancer
      3) Cryosurgery is the use of liquid nitrogen to freeze and kill cancer cells. This technique can sometimes be used instead of conventional surgery to destroy the tumor.
      4) Therapy should begin as soon as possible to avoid stiffness and improve mobility and, if amputation was unavoidable, to help the client learn how to use the prosthesis.
   e. Common types
      1) Osteosarcoma
         a) Tends to affect people between 10 and 30 years of age
         b) Makes up approximately 35% of all primary bone cancers
         c) Has an incidence rate that is twice as high in men as in women
         d) Starts most often in bones of the arms, legs, or pelvis
      2) Chondrosarcoma
         a) Tends to attack middle-aged adults; not often found in people younger than 20 years
         b) Originates in the cartilage cells
         c) Most common sites: pelvic bone, long bones, scapula
      3) Ewing's family of tumors

THE SPECIALTY PRACTICE OF REHABILITATION NURSING

a) Tend to occur in children and teenagers; not common in adults older than 30 years of age.

b) Occur most often in the Caucasian population and are extremely rare in African-American and Asian populations

c) About 60% of Ewing tumors start in bone, but others are found outside the bone in soft tissue.

d) Most common place is the pelvis

4) Fibrosarcoma

a) Originates in soft tissue around the bones (ligaments, tendons, fat, and muscle)

b) Tends to occur in older and middle-age adults

c) Originates most often in legs, arms, or jaw

G. Rehabilitation (Cancer.Net Editorial Board, 2009)

1. Can improve the quality of life for those with cancer (and their family) by

a. Improving strength

b. Encouraging independence and reducing reliance on caregivers

c. Helping the person to adjust to actual, perceived, and potential losses due to the disease and treatment

d. Reduce sleep problems

e. Decrease hospitalization

2. Cancer rehabilitation should include

a. Client and family education and counseling

b. Pain management

c. Nutritional counseling

d. Exercise programs to help build strength, endurance, and mobility

e. Smoking cessation education and support

f. Education for activities of daily living (ADLs) as well as cooking and basic housekeeping with assistive devices as indicated

3. The cancer rehabilitation team should include the oncologist.

H. Nursing Process

1. Assessment

a. History

1) Signs and symptoms of underlying disease and side effects of treatment

2) Pain quality, location, duration, intensity, relieving factors

3) Dietary evaluation with food preferences

4) Use of complementary therapies

5) Psychosocial evaluation (e.g., support systems, coping strategies)

b. Complete physical and functional assessment to determine the degree of loss of function

2. Plan of care

a. Nursing diagnoses

1) Risk of impaired skin integrity related to skin irritation during radiotherapy

2) Pain related to tumor causing pressure on nerves, metastases, and reaction from cancer therapy

3) Fatigue related to poor nutrition, disease progression, and reaction to cancer treatment

4) Risk of inadequate nutrition related to side effects of cancer therapy

5) Risk of infection related to effects of therapy on bone marrow production of white blood cells and platelets

6) Anxiety related to diagnosis, prognosis, treatment, and pain

7) Ineffective individual coping related to diagnosis, fear, treatment, and pain

8) Ineffective family coping related to diagnosis, treatment, and fear

9) Fear related to prognosis and possible death

10) Anticipatory grieving related to cancer diagnosis and prognosis

11) Spiritual distress related to cancer diagnosis and prognosis

b. Goals, according to phase of illness

1) Acute phase

a) Demonstrate healthy lifestyle and remain free of signs and symptoms of infection.

b) Identify and use effective strategies for coping with stressful situations and adjusting to illness.

c) Verbalize understanding of the disease process and significant implications.

d) Verbalize understanding of the treatment regimen and side effects.

e) Verbalize discomfort.

2) Intermittent or chronic phase

a) Verbalize understanding of the prevention and management of side effects of the treatment regimen.

b) Maintain maximal level of function.

c) Demonstrate safety in mobility and use assistive devices as needed.

d) Verbalize understanding of diet management, maintain present weight, and maintain fluid hydration.

e) Verbalize discomfort.

3) Palliative phase
   a) Maintain a desired level of comfort.
   b) Verbalize wishes and declare preferences regarding treatment options.
   c) Experience a dignified and comfortable death.

3. Interventions
   a. Acute phase: To attain remission and prevent and control side effects of treatment
      1) Educate the client and family about the diagnosis, prognosis, treatment, side effects and symptoms, nutritional needs, risk of injury caused by immunosuppression medication, prevention of infections, and support groups.
      2) Provide emotional support by helping the client and family express grief.
      3) Minimize infection and use strategies to prevent infection.
      4) Provide education on pain relief measures and complications.
      5) Maximize comfort and provide pain relief with prescribed analgesics, accepting the client's report of pain, using a consistent method or scale to evaluate pain, and providing nonpharmacological methods of pain control (imagery, distraction, relaxation, music).
      6) Assess psychological response to situations and provide emotional support by helping the client and family express grief.
      7) Ensure adequate hydration and nutrition with vitamin supplements.
   b. Intermittent or chronic stage: To address side effects of treatment and complications
      1) Provide assistive devices for use in performing ADLs.
      2) Balance rest with activities to conserve energy.
      3) Prevent infection, adhering to strict handwashing protocols, maintaining aseptic technique, and monitoring for signs and symptoms of infection, administering antimicrobial therapy as needed.
      4) Assess response to pain management and maintain comfort.
   c. Palliative and end-of-life care: To provide comfort, emotional support, and symptom management and promote peaceful death
      1) Neither hasten nor postpone death.
      2) Assist with end-of-life comfort measures in a suitable care setting and with appropriate services (e.g., hospice).
      3) Help the client achieve as full a life as possible with relief from pain and other symptoms; administer pain medication to relieve pain and discomfort, antianxiety medication for anxiety and restlessness, antiemetics for nausea and vomiting.
      4) Offer support systems to help the client live as actively as possible until death.
      5) Promote a calm environment.
      6) Provide emotional and spiritual support to the client and significant others.
      7) Maintain the client's dignity and spiritual beliefs and wishes throughout the dying process.
      8) Educate the client and significant others about the dying process.
      9) Provide bereavement counseling for significant others.

   4. Evaluation: Modify care according to the client's response to nursing interventions, focusing on quality of life and comfort.

IV. Obesity
   A. Overview (Uwaifo & Arioglu, 2010)
      1. Obesity has become a public health crisis in the United States and the rest of the developed world.
      2. Obesity represents a state of excess storage of body fat.
         a. Grade 1 overweight (also called overweight) is identified by a BMI of 25–29.9 kg/m².
         b. Grade 2 overweight (commonly called obesity) is identified by a BMI of 30–39 kg/m².
         c. Grade 3 overweight (commonly called morbid obesity) is identified by a BMI of 40 kg/m² or above.
      3. Obesity occurs when more calories are taken in than are burned through activity and exercise.
      4. A waist circumference more than 25 inches for women and 30 inches for men indicates obesity.
      5. In children overweight is indicated by being at the 85th percentile, and obesity is indicated by the 95th percentile for age- and sex-matched control subjects.
      6. Genetics and environment appear to affect the development of obesity.
      7. Prevention and treatment of overweight and obesity are challenging.
      8. Overweight and obesity have been shown to increase the likelihood of certain diseases and health problems.
      9. Modest weight loss can improve or prevent health problems associated with obesity.

10. Obesity is associated with a substantial increase in morbidity and mortality rates.
11. Overall trends in obesity may be associated with a reduced longevity of the population in the next few years.
12. Age at onset, duration of obesity, severity of obesity, amount of central adiposity, other comorbidities, sex, and level of cardiorespiratory fitness modulate the morbidity and mortality associated with obesity.
13. Research shows that initial weight loss is the strongest factor for predicting weight loss treatment outcomes (Elfhag & Rossner, 2010).

B. Prevalence, Incidence, and Trends (Flegal, Carroll, Ogden, & Curtin, 2010; Uwaifo & Arioglu, 2010)
1. 100 million adults in the United States are overweight or obese (35% of women and 31% of men 19 years or older).
2. Prevalence in children increased to 15%–25% in children during the last few years; adults remain at 30%–50%.
3. Approximately 300,000 deaths per year may be attributable to obesity (CDC, 2010).
4. Population-based strategies that improve social and physical environmental contexts for healthful eating and physical activity are helpful for the entire population.
5. Pima Indians of Arizona and other Native-American populations have a particularly high prevalence of obesity.
6. Polynesians, Micronesians, Anurans, Maoris of the West and East Indies, African Americans in North America, and the Hispanic populations in North America have high predispositions to obesity.

C. Symptoms Associated with Obesity (Mayo Clinic, 2009)
1. Difficulty sleeping
2. Snoring
3. Sleep apnea
4. Pain in the back or joints
5. Excessive sweating
6. Always feeling hot
7. Rashes or infection in folds of the skin
8. Feeling out of breath with minor exertion
9. Daytime sleepiness or fatigue
10. Depression

D. Comorbidities (Uwaifo & Arioglu, 2010): Just about every body system is affected by obesity. Examples include the following:
1. Cardiovascular: Hypertension, coronary artery disease, cardiomyopathy, accelerated atherosclerosis, pulmonary hypertension of obesity

2. CNS: Stroke, idiopathic intracranial hypertension
3. Gastrointestinal tract: Cholecystitis, cholelithiasis, nonalcoholic steatohepatitis, fatty liver infiltration, reflux esophagitis
4. Respiratory tract: Obstructive sleep apnea, Pickwickian syndrome, predisposition to respiratory infections, increased incidence of bronchial asthma
5. Malignancies: An association with endometrial, prostate, gall bladder, breast, and colon cancer
6. Psychological: Social stigmatization, depression
7. Orthopedic: Osteoarthrosis, chronic lumbago
8. Metabolic: Insulin resistance; hyperinsulinemia, type 2 diabetes, high total cholesterol, high triglycerides, normal or elevated LDL, low HDL
9. Reproductive: Anovulation, early puberty, infertility, hyperandrogenism and polycystic ovaries in women and hypogonadotrophic hypogonadism in men
10. Obstetric and perinatal: Pregnancy-related hypertension, fetal macrosomia, and pelvic dystocia
11. Stress incontinence
12. Cutaneous: Bacterial or fungal infection, hirsutism, increased risk for cellulitis, carbuncles
13. Extremities: Venous varicosities, lower extremity venous, or lymphatic edema
14. Reduced mobility
15. Difficulty maintaining personal hygiene

E. Known Causes and Theories of Obesity (Peckenpaugh, 2010)
1. Caloric imbalance
2. Diet quality or composition and eating habits
3. Hormonal imbalance
4. Genetics and gender differences
5. Altered metabolism

F. Secondary Causes of Obesity (Uwaifo & Arioglu, 2010)
1. Hypothyroidism
2. Cushing's syndrome
3. Insulinoma
4. Hypothalamic obesity
5. Polycystic ovarian syndrome
6. Genetic syndromes such as Prader-Willi, Alström's, Bardet-Biedl, Cohen's, Börjeson-Forssman-Lehmann, and Fröhlich's syndrome; growth hormone deficiency
7. Oral contraceptive use
8. Pregnancy
9. Medications such as phenothiazines, sodium valproate, carbamazepine, tricyclic antidepressants, lithium, glucocorticoids, megestrol acetate, thiazolidinediones, sulfonylureas, insulin, adrenergic antagonists, serotonin antagonists

10. Smoking cessation
11. Eating disorders such as binge eating, bulimia nervosa, night eating disorder
12. Hypogonadism
13. Pseudohypoparathyroidism
14. Tube feeding-related obesity

G. Assessment of Developing Obesity (Uwaifo & Arioglu, 2010)
1. Evaluate the following:
   a. Metabolic factors
   b. Genetic factors
   c. Level of activity
   d. Behavior
   e. Endocrine factors
   f. Race, sex, age factors
   g. Ethnic and cultural factors
   h. Socioeconomic status
   i. Dietary habits
   j. Smoking cessation
   k. Pregnancy and menopause
   l. Psychologic factors
   m. History of gestational diabetes
   n. Evaluation for the aforementioned secondary causes
2. Consider the following clinical problems that might have similar findings: Dercum's disease, partial lipodystrophies; mesomorphic body states, anasarca (severe edema).
3. Laboratory tests: With no comorbidities, tests will be normal, but comorbid problems should be ruled out.
   a. Full lipid panel: At a minimum, test fasting cholesterol, triglycerides, and HDL cholesterol levels. These levels may be normal or the typical dyslipidemia associated with metabolic syndrome X may be found. This is characterized by low HDL, elevated LDLs, normal to marginally elevated total cholesterol, and elevated fasting triglyceride concentrations.
   b. Hepatic panel: This test is expected to yield normal results, but findings may be abnormal (e.g., elevated transaminase levels in the setting of nonalcoholic steatohepatitis or fatty infiltration of the liver).
   c. Thyroid function: The results are typically normal, but checking them to detect primary hypothyroidism (characterized by elevated serum thyrotropin and normal or low levothyroxine or triiodothyronine levels) is worthwhile. Hypothyroidism rarely causes more than mild obesity.
   d. Fasting glucose and A1c: Obesity and insulin resistance go hand in hand.

H. Treatment
1. Weight loss goals (Flegal et al., 2010)
   a. An initial goal of 5%–10% of body weight should be attainable.
   b. Clients often have unrealistic goals of 24%–38% weight loss, which tend to be unattainable.
2. Dietary changes: Work with dietitian to decide best dietary changes.
3. Starvation diets
   a. Starvation should be avoided and is not validated as an effective method of achieving substantial and sustained weight loss. Starvation is a caloric intake of less than 200 kcal/d.
   b. Starvation is potentially dangerous and can lead to starvation ketosis; electrolyte imbalances; and vitamin, mineral, and other micronutrient deficiencies.
   c. Very-low-calorie diets (VLCDs) are best used in an established, comprehensive program.
   d. VLCDs involve reducing caloric intake to 800 kcal/d or less. When used in optimal settings, they can achieve weight loss of 1.5–2.5 kg/wk, with a total loss of as much as 20 kg over 12 weeks.
   e. VLCDs are associated with profound initial weight loss, much of which is from lean mass loss during the first few weeks. However, this weight loss rapidly ceases.
   f. Compliance beyond a few weeks is poor, and close supervision is needed to avoid complications.
4. Conventional diets
   a. Classified as balanced, low-calorie diets (or reduced portion sizes); low-fat diets; low-carbohydrate diets; midlevel diets (e.g., Zone diet, in which the three major macronutrients [fat, carbohydrate, protein] are eaten in similar proportions of 30%–40%); and fad diets.
   b. Balanced low-calorie diets or reduced-portion diets are the types that dietitians and other weight management professionals most commonly prescribe.
5. Increased physical activity
   a. Exercise is vital to any weight management program because it helps build muscle mass and increase metabolic activity of the whole body mass.
   b. Exercise helps reduce body fat proportions and decreases the amount of compensatory muscle mass loss.

c. Consistent moderate exercise is important in maintaining weight and improving overall cardiorespiratory fitness.

d. Clients should undergo cardiovascular and respiratory screening before undergoing any exercise program.

6. Behavior changes: The effectiveness depends on both a highly motivated client and a dedicated counselor who is willing to maintain long-term follow-up.

7. Prescription medications

a. Not many medications are available for the treatment of obesity, and those that are available have minimal long-term effectiveness.

b. Caution must be taken when using medications for weight loss.

8. Weight loss surgery: Comorbidities must be stabilized and adequately treated before surgery.

I. Maintaining Weight Loss (Ross, 2009)

1. Maintaining weight loss is a challenge for many.

2. Continued contact with a healthcare provider is helpful.

3. Behavioral factors are associated with sustained weight loss.

4. Exercise specialists and dietitians can provide support.

5. Simple programs including self-weighing, increased physical activity, and reduced calories can be effective.

6. Self-weighing combined with face-to-face contact and continued dialogue is helpful.

J. Current Basic Research

1. Leptin (Uwaifo & Arioglu, 2010)

a. 16-kDa protein produced predominantly by white adipose tissue

b. Myriad functions in carbohydrate, bone, and reproductive metabolism

c. In weight regulation, it signals satiety to the hypothalamus.

d. Higher circulating leptin levels are associated with a higher risk of congestive heart failure and cardiovascular disease

e. Leptin levels do not predict cardiovascular disease.

f. Research is continuing.

2. Thrifty gene hypothesis (Neal)

a. There is a mismatch between today's environment and energy-thrifty genes that multiplied in the past under different environmental conditions when food sources were not predictable.

b. The same genes that helped our ancestors survive occasional famines are now being challenged by the availability of food.

K. Rehabilitation

1. Research

a. An excessive BMI does not prevent gains during inpatient rehabilitation after knee arthroplasty; however, these gains are made less efficiently and at a higher cost than those made when the BMI is low (Vincent & Vincent, 2008).

b. Obese people with chronic obstructive pulmonary disease in pulmonary rehabilitation programs benefit at the same rate as normal-weight people (Greening, 2010; Sava, Laviolette, & Maltais, 2009).

c. Obese people with chronic low back pain showed a higher degree of spinal impairment and increased lumbar lordosis. Rehabilitation should include strengthening of lumbar and abdominal muscles and mobility exercises for the thoracic spine and pelvis (Vismara et al., 2010).

d. In a retrospective study, morbidly obese rehabilitation clients needed a longer length of stay to achieve Functional Independence Measure gains comparable to those of the nonmorbidly obese. They also had a higher rate of discharge to home and a higher rate of return to acute hospitalization than the nonobese population (Thananopavarn, Carrion-Jones, Nunez, Slayton, & Wong, 2007).

2. Rehabilitation nursing key requirements

a. Provide bariatric furniture and equipment (e.g., commodes, wheelchairs, beds, walkers).

b. Know your facility's safe client handling policy.

c. Increase the number of staff to assist with procedures, transfers, and moves.

d. Use bariatric lifts and assistive devices for your safety and that of the client.

e. Use blood pressure cuffs that are large enough for your client.

f. Perform frequent skin inspections, turning, and positioning. Remember to keep skin creases clean and dry.

g. Treat your client with dignity and respect.

L. Plan of Care: In addition to the rehabilitation plan of care, the client who is obese has the following needs (Harris, 2008):

1. Nursing diagnoses

a. Ineffective individual coping related to denial and depression

b. Knowledge deficit related to causes of weight gain and treatments for obesity

c. Self-care deficits related to the following:
   1) Physical, social, economic, and psychological barriers and limitations
   2) Lack of knowledge about complications of obesity
   3) Lack of financial and social support systems
   4) Lack of knowledge about follow-up needs and prevention of further complications related to the disease process
d. Altered nutritional intake (more than a body needs) related to lack of awareness about serving sizes, limited self-discipline, and non-compliance with dietary guidelines
e. Activity intolerance related to sedentary lifestyle

2. Goals
   a. State barriers to and develop methods of effective coping to avoid overeating.
   b. Verbalize an understanding of the relationship between weight loss, weight control, and exercise.
   c. Lose 1 pound per week.
   d. Identify behavioral modification strategies to avoid overeating.
   e. Practice selecting proper serving sizes of favorite foods.
   f. Identify individual concerns with and compensate for sexual dysfunction.
   g. Identify and obtain needed adaptive equipment.
   h. Exercise at least 30 minutes 5 days per week.

3. Interventions
   a. Teach coping strategies (e.g., stress management, humor, breathing exercises, support groups).
   b. Discuss current eating habits and strategies to reduce calorie intake.
   c. Promote identification and selection of proper food choices.
   d. Discuss cues that promote eating. Identify strategies to eliminate or reduce these cues.
   e. Teach the strategy of keeping a food diary to monitor dietary pattern changes.
   f. Discuss the role of exercise in weight loss and maintenance.
   g. Instruct the client to keep an exercise record to document time and intensity of exercise.
   h. Teach survival skills and suggest follow-up education and self-management support as needed after discharge from the hospital.
   i. Discuss follow-up care, lifestyle, and behavior modification strategies to promote successful weight loss.

V. **Advanced Practice for Specific Disease Processes That Warrant Rehabilitation Interventions**
   A. Clinician
      1. The goal of treatment is to prevent the onset of disease process or injury through education about healthy living, reduction of risk factors, support and treatment of symptoms, and prevention of further complications.
      2. Assess history, clinical presentation, and current treatment.
      3. Complete a physical examination.
      4. Assess effectiveness of treatment and medications.
      5. Assess psychosocial and economic factors that may influence the management of the disorder or injury.
      6. Assess coping mechanisms and available support systems.
      7. Follow up with the client as needed according to the progression of the disease, complications, and effects of current treatment.
      8. Role model use of evidence in practice.
   B. Educator
      1. Educate the client, family, and significant others about the disease process, course, signs and symptoms, and treatment options.
      2. Provide education about prescribed medications and adverse effects.
      3. Discuss prevention strategies, emphasizing the need to reduce risk factors that can be changed.
      4. Educate and encourage participation in local and national support groups.
      5. Teach the client, family, and significant others to assist with active and passive exercises to prevent further complications and maintain independence in mobility and ADLs.
      6. Teach the importance of eating a nutritious diet according to the disorder and injury.
      7. Encourage regular rest periods and daily activity and teach the client to balance rest with activity to prevent fatigue.
   C. Leader
      1. Provide in-service education to interdisciplinary staff in acute care about specific disease processes, clinical manifestations, interventions, and treatment options.
      2. Provide community education about disease prevention, healthy living, specific disease processes, treatment options, and prevention of further complications.
      3. Update protocols and procedures and implement changes in practice reflecting evidence-based practice.

4. Participate in research and translate research into practice.
5. Keep abreast of current literature and disseminate appropriate articles to clinical staff.
6. Actively participate in specialty nursing organizations focusing on policy and practice.
7. Consider implementing journal clubs.

D. Consultant
1. Refer to or consult with a specialist (neurologist, urologist, oncologist, burn specialist, HIV and AIDS specialist, endocrinologist, obesity surgeon) for an evaluation and complete workup.
2. Function as a liaison with community health professionals.
3. Refer to a national organization or chapters for education and support.
   a. American Diabetes Association: www.diabetes.org
   b. American Association of Diabetes Educators: http://aadenet.org/
   c. National Diabetes Education Program: www.ndep.nih.gov/
   d. CDC National Diabetes Fact Sheets: www.cdc.gov/diabetes/pubs/factsheet.htm
   e. National Association of People with AIDS: www.napwa.org/
   f. CDC HIV/AIDS: www.cdc.gov/hiv/
   g. American Cancer Society: www.cancer.org/
   h. American Association for Cancer Research: www.aacr.org/
   i. National Cancer Institute: www.cancer.gov/
   j. The American Obesity Association: www.obesity.org/
4. Refer to and collaborate with the rehabilitation team for therapy.
5. Refer the client and family for psychological counseling to help them cope with the diagnosis and prognosis.
6. Serve as a client and family advocate.
7. Serve as a resource to staff.

E. Researcher (Levin & Feldman, 2006)
1. Review current research on significant diagnostic categories.
2. Participate in clinical research studies as appropriate and available.
3. Help staff nurses develop research questions.
4. Serve as a mentor for staff nurses regarding quality improvement, evidence-based practice, and research.
5. Locate evidence for staff nurses to assist with bedside research.

6. Facilitate system change to support use of evidence-based practice.
7. Support research at the bedside (or clinic).

References

About.com: Cancer. (2007). *Grilling and cancer.* Retrieved August 5, 2010, from http://cancer.about.com/od/foodguide/a/grillingmeat.htm.

American Cancer Society. (2010). *Signs and symptoms of cancer.* Retrieved July 25, 2011, from www.cancer.org/cancer/cancerbasics/signs-and-symptoms-of-cancer

American Cancer Society. (2011). *Cancer facts and figures 2011.* Retrieved July 25, 2011, from www.cancer.org/acs/groups/content/@epidemiologysurveillance/documents/document/acspc-029771.pdf

American Diabetes Association. (2010a). Diagnosis and classification of diabetes mellitus. *Diabetes Care, 33,* S62–S69.

American Diabetes Association (ADA). (2010b). Standards of medical care in diabetes: 2010. *Diabetes Care, 33,* S11–S61.

Amylin Pharmaceuticals, Inc. (2010). Byetta (exenatide injection) [package insert]. San Diego, CA: Amylin Pharmaceuticals, Inc. Retrieved February 18, 2007, from http://pi.lilly.com/us/byetta-pi.pdf.

Avert.org. (2010). *HIV types, subtypes groups and strains.* Retrieved on July 26, 2010, from www.avert.org/hiv-types.htm.

Bailey, C., & Barnett, A. (2010). Inhaled insulin: New formulation, new trial. *Lancet, 375*(9733), 2199–2201.

Cancer.Net Editorial Board. (2009). *Rehabilitation.* Retrieved August 6, 2010, from www.cancer.net/patient/Survivorship/Rehabilitation.

Centers for Disease Control and Prevention. (2006). *MMWR recommendations and reports.* Retrieved July 25, 2011, from www.cdc.gov/mmwr/preview/mmwrhtml/rr5514a1.htm.

Centers for Disease Control and Prevention. (2007a). *HIV Counseling with rapid tests.* Retrieved July 25, 2011, from www.cdc.gov/hiv/topics/testing/resources/factsheet/rt_counseling.htm.

Centers for Disease Control and Prevention. (2007b). *National diabetes fact sheet: General information and national estimates on diabetes in the United States, 2007.* Retrieved June 29, 2010, from www.cdc.gov/diabetes/pubs/pdf/ndfs_2007.pdf.

Centers for Disease Control and Prevention. (2009). *HIV-AIDS in the United States. CDC HIV/AIDS facts.* Retrieved July 14, 2010, from www.cdc.gov/hiv/resources/factsheets/us.htm.

Centers for Disease Control and Prevention. (2010). *Obesity prevention.* Retrieved July 15, 2010, from www.thecommunityguide.org/obesity/index.html.

Chitre, M. M., & Burke, S. (2006). Treatment algorithms and the pharmacological management of Type 2 diabetes. *Diabetes Spectrum, 19,* 249–255.

Diabetes Health. (2006, June). Your complete insulin reference guide from *Diabetes Health. Diabetes Health,* 38–41.

Diabetes Mall. (2010). *Diabetes medications.* Retrieved July 19, 2010, from www.diabetesnet.com/diabetes_information/diabetes_medications.php#ixzz0uB5nDGd2.

Elfhag, K., & Rossner, S. (2010). Initial weight loss is the best predictor for success in obesity treatment and sociodemographic liabilities increase risk for drop-out. *Patient Education and Counseling, 79,* 361–366.

Fan, H. Y., Conner, R. F., & Villarreal, L. P. (2011). *AIDS science and society* (6th ed.). Sudbury, MA: Jones & Bartlett.

Fayed, L. (2009). *Top 10 ways to prevent cancer.* Retrieved August 12, 2010, from http://cancer.about.com/od/causes/tp/topreventcancer.htm.

Feigenbaum, K. (2006). Treating gastroparesis. *Diabetes Self-Management, 23*(5), 24–32.

Flegal, K. M., Carroll, M. D., Ogden, C. L., & Curtin, L. R. (2010). Prevalence and trends in obesity among US adults, 1999–2008. *JAMA, 303*(3), 235–242.

Genuth, S. (2006, January–February). Insights from the Diabetes Control and Complications Trial/Epidemiology of Diabetes Interventions and Complications study on the use of intensive glycemic treatment to reduce the risk of complications of Type 1 diabetes. *Endocrine Practice, 12*(Suppl. 1), 34–41.

Greening, N. (2010). *The effects of pulmonary rehabilitation on extreme obesity in COPD.* American Thoracic Society Meeting, New Orleans. Retrieved August 10, 2010, from www.medpagetoday.com/MeetingsCoverage/ATS/20147.

Harris, H. (2008). Nursing care of the morbidly obese patient. *Nursing Made Incredibly Easy, 6*(3), 34–43.

Health-Disease.org. (2011). *Acquired immunodificiency syndrome—Causes and treatment.* Retrieved July 28, 2011, from www.health-disease.org/immune-disorders/acquired-immunodificiency-syndrome.htm.

Joint United Nations Programme on HIV/AIDS (UNAIDS). (2009). *09 AIDS epidemic update.* www.unaids.org/en/KnowledgeCentre/HIVData/EpiUpdate/EpiUpdArchive/2009/default.asp

LaSalle, J. (2006). New insulin analogs insulin detemir and insulin glulisine. *Practical Diabetology, 25*(3), 34–44.

Leahy, J. L., Clark, N. G., & Cefalu, W. T. (Eds.). (2000). *Medical management of diabetes mellitus.* Burlington: University of Vermont College of Medicine.

Levin, R., & Feldman, H. (Ed.). (2006). *Teaching evidence based practice in nursing.* New York: Springer.

Lewis, S. M., Heitkemper, M. M., & Dirksen, S. R. (2004). *Medical-surgical nursing: Assessment and management of clinical problems* (6th ed.). St. Louis: Mosby.

Lifeclinic. (2010). *Devices for taking insulin.* Retrieved August 10, 2010, from www.lifeclinic.com/focus/diabetes/supply_syringes.asp.

Martz, K., Keresztes, K., Tatschl, C., Nowotny, M., Dachenhausen, A., Brainin, M., et al. (2006). Disorders of glucose metabolism in acute stroke patients: An underrecognized problem. *Diabetes Care, 29,* 792–797.

Mayo Clinic. (2009). *Obesity.* Retrieved July 15, 2010, from www.mayoclinic.com/health/obesity/DS00314.

Mayo Clinic. (2010). *Spinal tumor.* Retrieved August 7, 2010, from www.mayoclinic.com/health/spinal-tumor/DS00594.

McKennon, S. A., & Campbell, R. K. (2007). The physiology of incretin hormones and the basis for DPP-4 inhibitors. *The Diabetes Educator, 33*(1), 55–46.

Meriter Health Services. (2010). Prandase (acarbose) [product monograph]. Toronto, ON: Bayer. Retrieved August 16, 2011, from http://meriter.staywellsolutionsonline.com/RelatedItems/26,2.

Monahan, F. D., Sands, J. K., Neighbors, M., Marek, J. F., & Green, C. J. (2007). *Phipps' medical-surgical nursing: Health and illness perspectives* (8th ed.). St. Louis: Mosby Elsevier.

Muscat, J. E., Malkin, M. G., Thompson, S., Shore, R. E., Stellman, S. D., McRee, D., et al. (2000). Handheld cellular telephone use and the risk of brain cancer. *Journal of the American Medical Association, 284,* 3001–3007.

National Cancer Institute. (2006). *Gene therapy for cancer: Questions and answers.* Retrieved December 2, 2006, from www.cancer.gov/cancertopics/factsheet/Therapy/gene.

National Cancer Institute. (2008a). *Bone cancer questions and answers.* Retrieved August 8, 2010, from www.cancer.gov/cancertopics/factsheet/sites-types/bone.

National Cancer Institute. (2008b). *Bone marrow transplantation and peripheral blood stem cell transplantation.* Retrieved August 8, 2010, from www.cancer.gov/cancertopics/factsheet/Therapy/bone-marrow-transplant.

National Cancer Institute. (2009). *What is cancer?* Retrieved June 29, 2010, from www.cancer.gov/cancertopics/what-is-cancer.

National Cancer Institute. (2010a). *Acupuncture (PDQ).* Retrieved August 9, 2010, from www.cancer.gov/cancertopics/pdq/cam/acupuncture/HealthProfessional/allpages#Section_1.

National Cancer Institute. (2010b). *Adult brain tumors treatment (PDQ).* Retrieved August 6, 2010, from www.cancer.gov/cancertopics/pdq/treatment/adultbrain/HealthProfessional.

National Cancer Institute. (2010c). *Bone cancer.* Retrieved August 6, 2010, from www.cancer.gov/cancertopics/types/bone.

National Cancer Institute. (2010d). *Cancer prevention overview.* Retrieved June 29, 2010, from www.cancer.gov/cancertopics/pdq/prevention/overview/healthprofessional.

National Cancer Institute. (2010e). *Cancer trends progress report: 2009/2010 update.* Retrieved June 29, 2010, from http://progressreport.cancer.gov/highlights.asp.

National Cancer Institute (NCI). (2011). *Common cancer types.* Retrieved July 28, 2011, from www.cancer.gov/cancertopics/types/commoncancers.

Odegard, P. S. D., Setter, S. M., & Iltz, J. L. (2006). Update in the pharmacologic treatment of diabetes mellitus focus on pramlintide and exenatide. *The Diabetes Educator, 32,* 693–712.

Panel on Antiretroviral Guidelines for Adults and Adolescents. (2009, December 1). *Guidelines for the use of antiretroviral agents in HIV-1-infected adults and adolescents.* Department of Health and Human Services, pp. 1–161. Retrieved July 10, 2010, from www.aidsinfo.nih.gov/ContentFiles/AdultandAdolescentGL.pdf.

Peckenpaugh, N. J. (2010). *Nutrition essentials and diet therapy* (11th ed.). Philadelphia: Saunders.

Ross, R. (2009). The challenge of obesity treatment: Avoiding weight regain. *Canadian Medical Association Journal, 180*(10), 997.

Sava, F., Laviolette, L., & Maltais, F. (2009). Impact of obesity on functional status and response to rehabilitation in patients with COPD. *American Journal of Respiratory and Critical Care Medicine, 179.*

Thananopavarn, P., Carrion-Jones, M., Nunez, A., Slayton, S., & Wong, D. (2007). *Inpatient rehabilitation trends in the morbidly obese population.* Archives of Physical Medicine and Rehabilitation, 88.

Unwin, N., Whiting, D., Gan, D., Jacqmain, O., & Ghyoot, G. (Eds.). (2009). *IDF diabetes atlas.* Retrieved July 5, 2010, from www.diabetesatlas.org/content/diabetes.

Uwaifo, G. I., & Arioglu, E. (2010). *Obesity.* Retrieved July 15, 2010, from http://emedicine.medscape.com/article/123702.

Vincent, H., & Vincent, K. (2008). Obesity and inpatient rehabilitation outcomes following knee arthroplasty: A multicenter study. *Obesity, 16,* 130–136.

Vismara, L., Menegoni, F., Zaina, F., Galli, M., Negrini, S., & Capadaglio, P. (2010). Effect of obesity and low back pain on spinal mobility: A cross sectional study in women. *Journal of NeuroEngineering and Rehabilitation.* Retrieved August 9, 2010, from www.jneuroengrehab.com/content/7/1/3.

Vogel, W. H., Wilson, M. A., & Melvin, M. S. (2004). *Advanced practice oncology and palliative care guidelines.* Philadelphia: Lippincott Williams & Wilkins.

Zingman, B. (2010). *Diagnosis and management of acute HIV infection.* Retrieved July 21, 2010, from www.medscape.com/viewarticle/724634.

Suggested Reading

Centers for Disease Control and Prevention. (2008). *National diabetes fact sheet: General information and national estimates in diabetes in the United States, 2007.* Atlanta, GA: Author.

Suggested Resources

Centers for Disease Control and Prevention. (2010). *Basic information about HIV and AIDS.* Retrieved July 15, 2010, from www.cdc.gov/hiv/topics/basic/print/index.htm.

U.S. Department of Health and Human Services. (2006a). *HIV and its treatment: What you should know—Health information for patients.*

U.S. Department of Health and Human Services. (2006b). *Recommended HIV treatment regimens.* Retrieved December 2, 2006, from www.aidsinfo.nih.gov/ContentFiles/RecommendedHIVTreatmentRegimens_FS_en.pdf.

CHAPTER 17
A Lifespan Perspective on Individuals and Families

Mindi Miller, PhD MSN MA RN CRRN

A rich multidisciplinary history of theory building addresses human growth across the lifespan. Numerous interdisciplinary models depict aspects of physical, cognitive, emotional, and social development. Family concepts are tied to cultural beliefs and relationship values. In short, human growth and development involves a fluctuating milieu through which assorted tasks are accomplished. Choices and behavioral patterns lead to successful or unsuccessful management of life and its circumstances. Issues of compliance and independence correlate with personality traits, learning preferences, and moral decision making.

Nurses select and create theories to improve quality of life for their clients. Holistic care incorporates the client's development needs, social networks, and lifestyle preferences. Nurses plan interventions and perform research to measure outcomes related to various theories. As described within the Gestalt theory developed by Max Wertheimer in the 1920s, the whole is greater than the sum of its parts. Pieces and parts fit together to produce thoughts, actions, and structures, such as family units (Ellis, 1938; Goodman, 2009). Theories such as the Gestalt theory are invaluable to healthcare providers. A theory is more than a speculation; theories become methods for discovering the "whole." This chapter provides highlights from diverse viewpoints and models that can be applied to rehabilitation nursing. Key content includes the following:

- An overview of interdisciplinary philosophies and models related to lifelong growth and development.
- A summary of nursing theories applicable to rehabilitation nursing.
- A review of theories to better address healthcare challenges for age-specific clients.
- Examples of applicability of diverse frameworks to better understand and care for rehabilitation clients with complex needs.

I. Developmental Theories
   A. Overview
     1. Theories provide systematic statements to explain human phenomena.
     2. Models provide structure for testing new hypotheses about human growth and development.
     3. Theories can be organized in a variety of ways, although traditional headings are psychoanalytic, learning, cognitive, behavioral, and interactive (Boyd & Bee, 2006).

     4. Models that relate to milestones of age, personality, multiple intelligence, social interaction, family function, and moral development add to the mix of traditional conceptual frameworks (Shenk, 2009; Townsend, 2010).
     5. Nursing assessment, diagnosis, intervention, outcomes, and resultant reevaluation depend on a firm understanding of interdisciplinary theories (see a summary of individual development and functional theories in **Table 17-1**).
   B. Intrapsychic (Psychoanalytic) Theories
     1. Sigmund Freud (1856–1939), the early and long-dominant theorist in the field of personality development, is responsible for intrapsychic theory.
       a. People experience conflict between their natural instincts and society's restrictions on them.
       b. Conflict experienced in childhood influences one's adult personality (Freud, 1959; Gay, 2006).
       c. Four phases occur within set timeframes.
       d. Fixation (oral, anal, phallic) may result if phases are not achieved successfully.
         1) Oral phase: First year of life
          a) Involves exploring the world orally, and the mouth, lips, and tongue are the center of existence for the infant.
          b) Begins development of the infant's personality, which depends on the mother's (or mothering person's or caretaker's) sense of personal security in self and satisfaction in the mother role.
          c) The infant experiences maternal feelings, leading to vulnerability (e.g., if the mother's anxiety is pervasive and the infant begins life with a deficit in adaptive abilities).
          d) Weaning from breastfeeding may be challenging.
         2) Anal phase: 18 months to 3 years of age
          a) This phase centers on buildup and release of tension in the orifices; involves experiencing pleasure in expelling urine and feces.
          b) It is challenging for parents' coping ability to allow their child to move away and seek freedom or a greater sense of self.

Table 17-1. Summary of Individual Development and Function Theories

Theory and Theorist*	Description	Periods			
		Infancy (0–12 months)	Birth–2 years old	Toddler (12–36 months)	2–7 years old
Intrapsychic (Freud, 1959)	Conflict between an individuals' natural instincts and society's restrictions on them experienced in childhood influence individuals' adult personality; children are thought to progress through four stages of psychosexual development (Glod, 1998; Whiting, 1997).	Oral	N/A	Anal	N/A
Interpersonal (Sullivan, 1956, 1971)	Repeated experiences between parents or caretakers and children lead to development of a good self and a bad self, which is the basis for healthy development; six stages represent processes by which an individual's identity develops in the context of relationships (Glod, 1998; Whiting, 1997).	Infancy	N/A	Childhood	N/A
Social Learning (Erikson, 1963)	Interaction between parents or caretakers and the child is essential to healthy psychological growth; each phase of normal development requires the individual to accomplish age-appropriate developmental tasks through eight phases of development from infancy to older adulthood (Glod, 1998).	Trust vs. mistrust	N/A	Autonomy vs. shame and doubt	N/A
Behavioral (Pavlov, 1927; Skinner, 1953)	Individuals' development is influenced by stimulus-response interaction; individuals' behavior is shaped through the consistency of responding; two attributes of the human brain—flexibility and plasticity—allow for a developmentally significant variety of adaptive sequences (Glod, 1998).	N/A	N/A	N/A	N/A
Interactional (Schaie, 1981)	Development of individuals in a progressive direction occurs when goodness of fit (consonance) exists; poorness of fit (dissonance) involves discrepancies between individuals and their environment, which results in distorted development and maladaptive functioning; starting with dependency in infancy, interference with development of independence in adolescence is likely to inhibit the establishment of interdependence in adulthood (Schaie, 1981; Whiting, 1997).	Dependency	N/A	N/A	N/A
Cognitive (Piaget, 1952)	Motor activity involving concrete objects results in the development of mental functioning; children move through four general periods of cognitive development in the same sequence although not according to the same timetable (Glod, 1998).	N/A	Sensorimotor	N/A	Preoperational

Major Points

• Human development is a complex, interactive, and multifaceted process that involves a variety of forces.

• Some older theories of development (Freud, 1959; Piaget, 1952) emphasize completion of development early in childhood.

• Other theories (Pavlov, 1927; Skinner, 1953) are not age-specific but allow for a developmentally significant diversity of adaptive sequences.

*Many theories (Erikson, 1963; Schaie, 1981; Sullivan, 1956, 1971) view individual development as a continuous process that unfolds throughout the lifespan rather than as a process that is limited to a few early years in relationships with limited numbers of people (Glod, 1998; Whiting, 1997).

| | | | | Periods | | | | |
Preschooler (3–5 years old)	School age (5–12 years old)	7–11 years old	11–15 years old	Childhood (1–12 years old)	Adolescence (12–18 years old)	Early adulthood (18–25 years old)	Adulthood (26–65 years old)	Older adulthood (older than 65 years old)
Phallic, oedipal	Latent and genital	N/A	N/A	N/A	N/A	N/A	N/A	N/A
Childhood, juvenile	Juvenile, preadolescence	N/A	N/A	N/A	Early to late adolescence	Adulthood	Adulthood (continues)	Adulthood (continues)
Initiative vs. guilt	Industry vs. inferiority	N/A	N/A	N/A	Identity vs. role confusion	Intimacy vs. isolation	Generativity vs. stagnation	Integrity vs. despair
N/A	N/A	N/A	N/A	N/A	N/A	N/A	N/A	N/A
N/A	N/A	N/A	N/A	Decreasing dependency	Dependency to independence	Inter-dependency (adulthood)	Inter-dependency (adulthood continues)	Inter-dependency (adulthood continues)
N/A	N/A	Concrete operational	Formal operational	N/A	N/A	N/A	N/A	N/A

c) It involves ambivalence related to complying with parental and societal values of elimination.
  i. Complying through proper elimination on the part of the infant
  ii. Complying through retention or inappropriate discharge of feces or urine by the infant, which brings retribution and further anxiety
  iii. Toilet training by the parents and the infant's corresponding response, which can govern adult personality
3) Phallic phase: 3 to 6 years of age
  a) Becomes aware of gender roles and how males and females differ
    i. Has romantic attraction to the parent of the opposite sex (Oedipus complex, boys, and Electra, girls)
    ii. Experiences rivalry with the same-sex parent or resolves guilt and fear by identifying with the same-sex parent
  b) Develops a conscience
    i. Represses sexual urges
    ii. Imitates sex-related behaviors and beliefs of the parent of the same sex
    iii. Child learns standards of society from parents.
4) Latent and genital phase: 6 to 12 years (latent) and puberty (genital)
  a) Learns to hide sexuality or sublimate urges with hobbies and sports
  b) Learns social rules while experiencing sexual gratification related to feelings toward others
  c) Involves responses during the preceding stages
  d) May cause serious adjustment problems if not accomplished and brought into adulthood (i.e., person is unable to turn away from the self to a more productive activity) and may produce sexual problems
  e) Brings out defensive measures used in earlier phases (e.g., denial and regression; Freud, 1959)
e. Other concepts developed by Freud include theories of personality and coping.
  1) Levels of awareness influence personality.

a) The conscious mind is aware of the current moment.
b) The preconscious mind pays attention to details that are brought to conscious awareness.
c) The subconscious mind drives behavior.
2) Transference: Projecting onto another person
  a) Paternal transference (e.g., father figure) to promote feelings of security or authority
  b) Maternal transference, symbolizing unconditional love, or fairy godmother or wicked witch
  c) Sibling transference, brother or sister role development to substitute absent parental influences
  d) Nonfamiliar transference, treating others as stereotyped or envisioned rather than actual
3) Components of personality interrelate feelings, thoughts, and behaviors.
  a) The id is pleasure seeking, with primitive (animal-like) drives that do not perceive reality.
  b) The ego (agent of adaptation) is aware of reality and identifies consequences of behaviors.
  c) The superego (self-evaluation) houses values and recognizes social morals of right and wrong.
4) Tension may result in various forms of anxiety.
  a) Reality anxiety is diminished by taking oneself out of an anxiety-producing situation.
  b) Fear of punishment is largely unconscious (from the id) and may result in neurotic anxiety.
  c) Moral anxiety from violating values or moral codes may result in feelings of guilt and shame.
5) Defense mechanisms and reality distortions result from conflicts between the id, ego, and superego.
  a) Denial: Believing something false as true
  b) Displacement: Placing emotions elsewhere, onto a substitute
  c) Intellectualization: Objectively analyzing an issue or situation
  d) Projection: Blaming feelings on others

e) Regression: Behavior younger than age or previous developmental phase

f) Repression: Unpleasant thoughts pushed into the subconscious

g) Sublimation: Redirecting bad or wrong urges into socially acceptable forms

f. Freud's phases are criticized by others for lacking research data to support suppositions, although his models of behavior show relevancy as metaphors that depict his observations (Gay, 2006).

g. Freud's models have served as a springboard for later theories and philosophies (Tauber, 2010).

2. Anna Freud (1895–1982) expanded her father's views, which differed from those of others during this time period, such as Carl Jung and Alfred Adler.

a. Anna's theories were more practical and concentrated on child psychology and the study of personality.

b. She standardized records of children, noting that adult labels did not apply to problems of children.

3. Alfred Adler (1870–1937) researched the significance of birth order.

a. Adler expanded theories of personality to include aspects of superiority, inferiority, and self-actualization.

b. He identified a connection between illness and handicaps with the person's self-image and personality.

4. Carl Jung (1875–1961) developed analytical (or Jungian) psychology.

a. Jung proposed the collective unconscious that devised psychic or mental patterns.

b. Dreams, religion, and other symbols influenced a person's view of the world.

C. Interpersonal Theories

1. Harry Stack Sullivan (1892–1949) developed the interpersonal theory associated with potential personality factor.

a. Sullivan's theory departed from Freudian concepts; Sullivan believed the personality is developed from interaction with social groups (Barton, 1996).

b. The term *integrating tendencies* describes behavior by which one person moves toward another person.

c. Healthy development is based on repeated experiences between parents or caretakers and children that lead to the development of a good self and a bad self.

d. Seven stages of development represent processes by which the person's identity develops in the context of relationships.

1) Infancy: Developing senses of sequential time and self-representations of good and bad

2) Childhood: Beginning to develop interpersonal relationships with peers, language skills, and gender identity

3) Preadolescence juvenile: Expanding interactions to social, group, and societal relationships

4) Preadolescence: Same-sex relationship with ability to form meaningful nondependent peer relationships

5) Early adolescence: Developing sexuality and gender identity

6) Late adolescence: Beginning to assume responsibility

7) Adulthood: Containing these interpersonal themes that continue to emerge in new relationships

2. Personality is shaped by relationships.

a. Difficulties in development are viewed as manifestations of disordered interpersonal relationships (Sullivan, 1956).

b. Psychotherapy aims to understand interactions to improve participation and to facilitate connections (Barton, 1996; Goodman, 2009).

3. Frieda Fromm-Reichmann (1889–1957) and Clara Mabel Thompson (1893–1958) wrote extensively on the topic of interpersonal development.

4. Both worked with Harry Sullivan to establish the William Alanson White Institute to train psychotherapists.

5. Both addressed cultural influences and humanistic aspects of psychoanalysis, concentrating on interpersonal relationships (Bradberry, 2007; Carducci, 2009).

D. Social Learning Theories

1. Erik Erikson (1902–1994) suggested that interactions between parent or caretaker and child are essential to healthy psychological growth (i.e., parents raise the child, and the child influences the parents).

a. Through satisfactory completion of the developmental task of each psychosocial stage, people become ready to move through the stages of development from infancy to adulthood (Erikson, 1963).

b. There are eight sequential psychosocial stages.
  1) Trust versus mistrust (infancy)
     a) Viewing the universe as reliable
     b) Seeing relationships as stable and available
  2) Autonomy versus shame and doubt (toddlerhood)
     a) Understanding control over one's body and thinking
     b) Understanding disappointment in self and others
  3) Initiative versus guilt (preschool years): Dealing with predominantly genital issues
  4) Industry versus inferiority (school age): Dealing with latency, school, and relationships outside the family
  5) Identity versus role confusion (adolescence)
     a) Clarifying personal identity
     b) Depersonifying internal representations
  6) Intimacy versus isolation (young adulthood)
     a) Rediscovering attachment
     b) Developing mature bonding
  7) Generativity versus stagnation (middle adulthood)
     a) Being creative and productive
     b) Carrying out parental responsibilities
  8) Integrity versus despair (older adulthood): Feeling a sense of completeness based on an integrated philosophy of one's unique life (Erikson, 1963)
2. Joan Erikson (1920–1997) continued her husband's work on the eighth and the new ninth stage (Erikson, Erikson, & Kivnick, 1986).
  a. Using notes and her own ideas, she articulated the gerotranscendence stage.
  b. In the ninth stage, people experience a change of focus, shifting values from materialistic things to life satisfaction goals.
  c. This theory is relevant to the aging population with longer life spans (Jarvis, 2001).
3. Albert Bandura (1925–present) theorized that behavior is learned by observing and modeling others.
  a. Social learning results from attention, retention, reproduction, and motivation.
  b. He developed an additional theory related to self-efficacy, a belief in one's own ability to manage situations and challenges (Bandura, 1997).

c. Theories of belief, choice, and behavior may have dual classifications between developmental and behavioral frameworks (Newman & Newman, 2009).
E. Significance for Rehabilitation
  1. Milestones of age and developmental tasks are taken into consideration within the treatment milieu.
  2. Psychoanalytic theories assist with identifying appropriate age-specific coping mechanisms when dealing with life-changing events.

II. Behavioral Theories
A. Overview
  1. Ivan Pavlov (1849–1936) and B. F. Skinner (1904–1990) studied how behavior is affected by its consequences.
  2. Behavior is reportedly developed through a stimulus-response interaction.
  3. Human behavior is derived largely from childhood experiences (Sigelman & Rider, 2009; Skinner, 1953).
B. Classical Conditioning Theory
  1. Conditioning occurs when a once-neutral stimulus becomes analogous with a response after they have been associated with each other (Pavlov, 1927).
  2. Derived in part from Pavlov's work with dogs, behavioral theory suggests that internal responses can be changed by modifying behavior.
  3. Classical conditioning results in automatic responses evoked by a stimulus.
C. Environmental Consequences of Behavior Theory
  1. Skinner's theory extends Pavlovian theory to human beings.
  2. Learning is influenced by the effect of individuals' behaviors.
  3. Behavior is shaped with positive and negative reinforcers, increasing or decreasing the likelihood that a given action will result or learning will occur (Skinner, 1953).
  4. His views have also been classified as learning theories.
D. Interactional Model
  1. K. Warner Schaie (1928–present) focused on development from young adulthood to older ages.
  2. He developed the concept of goodness of fit (consonance) versus dissonance (Schaie, 1981).
  3. Adult outcomes may be influenced by childhood events and adolescent experiences.
     a. Consonance involves having environmental demands and expectations in accord with one's capacity to respond.
     b. A sense of comfort or consonance makes optimal development possible.

c. Progression from dependence to interdependence occurs through developmental stages.

d. Adaptation corresponds with the demands of a child's chronological age and particular interests.
   1) Dependency in infancy (0–1 year of age)
   2) Decreasing dependency in childhood (1–12 years of age)
   3) Dependency conflict in early adolescence, with struggling toward independence in middle adolescence and independence achieved in late adolescence (older than 13 years of age)
   4) Interdependency achieved in adulthood (older than 21 years of age)

e. Dissonance (poorness of fit) involves discrepancies between the individual and the environment, resulting in distorted development or maladaptive functioning (Festinger, 1957).

E. Significance for Rehabilitation
   1. Conditioning and learned behavior may be helpful when redirecting clients toward healthy behaviors.
   2. Dissonance happens at many levels, such as conflicts between rational and emotional reactions to stress.

III. Cognitive Theories

A. Overview
   1. Cognitive theories are closely related to learning and behavioral theories.
   2. Constructivists such as John Dewey (1859–1952) believe learning occurs through exploration, whereas behaviorists believe concepts are learned from adults or teachers.
   3. Piaget's and Vygotsky's theories of development share similarities, although Piaget's theory leans toward psychology whereas Vygotsky's views are more sociocultural (Piaget, 1952; Vygotsky, 1978).

B. Piaget's Stages of Development
   1. Jean Piaget (1896–1980) studied the development of children's understanding, including how children evolve ways of knowing and how they develop right and wrong answers.
   2. He believed growth resulted from social and neurological maturity.
      a. Every child passes through stages of cognitive development in the same sequence, although not according to a given timetable.
      b. Every child develops strategies for interacting with the environment and knowing the environment's properties.

c. A gradual progression takes place from one period of cognitive development to another; acquisition of each new operation builds on existing ones.

d. Differentiation and complexity occur and are matched by increasing integration and coordination of schemata in this process of development.

e. Infants possess both fixed and flexible reflexes that enable them to develop abstract, intelligent behavior.

f. Children move through four general periods of cognitive development.
   1) Sensorimotor: Occurs from 0–2 years of age
      a) Development proceeds from reflex activity to representation and sensorimotor learning.
      b) Feelings and actions are inseparable.
      c) Sucking and touching actions by infants are innate at first.
      d) Infants begin to understand how personal behavior affects the world and become involved in trial-and-error actions.
   2) Preoperational: Occurs from 2–7 years of age
      a) Development proceeds from sensorimotor representation to prelogical thought.
      b) By maintaining stable and consistent images, children are able to create a representational world.
      c) Children begin to fantasize and use symbols to represent objects and feelings.
   3) Concrete operational: Occurs from 7–11 years of age
      a) Development proceeds from prelogical thought to logical, concrete thought.
      b) Rules are devised to govern behavior.
      c) Trial-and-error is replaced by the ability to problem solve.
   4) Formal operational: Occurs from 11–15 years of age
      a) Development proceeds from logical, concrete thought to logical solutions to all kinds of categories of problems.
      b) Reasoning and abstract conceptualizations are used to help guide future actions.

c) The ability to walk in another's shoes is gained.
d) Deductive logic is used (Piaget, 1952).

C. Vygotsky's Theoretical Framework
1. Lev Vygotsky (1896–1934) theorized that children build on previously learned experiences and ideas.
2. Social interaction provides means for step-by-step changes in a child's thought process and behavior.
3. Development varies between cultures and worldviews.
4. The four basic principles of the Vygotskian sociocultural theory are as follows:
   a. Children construct their knowledge.
   b. Development cannot be separated from social context.
   c. Learning leads to development.
   d. Language has a major role in mental development.

D. Significance for Rehabilitation
1. Building on previously learned tasks and developmental achievements may facilitate progress (e.g., starting from a point of success or known ability).
2. Developmental guidelines assist with planning reasonable steps toward restoration.

IV. **Moral Theories**
A. Overview
1. Greek philosophers discussed moral issues in terms of happiness and harmony, whereas later theories concentrated on ethical-moral issues of right and wrong.
   a. Socrates: Virtue means knowing the meaning of good and evil.
   b. Plato: Virtue means all parts of the soul are in harmony.
   c. Aristotle: Good is that which is done for its own sake.
      1) The goal of all activities is happiness.
      2) Happiness means doing well, flourishing.
      3) The highest good is self-sufficiency, lacking nothing (Myers, 2007).
2. Kohlberg's and Gilligan's viewpoints of moral development are an expansion of Piaget's theories.
3. Focus of theories concerns moral development in adolescence; can be applied to ethical situations. (See **Table 17-2** for a comparison of these theories.)

B. Levels of Moral Development
1. Lawrence Kohlberg (1927–1987) created three levels of moral development.
   a. Preconventional morality (selfishness)
   b. Conventional morality
   c. Postconventional morality: principles higher than rules (Kohlberg, 1976)
2. His model is based on research and extends from childhood through adulthood.
   a. Kohlberg's theories are based on responses to hypothetical moral dilemmas.
   b. Women were not included in study samples.
3. Kohlberg outlined six stages within his three levels of moral development, as identified from his observations.
   a. Stage 1: A punishment and obedience orientation in children age 5–6, in which decisions are based on avoidance of punishment by an authority figure

Table 17-2. A Comparison of Kohlberg's (1963, 1976) and Gilligan's (1982) Theories of Moral Development

	Kohlberg's Theory	Gilligan's Theory
Development of the self	Autonomy, individuality, independence	Connections with others, interdependence
Others	Objective concern for others; treats others fairly in terms of equality	Concern for others; helping, caring
Relationships	Reciprocity between separate individuals with a focus on fulfilling duties and obligations.	Responsiveness to others in the context of their situation and on their own terms.
Morality	Use of a "justice" approach: Moral problems are resolved by the use of impartial, abstract rules, principles, and standards of society, especially fairness.	Use of a "care" approach: Moral problems are resolved by reflecting or responding to the problem in the context of the individual; use of relativism and situational ethics; concern for maintaining relationships and interdependence.

Gilligan, C. (1982). *In a different voice: Psychological theory and women's development.* Cambridge, MA: Harvard University Press.
Kohlberg, L. (1963). Moral development and identification. In H. Stevenson (Ed.), *Child psychology.* Chicago: University of Chicago Press.
Kohlberg, L. (1976). Moral stages and moralization: The cognitive-developmental approach. In T. Lickona (Ed), *Moral development and behavior: Theory, research and social issues.* New York: Holt, Rinehart & Winston.

b. Stage 2: Instrumental/relativist orientation in children age 7–10, quid pro quo ("scratch my back, I'll scratch yours")
   1) Decisions are based on perceived benefits to self in return for agreeing to a rule.
   2) The focus is on reciprocity (i.e., the right action consists of satisfying one's own needs by seeking out rewards for good behavior).
c. Stage 3: Good boy/nice girl orientation in early adolescence, in which decisions are based on seeking approval and on helping and pleasing others
d. Stage 4: Law-and-order views in adolescents to young adulthood, in which decisions are based on adhering to rules for the sake of maintaining social order
e. Stage 5: Social contract, legalistic orientation in adults
   1) Decisions are based on justice and fairness to others.
   2) The emphasis is on the possibility of changing laws to maintain social utility.
f. Stage 6: A universal ethical principle orientation in adults, in which decisions are based on a person's self-chosen ethical principles, such as the universal principles of justice, equality of human rights, and respect for the individuality of human beings as people

C. Gender Studies
1. Carol Gilligan (1936–present) conducted research that included female participants.
2. Her study focused on female adolescents, which differed from Kohlberg's work based on all-male subjects.
   a. Consists of broad developmental patterns of orientation to care
   b. Does not address a stage hierarchy
3. Basic elements of moral judgment (Gilligan, 1982) include a definition and development of the self.
   a. Individuals define themselves in terms of their ability to form meaningful relationships or connections with others.
   b. Also define themselves in terms of their ability to care for others
   c. A description of others is identified in relation to the self.
   d. The self's interdependence with others is crucial.
   e. Moral decision making is based on the context of the situation, although exceptions to rules are allowed. (See a comparison of Kohlberg's and Gilligan's theories in Table 17-2.)

D. Significance to Rehabilitation
1. Concepts of right, wrong, good, and bad highlight areas where clients and families may experience conflict.
2. Negative emotions, such as guilt, may be obviated or minimized when articulated and addressed.
3. Moral and ethical issues may be pertinent to choices of care and discussions of quality of life.

V. **Personality Theories**
A. Overview: Personality is a branch of psychology that investigates human nature and individual differences.
1. Many theories have an element of personality within their framework.
2. Early life experiences may be significant in terms of attitudes and actions, yet behaviors may have no obvious connection or correlation with the theories that attempt to explain personality.
3. Personality types (e.g., introvert or extrovert) and personality traits (e.g., shy or creative) are defined differently.

B. Personality Assessment
1. Multiple personality tests have been developed, such as the 1921 Rorschach inkblot test and the Myers-Briggs Type Indicator, yet theories abound about environment, heredity and DNA, social factors, and birth order, and a host of other variables fuel the debates (McGhee, Ehrler, & Buckhard, 2008).
2. A newer theory emerges that describes potential survivor types, or a Survivor IQ, that may predict who is more likely to live through catastrophic events (Sherwood, 2010).

C. Maslow's Hierarchy
1. Abraham Maslow (1908–1970) developed the idea of self-actualization.
2. A hierarchy of needs is listed in five layers, with the most important physiological human needs identified as air, water, food, and sex.
3. Safety and security needs are next in Maslow's hierarchy; they include concepts of shelter (home), job security, and monetary security (e.g., insurance and retirement plans).
4. Love and belonging follows safety and includes family, work, and community belongingness; negativity may result in loneliness (Maslow, 1954).
5. Esteem needs include two types: respect from others and a sense of achievement and self-respect. If they are not achieved, inferiority complexes develop.
6. Self-actualization allows people to achieve their potential, and homeostasis results (Maslow, 1971).

D. Fully Functioning Person: Carl Rogers (1902–1987) developed the fully functional person philosophy, with five basic categories that have elements of personality in each category.
  1. Openness to experience: The antithesis of defensiveness
     a. Able to accept reality
     b. In touch with personal feelings and values
  2. Existential living: Living in the here and now
     a. Tendency to be balanced and not living in the past or future
     b. Sees dreams and memories for what they are, not what they should have been
  3. Organismic trusting: Self-trust with a tendency for self-actualization
  4. Experiential freedom: People feel free to make available choices.
  5. Creativity: People feel obligated to help others feel actualized.
     a. Joy in doing a job well-done
     b. Similar concepts to Erikson's generativity (Rogers, 1980)
E. Multiple Intelligences
  1. Howard Gardner (1943–present) conceptualized more than one IQ or intelligence in an individual.
  2. Gardner's multiple intelligence categories include interpersonal/intrapersonal, kinesthetic, linguistic, logical/math, naturalist, musical, moral, and spatial intelligence.
  3. His theory is similar to some learning theories; he suggests using different methods (such as a preferred learning approach) to capture the intelligence for maximum expertise and growth (Gardner, 1993).
F. Significance for Rehabilitation
  1. The optimal treatment plans correlate client learning styles, personality traits, and innate abilities and preferences.
  2. Client responses are linked to their self-actualization issues and ability to focus on priorities.
  3. Individual needs and expectations are housed within the scope of their personae and values of self.

VI. **Family Development and Function Theories (Table 17-3)**
A. Overview
  1. The family is a group of people in varying stages of growth.
     a. Patterns of changes occur, and like the individual, the family unit progresses through stages of growth and development.

b. Family life stages of development can be useful to rehabilitation nurses who are assessing and intervening with families across the lifespan.
c. Attachment theories provide a guide for assessing support systems and relationship risks (Becker, 1974; Bowlby, 1969).
  2. The needs of the family can be anticipated, depending on the family's developmental stage (Anderson, 2000).
B. Ruth Evelyn Millis Duvall (1906–1998) was a pioneer in applying developmental theories to the study of families.
  1. Basic tasks of families occur during the family life cycle, including the following:
     a. Physical maintenance: Keeping the family together
     b. Allocating resources: Meeting the family's needs and allocating goods, facilities, space, and authority
     c. Division of labor: Dividing the work within the family
     d. Socialization of family members: Teaching family members active participation in society
     e. Providing for reproduction: Recruitment and release of family members
     f. Maintaining order: Keeping structure and organization within the family
     g. Placing family members into society
     h. Maintaining motivation and morale: Giving encouragement and affection
        1) Meeting personal and family crises
        2) Refining a philosophy of life and a sense of family loyalty through use of rituals
  2. Stages of family development
     a. Marriage and the joining of families
        1) Establishing an identity as a couple
        2) Establishing relationships with extended families
        3) Making decisions about parenthood
     b. Families with infants
        1) Maintaining the couple's relationship while bonding with and integrating the infant into the family
        2) Maintaining the couple's relationship while assuming the parenting role
     c. Families with preschool-age children
        1) Teaching socialization to children
        2) Learning to adjust to the children being with babysitters or other adult caregivers
     d. Families with school-age children
        1) Helping the children develop peer relationships

2) Adjusting to longer periods of separation by parents and children

e. Families with teenagers
   1) Adjusting to increased autonomy, which the children are developing
   2) Focusing on midlife issues

f. Families as launching centers
   1) Adjusting to the children leaving home and becoming independent adults
   2) Adjusting the couple's relationship as they need to do less parenting

g. Families of middle years (empty nesters)
   1) Adjusting to living alone again as a couple as the last child leaves home
   2) Beginning to prepare for retirement
   3) Developing new relationships with adult children and grandchildren

h. Families in retirement (retirement to death)
   1) Beginning to prepare for death of spouse
   2) Adjusting to loss of family members and friends (Duvall, 1977)

C. Family Life Cycle Theory: Joan Stevenson-Hinde (1977) based this theory on the length of a couple's relationship.
   1. The emerging family (years 1–10 of the relationship)
      a. Initiating work and career paths by the couple
      b. Deciding and having children
   2. The crystallizing family (years 11–24 of the relationship)
      a. Dealing with adolescent children, a two-way relationship between parents and children
      b. Launching children into independent status
      c. Continuing to grow as a couple
      d. Beginning participation in community life by the couple
   3. The integrating family (years 26–40 of the relationship)
      a. Renewing and enhancing the couple's relationship
      b. Continuing work roles by the couple
      c. Developing leisure activities by the couple
      d. Making adjustments on the part of the children to aging parents
   4. The actualizing family (more than 40 years of living together)
      a. Continuing development by the couple
      b. Dealing with aging, chronic illness and disease, dying spouse or parents, and death
      c. Grieving and continuing to grow if one partner dies (Stevenson, 1977)

D. Attachment Theories
   1. John Bowlby (1907–1990) developed a theory of attachment to explain the crying and distress infants show when separated from their parents.
   2. Adult attachment theories postulate adaptive and nonadaptive behaviors related to security and intimacy factors.
   3. Three implications of adult attachment theory
      a. Adult needs for attachment are similar to infant/caregiver relationships.
      b. Romantic relationships are attachment relationships.
      c. Early childhood experiences reflect on adult feelings of security and insecurity (Bowlby, 1969).

E. Significance for Rehabilitation
   1. Theories such as Duvall's and Stevenson's that describe family life stages can be useful for those who study families and for practicing rehabilitation nurses because the needs of the family can be anticipated depending on the stage of the family.
   2. Because the life cycles defined by Duvall and Stevenson are based on the traditional nuclear family, caution is needed when rehabilitation nurses assess and assist nontraditional families.
   3. Family function theories cannot be used to describe many of the families in today's society that reflect different lifestyles and forms (divorce, alternative marriage, single parenting), yet the tasks may be similar (e.g., child rearing), and elements of these theories apply to rehabilitation.
   4. Support from relationships may influence feelings of well-being when attachment promotes security.

VII. Nursing Theories and Conceptualizations
   A. Overview
      1. Nursing as a profession uses different categories to structure its discipline-specific knowledge.
      2. The foundation (metaparadigm) branches into grand and middle-range theories.
      3. There are different ways to categorize conceptual models and theories, including an approach to earmark areas pertinent to rehabilitation nursing.
      4. Since Nightingale's time, theories have emerged that relate to interactions, systems, and developmental concepts.
   B. Metaparadigms: Generalized, global perspectives (e.g., the bio-psycho-social-spiritual or human-environment-wellness nursing models)
      1. Metaparadigms and metatheories are abstract and difficult to research (Fawcett & Garity, 2009).
      2. Grand, middle-range, and practice theories may all be part of a comprehensiveness paradigm.

Table 17-3. Summary of Family Development and Function Theories

Theory	Description	Periods		
		Stage 1	**1–10 years**	**Stage 2**
Duvall's (1977) Family Life Cycle	Family development is an 8-stage division that allows differentiation of the family's changes over time and an analysis of the relationship between the family and the individual's developmental tasks. These cycles begin with the establishment of the marital relationship and are based primarily on the age or school placement of the eldest child. Successful accomplishment of the tasks in each stage promotes growth and provides a basis for success in the next developmental stage. On the other hand, failure to successfully complete each stage's developmental tasks may result in unhappiness, societal disapproval, and difficulties in accomplishing the tasks in the next stage (Hogarth & Weeks, 1997; Young-blood, 1999).	Marriage and the joining of families	N/A	Families with infants
Stevenson's (1977) Family Life Cycle	Four stages of family development are identified that are based on the couple's relationship over time. Success or failure of the family depends on the developmental tasks accomplished in each stage beginning in the first year of the relationship. The last stage ends with the death of one partner and the remaining partner grieving and continuing to grow (Hogarth & Weeks, 1997; Stevenson, 1977).	N/A	The emerging family	N/A

Major Points

- Family life cycle is defined as the existence of a nuclear family unit (i.e., mother, father, child) from its inception to its dissolution.
- Family life cycle stages are viewed as the amount of time needed to complete each stage of family development.
- The family is a task-performance group that also has specific stage-related behaviors.
- A family evolves over time. The life history of a family is divided into expected stages of development.
- Each stage of development is characterized by relevant tasks and predictable crises associated with the achievement or nonachievement of specific developmental tasks.
- The life cycles defined by Duvall (1977) and Stevenson (1977) are based on a traditional nuclear family form. Neither theory reflects today's lifestyle changes and various types of families (e.g., divorce, alternative marriage, single parenting).
- Duvall's theory assumes that an intact family (i.e., marriage and children) has universal tasks as well as specific developmental tasks that must be accomplished by the family at eight different stages.
- Stevenson's four stages of family development are based on the length of the couple's relationship and specific developmental task completion throughout the relationshiop (Carter & McGoldrick, 1989; Youngblood, 1999).

3. Rehabilitation nurses use dimensions of person, environment, and nursing to provide restorative care.

C. Philosophies: Relate to beliefs and values about nursing

1. Nursing is generally believed to be an art and a science.
2. In rehabilitation, nurses value holistic care and develop interventions to meet the client's multiple needs (e.g., medical, vocational, educational, and interpersonal challenges).
3. Examples of early nurse philosophers are Virginia Henderson, Florence Nightingale, and Ernestine Weidenbach (Meleis, 2007).

D. Conceptual Frameworks (or Models): Ideas rather than tested concepts

1. In the mid 1850s, Florence Nightingale presented her nursing views that provided a foundation for future nursing theories (Nightingale, 1860).
2. Conceptual models offer structure and rationale for arranging concepts into consistent actions.
   a. Conceptual frameworks identify intuitive insights, expectations, and deductions.
   b. Conceptual frameworks are good tools for organizing areas of concern identified by rehabilitation clients and families.

E. Grand Nursing Theories: Less abstract but broad enough to provide a foundation for middle-range theories.

1. Grand theories offer traditional suppositions and congruent views to help focus nursing practice.
2. Because these theories are grand (inclusive), they are pertinent to most areas of nursing practice.

				Periods				
Stage 3	**Stage 4**	**Stage 5**	**Stage 6**	**11–25 years**	**Stage 7**	**26–40 years**	**Stage 8**	**More than 40 years**
Families with preschool-age children	Families with school-age children	Families with teenagers	Families as launching centers	N/A	Families of middle years (empty nesters)	N/A	Families in retirement (retirement to death)	N/A
N/A	N/A	N/A	N/A	The crystallizing family	N/A	The integrating family	N/A	The actualizing family

3. Holistic care is an example of how broad concepts are applied for the purpose of providing well-rounded care that promotes quality of life.
4. Well-known grand theorists include Myra Levine (conservation model), Betty Neuman (systems model), and Dorothea Orem (self-care model). Grand theories are particularly useful when planning nursing care for rehabilitation clients.
5. **Table 17-4** highlights early theorists and their relevance to restorative care.

F. Middle-Range Nursing Theories: Contain testable variables that have potential to contribute to evidence-based nursing practice
   1. Middle-range theories are more concrete and describe situations or phenomena.
      a. These theories explain relationships and commonalities between concepts.
      b. Middle-range theories are practical for research and practice applications.
   2. Middle-range theories are particularly pertinent to rehabilitation nursing.
   3. Commonly used theorists include Katharine Kolcaba (comfort theory), Nola Pender (health promotion), and Jean Watson (caring theory).

G. Nursing Theory: Can be depicted as a tree, with roots and branches
   1. The metaparadigm of person, environment, health, and nursing represents the roots.
   2. Florence Nightingale's work forms the trunk of the tree.
   3. The branches are shaped by three theory types: interactive with Henderson and Peplau, systems with Neuman and Roy, and development with Rogers, Leininger, and Watson (Tourville & Ingalls, 2003).

Table 17-4. Selected Historical Views Significant to Rehabilitation

Nurse Theorists	Philosophies, Theories, and Models	Key Concepts	Applicability to Restorative Care
Abedellah, Faye (1919–Retired)	Philosophy: Nursing care tailored toward client problems	Three areas of nursing focus: Physical, social, and emotional; developed typology of outcomes	Nurses promote goals to maximize community resources.
Hall, Lydia (1926–1996)	Model: Care, core, and cure	Nurse-directed interventions to prevent fragmented care	Nurse as team leader; model initially used at Loeb rehabilitation center in New York
Henderson, Virginia (1897–1996)	Philosophy: Synopsis of nursing definition: To assist individual, sick or well, for health or its recovery	Nursing activities related to survival (e.g., air, food, sleep), clothing, hygiene, posture, play, work, worship, learn, communicate, safety	Substitutive nursing care (doing for), supplementary (helping), complementary (working with)
Johnson, Dorothy (1919–1999)	Behavior system model: Subsystems house motivation, predisposition, choice, and action components	Nursing diagnosis and treatment aimed at classifying and determining problem to evaluate balance	Nurses direct restoration and attainment of behavioral system balance and stability for clients.
Kenny, Elizabeth (1880–1952)	Philosophy: Unique interventions based on independent nursing assessments	Interdisciplinary model emerged from independent nursing care of people with polio	Kenny Institute in Minneapolis based on principles of muscle rehabilitation
King, Imogene (1923–2007)	Open system theory of adjustments to stressors; contributed to North American Nursing Diagnosis Association	Personal, interpersonal, and social systems are open and interacting; focus on goal attainment	Dynamic nurse-client dyad with mutual and purposeful goal setting
Leininger, Madeleine (1923–2007)	Model and theory: Transcultural nursing	Theory for providing culturally congruent nursing care; care is the essence of nursing	Caring is universal; nurses assess transcultural variables (i.e., values of self-care).
Levine, Myra (1920–1996)	Conceptual model of conservation; sought ways to teach nursing rather than theory development	Principles: Energy, structural integrity, personal integrity, social integrity; environments: perceptual, operational, conceptual	Conservation, redundancy, and therapeutic intention for promoting client integrity and holism
Neuman, Betty (1924–Retired)	Healthcare systems model: Prevention as an intervention	Optimal client stability; health is relative and remains in state of flux	Primary, secondary, and tertiary prevention practiced; help clients maximize their defenses
Nightingale, Florence (1820–1910)	Philosophy: Did not articulate a theory per se; writings described theory concepts	Emphasized clean and quiet environment, ventilation, warmth, and sunlight	Encouraged use of one's own powers; nurses help clients obtain the best condition possible so nature can cure
Orem, Dorothea (1914–2007)	Grand theory: Self-care and self-directed care	Wholly and partially compensatory; supportive	Nursing focus toward clients helping themselves; promotion of assistive devices and aids to obtain independence
Orlando, Ida Jean (1926–2007)	Nurse-client relationship	Nursing process followed to meet client's immediate needs	Nurses explore meanings behind client behaviors; determine nature of distress unique to the client
Peplau, Hildegard (1909–1999)	Psychodynamic nursing; nurse-client relationship	Client makes use of the nurse; four phases of relationship: orient, identify, exploit, and resolution	Nursing roles: Counselor, leader, resource person, teacher

continued

THE SPECIALTY PRACTICE OF REHABILITATION NURSING

Table 17-4. Selected Historical Views Significant to Rehabilitation *continued*

Nurse Theorists	Philosophies, Theories, and Models	Key Concepts	Applicability to Restorative Care
Rogers, Martha (1914–1994)	Nursing focused on compassion; learned profession	Four-dimensional energy field; pattern and organization of characteristics and behaviors; knowledge of parts not predictive	Nurses promote change and facilitate order during rehabilitation of sick and disabled people.
Travelbee, Joyce (1926–1973)	Human-to-human relationship model; care of the whole person	Inductive theory; uses specific nursing situations to create ideas; humanistic approach	Positive nurse-client relationship brings favorable client outcomes
Weidenbach, Ernestine (1900–1996)	Philosophy: Clinical nursing is a helping art	Assess client's ability to resolve problems and identify when help is needed.	Concepts of maternal-child nursing are applicable to family units and their rehabilitation needs.

Fawcett, J. (2005). *Contemporary nursing knowledge: Analysis and evaluation of nursing models and theories* (2nd ed.). Philadelphia: F. A. Davis.
Meleis, A. I. (2007). *Theoretical nursing: Development and progress* (4th ed.). Philadelphia: Lippincott Williams & Wilkins.

H. Classification: Various theorists contribute to restorative concepts, although their classifications vary and may be difficult to identify.
  1. Theories may be classified in multiple areas.
     a. Sister Roy's adaptation model is both a grand theory and a middle-range theory, depending on its application.
     b. Margaret Newman's theory of health as expanding consciousness discusses the meaning of life, even when life changes, a theory that has been classified as both grand and middle range.
  2. Various practice models may share dual classifications.
     a. Madeline Leininger's transcultural nursing model is anthropological and caring.
     b. Humanistic models such as Patricia Benner's Novice to Expert Theory have strong ties to social psychology theories.
     c. Practice models by Rosemary Parse or by Josephine Paterson and Loretta Zderad share humanistic approaches.
     d. Imogene King's framework fits into both interaction and system models.
     e. Martha Roger's unitary theory (an energy field model) presents elements of growth and change, initially considered radical and later described as nontraditional.
  3. Rehabilitation nursing continues to be influenced by the expansion of theory-based practice and evidence-based research.
  4. Multiple classifications of theories show versatility of application, which is especially important to changes that occur during rehabilitation.
  5. Age-specific nursing theories are helpful when practicing rehabilitation across the lifespan, such as Anne Casey's nursing model for children and families and Dorothea Orem's self-care model for adults.
  6. Theories can be shared by healthcare providers to promote restorative care, including long-used and improved theories from psychosocial disciplines, as previously reviewed.

I. Significance for Rehabilitation
  1. Nursing theories built on a wide range of interdisciplinary frameworks and models.
  2. Nursing models and theories outline the needs of clients and family to promote recovery and quality of life.
  3. Nurses use theory foundations based in history (perhaps more than realized) on a daily basis.
  4. Rehabilitation nursing continues to discover new theories.
  5. The nursing profession continues to develop models and test associated theories to provide evidence-based care for optimal client outcomes (Schmidt & Brown, 2009).
  6. A holistic approach to nursing care requires a Gestalt approach, through which the whole of the client, not just the parts, can be restored and rehabilitated.
  7. **Table 17-5** shows the juxtaposition of theories and the nursing process for developing a plan of care for a rehabilitation client.

VIII. Theory Application to Advanced Practice
  A. Clinician
    1. The clinician uses developmental theories to link the determinants of health and illness across the lifespan (Hoeman, 2008; Jarvis, 2008).

Table 17-5. A Gestalt Nursing Approach for Restorative Care

Case Synopsis	Nursing Process Examples	Theory-Based Considerations
Client T.S. had a bowel obstruction and spontaneous rupture that resulted in spillage of stool and barium (from her earlier gastrointestinal study) outside the intestines and throughout the abdomen. Two fistulas resulted, with openings that expelled feces from the intestinal area to colostomy bags attached to the outside of the client's abdomen. This health problem was a surprise to T.S., giving her little time to adjust to the situation. Fistula care resembled colostomy care, with wafers, bags, and emptying procedures. The intestinal obstruction and subsequent complications resulted in physical and emotional distress for T.S.	FHP: Coping-stress tolerance S: "I can't believe this is happening." O: Open fistulas managed with ostomy bags ND: Coping, ineffective, denial NIC: Assess T.S.'s usual coping strategies, and explore the situation with T.S. NOC: T.S. identifies her own maladaptive coping behavior; acknowledges the situation, and verbalizes available support. FHP: Self-perception S: "I have waste oozing from my abdomen; this is disgusting; it's worse than being a baby." ND: Disturbed body image. NIC: Encourage T.S. to express feelings; clarify any misconceptions (i.e., prognosis). NOC: T.S. demonstrates enhanced body image and self-esteem, as evidenced by her ability to look at and care for the altered body area and function with ostomy care.	Coping challenges may occur across the lifespan. Coping mechanisms will vary, depending on developmental stage (i.e., Erikson). Multiple theories address defense mechanisms, such as denial and repression. Health issues related to elimination may have Freudian connotations. Fully functioning individuals (described by Carl Rogers) will accept reality and adjust. Dissonance (e.g., Schaie's theory) may occur when the person and the environment are not in sync.
Over 6 weeks, T.S. underwent three laparoscopies as surgeons tried to remove the barium and repair the fistulas. Her activity tolerance grew worse instead of better. T.S. was referred to rehabilitation.	FHP: Activity-exercise S: "I'm too weak to do anything for myself; this is so embarrassing." ND: Self-care deficit syndrome NIC: Assist T.S. in accepting the necessary amount of dependence; set realistic goals with T.S. NOC: Demonstrates total self-care by target date	Numerous variables may interrelate, such as dependency and self-perception issues when facing a rehabilitation challenge. Holistic care addresses diverse needs of clients and families. Physical needs may outweigh emotional needs, as outlined in Maslow's theory.
Apart from her general debilitation, T.S. exhibited anger and frustration, especially related to her ostomy care.	FHP: Cognitive-perceptual S: "I can't get these (curse word) bags to stop leaking. What can I do?" O: Stool on abdomen and bed; open areas on wafer ND: Knowledge, readiness for enhanced NIC: Support self-directed, self-designed learning; allow adequate time for integration; ensure that necessary supplies are available so the environment is conducive to learning. NOC: T.S. will demonstrate motivation to learn; will verbalize understanding and perform skill of ostomy self-care.	Cognitive and learning theories have implications for health education. Abilities vary, as do preferences and personalities for developing coping strategies. The multiple intelligence model (Gardner) is applicable as learning strategies are assessed and client strengths are identified. Formal health assessments may ask clients about their preferred learning style.
T.S. had recently moved to be near her elderly mother. T.S. became sick before she fully relocated, which resulted in her being unemployed. She did not want to move in with family, but medical bills had depleted her down payment for a home.	FHP: Coping-stress tolerance S: "I'm homeless and jobless, and I'm really mad and don't know what to do." ND: Resilience, impaired individual NIC: Emotional support; referral and counseling, if needed. Encourage client to evaluate options. NOC: Appraise support systems; relate available community resources.	Adaptation models help identify psychosocial problems and potential solutions. Nursing theories have elements of earlier philosophies of human growth and development. A combination of philosophies and interdisciplinary models provide a Gestalt approach to care.

FHP, functional health pattern; ND, nursing diagnosis; NIC, Nursing Intervention Classification; NOC, Nursing Outcomes Classification; O, objective; S, subjective.

Carpenito-Moyet, L. J. (2010). *Handbook of nursing diagnosis* (13th ed.). Philadelphia: Lippincott Williams & Wilkins.

Doenges, M. E., Moorhouse, M. F., & Murr, A. C. (2010). *Nursing diagnosis manual: Planning, individualizing, and documenting client care* (3rd ed.). Philadelphia: F. A. Davis.

Johnson, M., Bulechek, G., Dochterman, J. M., Mass, M., Moorhead, S., Swanson, E., et al. (2005). *NANDA, NOC and NIC linkages.* St. Louis: Mosby.

a. Provides a construct for interpreting how clients' and families' experiences in their early years influence their later health and functioning

b. Aids in understanding clients' and families' health and well-being for nurses providing direct care

2. Applies developmental theories and tasks across the lifespan to provide paradigms for clinical issues.

a. Assesses and diagnoses healthcare needs

b. Plans, implements, and evaluates proactively health and illness interventions when working with clients and families in various settings

B. Educator

1. The educator reviews developmental theories and tasks of clients and families when teaching.

a. Determines the most appropriate teaching strategy based on the developmental stage or life point of the client and family

b. Plans and implements educational interventions, such as choosing the best presentation method or teaching material to fit the needs of the client and family

c. Evaluates informal and formal educational programs related to developmental needs of the client and family (Hamric, Spross, & Hanson, 2009)

2. The educator considers theories and tasks of clients and families when teaching professional and nonprofessional staff members.

a. Assesses client and family readiness for learning

b. Plans and implements educational content, such as in-service offerings

c. Evaluates informal and formal educational offerings

C. Leader and Consultant

1. The consultant applies developmental theories and frameworks as a foundation for integrating child and adult health policies by emphasizing the potential for social and biological processes early in life to find clinical expression in adult-onset disease.

2. The consultant applies this knowledge to reduce the heavy human and economic costs of healthcare and to actively participate in healthcare policy making.

D. Researcher

1. The researcher identifies and expands theoretical frameworks to depict or explain relationships between concepts of interest in a study.

2. The researcher uses theories to form research designs or to participate in studies that nurse scientists develop and direct, such as the following:

a. Improving the health and well-being of children

b. Examining the effects of environmental influences on the health and development of children and adults

c. Defining natural and human-made environmental factors that result in rehabilitation risks that may be prevented or minimized when identified by research data

1) Biological and chemical factors
2) Hazards in physical surroundings
3) Social risk factors
4) Risk-taking behaviors

3. Critically appraises and synthesizes evidence

a. Analyzes how these elements interact with each other and the helpful or harmful effects they might have for clients across the lifespan

b. Studies children and adults through their different phases of growth and development to better understand health and disease

c. Contributes to best practices as determined by theory-based research (Barker, 2009; Derstine & Hargrove, 2001)

Acknowledgment

I would like to acknowledge Linda L. Pierce, PhD CNS RN CRRN FAHA, for her work on this chapter in the previous edition.

References

Anderson, K. H. (2000). The family health system approach to family systems nursing. *Journal of Family Nursing, 6*(2), 103–117.

Bandura, A. (1997). *Self-efficacy.* New York: W. H. Freeman.

Barker, A. M. (Ed.). (2009). *Advanced practice nursing: Essential knowledge for the profession.* Boston: Jones & Bartlett.

Barton, E. F. (1996). *Harry Stack Sullivan: Interpersonal theory and psychotherapy.* London: Routledge.

Becker, M. H. (Ed.). (1974). *The health belief model and personal health behavior.* Thorofare, NJ: Slock.

Bowlby, J. (1969). *Attachment and loss.* New York: Basic Books.

Boyd, D., & Bee, H. (2006). *Lifespan development* (4th ed.). Upper Saddle River, NJ: Pearson.

Bradberry, T. (2007). *The personality code.* New York: Putnam.

Carducci, B. J. (2009). *The psychology of personality.* Malden, MA: Wiley-Blackwell.

Carpenito-Moyet, L. J. (2010). *Handbook of nursing diagnosis* (13th ed.). Philadelphia: Lippincott Williams & Wilkins.

Carter, B., & McGoldrick, M. (1989) *The changing family life cycle: A framework for family therapy.* Needham Heights, MA: Allyn & Bacon.

Derstine, J. B., & Hargrove, S. D. (2001). *Comprehensive rehabilitation nursing.* Philadelphia: W. B. Saunders.

Doenges, M. E., Moorhouse, M. F., & Murr, A. C. (2010). *Nursing diagnosis manual: Planning, individualizing, and documenting client care* (3rd ed.). Philadelphia: F. A. Davis.

Duvall, E. (1977). *Marriage and family development* (5th ed.). Philadelphia: Lippincott.

Ellis, W. D. (1938). *Source book of gestalt psychology*. New York: Harcourt, Brace & Company.

Erikson, E. (1963). *Childhood and society* (2nd ed.). New York: W. W. Norton.

Erikson, E. H., Erikson, J. M., & Kivnick, H. Q. (1986). *Vital involvement in old age*. New York: W. W. Norton.

Fawcett, J. (2005). *Contemporary nursing knowledge: Analysis and evaluation of nursing models and theories* (2nd ed.). Philadelphia: F. A. Davis.

Fawcett, J., & Garity, J. (2009). *Evaluating research for evidence-based nursing practice*. Philadelphia: F. A. Davis.

Festinger, L. (1957). *Theory of cognitive dissonance*. Stanford, CA: Stanford University Press.

Freud, S. (1959). Inhibitions, symptoms, and anxiety. In J. Strachey (Ed.), *The standard edition of the complete psychological works of Sigmund Freud* (Vol. 18, pp. 1–64). London: Hogarth.

Gardner, H. (1993). *Multiple intelligences: The theory in practice*. New York: Basic Books.

Gay, P. (2006). *Freud: A life for our times*. New York: W. W. Norton.

Gilligan, C. (1982). *In a different voice: Psychological theory and women's development*. Cambridge, MA: Harvard University Press.

Glod, C. (1998). Developmental and psychological theories of mental illness. In C. Glod (Ed.), *Contemporary psychiatric–mental health nursing* (pp. 64–72). Philadelphia: F. A. Davis.

Goodman, C. J. (2009). *A history of modern psychology* (3rd ed.). Somerset, NJ: Wiley.

Hamric, A. B., Spross, J. A., & Hanson, C. M. (2009). *Advanced practice nursing: An integrative approach* (4th ed.). St. Louis: Saunders-Elsevier.

Hoeman, S. P. (2008). *Rehabilitation nursing: Prevention, intervention, and outcomes* (4th ed.). St. Louis: Mosby-Elsevier.

Hogarth, C., & Weeks, S. (1997). Families and family therapy. In B. Johnson (Ed.), *Psychiatric–mental health nursing: Adaptation and growth* (4th ed., pp. 277–298). Philadelphia: Lippincott.

Jarvis, C. (Ed.). (2008). *Physical examination & health assessment* (5th ed.). Philadelphia: W. B. Saunders.

Jarvis, P. (2001). *Learning in later life*. London: Kogan Page.

Johnson, M., Bulechek, G., Dochterman, J. M., Mass, M., Moorhead, S., Swanson, E., et al. (2005). *NANDA, NOC and NIC linkages*. St. Louis: Mosby.

Kohlberg, L. (1963). Moral development and identification. In H. Stevenson (Ed.), *Child psychology*. Chicago: University of Chicago Press.

Kohlberg, L. (1976). Moral stages and moralization: The cognitive-developmental approach. In T. Lickona (Ed.), *Moral development and behavior: Theory, research and social issues*. New York: Holt, Rinehart & Winston.

Maslow, A. (1954). *Motivation and personality*. New York: Harper.

Maslow, A. (1971). *The farther reaches of human nature*. New York: Viking.

McGhee, R. L., Ehrler, D., & Buckhalt, J. (2008). *Manual for the five factor personality inventory*. Austin, TX: Pro Ed, Inc.

Meleis, A. I. (2007). *Theoretical nursing: Development and progress* (4th ed.). Philadelphia: Lippincott Williams & Wilkins.

Myers, S. S. (2007). *Ancient ethics*. New York: Routledge.

Newman, B. M., & Newman, P. R. (2009). *Theories of human development*. Mahwah, NJ: Erlbaum.

Nightingale, F. (1860). *Nursing: What it is, and what it is not*. New York: D. Appleton.

Pavlov, I. (1927). *Conditioned reflexes: An investigation of the physiological activity of the cerebral cortex*. New York: Oxford University Press.

Piaget, J. (1952). *Origins of intelligence in children*. New York: International Universities Press.

Rogers, C. (1980). *A way of being*. Boston: Houghton Mifflin.

Schaie, K. (1981). Psychological changes from midlife to early old age: Implications for the maintenance of mental health. *American Journal of Orthopsychiatry, 51*(4), 199–218.

Schmidt, N. A., & Brown, J. M. (2009). *Evidence-based practice for nurses: Appraisal and application of research*. Sudbury, MA: Jones & Bartlett.

Shenk, J. W. (2009, June). What makes us happy? *Atlantic Monthly, 36–54.*

Sherwood, W. R. (2010). *The survivors club*. New York: Grand Central Publishing.

Sigelman, C. K., & Rider, E. A. (2009). *Life-span human development* (6th ed.). Belmont, CA: Wadsworth Cengage Learning.

Skinner, B. F. (1953). *Science and human behavior*. New York: Macmillan.

Stevenson, J. (1977). *Issues and crises during middlescence*. New York: Appleton-Century-Crofts.

Sullivan, H. (1956). *Clinical studies in psychiatry*. New York: Norton.

Sullivan, H. (1971). *The fusion of psychiatry and social science*. New York: Norton.

Tauber, A. I. (2010). *Freud the reluctant philosopher*. Princeton, NJ: Princeton University Press.

Tourville, C., & Ingalls, K. (2003). The living tree of nursing theories. *Nursing Forum, 38*(3), 21–30, 36.

Townsend, M. C. (2010). *Essentials of psychiatric mental health nursing: Concepts of care in evidence-based practice* (5th ed.). New York: F. A. Davis.

Vygotsky, L. S. (1978). *Mind in society*. Cambridge, MA: Harvard University Press.

Whiting, S. (1997). Development of the person. In B. Johnson (Ed.), *Psychiatric–mental health nursing: Adaptation and growth* (4th ed., pp. 357–373). Philadelphia: Lippincott Williams & Wilkins.

Youngblood, N. (1999). Family-centered care. In P. Edwards, D. Hertzberg, S. Hays, & N. Youngblood (Eds.), *Pediatric rehabilitation* (pp. 129–143). Philadelphia: W. B. Saunders.

CHAPTER 18

Pediatric Rehabilitation Nursing

Dalice Hertzberg, MSN RN FNP-C • Lyn Sapp, MN RN CRRN

This chapter brings together a unique body of knowledge specific to the care of children and adolescents with disabilities and chronic conditions and their families. It provides a reference for nurses in a variety of settings across the continuum of care, from hospital to home and community. The emphasis is on the roles of the pediatric rehabilitation nurse in relation to care coordination and provision, health teaching and promotion, leadership, collaboration, advocacy, and professional practice.

Family-centered care and developmental assessment and intervention are addressed in this chapter in an interdisciplinary approach. Specific diagnoses are outlined, including accidents and trauma, congenital diseases and birth defects, and chronic conditions. Long-term planning, including community services, home health care, school, and early intervention programs and transition to adulthood are presented.

I. **Overview**
   A. Definitions
      1. Pediatric rehabilitation nursing: "Pediatric rehabilitation nursing is the specialty practice committed to improving the quality of life for children and adolescents with disabilities and their families. The mission is to provide, in collaboration with the interdisciplinary team, a continuum of nursing care from onset of injury or illness to productive adulthood. The goal of the rehabilitation process is for children, regardless of their disability or chronic illness, to function at their maximum potential and become contributing members of both their families and society" (Association of Rehabilitation Nurses [ARN], 2007, pp. 1–2).
      2. Habilitation: Enabling children with congenital or early-onset disabling conditions to develop their physical, intellectual, and social abilities to reach their potential in self-care and community participation (Ronen et al., 2009)
      3. Rehabilitation: Relearning skills and abilities after trauma or disease to meet age-related developmental expectations
   B. Roles of the Pediatric Rehabilitation Nurse
      1. Advocacy
      2. Coordination of care
      3. Leadership and consulting
      4. Care provision

   5. Health teaching and promotion
   6. Team participation
   7. Research
   8. Professional practice, education, and evaluation (ARN, 2007, pp. 1–2)
   C. Practice Settings
      1. Pediatric rehabilitation hospitals (inpatient and outpatient)
      2. Pediatric rehabilitation units in rehabilitation hospitals
      3. Subacute and postacute rehabilitation units
      4. Day treatment programs
      5. Freestanding pediatric outpatient therapy centers
      6. Outpatient primary care and specialty clinics
      7. Health department outpatient services
      8. State children's rehabilitation services
      9. School or child care centers
      10. Home health agencies
      11. Family homes
   D. General Principles
      1. Family-centered care: A philosophy of care that recognizes the role of the family in the lives of children
         a. All children are part of a family, even if the family is not considered traditional in American culture.
         b. Including the family in care ensures that family members and the child receive support in coping with the child's disability or chronic illness.
      2. Community-based delivery systems: Services that are delivered in the child's environment (e.g., early intervention center, medical home, school, day care, pediatric outpatient therapy center, home)
      3. Medical home concept: "A medical home is not a building, house, or hospital, but rather an approach to providing health care services in a high-quality and cost-effective manner" (American Academy of Pediatrics [AAP], 2010). Pediatric healthcare professionals and parents act as partners in a medical home to identify and access all the medical and nonmedical services needed to help children and their families achieve the maximum potential for the child. A medical home for a child usually is part of a pediatric primary care

office but may be part of a comprehensive outpatient program.

4. Human development
    a. Pediatric rehabilitation nurses must have in-depth knowledge of developmental theories, normal development, and related assessment skills and knowledge of interventions that promote developmental milestones. (Refer to Chapter 17 for more information about developmental theories.)
    b. Understanding family life stages of development is useful in assessing and intervening with children and families.

5. Developmental levels: The child's developmental level should be considered in determining the rehabilitation plan and interventions.
    a. Infant and toddler (1–3 years old)
    b. Preschooler (3–5 years old)
    c. School-age child (6–12 years old)
    d. Adolescent (12–21 years old)

6. Assessment: Each child and family should be assessed in the following areas:
    a. Birth history
    b. Developmental history
    c. Current developmental level and expected level of development for the child's age
    d. The impact of the child's disability on his or her developmental level
    e. Plans for important service system transitions (according to age)
        1) Neonatal intensive care unit to home, in the case of congenital disability or prematurity
        2) Early intervention, Part C of the Individuals with Disabilities Education Act, to preschool
        3) Preschool to grade school programs, then middle school and high school
        4) High school to secondary school, vocational program, or independent living
    f. Plans for pediatric healthcare system transition to adult healthcare system
    g. Family assessment to determine strengths and areas for assistance or support

7. Interventions: Physical, emotional, social, cultural, educational, developmental, and spiritual dimensions are all considered in a holistic approach to care.
    a. Focus on helping the child meet his or her developmental milestones as much as possible.
    b. Investigate alternative ways to achieve tasks if developmental milestones cannot be met through therapy or assistive devices.

    c. Anticipate upcoming developmental challenges and plan ahead for age-appropriate interventions.
    d. Facilitate adaptation to the disability and treatment.
    e. Promote community integration.
    f. Provide resources and referrals to meet transitional needs when the child is no longer eligible for pediatric services.
    g. Incorporate appropriate recreational activities, toys, and fun as well as therapeutic interventions. Play, the means by which children learn about the world, is an integral part of the rehabilitation plan.

8. Family interventions
    a. Provide family emotional support.
    b. Facilitate family adaption to the child's disability.
    c. Educate family members about the child's disability and how to promote independence.
    d. Promote changes in family roles and responsibilities.
    e. Provide care management and resources.
    f. Enable families to manage their child's care and to advocate for the child's needs.

9. Interdisciplinary team approach (nursing, medicine, physical and occupational therapy, speech, nutrition, psychology, education, social work, orthotics, medical subspecialties [e.g., neurology], and support services [e.g., vision and dental])
    a. Recognize the child's intellectual and physical abilities.
    b. Coordinate the plan of care to maximize potential.
    c. The family plays a vital role in advocating for the child and is a core part of the rehabilitation team.
    d. Provide parent education and training.
    e. Work collaboratively with other team members to promote optimal treatment outcomes and quality of life.

10. Pediatric rehabilitation differs from rehabilitation of adults. Children are not small adults; differences are related to developmental and physiological immaturity.
    a. Rapid changes in size of organs and in neurological development necessitate frequent monitoring in infants, toddlers, and preschoolers.
    b. Emergency equipment must be sized for the age of the child; small airways are more vulnerable to injury with invasive procedures such as intubation.

c. Young children's renal and hepatic function is still developing, so they need adjustments in medication dosing until about 16 years of age.

d. Age- and growth-related vulnerabilities influence biomechanical response to injury (e.g., the amount of cartilage in children's bones results in more "greenstick" type fractures; fractures involving the epiphyseal growth plate may cause lifelong deformity if not treated appropriately).

11. Prevention of secondary conditions: A secondary condition is any condition that develops as a result of a primary disability (Centers for Disease Control and Prevention, 2010). Secondary conditions in children include the following:

a. Joint contractures

b. Obesity, which increases risk of hypertension, hyperlipidemia, type 2 diabetes, mobility problems, fatigue, pain, and pressure sores (Rimmer, Rowland, & Yamaki, 2007)

c. Respiratory disorders

d. Spasticity

e. Communication problems

f. Swallowing disorders and nutritional deficits

g. Emotional problems, depression, school problems, and social isolation

II. Specific Pediatric Diagnoses

A. Accidents: Traumatic and acquired conditions

1. Traumatic brain injury (TBI)

a. Definition: An insult to the brain from non-congenital trauma, associated with an altered state of consciousness, causing permanent neurologic impairment (Dawodu, 2007)

1) Children may experience deficits in physical, psychosocial, and cognitive functioning.

2) Children differ from adults with TBI. Physiological differences in children lead to differences in acute care management.

a) Response to injury, such as more diffuse cerebral edema after injury, makes acute management of elevated intracranial pressure paramount.

b) Maintenance of adequate cerebral perfusion is critical to a more positive outcome in children (Hackbarth et al., 2002).

c) Characteristics of injury, such as delays in treatment, particularly in young children, can lead to increased ischemic injury.

d) Causes of injury differ (e.g., in young children falls and child abuse are likely causes, motor vehicle accidents are common causes in older children, and sports-related head injuries are more prevalent in adolescents and young adults).

e) Outcomes of injury are affected in part by age at the time of injury; infants are more likely to have worse outcomes (Dawodu, 2007; Giza, Mink, & Madikians, 2007).

3) Differences between children and adults lead to differences in rehabilitation management and outcome.

a) Children are more likely to survive TBI than adults.

b) Predictors of outcome in children and adolescents include Glasgow Coma Scale rating, intracranial pressure, length of time in a coma, and severity of injury (Chung et al., 2006; Fay et al., 2009; Giza et al., 2007).

c) Children continue to grow and develop after TBI; this puts them at an additional disadvantage with regard to future learning.

d) There is even more impact on the family because caregiving often is extended beyond childhood.

e) The cost to family and society is higher because the child with TBI generally has more years to live.

f) The school system and special education are critical pieces in the rehabilitation of children with TBI.

b. Epidemiology

1) TBI in children from birth to 14 years of age results in 2,685 deaths, 37,000 hospitalizations, and 435,000 emergency department visits (National Center for Injury Prevention and Control [NCIPC], 2006).

2) Of children with head injury, about 30,000 experience long-term disability (NCIPC, 2006; National Dissemination Center for Children with Disabilities, 2006).

3) Adolescents, young adults, and very young children are at highest risk for TBI.

4) As with adults, males are more likely to experience TBI than females.

c. Outcomes of TBI in children

1) Speech and language disorders
2) Motor deficits
3) Dysphagia and feeding problems; some children need gastrostomy feedings temporarily or in the long term
4) Behavioral problems: Impulsivity, secondary attention deficit disorder, aggression, and personality changes
5) Cognitive deficits (executive function disorders, processing disorders, memory deficits) leading to a need for special education and school services
6) Social problems, caused in part by cognitive deficits and behavioral disorders
7) Seizure disorder
8) Vision and hearing deficits

d. Assessment
1) Physical assessment for common postinjury problems
    a) Neurologic deficit: Level of consciousness, intracranial pressure, Glasgow Coma Scale (Chung et al., 2006), Rancho Los Amigos Scale
    b) Respiratory deficit: Adequate oxygenation; some children need tracheostomy or ventilation initially, and those with more severe injury may be discharged on mechanical ventilation
    c) Cardiovascular: Hemodynamic instability
    d) Endocrine deficit (e.g., syndrome of inappropriate antidiuretic hormone, diabetes insipidus, hyperglycemia)
    e) Gastrointestinal and nutritional assessment: Nasogastric tube, gastrostomy tube, oral stimulation, oral feedings, choking risk (Blissit, 2006)
2) Developmental assessment: Cognitive abilities, premorbid functioning
3) Functional assessment: WeeFIM™ instrument (Rice et al., 2005; refer to Chapter 22)
4) Communication and language
5) Family assessment: coping, guilt, ability to care for child, financial concerns, siblings

e. Rehabilitation issues
1) Independence level appropriate for developmental level
2) Cognitive rehabilitation
3) Speech and language therapy
4) Prevention of further injury and complications
5) Family involvement
6) Behavioral problems, personality changes, need for increased supervision
7) Special education, integration into school, planning with school staff
8) Discharge planning: Daily care of child at home, therapy and medical appointments, equipment and planning for an emergency, respite care, community resources
9) Community integration

f. Family and child education topics
1) Methods of promoting development and independence; "normalization"
2) Use and care of equipment and assistive devices
3) Prevention of further injury and use of protective equipment
4) Behavior modification strategies
5) Service coordination and advocacy
6) Teaching strategies that may include play therapy

2. Stroke from arteriovenous malformation (AVM) in the brain: AVM is a defect in the circulatory system believed to arise during embryonic or fetal development or soon after birth. Approximately 2%–4% of all AVMs may hemorrhage, resulting in hemorrhagic stroke (National Institute of Neurological Disorders and Stroke [NINDS], 2009a). Posthemorrhage care is similar to head injury care in terms of assessment, rehabilitation issues, outcomes, and client and family education.

3. Nonaccidental TBI has become a leading cause of death in infants and toddlers. These children present with injuries requiring neurosurgical management and operative interventions. Children in this age group often have significantly worse injuries and outcomes than those whose trauma was accidental. With aggressive intervention, many can make significant improvements (Adamo, Drazin, Smith, & Waldman, 2009).

4. Spinal cord injury (SCI), traumatic and acquired (Refer to Chapter 12 for an in-depth discussion of SCI.)
    a. Types
    1) Traumatic: Before puberty, children have unique physical and developmental characteristics that distinguish them from adults. These characteristics predispose them to SCI from lap-belt injuries, injuries related to birth and child abuse, SCI without radiologic abnormalities (more common in children younger than 8 years old), delayed onset of neurologic deficits,

high cervical injuries, and potential for additional common associated brain, chest, and limb injuries (Launay, Leet, & Sponseller, 2005; Martin, Dykes, & Lecky, 2004; Vogel, Hickey, Klaas, & Anderson, 2004). Injuries occur at all ages, including in utero, during delivery, and throughout childhood (Brand, 2006; Massagli, 2000; Vogel et al., 2004).

2) Acquired
   a) Transverse myelitis: A neurological disorder caused by inflammation across both sides of the spinal cord. It may involve one level or a segment of the spinal cord. No effective treatment is available at this time. One-third of those affected have full recovery, one-third have partial recovery, and one-third may have no recovery (NINDS, 2010). Use spinal cord injury care for assessment, rehabilitation, and education for child and family.
   b) Spinal cord tumor: Various tumor types may entwine the spinal cord, presenting similar problems and care needs as other types of SCI. In addition to basic SCI care, considerations include surgical and chemotherapy treatments and the effects of these interventions (e.g., nadir), no rectal treatments (for risk of bleeding and infection), fatigue, palliative options, and child and family preferences. (See "Cancer" later in this chapter for more information.)

b. Assessment components
   1) Health history
   2) Functional and cognitive levels
   3) Spinal stability
   4) Developmental levels: Rehabilitation goals are dynamic, to be adjusted with growth and development of the child.
   5) Skin integrity
   6) Bladder and bowel function
   7) Psychosocial issues
   8) Family history
   9) Respiratory status (especially in tetraplegia and upper-level thoracic injury)
   10) Home environment accessibility
   11) Pain: Types of pain with SCI may be acute traumatic (postinjury), neuropathic, repetitive use (upper-limb discomfort from propelling a wheelchair), and related to

muscles spasms (spasticity). (See Chapter 15 for more pain descriptions, assessment, and interventions.)

c. Rehabilitation issues
   1) Neurogenic bladder and bowel management
   2) Skin care: Adolescents may be at risk for pressure ulcers, which are related to body image and peer embarrassment; the challenge of taking time to check skin; and distraction by teen activities (Vogel et al., 2004).
   3) Mobility: Immobilization and spine stabilization with bracing, functional-dependent to independent-mobility activities (power mobility for children as young as 3 years of age)
   4) Pulmonary function, mechanical ventilation (if injury is at C3 and above): Infants and younger children with tetraplegia are at risk of incipient respiratory failure. Sleep studies are recommended when there is a history of excessive daytime sleepiness or prominent snoring (Vogel et al., 2004).
   5) Risk for heterotopic ossification
   6) Risk for autonomic dysreflexia (injuries at level T6 and above): 20–40 mm Hg above baseline in adults, 15–20 mm Hg above baseline in adolescents, 15 mm Hg above baseline in children (Vogel et al., 2004). Recommendation: The child should wear a medical alert bracelet and have an autonomic dysreflexia information card and care supplies in his or her school backpack.
   7) Risk for spasticity and contractures: Range of motion and splinting for pediatrics
   8) Risk for sexual dysfunction
   9) Risk for osteopenia
   10) Risk for deep vein thrombosis: Prophylactic treatment follows adult practice.
   11) Prevention of further injury
   12) Plans for return to home, school, and community
   13) Orthopedic complications: Scoliosis and hip instability
   14) Hypercalcemia
   15) Latex sensitivity related to longevity of exposure. It is best to be in a latex-free environment to prevent development of latex sensitivity and allergy (Vogel et al., 2004).

16) Pain issues related to trauma, recovery, neuropathic pain: Use appropriate pain assessment tools, medication, and therapy approaches.

d. Client education topics: Dramatic developmental changes occur as children grow. Developmentally appropriate educational methods and family-centered care are essential because of dependency on caregivers. An individualized educational SCI program is essential, incorporating parental and child education adjustment from dependence to independence as the child grows into adulthood (Vogel et al., 2004).

1) Bladder and bowel program: Self-clean intermittent catheterization (depending on fine motor abilities and injury considerations) can be taught as early as 5 years of age. Bowel programs are initiated at about 3 years of age, transitioning to independence and directing caregivers in late school age to adolescence (Massagli, 2000; Vogel et al., 2004).

2) Skin care

3) Autonomic dysreflexia (if injury is at T6 or above)

4) Medications

5) Community reintegration strategies

6) Sexuality: Effects on sexual function in children are similar to those in adults with SCI (pregnancy, fertility, erectile dysfunction, and ejaculation dysfunction). Education with parents and the child or adolescent is similar to that of children without SCI and as developmentally appropriate (Vogel et al., 2004).

7) Emotional support: Sense of hope is important throughout rehabilitation and at all ages (Lohne & Severinsson, 2004).

5. Burns

a. Definitions

1) The loss of any of the three layers of skin by fires; scalds (including immersion or splashing by hot liquids, grease, and steam); contact (touching a hot object or substance); and chemical, electrical, or radiation burns (Weed & Berens, 2005)

2) Classification

a) First degree: Superficial

b) Second degree: Partial thickness

c) Third degree: Full thickness

d) Some centers include fourth degree, which includes muscles and bone (Weed & Berens, 2005).

3) Classifications in children

a) Mild or minor: Ten percent of total body surface area (TBSA) partial thickness and less than 2% full thickness unless eyes, ears, face, or perineum is involved

b) Moderate: Ten percent to 20% TBSA regardless of depth and 2%–10% TBSA full thickness unless the eyes, ears, face, or perineum is involved

c) Major: More than 20% TBSA partial thickness; more than 10% TBSA full thickness; all burns involving the face, eyes, ears, feet, and perineum; all burns that are electrical or involve inhalation injury; all burns with ancillary injury (e.g., fracture, tissue trauma; Weed & Berens, 2005)

4) Further studies and informational demographics are tracked through research burn model system databases (Klein et al., 2007).

b. Assessment components

1) Skin integrity: Consider a photo journal.

2) Respiratory condition

3) Mobility and functional levels (e.g., WeeFIM™)

4) Pain assessment scales must be chosen according to communication and developmental abilities. Scales include pain intensity self-report (e.g., 0–10, Faces, Oucher, Visual Analogue Scale, Poker Chip Tool) via questionnaires and diaries and behavior observation scales for assessing pain and behavioral distress (e.g., procedural-based; Children's Hospital of Eastern Ontario Pain Scale [CHEOPS], Face, Legs, Activity, Cry, Consolability [FLACC], COMFORT; Cohen et al., 2008; Stoddard et al., 2002).

5) Nutrition

6) Self-image

7) Developmental level (using Battelle Developmental Inventory)

8) Family history and coping

9) Sleep (itching, splinting, and night terrors may be common)

c. Rehabilitation issues and interventions: Children are more likely than adults to develop hypertrophic scars and keloids as a result of vigorous healing; compliance may be challenged by uncomfortable and unsightly treatment modalities and extreme social pressure for acceptance by peers (Passaretti & Billmire, 2003).

1) Potential for infection (e.g., skin, respiratory, mild restrictive disease in thermal burns; exercise or activity improves pulmonary function; Suman, Mlcak, & Herndon, 2002)

2) Burn locations most challenging to functional ability: Axillary, neck, flexion areas, bottoms of feet

3) Comfort level and pain management: Pharmacological (narcotic, nonnarcotic, anti-itching, and antianxiolytic formulations), cognitive/behavioral therapy, relaxation training, hypnosis, reassurance, parental support, guided imagery, biofeedback, distraction, therapeutic touch, art, music, and play therapy (Stoddard et al., 2002)

4) Nutrition deficit related to hypermetabolic state for as long as 1 year after burn injury; enteral or parenteral nutrition for supplementation should be considered at a rate of 1.4 times resting energy expenditure in pediatric population (Gordon, Gottschlich, Helvig, Marvin, & Richard, 2004; Pereira, Murphy, & Herndon, 2005)

5) Pressure garments: Average length of wearing is 1–2 years after acute burn, while scarring is still in inflammatory stage (Passaretti & Billmire, 2003).

6) Restoration of self-image

7) Elimination pattern: Toileting is complicated by difficult-to-remove pressure garments or splints; decreased mobility and pain medications increase the risk of constipation.

8) Contracture management and surgeries for function or cosmesis: Scar contraction, joint contractures, muscle shortening, and growth restriction in pediatrics; physical and occupational therapy, splinting, massage, pressure garments, and surgical evaluation during the child's growing years (Passaretti & Billmire, 2003; Vehmeyer-Heeman, Lommers, Van den Kerckhove, & Boeckx, 2005)

9) Risk for pressure ulcers is related to immobility, significant edema, nutrition alterations, injuries or operative procedures, moisture imbalance, splinting, and pressure garments. Consider a pressure-reducing mattress, frequent turning (more often than every 2 hours), nutrition support, skin emollients and protective moisture barriers, and skin checks with splint and pressure garment removal (Gordon et al., 2004).

10) Risk for long bone fractures: Increased incidence in children younger than 3 years of age and with burns more than 40% TBSA (potential contributory factors: hormonal changes after burn, depressed vitamin D status, inadequate protein intake, decreased weight-bearing activity, opposition to physical therapy; Mayers, Gottschlich, Scanlon, & Warden, 2003)

11) Medication management: Potential treatment of hypermetabolic state (in children with more than 40% TBSA burns) with insulin, anabolic steroids, catecholamine antagonists, and anabolic and anticatabolic agents (Pereira et al., 2005; Przkora et al., 2006)

12) School reintegration: Potential compliance resistance necessitating assistance from school therapists for ongoing therapeutic management or a behavior management program (Pidcock, Fauerback, Ober, & Carney, 2003)

d. Client education topics
1) Importance of prevention of complications, contractures, loss of function, and ongoing exercise and therapy
2) Care and use of pressure garments
3) Signs and symptoms of infection
4) Skin and wound care
5) Social reintegration strategies
6) School and community reintegration strategies, camp opportunities
7) Psychosocial and behavioral interventions
8) Personal care
9) Nutrition
10) Pain and itching management
11) Medications
12) Home environment and safety as indicated; prevention of further injury

6. Limb deficiency
a. Definition: The absence of one or more limbs, caused by congenital conditions, trauma or

accidents, tumors, or diseases. Congenital amputations in children account for 60% of amputations, and acquired amputations account for about 40% of all amputations (Beaty, 2007). Acquired amputations most commonly result from trauma, with tumors occurring less frequently, and infection causing the remainder.

1) Congenital: May be spontaneous, related to prenatal infection or teratogen exposure during the first trimester, or genetic. Other associated congenital anomalies are likely, including genitourinary defects, cardiac defects, and cleft palate (Eilert, 2007)

   a) A terminal limb deficiency exists when there are no body parts distal to the deficiency.

   b) An intercalary limb deficiency exists when a middle limb portion is missing but distal structures are present (Beaty, 2007).

   c) Upper extremity: Below-elbow transverse arrest (most common), humeral deficiency, longitudinal arrest, failure of differentiation (i.e., synostosis), constriction or amniotic band syndromes, cleft hand, phocomelia (distal portion of extremity appears to attach directly to body), and amelia (missing limb; Kozin, 2004; Morrissy, Giavedoni, & Coulter-O'Berry, 2006)

   d) Lower extremity: Fibular hemimelia (missing fibula; most common), tibial hemimelia, proximal femoral focal deficiency (Morrissy et al., 2006; Mosca, 2006)

   e) Digits: Syndactyly (fused), adactylia (absent)

2) Acquired

   a) Trauma: Leading cause is lawn mower accidents, followed by motor vehicle and farm machinery accidents, gunshot wounds, fire or other burns, and amputations from triggered landmines (in war-torn countries; Morrissy et al., 2006)

   b) Malignancies or tumors

   c) Diseases (e.g., meningococcemia: Decreased tissue perfusion leading to amputation)

3) Amputation terminology

   a) Trans: Amputation across axis of long bone

   b) Disarticulation: Amputation through joint

   c) Partial: Amputation distal to the wrist or ankle joint

   d) Van Ness rotationplasty: Generally used after osteosarcoma around the knee joint, or congenital short femur, where the foot and ankle are preserved, rotated 180 degrees, and reattached to the distal femur, making a functional joint (Hillman, Weist, Fromme, Volker, & Rosenbaum, 2007)

b. Assessment components

1) Developmental level

2) Musculoskeletal system

3) Mobility: Ambulation and use of prosthesis

4) Skin integrity or residual limb care

c. Rehabilitation issues

1) Developmental and independence level

2) Function of limb: The goal is for the most functional support. Varying degrees of limb difference and function may occur with or without use of a prosthesis (Shida-Tokeshi et al., 2005); cosmesis, function, and comfort contribute to prosthetic wear; this is a team decision with limb deficiency clinic practitioners, the client, and family.

3) Prosthetic management: Consult with a physical or occupational therapist and prosthetist experienced in pediatric limb deficiencies (Gitter & Bosker, 2005); secure funding and long-term planning to allow frequent refittings and new prostheses related to growth:

   a) Upper extremity: Cosmetic, body powered, myoelectric, hybrid (with control cable system for function)

   b) Lower extremity: Function, above knee, below knee, special types of feet for various functions (Morrissy et al., 2006; Mosca, 2006)

   c) Acquired amputations across the diaphyseal plate may result in an irregular stump as the limb grows (Heck, 2007).

4) Mobility: Ambulation and prosthesis introduction at developmentally appropriate milestones, more likely to succeed and incorporate prosthesis into new tasks

   a) Upper extremity: Introduce a prosthesis when the child has developed sitting balance (approximately 6 months of age).

b) Lower extremity: When the child has had an amputation before learning ambulation, introduce the prosthesis during pulling to stand and beginning walking motions (approximately 9–14 months; Eilert, 2007; Gitter & Bosker, 2005).

5) Skin or residual limb management: Monitor for pressure areas, bony prominences, rashes from excessive moisture and heat (confinement in prosthesis), surgical incisions for newer amputations, stump care, and skin breakdown at amputation terminal ends related to bony overgrowth at the distal end of the residual limb (Gitter & Bosker, 2005; Mosca, 2006).

6) Pain management
   a) The most common causes and contributors of pain are postoperative surgical incision pain, anxiety, bony overgrowth (most common in children who have had amputation through a long bone, especially in a lower extremity).
   b) Phantom pain: Few children experience this phenomenon, especially if amputation occurred before 4 years of age (Morrissy et al., 2006).

7) Self-esteem and self-concept
   a) Facilitate networking with other parents and children with limb deficiencies or differences; networking is often available through limb deficiency specialized outpatient clinics.
   b) Talk to parents, teachers, and peers to facilitate communication about differences, reactions, and responses as developmentally appropriate and ready (Morrissy et al., 2006).
   c) Adaptations for activities and sports are critical for emotional, physical, self-esteem, and social development.

d. Provide support network resource information.
   1) Amputee Resource Foundation of America: www.amputeeresource.org
   2) National Amputation Foundation: www.nationalamputation.org
   3) I-Can International Child Amputee Network: www.child-amputee.net

7. Client education topics
   a. Use and care of equipment or prosthesis
   b. Residual limb wrapping or "stump sock" and skin care
   c. Pain management
   d. Community reintegration strategies, resources, and supports
   e. Therapy and prosthetic centers
   f. Safety and community education prevention
   g. For congenital deficiencies, genetic counseling (for the parents or the child; Morrissy et al., 2006)
   h. Emotional and social support: Review support systems to deal with family distress, shock, and possible feelings of guilt (in trauma and congenital events; Morrissy et al., 2006; Mosca, 2006).

B. Cancer: Cancer is the fourth leading cause of death in children, behind unintentional injuries, homicides, and suicides. Treatment modalities have improved such that the 5-year survival rate is greater than 75% (better than in adults). Most common malignancies are acute lymphocytic leukemia, acute myeloid leukemia, brain tumors (most common of solid tumors in children), lymphomas, neuroblastomas, bone tumors, retinoblastomas, hepatic tumors, and Langerhans cell histiocytosis (American Cancer Society, 2009; Maloney et al., 2007).

1. Brain tumors: Rehabilitation needs during and after intervention
   a. Behavioral and cognitive function impairments, short- and long-term memory problems, similar to those of acquired brain injury (Poggi et al., 2005; Vargo & Gerber, 2005)
   b. Dysphagia, treatment similar to that of stroke
   c. Weakness and often gait disturbance
   d. Visual/perceptual impairment
   e. Increased incidence of seizures

2. General cancer care and rehabilitation nursing: assessment and monitoring
   a. Developmental level
   b. Family assessment
   c. Community resources
   d. Functional ability related to disease progression
   e. Complications: Growth, endocrine, cardiopulmonary, renal, neuropsychological, secondary malignancies
   f. Monitoring laboratory results for nadir (lowest point of white and red blood cell count and platelet count after chemotherapy) and need for protective precautions

3. Rehabilitation issues
    a. Pain management
    b. Independence level related to developmental level
    c. Disease progression
    d. Coping
    e. Self-image (especially with chemotherapy effects, amputation, scarring, alopecia)
    f. Fatigue
    g. Integration of rehabilitation and cancer treatment and palliative care plan
    h. Skin integrity, especially with radiation
4. Client education topics
    a. Use and care of equipment and assistive devices
    b. Medication regimen
    c. Pain management techniques
    d. Energy conservation
    e. Community reintegration strategies
C. Congenital Diseases and Birth Defects
1. Myelodysplasia or myelomeningocele (spina bifida)
    a. Definition: A condition in which the neural tube fails to close during the first 3–4 weeks of fetal development, resulting in incomplete closure of the spinal column. The opening in the spine may be at any level, but thoracic and lumbar levels are most common. There are different types of spina bifida.
        1) Myelomeningocele: The most severe form. The spinal cord and meninges protrude from the opening in the spine; they may be covered with a sac or be open.
            a) Hydrocephalus occurs in about 80% of cases.
            b) Motor and sensory nerves below the level of the lesion are affected, resulting in paraplegia, neurogenic bowel and bladder, and lack of sensation.
        2) Meningocele: Meninges protrude from the open spine. Motor and sensory nerves below the level of the lesion may be affected.
        3) Spina bifida occulta: An abnormal opening in the spinal column, without any nerve tissue protruding, and completely covered by skin
            a) There may be a patch of hair covering the site but no unusual appearance.
            b) There usually is no disability (NINDS, 2009b; Spina Bifida Association of America [SBAA], 2010).
    b. Cause and incidence
        1) The exact cause is unknown but is thought to be multifactorial, involving genetics and environment.
        2) Folic acid supplementation in women of childbearing age significantly reduces the risk of a neural tube defect.
        3) Women who take valproic acid for seizures are more likely to have a child with a neural tube defect (Koren, Nava-Ocampo, Moretti, Sussman, & Nulman, 2006).
        4) Occurrence is 7 out of every 10,000 births in the United States (SBAA, 2010).
    c. Outcomes
        1) Cognitive deficits: Children with hydrocephalus are more likely to be affected, with problems ranging from learning disabilities to mental retardation.
            a) Motivation is a significant problem and stems in part from executive function deficits.
            b) Depression and anxiety are common but may also be signs of shunt malfunction or infection, so organic causes must be ruled out before treatment (Oddson, Clancy, & McGrath, 2006; SBAA, 2010).
        2) Neurogenic bowel and bladder
            a) Timed voiding, clean intermittent catheterization, and continent stomas that may be catheterized (e.g., the Mitrofanoff procedure) are some management methods.
            b) Urinary tract infections are common and may damage ureters and kidneys (Clayton & Brock, 2010).
            c) Infants are assessed at birth and regularly thereafter for reflux and kidney damage (Snodgrass & Garagallo, 2010).
            d) Bowel programs focus on preventing constipation and maintaining continence. Bowel programs are among the most frustrating tasks for children and parents (Sawin & Thompson, 2009).
            e) Use of the antegrade continence enema has contributed to increased continence in a flaccid bowel; however, it requires major abdominal surgery and placement of a cecostomy, an artificial opening to the intestine (Sawin & Thompson, 2009).

3) Hydrocephalus: A ventriculoperitoneal shunt may be necessary to control hydrocephalus. Shunts may malfunction, become infected, or need revision for growth.

4) Sensory deficits: Sensation is partially or completely lost below the level of the lesion.

5) Mobility: Depending on the level of the lesion and the muscles enervated, braces, crutches, a walker, or a wheelchair may be used. Children who are able to walk short distances with crutches and braces when they are small often move to wheelchair mobility in adolescence when they are older and heavier (Verhoef et al., 2006).

6) Latex allergy is very common in people with spina bifida and ranges from mild to very severe (Pollart, Warniment, & Mori, 2009).

7) Neurologic complications: Although these do not occur in every person, they may significantly affect function and long-term outcome.

   a) Tethered spinal cord: The spinal cord is "caught" and cannot move as the child grows.

   b) Symptomatic Chiari malformation: A brain malformation associated with hydrocephalus that becomes symptomatic in about one-third of children with spina bifida (SBAA, 2010)

8) Orthopedic problems

   a) Hip dysplasia

   b) Clubfoot

   c) Scoliosis and kyphosis

d. Nursing assessment and interventions

1) Developmental and cognitive assessment

2) Neurologic assessment

   a) Presence of neurologic complications

   b) Signs of shunt malfunction

3) Bladder and bowel function

   a) Signs of urinary tract infection

   b) Constipation

   c) Child's readiness to begin self-care

4) Skin integrity: Prevention and management of pressure ulcers (Butler, 2006)

5) Orthopedic concerns

   a) Preoperative and postoperative surgical repair

   b) Use of braces and mobility devices

6) Latex allergies: Prevention and treatment

7) Visual perceptual deficits

8) Cardiopulmonary function: May be compromised in children with high thoracic lesion levels or with symptomatic Chiari malformation

9) Nutritional status: Adequate growth and development, prevention of obesity

10) Ability to perform activities of daily living (ADLs)

11) Self-concept and self-esteem: Participation in adaptive sports can be helpful (Leger, 2005).

12) Family assessment: Ability to care for child, stressors, support systems

e. Rehabilitation issues

1) Promotion of development, attainment of milestones as much as possible

2) Self-care as appropriate for age, ability to perform ADLs

3) Independence level related to growth and developmental level (Greenley, 2010)

4) Promotion of mobility and upright position

5) Bowel and bladder management

6) Skin care

7) Special education

8) Community inclusion (Lomax-Bream, Barnes, Copeland, Taylor, & Landry, 2007)

9) Transition to adult health care

f. Family and child education topics

1) Bladder and bowel program (Mason, Tobias, Lutkenhoff, Stoops, & Ferguson, 2004)

2) Skin care and pressure-relief techniques

3) Use and care of equipment and orthoses

4) Promotion of independence and ADLs at home and school (Greenley, Coakley, Holmbeck, Jandasek, & Wills, 2006)

5) Transfers and ambulation (if appropriate to level of lesion)

6) Service coordination and advocacy

2. Diseases related to muscular dystrophy: Most children with a progressive neuromuscular condition are cared for and followed in an outpatient setting. Inpatient rehabilitation services may be sought for postoperative endurance or for a secondary condition unrelated to the reason for the rehabilitation admission (e.g., car accident). The rehabilitation nurse may be called on for consultation to acute care inpatient surgical services.

   a. Types and definitions (Muscular Dystrophy Association [MDA], 2007)

1) Duchenne muscular dystrophy. Occurrence in males is caused by the absence of dystrophin. Age of recognition: 2–6 years, progresses rapidly. Genetics: X-linked recessive. Most common.

   a) Medical and mobility issues: Wheelchair use often by age of 9, gross motor strength significantly affected, able to do some fine motor independent skills with setup. Most often warrants surgical intervention for heel cord releases, scoliosis corrective spine surgery, respiratory support; cardiomyopathy is common (in the late teen years).

   b) Lifespan: Without intervention, late teens or early 20s; often into 30s or longer with respiratory support and cardiac interventions

2) Becker muscular dystrophy: A condition similar to but less severe than Duchenne, caused by insufficient production of dystrophin (X-linked recessive).

   a) Medical and mobility issues: Often ambulatory through the teen years

   b) May consider using a wheelchair for long distances

   c) Lifespan: Into late adulthood, may need cardiac intervention

3) Congenital muscular dystrophy: A group of genetic, degenerative diseases affecting voluntary muscles. Onset at or near birth. Progression and disability vary; often seen as generalized muscle weakness. Autosomal recessive.

4) Myotonic dystrophy: Affects generations, progressively more involved with each generation. Generalized weakness, muscle wasting, myotonia, developmental disability appear in children. Caused by a repeated section of DNA on chromosome 19, autosomal dominant, medical and mobility problems, often ambulatory into the late teens, wheelchair for long distances.

5) Limb girdle muscular dystrophy: Mutation of different genes affecting proteins for muscle function. Presents as weakness and wasting of muscles around shoulders and hips. Can be autosomal dominant or autosomal recessive. May look similar in functional challenges to Duchenne but is less severely progressive.

6) Facioscapulohumeral muscular dystrophy: Missing area of chromosome 4, onset usually by age 20. Weakness of eye and mouth muscles, shoulders, upper arms, and lower legs. Autosomal dominant.

7) Spinal muscular atrophy (SMA). Definition: Deficiency of motor neuron protein SMN on chromosome 5. Loss of motor neuron nerve cells in the spinal cord, resulting in loss of voluntary muscle control. Mental, emotional, and sensory development are normal in SMA. All types are autosomal recessive (MDA, 2010). A support network is available at www.fsma.org, Families of Spinal Muscle Atrophy.

   a) Type 1: Infantile (Werdnig-Hoffman), onset birth to 6 months. Rapid progression, often leading to death in the first 1–2 years of life. Increased longevity with respiratory ventilation and nutritional support.

   b) Type 2: Intermediate, onset 6–18 months. Weakness in central core muscles: shoulders, hips, thighs, upper back; wheelchair dependent. At risk for respiratory compromise. Lifespan can be into childhood, teens, young adulthood.

   c) Type 3: Mild (Kugelberg-Welander), onset after 18 months. Often presents after the child has started walking. Slower progression. Walking ability often maintained at least until adolescence. Lifespan usually not affected, but respiratory function and spinal curvature should be assessed regularly.

   d) Type 4: Adult-onset SMA, onset in adulthood. Mildest type of SMA (NINDS, 2008).

8) Charcot-Marie-Tooth (CMT; MDA, 2007): Neurological damage to peripheral nerves. Caused by defects in axons or in genes for proteins found in myelin. Onset birth to adulthood. Different forms of CMT: autosomal dominant, autosomal recessive, and X-linked. Slowly progressive, often see muscle weakness, wasting, loss of sensation in periphery.

9) Friedreich's ataxia: Genetic defect to frataxin protein, diminishing energy production in mitochondria, resulting in damage to peripheral nerves and cerebellum. Affects all ages as young as 2

years old. Most characterized by ataxia, loss of sensation, cardiac involvement, difficulty with speech and swallowing, diabetes. A support network is available at www.ataxia.org, National Ataxia Foundation.

    10) Leukodystrophy (NINDS, 2007): Different types, genetic related, progressive degeneration of white matter of the brain from decreased growth and development of myelin sheath. Varies in prognosis, often quite debilitating, life-limiting.

  b. Assessment components
    1) Developmental level
    2) Respiratory status
    3) Cardiovascular
    4) Scoliosis
    5) Assistive, orthotic mobility devices
    6) Medication history (especially corticosteroid use)
    7) Skin integrity
    8) Nutrition and fluid intake
    9) Seizures (in leukodystrophy)
    10) Bladder and bowel function (retain sensation, decrease in motor control, and decrease in motility as disease progresses)
    11) Psychosocial
    12) Home environment accessibility
    13) Family history and genetics

  c. Rehabilitation issues
    1) Pulmonary management and support
    2) Corticosteroid precautions (Moxley et al., 2005)
    3) Maintenance of intact skin
    4) Toileting
    5) Assistance with ADLs depending on severity and progression of condition
    6) Seizure management (as applicable)
    7) Maintain independence as much as possible
    8) Accessibility of home environment

  d. Client education topics
    1) Pulmonary and cardiovascular maintenance and precautions
    2) Maintenance of skin integrity
    3) Range-of-motion exercises
    4) Use of assistive, orthotic, and mobility devices
    5) Nutrition and fluid intake
    6) Home environment modifications
    7) Medication management
    8) Mobility
    9) Community integration strategies

3. Joint and orthopedic conditions
  a. Common types of disabling orthopedic conditions that may necessitate rehabilitation
    1) Legg-Calvé-Perthes disease is a condition most common in males in which the femoral head develops avascular necrosis.
      a) May occur at any age but usually between 3 and 9 years of age
      b) Cause is unknown, but various factors such as attention deficit hyperactivity disorder (ADHD), delayed skeletal age, metabolic factors, and mechanical dysfunction may play a role in its development.
      c) Treatment includes bed rest with periodic mobilization, abduction bracing, biphosphate medications, or surgery (McQuade & Houghton, 2005).
    2) Osteogenesis imperfecta (OI) is a metabolic bone and connective tissue disease that results in brittle bones; it is commonly associated with fractures that can occur with normal movement and care of the child with this condition. Fractures that are characteristic of this condition often are mistaken for child abuse (Paterson & McAllion, 2006).
      a) Cause is a dominant genetic mutation.
      b) There are many different types of OI, from very mild to lethal.
      c) OI is present from conception, but, depending on the severity, it may be diagnosed at birth or late in life.
      d) Approximately 50,000 people in the United States have OI.
      e) In most types, more fractures occur in childhood, then become less frequent with age.
      f) Treatment varies with severity. Special handling techniques for children more significantly affected reduce the number of fractures. Frequent surgery may be needed to repair bone deformities (Osteogenesis Imperfecta Foundation, 2006; Shapiro & Sponsellor, 2009).
    3) Leg length discrepancy: Inequality of the leg lengths, usually more than 2 cm, which may be the result of congenital malformations of the fibula, infections, trauma affecting the epiphyses, or neurologic disorders such as poliomyelitis

a) Discrepancies of 2–4 cm may be treated using lifts in the shoe.

b) Greater discrepancies may be treated with a surgical procedure to slow down the growth of the longer leg.

c) Larger discrepancies may be treated with leg-lengthening surgery, often using an external fixator that extends the ends of the bone and soft tissues over a period of weeks (American Academy of Orthopedic Surgeons, 2007).

4) Juvenile rheumatoid arthritis: A chronic inflammation that involves the connective tissue, joints, and viscera, which begins before the age of 16.

5) Achondroplasia: A skeletal dysplasia causing short stature and bony deformities.

a) The cause is genetic, occurring in 1 out of 30,000 live births.

b) Developmental delays, kyphosis, flexion contractures of joints, bowed legs, other hip and spine problems, and characteristic bowed forehead are associated with achondroplasia.

c) Treatment includes physical therapies, bracing, and surgical treatment (Amirfayz & Gargan, 2005).

6) Arthrogryposis multiplex congenita: Congenital joint contractures, decreased fetal movement in utero related to a variety of reasons and conditions, most often associated with motor neuron involvement (amyoplasia). There is limited function of upper and lower extremities (Defendi, 2009).

b. Nursing assessment and interventions

1) Developmental milestones and self-care ability

2) Level of disability related to diagnosis

3) Pain assessment and management preoperatively and postoperatively

4) Preoperative and postoperative nursing care (Ireland, 2006)

5) Mobility, use, and care of equipment and assistive devices

6) Ability to perform ADLs; self-care

7) Family

a) Medical history and genetics

b) Coping and adaptive skills

c) Ability to care for child

8) Discharge planning, service coordination, and case management (Faux & Nehring, 2010)

c. Rehabilitation issues

1) Promotion of maximum independence level based on severity of the diagnosis

2) Mobility

3) Joint protection

4) ADL modification

5) Safety

6) Psychological implications such as developmental regression, avoidance behavior, depression, social isolation (e.g., of prolonged bed rest, disability, painful procedures)

7) Community integration and school attendance (Selekman & Vessey, 2010)

d. Family and child education topics

1) Medication regimen

2) ADLs

3) Safety

4) Mobility versus joint protection

5) Pain management

6) Use and care of equipment and assistive devices

7) Community resources (Sullivan-Bolyai, Knafl, Sadler, & Gilliss, 2004)

4. Cerebral palsy (CP)

a. Definition: A mild to severe condition that results from damage to the developing brain that produces a permanent but nonprogressive abnormality of muscle coordination, balance, and purposeful movement. CP is the most common childhood disability and usually is detected by the time the child is 3 years old. The terms used to describe CP relate to extremity involvement: monoplegia, diplegia, hemiplegia, quadriplegia.

b. Types of CP

1) Spastic: Hyperactive reflexes, increased muscle tone, muscle spasms, motor weakness, persistent reflexes

2) Athetoid: Abnormal involuntary movements, facial grimacing, dystonic movements, poor speech, distorted posturing

3) Ataxia: Hypotonia, floppy muscle tone, impaired balance and coordination, unsteady gait

4) Mixed: Combination of several types

c. Assessment must be highly individualized and reflect the child's age, level of involvement, and associated problems (Edwards, 2001).

1) Developmental level

2) Cognitive level
3) Communication and speech
4) Ability to perform ADLs
5) Feeding pattern
6) Toileting
7) Muscle function
8) Ambulation
9) History of seizure disorders and other associated conditions
10) Vision and hearing
11) Skin integrity
12) Learning disability

d. Rehabilitation issues: Additional problems and symptoms may develop as the child progresses and grows (Edwards, 2001).
   1) Neurodevelopmental and sensory therapies
   2) Independent living skills
   3) Positioning and therapeutic handling (depending on severity)
   4) Feeding problems
   5) Communication
   6) Seizure management
   7) Spasticity management
   8) Motor control
   9) Assistive technology
   10) Social and sexual relationships
   11) Surgery and nonsurgical procedures: Orthopedic procedures, intrathecal baclofen, dorsal rhizotomy, peripheral neurotomy (Steinbok, 2006)

e. Family and child education topics
   1) Skin assessment and care
   2) Exercise and fitness programs
   3) Medications
   4) Spasticity management techniques
   5) Self-care
   6) Feeding and nutrition
   7) Bowel and bladder management
   8) Community integration strategies: School, leisure activities, transportation, independent living arrangements

D. Chronic Illnesses
   1. Bronchopulmonary dysplasia
      a. Definition: A range of conditions characterized by scarring or fibrosis of immature lung tissue that occur in premature infants. Also known as chronic lung disease of infancy, it can last throughout childhood and into adulthood. Contributing factors include the following:
         1) Prematurity, and maternal factors such as preeclampsia and chorioamnionitis

2) Mechanical ventilation and oxygen in response to severe respiratory distress syndrome caused by pneumonia, sepsis, meconium aspiration, or fluid overload
3) Infection and inflammation
4) Patent ductus arteriosus
5) Possible genetic influences (Abman, Mourani, & Sontag, 2008)

b. Cause and incidence
   1) Thought to be caused by exposure of the immature alveoli and microvasculature of the lungs to trauma from mechanical ventilation, high oxygen concentrations, and respiratory distress itself. The resulting decrease in oxygenation affects the lungs, heart, and brain.
   2) May be related to abnormal signaling within the alveoli that fails to repair damage (Cerny, Torday, & Rehan, 2008)
   3) Occurs most commonly in premature infants with a birth weight of less than 1,250 grams and at fewer than 30 weeks' gestation
   4) The occurrence can be reduced by the use of glucocorticoid and surfactant treatment (Baveja & Christou, 2006).
   5) Incidence ranges from 17% to 57% because multiple factors influence its development (Driscoll & Davis, 2007).

c. Commonly associated complications
   1) Airway complications such as stenosis, granuloma, scarring, tracheomalacia, and frequent infections
   2) Growth retardation and poor weight gain; vitamin deficiencies
   3) Gastroesophageal reflux
   4) Cardiac conditions such as pulmonary hypertension and cor pulmonale
   5) Seizures
   6) Retinopathy of prematurity and other ophthalmic complications
   7) Frequent ear and sinus infections
   8) Renal calcification from long-term use of diuretics
   9) Lack of patency of tracheostomy and gastrostomy tubes; inflammation and infection of stomas
   10) Developmental delays including cognitive disability, gross and fine motor deficits, speech and language problems, visual/motor integration disorders, ADHD, and behavioral problems (Anderson & Doyle, 2006)

11) Long-term outcomes may include all of the above, as well as chronic pulmonary disease with risk of respiratory failure in adolescence and adulthood and long-lasting cardiac disorders (Doyle et al., 2006).

d. Nursing assessment and interventions
1) Respiratory assessment: Adequacy of ventilation, function of assistive technology, patency of tracheostomy and suctioning or replacement when necessary, early identification of infection and treatment, respiratory medications.
2) Developmental level in all domains; promote attainment of developmental milestones. Assess self-care skills and ADLs in the older child.
3) Cardiac assessment: Pulse, blood pressure, symptoms of heart failure, cardiac medications
4) Oral feeding if possible, maintenance of gastrostomy tube and tube feedings, promote good nutrition; evaluate for anemia and other deficiencies, monitor growth and gastroesophageal reflux, administer medications as appropriate
5) Skin care: Assess stomas for irritation, granulomatous tissue, and leakage.
6) Appropriate screenings: Vision, hearing, dental, developmental
7) Health promotion and prevention: Immunizations, need for palivizumab (Synagis) to prevent respiratory syncytial virus (Parmigiani et al., 2009)
8) Discharge planning
9) Family stress and coping skills, ability to manage child's needs

e. Rehabilitation issues
1) Developmental interventions including physical therapy, occupational therapy, speech therapy, and recreational therapy; promotion of independence as appropriate for age (Anderson & Doyle, 2006)
2) Respiratory management with pulmonary specialists to ameliorate impact of long-term ventilation or tracheostomy on development; chest physiotherapy
3) Early intervention, special education, and school inclusion (Clements, Barfield, Kotelchuck, Lee, & Wilbur, 2006)
4) Behavioral problems

f. Family and child education topics
1) Management of technology in the home and community: Troubleshooting the ventilator, suctioning and changing the tracheostomy, administering tube feedings, changing the gastrostomy tube
2) Medication management: Administration, side effects
3) Prevention of complications and health maintenance
4) Promoting independence in self-care in the child (Rehm & Bradley, 2005)
5) Negotiating with caregivers in the home, service coordination, school liaison
6) Safety at home, at school, and in the community
7) Maintenance of family equilibrium, dealing with siblings

2. Technology dependence
a. Definition: Children who are technology dependent are defined as those who use "a medical device to compensate for the loss of a vital bodily function and substantial and ongoing nursing care to avert death or further disability" (Office of Technology Assessment, 1987, p. 3).
1) Examples include children with a tracheostomy or gastrostomy tube or who need home oxygen, mechanical ventilation, or other medical devices such as colostomies or intravenous fluid pumps; they may need more than one device.
2) They need high-tech care from parents or caregivers who have been specially trained or from nurses.
3) Up to 40% of children discharged from one urban pediatric hospital were technology dependent (Feudtner et al., 2005).
4) In one state, fewer than 1% of children birth through 19 years of age were found to be medically fragile and used technology; however, these children used almost 7% of the Medicaid dollars allocated for that age group (Buescher, Whitmire, Brunssen, & Kluttz-Hile, 2006).

b. Nursing assessment of the child
1) Developmental and cognitive level
2) Language skills and communication methods
3) Age-appropriate ability to perform ADLs and assistance needed
4) Frequent physiological assessment, particularly respiratory system, gastrointestinal

system, genitourinary system, skin integrity, musculoskeletal system
5) Ability to eat; nutrition
6) Toileting and bowel and bladder management; signs of urinary tract infection, constipation
7) Ambulation or form of mobility
8) Psychosocial issues
9) Hospital discharge planning and assessment
   a) Equipment and supply assessment: Appropriate for child, in good working order, sufficient supplies (e.g., suction catheters, gloves)
   b) Home assessment: Accessibility, enrichment of the environment (e.g., books, toys), cleanliness, safety; presence of an emergency backup plan for equipment or power failure, notification of emergency responders (e.g., child with a tracheostomy or using a ventilator), notification of public utility services (e.g., need for immediate attention to resumption of electrical service); availability of home nursing care, therapy, and medical care in the home community
   c) School assessment: Accessibility, plan for care while the child is in school, equipment and supplies, individualized educational plan, appropriate caregiver training (e.g., school nurse, licensed practical nurse, or designated caregiver; Earle, Rennick, Carnavale, & Davis, 2006; Hewitt-Taylor, 2005)
c. Nursing assessment of family and family issues
   1) Family stress and coping skills; sibling stress
   2) Ability to meet child's needs; role confusion of parent role versus high-tech caregiver role
   3) Family and caregiver skill assessment
   4) Financial stress
   5) Social isolation (Kirk, Glendinning, & Callery, 2005)
   6) Accessible transportation for medical services and recreational activities
   7) Fatigue and burnout
   8) Intrusiveness of technology and nursing care in the home (Rehm & Bradley, 2005)
d. Rehabilitation nursing interventions
   1) Plan for discharge.

2) Promote community integration and independence as appropriate for the child's developmental level and functional abilities.
3) Ensure safety in the home, community, and school.
4) Provide expert clinical nursing.
5) Offer family support and referrals as needed and community resources.
e. Family and child education topics
   1) Operation and maintenance of assistive technology
   2) Clinical care of child
   3) Promotion of independence in self-care
   4) Community integration
   5) Training of community service providers (Reeves, Timmons, & Dampier, 2006).

III. **Long-Term Planning: Community Services for Children and Youth with Disabilities**
A. Philosophy of Inclusion
   1. Inclusion is a philosophical viewpoint that asserts that children with disabilities are an integral part of the community and should participate with their peers in typical activities such as school.
   2. Inclusion may occur in playgroups, school, recreation, social activities, and work.
   3. In the school setting inclusion means that children with disabilities should receive educational services in a typical classroom in which other children without disabilities are schooled (Wisconsin Education Association Council, 2007).
B. School Programs
   1. The Individuals with Disabilities Education Act (IDEA Reauthorization 2004, final regulations published August 14, 2006) ensures that all children and youth ages 3–21 years receive a free, appropriate public education.
   2. Education and special education services should be delivered in the least restrictive environment, as similar to settings for children without disabilities as possible.
   3. Children who need special education are entitled to receive an individualized education plan that is reviewed yearly to best meet the child's educational needs.
   4. Children with disabilities may also receive related services through the school (e.g., physical therapy, occupational therapy, speech therapy, nutrition, other health-related services), as mandated by IDEA, if those services are necessary for learning.
   5. Child Find is a system each school district has in place to identify children who are eligible for

special education services (U.S. Department of Education, 2007).

6. The No Child Left Behind legislation, passed in 2001, set high standards for the education of all children and requires accountability from schools in the areas of reading and math. Children are tested on a regular basis to determine whether their education meets standards. Children with disabilities that hinder learning may receive alternative testing or may be excluded from testing. The legislation is up for reauthorization in 2011 (National Education Association, 2010).

C. Early Intervention

1. Part C of IDEA provides for early educational services for young children with or at risk for disabilities from birth to 3 years of age.

2. Eligible children and their families receive an individualized family service plan that includes interventions to eliminate or reduce the developmental delay or disability and offer family support.

3. Early intervention services may include speech and language, physical or occupational therapy, psychological services, service coordination, social work, vision screening, and medical services (U.S. Department of Education, 2007).

D. Other Legislation Affecting Children with Disabilities

1. Rehabilitation Act: Provides for supportive services in school for children with physical disabilities who do not qualify for special education

2. Title V of the Social Security Act was passed in 1935 and established the Maternal and Child Health Bureau to provide public health services for mothers and children, as well as disabled children (U.S. Department of Health and Human Services, 2007).

3. The Children's Bureau was established in 1912 to promote child welfare. The Child Abuse Prevention and Treatment Act was passed in 1974 and reauthorized in 2003 (Child Welfare Information Gateway, 2007).

4. Americans with Disabilities Act of 1990 (Refer to Chapter 1.)

5. Vocational Rehabilitation Act

E. Home Health Care

1. Children who are technology dependent as a result of prematurity, illness, or injury often need skilled care at home and at school.

2. Living at home is much better for the child's developmental, psychological, and social well-being than living in an institution.

3. Medicaid is the primary payer for home health care, with private health insurance covering only

about 1% of costs. Medicaid's low reimbursement rate makes it difficult to locate qualified agencies to provide specialized pediatric care in the home (AAP Committee on Child Health Financing, Section on Home Care, 2006; Musheno, 2010).

4. Although the assistance of home health is welcomed, the intrusiveness of strangers in the home on a daily basis may be stressful (Hewitt-Taylor, 2005).

5. Many families' insurance does not cover home health care and families are forced to provide skilled nursing care without assistance, which may put extreme stress on them.

a. In these cases, respite care, which gives families a break, can be very useful (Neufield, Query, & Drummond, 2001).

b. The Division of Developmental Disabilities in each state may have respite care funding available.

F. Health Promotion and Prevention

1. Children with disabilities need a "medical home" to coordinate specialty care and ensure well care (AAP Council on Children with Disabilities, 2005). Most recently the "Family-Centered Medical Home" (AAP, 2010) is described as a model in which the pediatric healthcare team (not just one pediatrician) partners with the family to ensure that all the medical and nonmedical needs of the child are met.

2. Developmental screening (identification of children who need in-depth assessment related to developmental delays) is the responsibility of the primary healthcare provider.

3. All children need immunizations and health screening, and children with disabilities may need specific preventive activities such as prevention of secondary conditions (AAP Council on Children with Disabilities, 2005, 2006).

4. Health promotion for children with disabilities includes good nutrition, physical activity, friendships, and positive social interaction.

G. Transition to Adulthood and Independent Living Situations (**Figure 18-1**)

1. School-to-work transition services are provided by the school system, which links with vocational education (Betz, 2007).

2. Youth with disabilities must also transition health care from pediatric to adult providers.

a. Many adult healthcare providers are unfamiliar with the health consequences of growing up with a pediatric disability.

b. Pediatric providers are unfamiliar with adult health issues (American Academy of Pediatrics,

American Academy of Family Physicians, American College of Physicians, & American Society of Internal Medicine, 2002).

3. Primary factors in successful transition and independent living models
   a. Attitude and attributes of the youth and family
   b. Self-care skills
   c. Availability of resources in the community, such as independent living services, accessible transportation, knowledgeable health and education providers, and supported employment
   d. Ability of the youth to perform ADLs and self-care independently or direct others to do so, or if youth is unable to make decisions, guardianship
   e. Independent mobility
   f. Healthcare needs
   g. Living arrangements (e.g., where, with whom, community options, housekeeping skills)
   h. Housing (e.g., adaptations needed, ability to maintain a home)
   i. Recreation and leisure activities
   j. Social skills
   k. Cognitive abilities and communication skills
   l. Job skills
   m. Financial management strategies
   n. Legal issues (http://depts.washington.edu/healthtr/, December 2008)

H. Vocational Rehabilitation and Higher Education
   1. State and local vocational rehabilitation offices work closely with schools-in-transition programs and local employers.
   2. Youth with disabilities who have academic capabilities may go on to higher education.
      a. Many city and community colleges and universities are reaching out to young adults with disabilities.
      b. Vocational rehabilitation offices may provide assistive technology to aid youth in educational pursuits.
   3. Although not all children have the potential to be working members of society, many are overlooked simply because of lack of information about potential options (Adolescent Youth Transition Project, 2006; Betz, 2007).

IV. **Trends and Future Directions**
A. Health Care
   1. Healthcare reform legislation, the Patient Protection and Affordable Care Act, was enacted in March 2010 and is scheduled for implementation over the next 3 years. However, a number of its provisions remain controversial, and rules and regulations have not been established. Currently, provisions that may affect children with disabilities include the following:
      a. Expand Medicaid and Child Health Plan eligibility and increase Medicaid payment for services to primary healthcare providers (e.g. family practice, pediatricians) to increase access to care for many children.
      b. Improve access to health care for people with preexisting conditions (e.g. children with disabilities) whose families must change jobs or insurance.
      c. Prohibit health insurance plans from placing a lifetime limit on coverage. Currently, for example, premature infants with multiple medical complications often reach their lifetime limits on insurance funding before they are discharged to home for the first time.
      d. Improve funding of preventive care for children and youth.
      e. More funding for training of future and existing healthcare providers, particularly in chronic care (Musheno, 2010).
   2. Technology is more readily available to preserve and improve life but at increasing expense. As a result, funding may be more scarce.
   3. There will be a greater emphasis on quality and safety, tracking the impact of nursing care on outcomes.
   4. Emphasis on research and evidence-based practice addresses new ideas and validates current practice.
   5. With nursing shortages, there is increased need for education in pediatrics and rehabilitation for nurses practicing with children and adolescents in a variety of settings.
   6. Quality of life and end-of-life decision making incorporating rehabilitation and developmental principles will be important, as will more nursing research to identify better treatment options.
   7. Collaborative, interdisciplinary service models will continue to evolve, with growth in nonhospital settings.
   8. Incidence of orthopedic and sports-related injuries will increase.
   9. Genetics and stem-cell research will link diseases to certain genes, with potential for new treatment options.
B. Community
   1. There will be less hospital-based care with shorter stays and more outpatient, community, and home-based care.
   2. There will be a greater need for accommodations for children who are technology dependent in schools and in the community.

Please note: The following recommendations are based on the child's developmental age and ability.

Birth–3 Years Old
- Encourage your child to assist with activities.
- Allow your child enough time to complete tasks.
- Talk with your child about his or her condition and abilities.

3–5 Years Old
- Teach your child about his or her special healthcare needs.
- Encourage your child to participate in self-care.
- Help your child to interact socially in various settings.
- Assign household chores or responsibilities particular to him or her.

6–12 Years Old
- Continue to assess your child's knowledge of his or her disability and provide additional information.
- Continue to teach your child self-care skills while addressing his or her special needs.
- Encourage his or her attempts to participate in self-care.
- Encourage hobbies and time for play.
- Allow your child to relate his or her experiences about the disability.
- Allow your child to participate in decision making by offering choices.
- Continue to assign appropriate chores or household duties that affect the child and the entire family.
- Help your child to interact with healthcare providers (allow him or her to speak directly to the doctor, nurse, or therapist).
- Talk about career options, interests, and abilities related to career choices.
- Take your child to work with you.

13–18 Years Old
- Help your teenager to develop self-awareness by focusing on interests, talents, and abilities.
- Continue to support your teenager's attempts to identify career choices.
- Continue to assess your teenager's knowledge and perception of his or her disability while providing additional information as needed.
- Continue to assist and encourage your teenager's attempts to do self-care.
- Encourage your teenager to do volunteer work or find part-time employment.
- Continue to assign chores and discuss the importance of family responsibilities.
- Obtain information about your teenager's state vocational rehabilitation program and school transition program.
- Discuss a plan for adult living, including healthcare services.
- Apply for SSI and Medicaid, if appropriate, at age 18 if previously denied for financial reasons.
- Discuss adult healthcare financing with your teenager.
- Discuss sexuality with your teenager, including how his or her disability may affect future health, career options, marriage, and the ability to have children.
- Encourage your teenager to speak freely with healthcare providers.
- Begin to look for adult care providers while allowing your teenager to participate in the decision-making process.
- Help your teenager keep a record of appointments, medications, and medical history (surgeries, treatments, hospitalizations, and allergies).
- Allow your teenager to make his or her own appointment, call for medication refills and supplies.
- Teach your teenager how to have medical information sent.

19–21 Years Old
- Identify an adult healthcare provider with your young adult.
- Transfer medical record to the adult care provider.
- Assist the young adult with finalizing adult healthcare financing and insurance options.
- Assist your young adult to schedule an appointment with adult care provider while still under pediatric care to ensure that the transfer to adult care will be uninterrupted and complete.
- Remain as a resource, support system, and safety net for your young adult as he or she assumes the responsibility of self-care.

From "Unique issues in pediatric spinal cord injury," by L. C. Vogel, K. J. Hickey, S. J. Klaas, & C. J. Anderson, 2004, *Orthopaedic Nursing, 23*(5), 300–308. Copyright 2004 by Lippincott Williams & Wilkins. Reprinted with permission.

3. There will be an increased need for home care education and for training caregivers in various settings.
4. Foster parents will be more likely to accept medically fragile children if they have a good medical home.
5. Legislation and litigation will continue to be a means to provide services to the pediatric population at the state and federal levels.

V. **Advanced Practice Nurses (APNs) in Pediatric Rehabilitation**
A. Qualifications: The APN has acquired the knowledge and practice experience for specialization, expansion, and advancement of pediatric rehabilitation nursing practice.
B. Characteristics of Graduate Nursing Education
1. Graduate nursing education prepares the APN to use critical thinking and decision-making skills to assess, plan, intervene, and evaluate the health and illness experiences of clients, families, and communities.
2. Core competencies include the following:
   a. The ability to critically assess research and to integrate research findings into evidence-based care
   b. The ability to provide cost-effective care and take part in designing and implementing healthcare systems
   c. The ability to assess and evaluate ethical dilemmas that affect care
   d. The ability to integrate the APN role into practice
   e. The ability to appreciate and evaluate nursing and other theories in the context of client care and systems of care
   f. The ability to apply knowledge about health disparities and cultural diversity to the care of clients, families, and communities
   g. The ability to maximize health and health promotion for clients, families, and communities (AACN, 2010)
C. Broad Range of Titles and Variety of Settings
1. Clinical nurse specialists
   a. More likely to work in an acute care setting but may also work in community agencies such as health department program for children with special needs
   b. Broad range of responsibilities, such as coordination of care, client education, and nursing education (Sparacino & Cartwright, 2009)
   c. Use nursing diagnosis to assess, plan, and intervene
2. Nurse practitioners

a. Usually provide routine health care, preventive care, immunizations, and minor illness care
b. Are prepared to diagnose and manage acute, episodic, and chronic illnesses
c. May specialize, providing care alongside medical subspecialists such as neurologists
d. Often provide care in community medical practices or outpatient settings (Anderson & O'Grady, 2009).
D. Scope of Practice
1. Autonomous practice and ability to bill for services
2. Advanced delivery of care in a specific specialty area (e.g., pediatric nurse practitioner, acute care clinical nurse specialist)
3. Complexity of situations or conditions managed
4. Leadership in the interdisciplinary team
5. In-depth understanding of interacting pathophysiologic and psychosocial changes associated with chronicity and disability (American Academy of Nurse Practitioners [AANP], 2010; American Medical Association, 2009)
E. Advanced Practice Roles
1. Clinician
   a. Facilitates the design and implementation of the individualized plan of care and the transition from the hospital to home and community
   b. Assesses health needs; develops diagnoses; plans, implements, and manages care; and evaluates outcomes of care
2. Educator
   a. Provides health education for professionals and consumers about the needs of children with disabilities and their families
   b. Bases teaching methods on developmental level, functional ability, learning needs and abilities, and sociocultural factors
3. Leader and consultant
   a. Serves as a model for child, adolescent, and family advocacy through direct intervention
   b. Promotes community and government knowledge of pediatric rehabilitation issues and works to influence policy-making bodies to improve care
   c. Involves stakeholders in the decision-making process and considers factors related to safety, effectiveness, cost, and impact on practice
   d. Provides consultation to influence the plan of care, enhances the practice of team members, and affects resource use

4. Researcher
   a. Participates in research and quality-improvement projects and is responsible for providing evidence-based care
   b. Critically evaluates current practice and uses scientific findings to improve client care outcomes
   c. Identifies research questions and disseminates relevant research findings to various constituencies

References

Abman, S. A., Mourani, P. M., & Sontag, M. (2008). Bronchopulmonary dysplasia: A genetic disease. *Pediatrics, 122,* 658–659.

Adamo, M. A., Drazin, D., Smith, C., & Waldman, J. (2009). Comparison of accidental and nonaccidental traumatic brain injuries in infants and toddlers: Demographics, neurosurgical interventions, and outcomes. *Journal of Neurosurgery. Pediatrics, 4,* 414–419.

Adolescent Youth Transition Project. (2006, June). Working together for successful transition. *Washington State adolescent transition resource notebook.* Publication no. 970-110. Retrieved June 22, 2007, from http://depts.washington.edu/healthtr/.

American Academy of Colleges of Nursing. (2010). *Essentials of nursing education.* Retrieved August 18, 2011, from www.aacn.nche.edu/education/essentials.htm.

American Academy of Pediatrics, American Academy of Family Physicians, American College of Physicians, & American Society of Internal Medicine. (2002). A consensus statement on health care transitions for young adults with special health care needs. *Pediatrics, 110*(6), 1304–1307.

American Academy of Nurse Practitioners. (2010). *Standards of practice for nurse practitioners.* Retrieved September 20, 2011, from www.aanp.org/NR/rdonlyres/FE00E81B-FA96-4779-972B-6162F04C309F/0/2010StandardsOfPractice.pdf.

American Academy of Orthopedic Surgeons. (2007). *Leg length discrepancy.* Retrieved September 20, 2011, from http://orthoinfo.aaos.org/topic.cfm?topic=a00259.

American Academy of Pediatrics. (2010). *Medical home fact sheet.* Retrieved September 20, 2011, from www.medicalhomeinfo.org/.

American Academy of Pediatrics Committee on Child Health Financing, Section on Home Care. (2006). Financing of pediatric home health care. *Pediatrics, 118*(2), 834–838.

American Academy of Pediatrics Council on Children with Disabilities. (2005). Care coordination in the medical home: Integrating health and related systems of care for children with special health care needs. *Pediatrics, 116*(5), 1238–1244.

American Academy of Pediatrics Council on Children with Disabilities. (2006). Identifying infants and young children with developmental disorders in the medical home: An algorithm for developmental surveillance and screening. *Pediatrics, 118*(1), 405–420.

American Cancer Society. (2009, May 19). *Detailed guide: Cancer in children.* Retrieved September 20, 2011, from www.cancer.org/Cancer/CancerinChildren/DetailedGuide/cancer-in-children-ref.

American Medical Association. (2009). *AMA Scope of Practice Data Series. A resource compendium for state medical associations and national medical societies. Nurse practitioners.* Chicago: Author.

Amirfayz, R., & Gargan, M. (2005). Achondroplasia. *Current Orthopaedics, 19*(6), 467–470.

Anderson, A. R. & O'Grady, E. T. (2009). The primary care nurse practitioner. In A. B. Hamric, J. A. Spross, & C. M. Hanson (Eds.), *Advanced practice nursing: An integrative approach* (4th ed., pp. 380–402). Philadelphia: Saunders.

Anderson, P. J., & Doyle, F. W. (2006). Neurodevelopmental outcome of bronchopulmonary dysplasia. *Seminars in Perinatology, 30*(4), 227–232.

Association of Rehabilitation Nurses. (2007). *Pediatric rehabilitation nursing role description* [Brochure]. Skokie, IL: Author.

Baveja, R., & Christou, H. (2006). Pharmacological strategies in the prevention and management of bronchopulmonary dysplasia. *Seminars in Perinatology, 30*(4), 209–218.

Beaty, J. H. (2007). Congenital anomalies of the lower extremity. In S. T. Canale & J. H. Beaty (Eds.), *Campbell's operative orthopedics* (Vol. II, 11th ed., pp. 1063–1250). Philadelphia: Mosby.

Betz, C. L. (2007). Facilitating the transition of adolescents with developmental disabilities. Nursing practice issues and care. *Journal of Pediatric Nursing, 22*(2), 103–115.

Blissit, P. A. (2006). Care of the critically ill patient with penetrating head injury. *Critical Care Nursing Clinics of North America, 18*(3), 321–332.

Brand, M. (2006). Focus on the physical series: Part 1. Recognizing neonatal spinal cord injury. *Advances in Neonatal Care, 6*(1), 15–24.

Buescher, P. A., Whitmire, J. T., Brunssen, S., & Kluttz-Hile, C. E. (2006). Children who are medically fragile in North Carolina: Using Medicaid data to estimate prevalence and medical care costs in 2004. *Maternal and Child Health Journal, 10*(5), 461–466.

Butler, C. T. (2006). Pediatric skin care: Guidelines for assessment, prevention and treatment. *Pediatric Nursing, 32*(5), 112–116.

Centers for Disease Control and Prevention. (2010). *Disability and health.* Retrieved August 27, 2010, from www.cdc.gov/ncbddd/disabilityandhealth/relatedconditions.html.

Cerny, L., Torday, J. S., & Rehan, V. K. (2008). Prevention and treatment of bronchopulmonary dysplasia: Contemporary status and future outlook. *Lung, 186,* 75–89.

Child Welfare Information Gateway. (2007). *About CAPTA: A legislative history.* Retrieved June 22, 2007, from www.childwelfare.gov/pubs/factsheets/about.cfm.

Chung, C. Y., Chen, C. L., Cheng, P. T., See, L. C., Tang, S. F., & Wong, A. M. (2006). Critical score of Glasgow Coma Scale for pediatric traumatic brain injury. *Pediatric Neurology, 34*(5), 379–387.

Clayton, D. B., & Brock, J. W. (2010). Congenital anomalies. The urologist's role in the management of spina bifida: A continuum of care. *Urology, 76,* 32–38.

Clements, K. M., Barfield, W. D., Kotelchuck, M., Lee, K. G., & Wilbur, N. (2006). Birth characteristics associated with early intervention referral, evaluation for eligibility, and program eligibility in the first year of life. *Maternal and Child Health Journal, 19*(5), 433–441.

Cohen, L., Lemanek, K., Blount, R. L., Dahlquist, L. M., Lim, C. S., Palermo, T. M., et al. (2008). Evidence-based assessment of pediatric pain. *Journal of Pediatric Psychology, 33*(9), 939–955. Retrieved December 12, 2010, from www.medscape.com/viewarticle/584206_3.

Dawodu, S. T. (2007). *Traumatic brain injury: Definition, pathophysiology, epidemiology.* Retrieved June 22, 2007, from www.emedicine.com/PMR/topic212.htm.

Defendi, G. L. (2009). *Achondroplasia.* Medscape.com. Retrieved September 20, 2011, from http://emedicine.medscape.com/article/941280-overview.

Doyle, L. W., Faber, B., Callanan, C., Freezer, N., Ford, G.W., & Davis, N. M. (2006). Bronchopulmonary dysplasia in very low birth weight subjects and lung function in late adolescence. *Pediatrics, 118*(1), 108–113.

Driscoll, W., & Davis, J. (2007). *Bronchopulmonary dysplasia.* Retrieved June 22, 2007, from www.emedicine.com/PED/topic289.htm.

Earle, R. J., Rennick, J. E., Carnavale, F. A., & Davis, G. M. (2006). "It's okay, it helps me to breathe": The experience of home ventilation from a child's perspective. *Journal of Child Health Care, 10*(4), 270–282.

Edwards, P. (2001). Pediatric rehabilitation nursing. In J. Derstine & S. Hargrove (Eds.), *Comprehensive rehabilitation nursing* (pp. 545–570). Philadelphia: W.B. Saunders.

Eilert, R. (2007). Orthopedics: Disturbances of prenatal origin—Congenital amputations & limb deficiencies. In W. W. Hay, M. Levin, J. M. Sondheimer, & R. R. Deterding (Eds.), *Current diagnosis & treatment in pediatrics* (18th ed., pp. 787–805). New York: McGraw-Hill.

Faux, S. A., & Nehring, W. M. (2010). Intellectual and developmental disabilities. In C. L. Betz & W. M. Nehring (Eds.), *Nursing care for individuals with intellectual and developmental disabilities: An integrated approach* (pp. 193–210). Baltimore, MD: Brookes.

Fay, T. B., Yeates, K. O., Wade, S., Drotar, D., Stancin, T., & Taylor, H. G. (2009). Predicting longitudinal patterns of functional deficits in children with traumatic brain injury. *Neuropsychology, 23*(3), 271–282.

Feudtner, C., Villareale, N. L., Morray, B., Sharp, V., Hays, R. M., & Neff, J. M. (2005). Technology-dependency among patients discharged from a children's hospital: A retrospective cohort study. *BMC Pediatrics, 5*(1), 8.

Gitter, A., & Bosker, G. (2005). Upper and lower extremity prosthetics. In J. A. DeLisa, G. B. M. Gans, N. E. Walsh, W. L. Bockenek, W. R. Frontera, et al. (Eds.), *Physical medicine & rehabilitation: Principles and practice* (4th ed.). Philadelphia: Lippincott Williams & Wilkins.

Giza, C. C., Mink, R. B., & Madikians, A. (2007). Pediatric traumatic brain injury: Not just little adults. *Current Opinion in Critical Care, 13*(2), 143–152.

Gordon, M., Gottschlich, M., Helvig, E., Marvin, J., & Richard, R. (2004). Review of evidence-based practice for the prevention of pressure sores in burn patients. *Journal of Burn Care & Rehabilitation, 25*, 388–410.

Greenley, R. N. (2010). Health professional expectations for self-care skill development in youth with spina bifida. *Pediatric Nursing, 36*(2), 98–102.

Greenley, R. N., Coakley, R. M., Holmbeck, G. N., Jandasek, B., & Wills, K. (2006). Condition-related knowledge among children with spina bifida: Longitudinal changes and predictors. *Journal of Pediatric Psychology, 31*(8), 828–839.

Hackbarth, R. M., Rzeszutko, K. M., Sturm, G., Donders, J., Kuldanek, A. S., & Sanfilippo, D. J. (2002). Survival and functional outcome in pediatric traumatic brain injury: A retrospective and analysis of predictive factors. *Critical Care Medicine, 30*(7), 1630–1635.

Heck, R. K. (2007). General principles of amputation. In S. T. Canale & J. H. Beaty (Eds.), *Campbells' operative orthopedics* (Vol. 1, 11th ed., pp. 562–639). Philadelphia: Mosby.

Hewitt-Taylor, J. (2005). Caring for children with complex and continuing health needs. *Nursing Standard, 19*(42), 41–47.

Hillmann, A., Weist, R., Fromme, A., Volker, K., & Rosenbaum, D. (2007). Sports activities and endurance capacity of bone tumor patients after rotationplasty. *Archives of Physical Medicine and Rehabilitation, 88*(7), 885–890.

Ireland, D. (2006). Unique concerns of the pediatric surgical patient: Pre-, intra-, and post-operatively. *Nursing Clinics of North America, 41*(2), 265–298.

Kirk, S., Glendinning, C., & Callery, P. (2005). Parent or nurse? The experience of being a parent of a technology-dependent child. *Journal of Advanced Nursing, 51*(5), 456–464.

Klein, M., Lezotte, D., Fauerbach, J., Herndon, D., Kowalske, K., Carrougher, G., et al. (2007). The National Institute on Disability and Rehabilitation Research burn model system database: A tool for the multicenter study of the outcome of burn injury. *Journal of Burn Care & Rehabilitation, 28*, 84–96.

Koren, G., Nava-Ocampo, A. A., Moretti, M. E., Sussman, R., & Nulman, I. (2006). Major malformations with valproic acid. *Canadian Family Physician, 52*, 441–442, 444, 447.

Kozin, S. (2004). Classification of limb anomalies in congenital disorders: Classification and diagnosis. In R.A. Berger & A. C. Weiss (Eds.), *Hand surgery* (pp. 1405–1423). Philadelphia: Lippincott Williams & Wilkins.

Launay, F., Leet, A., & Sponseller, P. (2005). Pediatric spinal cord injury without radiologic abnormality: A meta-analysis. *Clinical Orthopedics and Related Research, 433*, 166–170.

Leger, R. (2005). Severity of illness, functional status, and HRQOL in youth with spina bifida. *Rehabilitation Nursing, 30*(5), 180–187.

Lohne, V., & Severinsson, E. (2004). Hope after the first months after acute spinal cord injury. *Journal of Advanced Nursing, 47*(3), 279–286.

Lomax-Bream, L. E., Barnes, M., Copeland, K., Taylor, H. B., & Landry, S. H. (2007). The impact of spina bifida on development across the first 3 years. *Developmental Neuropsychology, 31*(1), 1–20.

Maloney, K., Greffe, B., Foreman, N., Porter, C., Graham, D., Sawczyn, K., et al. (2007). Neoplastic disease and brain tumors. In A. Hay, W. William, A. Levin, J. Myron, J. Sondheiver, et al. (Eds.), *Diagnosis & treatment in pediatrics* (18th ed., pp. 885–916). New York: McGraw-Hill.

Martin, B., Dykes, E., & Lecky, F. (2004). Patterns and risks in spinal trauma. *Archives of Diseases in Childhood, 89*(9), 860–865.

Mason, D., Tobias, N., Lutkenhoff, M., Stoops, M., & Ferguson, D. (2004). The APN's guide to pediatric constipation management. *The Nurse Practitioner: American Journal of Primary Health Care, 29*(7), 13–15, 19–23.

Massagli, T. (2000). Medical and rehabilitation issues in care of children with spinal cord injury. *Physical Medicine and Rehabilitation of North America, 11*(1), 169–182.

Mayers, T., Gottschlich, M., Scanlon, J., & Warden, G. (2003). Four-year review of burns as an etiologic factor in the development of long bone fractures in pediatric patients. *Journal of Burn Care & Rehabilitation, 24,* 279–284.

McQuade, M., & Houghton, K. (2005). Use of bisphosphonates in a case of Perthes disease. *Orthopaedic Nursing, 24*(6), 393–398.

Morrissy, R., Giavedoni, B., & Coulter-O'Berry, C. (2006). The child with a limb deficiency. In R. T. Morrissy & S. L. Weinstein (Eds.), *Lovell & Winter's pediatric orthopaedics* (6th ed., pp. 1330–1444). Philadelphia: Lippincott Williams & Wilkins.

Mosca, V. (2006). Lower limb: Lower limb deficiencies. In L. T. Staheli (Ed.), *Practice of pediatric orthopedics* (2nd ed., pp. 101–103). Philadelphia: Lippincott Williams & Wilkins.

Moxley, R., Ashwal, S., Pandya, S., Connolly, A., Florence, J., Mathews, K., et al. (2005). Practice parameter: Corticosteroid treatment of Duchenne dystrophy. *Neurology, 64,* 13–20.

Muscular Dystrophy Association. (2007). *Diseases.* Retrieved March 6, 2007, from www.mda.org/disease.

Muscular Dystrophy Association. (2010). *Facts about spinal muscular atrophy.* Retrieved August 9, 2010, from www.mdausa.org/publications/fa-sma-qa.html.

Musheno, K. (2010). *Patient Protection and Affordable Care Act: AUCD summary.* Retrieved September 20, 2011, from http://AUCD.org.

National Center for Injury Prevention and Control. (2006). *Traumatic brain injury.* Retrieved June 20, 2007, from www.cdc.gov/ncipc/tbi/TBI.htm.

National Dissemination Center for Children with Disabilities. (2006, May). *Traumatic brain injury, fact sheet 18, Susan's story.* Retrieved June 22, 2007, from www.nichcy.org/pubs/fact-she/fs18txt.htm.

National Institute of Neurological Disorders and Stroke. (2007). *NINDS leukodystrophy information page.* Retrieved March 6, 2007, from www.ninds.nih.gov/disorders/leukodystrophy/leukodystrophy.htm.

National Institute of Neurological Disorders and Stroke. (2008, June 9). *Spinal muscular atrophy fact sheet.* Retrieved August 18, 2011, from www.ninds.nih.gov/disorders/sma/detail_sma.htm.

National Institute of Neurological Disorders and Stroke. (2009a). *NINDS arteriovenous malformation information page.* Retrieved August 9, 2010, from www.ninds.nih.gov/disorders/avms/avms.htm.

National Institute of Neurological Disorders and Stroke. (2009b). *NINDS spina bifida information page.* Retrieved August 12, 2010, from www.ninds.nih.gov/disorders/spina_bifida/spina_bifida.htm.

National Institute of Neurological Disorders and Stroke. (2010). *NINDS transverse myelitis information page.* Retrieved August 9, 2010, from www.ninds.nih.gov/disorders/transversemyelitis/transversemyelitis.htm.

Neufield, S.M., Query, B., & Drummond, J.E. (2001). Respite care users who have children with chronic conditions: Are they getting a break? *Journal of Pediatric Nursing, 16*(4), 234–244.

Oddson, B. E., Clancy, C. A., & McGrath, P. J. (2006). The role of pain in reduced quality of life and depressive symptomology in children with spina bifida. *Clinical Journal of Pain, 22*(9), 784–789.

Office of Technology Assessment. (1987). *Technology-dependent children: Hospital v. home care—A technical memorandum* (report no. OTA-TM-H-38). Washington, DC: U.S. Government Printing Office.

Osteogenesis Imperfecta Foundation (OIF). (2006). *Osteogenesis imperfecta: A guide for medical professionals, individuals and families affected by OI.* Retrieved June 22, 2007 from www.oif.org.

Parmigiani, S., Pezzoni, S., Solari, E., Arena, V., De Martino, A., Allessandrini, C., et al. (2009). Palivizumab for prophylaxis of RSV infection: Five epidemic seasons' experience on adverse effects (2002–2007). *Journal of Perinatal Medicine, 37*(3), 304–305.

Passaretti, D., & Billmire, D. (2003). Management of pediatric burns. *Journal of Craniofacial Surgery, 14*(5), 713–718.

Paterson, C. R., & McAllion, S. J. (2006). Classical osteogenesis imperfecta and allegations of nonaccidental injury. *Clinical Orthopaedics and Related Research, 452,* 260–264.

Pereira, C., Murphy, K., & Herndon, D. (2005). Altering metabolism. *Journal of Burn Care & Rehabilitation, 26,* 194–199.

Pidcock, F., Fauerbach, J., Ober, M., & Carney, J. (2003). The rehabilitation/school matrix: A model for accommodating the noncompliant child with severe burns. *Journal of Burn Care & Rehabilitation, 24,* 342–346.

Poggi, G., Liscio, M., Galbiati, S., Adduci, A., Massimino, M., Gandola, L., et al. (2005). Brain tumors in children and adolescents: Cognitive and psychological disorders at different ages. *Psycho-Oncology, 14*(5), 388–395.

Pollart, S. M., Warniment, C., & Mori, T. (2009). Latex allergy. *American Family Physician, 80*(12), 1413–1420.

Przkora, R., Barrow, R., Jeschke, M., Suman, O., Celis, M., Sanford, A., et al. (2006). Body composition changes with time in pediatric burn patients. *Journal of Trauma Injury, Infections and Critical Care, 60,* 968–971.

Reeves, E., Timmons, D., & Dampier, S. (2006). Parents' experiences of negotiating care for the technology dependent child. *Journal of Child Health Care, 10*(3), 228–239.

Rehm, R. S., & Bradley, J. F. (2005). Normalization in families who are raising a child who is medically fragile, technology dependent and developmentally delayed. *Qualitative Health Research, 5*(6), 807–820.

Rice, S. A., Blackman, J. A., Braun, S., Linn, R. T., Granger, C. V., & Wagner, D. P. (2005). Rehabilitation of children with traumatic brain injury: Descriptive analysis of a nationwide sample using the WeeFIM. *Archives of Physical Medicine and Rehabilitation, 86*(4), 834–836.

Rimmer, J. H., Rowland, J. L., & Yamaki, K. (2007). Obesity and secondary conditions in adolescents with disabilities: Addressing the needs of an underserved population. *Journal of Adolescent Health, 41,* 224–229.

Ronen, G. M., Meaney, B., Dan, B., Zimprich, F., Stögmann, W., & Neugebauer, W. (2009). From eugenic euthanasia to habilitation of "disabled" children: Andreas Rett's contribution. *Journal of Child Neurology, 24,* 115–127.

Sawin, K. J., & Thompson, N. M. (2009). The experience of finding an effective bowel management program for children with spina bifida: The parent's perspective. *Journal of Pediatric Nursing, 24*(4), 280–291.

Selekman, J., & Vessey, J. A. (2010). School and the child with a chronic condition. In P. J. Allan, J. A. Vessey, & N. A. Schapiro (Eds.), *Primary care of the child with a chronic condition* (5th ed., pp. 42–59). St. Louis: Mosby/Elsevier.

Shapiro, J. R., & Sponsellor, P. D. (2009). Osteogenesis imperfecta: Questions and answers. *Current Opinion in Pediatrics, 21,* 709–716.

Shida-Tokeshi, J., Bagley, A., Molitor, F., Tomhave, W., Liberatore, J., Brasington, K., et al. (2005). Predictors of continued prosthetic wear in children with upper extremity prostheses. *Journal of Prosthetics and Orthotics, 17,* 119–124.

Simeonsson, R. J., & McDevitt, L. N. (Eds.). (1999). *Issues in disability & health: The role of secondary conditions and quality of life.* Chapel Hill: University of North Carolina, Frank Porter Graham Child Development Center.

Snodgrass, W. T., & Gargollo, P. C. (2010). Urologic care of the neurogenic bladder in children. *Urologic Clinics of North America, 37,* 207–214.

Sparacino, P. S., & Cartwright, C. C. (2009). The clinical nurse specialist. In A. B. Hamric, J. A. Spross, & C. M. Hanson (Eds.), *Advanced practice nursing: An integrative approach* (4th ed., pp. 349–374). St. Louis: Saunders.

Spina Bifida Association of America. (2010). *Fact sheet.* Retrieved August 12, 2010, from www.sbaa.org/site/c.liKWL7PLLrF/b.2642343/k.8D2D/Fact_Sheets.htm.

Steinbok, P. (2006). Selection of treatment modalities in children with spastic cerebral palsy. *Neurosurgical Focus, 12*(2), e4.

Stoddard, F., Sheridan, R., Saxe, G., King, B. S., King, B. H., Chedekel, D., et al. (2002). Treatment of pain in acutely burned children. *Journal of Burn Care & Rehabilitation, 23,* 135–156.

Sullivan-Bolyai, S., Knafl, K.A., Sadler, L., & Gilliss, C.L. (2004). Great expectations: A position description for parents as caregivers: Part II. *Pediatric Nursing, 30*(1), 52–56.

Suman, O., Mlcak, R., & Herndon, D. (2002). Effect of exercise training on pulmonary function in children with thermal injury. *Journal of Burn Care & Rehabilitation, 23,* 288–293.

U.S. Department of Education. (2007). *Individuals with Disabilities Education Act (IDEA).* Retrieved June 29, 2007, from http://idea.ed.gov/explore/home.

U.S. Department of Health and Human Services. (2007). *Maternal and Child Health Bureau.* Retrieved September 20, 2011, from http://mchb.hrsa.gov/about/index.html.

Vargo, M., & Gerber, L. (2005). Rehabilitation for patients with cancer diagnosis. In J. A. DeLisa, B. M. Gans, N. E. Walsh, W. L. Bockenek, W. R. Fontera, S. R. Geiringer, et al. (Eds.), *Physical medicine & rehabilitation: Principles and practice* (4th ed., pp. 1771–1794). Philadelphia: Lippincott Williams & Wilkins.

Vehmeyer-Heeman, M., Lommers, B., Van den Kerckhove, E., & Boeckx, W. (2005). Axillary burns: Extended grafting and early splinting prevents contractures. *Journal of Burn Care & Rehabilitation, 26,* 539–542.

Verhoef, M., Barf, H., Post, M., van Asbeck, F., Gooskens, A., Rob, H., et al. (2006). Functional independence among young adults with spina bifida in relation to hydrocephalus and level of lesion. *Developmental Medicine & Child Neurology, 48*(2), 114–119.

Vinck, A., Maassen, B., Mullaart, R., & Rotteveel, J. (2006). Arnold-Chiari II malformation and cognitive functioning in spina bifida. *Journal of Neurology, Neurosurgery & Psychiatry, 77*(9), 1083–1086.

Vogel, L., Hickey, K., Klaas, S., & Anderson, C. (2004). Unique issues in pediatric spinal cord injury. *Orthopedic Nursing, 23*(5), 300–308.

Weed, R., & Berens, D. (2005). Basics of burn injury: Implication for case management and life care planning. *Lippincott's Case Management, 10*(1), 22–29.

Wisconsin Education Association Council. (2007). *Special education inclusion.* Retrieved August 11, 2010, from www.weac.org/resource/june96/speced.htm.

CHAPTER 19
Gerontological Rehabilitation Nursing

Kristen L. Mauk, PhD DNP RN CRRN GCNS-BC GNP-BC FAAN • Usha K. Patel, APN MSN RN CRRN CWOCN

The rapid growth in the older adult population is beginning to have a major impact on the healthcare delivery system. Currently, one in every eight Americans is older than 65 years of age. Older adults (65+) numbered 38.9 million in 2008, an increase of 4.5 million (13%) in the past 12 years. The population age 65 and older accounted for 40 million people in 2010 (a 15% increase). Experts predict this number to increase to 55 million by 2020 (a 36% increase for that decade; Greenberg, 2009); this is particularly related to the Baby Boomer generation entering the older age group and a continued increased life expectancy. The oldest old—or frail older adults—will be the fastest-growing age group in the country. As a person's age increases, so does the likelihood of chronic illness and functional limitations. In light of these statistics, rehabilitation nurses must be prepared to meet the demands of an aging society. This can be accomplished only through special knowledge and training in the areas of gerontology and rehabilitation.

I. Theories of Aging

A. Biological (Lange & Grossman, 2010)
  1. Genes or biological clock: Each person has a genetic program that helps predetermine life expectancy.
  2. Wear and tear: The length of life is inversely related to the rate of living (i.e., the more wear and tear placed on the body, the faster one ages).
  3. Lipofuscin and connective tissue: This lipoprotein byproduct of metabolism increases with age, resulting in visible signs of aging.
  4. Free radicals: Unstable molecules damage cells, causing injury and signs of aging. Examples include tobacco smoke, herbicides and pesticides, radiation, and ozone.
  5. Stress: Aging is related to or influenced by life stress.
  6. Orgel: Errors in protein synthesis occur with aging, causing genes to mutate.
  7. Autoimmune or immunological: The body perceives old, irregular cells as hostile agents and begins to attack itself; the immune system becomes less effective with age.
  8. Nutritional: Length of life and age-related changes can be either positively or negatively influenced by nutritional intake.
  9. Environmental: Pollutants in one's surroundings, such as air and noise pollution or radiation adversely affect health and cause signs of aging.

B. Psychological
  1. Human needs (Maslow, 1954)
    a. Hierarchy of five basic needs that motivate human behavior
      1) Physiologic
      2) Safety and security
      3) Love and belonging
      4) Self-esteem
      5) Self-actualization
    b. Failure in self-growth may lead to feelings of failure and depression (Lange & Grossman, 2010).
  2. Individualism (Jung, 1960)
    a. Lifespan view of development versus need attainment
    b. Older adults engage in an inner search to evaluate their lives.
    c. Successful aging includes accepting the past and coping positively with changes.
  3. Lifespan development paradigm (Buhler, 1933)
    a. Life occurs in stages.
    b. Life satisfaction is related to goal achievement.
    c. Successful adaptation to changes in life may include a reevaluation of the older person's beliefs relative to societal expectations.
  4. Selective optimization with compensation (Baltes, 1987)
    a. Emerged from Buhler's work
    b. Successful aging comes from learning to cope with losses of aging through choices.
    c. Selective optimization with compensation suggests that as people age they make choices of activities and roles that provide the most satisfaction, and this in turn facilitates successful aging (Baltes & Baltes, 1990).

C. Sociological
  1. Activity theory: Older adults should remain active, occupied, and contributing to society to age positively and avoid the negative effects of advanced age (Havighurst, Neugarten, & Tobin, 1963).
    a. Research has shown a direct relationship between life satisfaction and activity in older adults (Lemon, Bengston, & Peterson, 1972).

b. Informal activities such as gathering with friends, having hobbies, and engaging in group activities provide more life satisfaction than solitary activities, and meaningful activities have also been correlated with successful aging and life satisfaction (Harlow & Cantor, 1996, Schroots, 1996; Vaillant, 2002).

2. Disengagement: Society and older adults mutually withdraw from one another as one ages; disengagement is thought to maintain social equilibrium (Cumming & Henry, 1961).

   a. This theory has been and continues to be challenged by numerous studies that support activity theory.

   b. The Harvard Aging Study, which followed three cohorts of more than 800 people each for more than 50 years, provides evidence that happiness in later life is more related to individual lifestyle choices than genetics, wealth, race, or other largely uncontrollable factors (Vaillant, 2002), raising questions about the validity of disengagement theory.

3. Continuity: Older adults continue with the same personality and behavior patterns they developed throughout their lives (Havighurst, Neugarten, & Tobin, 1968). There are four personality types of older adults.

   a. Integrated: Well adjusted, actively engaged

   b. Armored/defended: Continue activities and roles from middle age

   c. Passive/dependent: Disinterested or dependent on others

   d. Unintegrated: Fails to cope successfully with aging

   e. A study by Agahi, Ahacic, and Parker (2006) showed that active participation tends to decline over time and that previous life patterns predict involvement in activities in later life.

4. Gerotranscendence: Older adults move toward oneness with the universe by maintaining close relationships, accepting impending death, and remaining connected with people of other generations (Tornstam, 1994).

   a. Three main elements

      1) The cosmic level

      2) The self

      3) Social and individual relations

   b. A study investigating whether staff could recognize signs of gerotranscendence revealed that an interpretive framework for use in settings such as nursing homes would be of assistance in acceptance of these behaviors as a normal part of aging (Wadensten & Carlsson, 2001).

II. **Review of Normal Aging**

A. Cardiac and Circulatory System

   1. Decreased cardiac output

   2. Valvular changes that may result stenosis (Pugh & Wei, 2001) or heart murmurs

   3. Decreased ability to adapt to increased demands

   4. Age-associated changes across time may vary between individuals (Heineman, Hamrick-King, & Scaglione Sewell, 2010).

   5. Increased incidence of varicose veins

   6. Increased thickness of heart and arterial walls (Ferrari, Radaelli, & Centola, 2003)

   7. Increased systolic blood pressure (Heineman et al., 2010)

B. Respiratory System

   1. Decreased elasticity of the lungs

   2. Impaired gas exchange over time caused by a loss of elasticity and decreased surface area of alveoli

   3. Increased carbon dioxide retention caused by a less efficient system

   4. Less useful oxygen with each breath

   5. Reduced vital capacity but no change in total lung capacity (Krauss Whitbourne, 2002)

   6. Decreased blood oxygen level

C. Musculoskeletal System

   1. Decreased muscle mass (sarcopenia; Roubenoff, 2001) and related loss of muscle strength (Ivey et al., 2000)

   2. Changes in range of motion in joints

   3. Decreased overall height caused by compression of vertebrae over time

   4. Decreased bone density, leading to increased risk for fractures

   5. Decreased cartilage surface of joints, leading to possible limitations in range of motion

D. Genitourinary System

   1. In women

      a. Decreased estrogen with perimenopause and menopause (Hall, 2004)

      b. Average age for menopause, defined as occurring 1 year after the final menstrual period, is about 51 years (Hall, 2007)

      c. Ovaries atrophy, vagina shortens and narrows, uterus decreases in size, and supporting ligaments weaken (Digiovanna, 2000)

      d. Decreased vaginal lubrication, often leading to pain during sexual intercourse

      e. Stress incontinence (common but treatable)

      f. Other types of incontinence (common but not a normal part of aging)

   2. In men

THE SPECIALTY PRACTICE OF REHABILITATION NURSING

a. Testes decrease in size and weight, penis shows fibrous changes in erectile tissues by age 55 or 60 (Digiovanna, 2000).

b. No significant changes in sexual libido or previous patterns of behavior

c. Longer refractory times during phases of sexual intercourse

d. Less complete erections and less frequent orgasms

e. Enlarged prostate, resulting in clinical benign prostatic hyperplasia in 13% of men by age 60 and 23% by age 85 (Hafez & Hafez, 2004)

3. In both men and women

a. Decreased bladder capacity caused by bladder shrinkage and change in capacity and contractility (Digiovanna, 2000)

b. Increase in urinary frequency and nocturia (Asplund, 2004), which can affect sleep quality

E. Neurological System (Heineman et al., 2010)

1. Brain decreases in size and weight

2. Loss of 10% of functioning neurons over lifespan in both genders, but neuron loss may be less than previously thought (Peters, 2002)

3. Cognition

a. Some memory loss is common but should be distinguished from abnormalities such as those that occur with Alzheimer's disease.

b. Intelligence and ability to learn are not affected.

4. Proprioception (awareness of body position in space) may decrease with age, which can result in less coordination and balance, which could lead to falls.

5. Slower voluntary reflexes

6. Deep tendon reflexes still responsive

7. More difficulty responding to multiple stimuli

8. Decreased kinesthetic sense

9. Complaints of feeling tired (even if staying in bed longer) caused by sleep pattern changes such as a decrease in stage IV, rapid eye movement sleep

10. Decreased dopamine levels, which may contribute to Parkinsonian features such as abnormal gait

11. Spinal cord cells begin to decline around age 60 (Beers & Berkow, n.d.), and the spine may narrow, causing pressure on the spinal cord that over time can cause changes in sensation.

F. Sensory System

1. Vision

a. Presbyopia: Farsightedness or trouble focusing on near objects, caused by age-related changes in the shape of the eye that begin around age 40 (Digiovanna, 2000)

b. Decreased peripheral vision

c. The most common age-related eye diseases are cataracts (extremely common but highly treatable with surgery and intraocular lens implants), glaucoma, macular degeneration, and diabetic retinopathy (Jackson & Owsley, 2003).

d. Decreased tear production, which increases susceptibility to infections

e. Changes in depth perception

2. Hearing

a. Presbycusis: Decrease in hearing acuity, especially the ability to detect high-frequency tones and discern speech (Rees, Duckert, & Carey, 1999)

b. Impacted wax

c. Need for hearing aids, which may amplify extraneous noises

3. Smell: General decrease in acuity (Seiberling & Conley, 2004)

4. Taste: Atrophied taste buds, slight decrease in taste around age 60, and more exaggerated past age 70 (Seiberling & Conley, 2004)

5. Touch: Decreased ability to distinguish sensations and textures (Digiovanna, 2000)

6. Pain

a. Increased tolerance for pain

b. General decreased sensitivity to light touch

c. Increased pain threshold

G. Endocrine System

1. Changes in sex hormones

2. Decreased efficiency of the entire system

3. Changes in thyroid hormone production and glucose tolerance, which may warrant treatment (e.g., thyroid changes may lower the metabolic rate)

H. Hematological System

1. Anemia is common in 8%–44% of older adults (Nilsson-Ehle, Jagenburg, Landahl, & Svanborg, 2000), particularly iron deficiency and pernicious types.

2. Hypoalbuminemia

a. Serum albumin has been shown to be a predictor of geriatric rehabilitation outcomes (Aptaker, Roth, Reichhardt, Duerden, & Levy, 1994).

b. Albumin less than 3.5 g/dL may place a person at risk for poor outcomes, including pressure ulcers (Aptaker et al., 1994).

I. Immune System

1. Generally less efficient; immunosenescence is the aging of the immune system

2. Less effective T cells

3. Possibly less resistant to infections

4. Possible absence of typical symptoms of illness (e.g., elevated temperature with pneumonia)

J. Integumentary System

1. Skin (Plahuta & Hamrick-King, 2006)
   a. Becomes more wrinkled, thinner
   b. Loses elasticity
   c. Is dry, which may lead to itching
   d. Has greater potential for tears and bruising
   e. Decreased number of sweat glands, which may lead to impaired thermoregulation

2. Hair
   a. Pigment loss, resulting in what appears as gray or white hair
   b. Development of facial hair (in women)
   c. Thinning, balding (in men)

3. Nails: More brittle, changes in color and texture

4. Fat: Distributed more on the trunk and less on the arms and legs

K. Gastrointestinal System (Heineman et al., 2010)

1. Slowed absorption in intestines
2. Decreased digestive enzymes
3. Decreased saliva production
4. Decreased esophageal and intestinal peristalsis
5. Constipation
6. Weaker gag reflex or delayed swallowing, which can increase the risk of aspiration

L. Renal System

1. The kidneys shrink, with a potential loss of up to half of functioning nephrons (Minaker, 2004).
2. Decreased glomerular filtration rate, related in part to changes in blood flow (Digiovanna, 2000)
3. There is less effective filtration of wastes, which may allow medications to stay in the body longer and increase the risk of side effects.

III. **Aging and Disability: Acquiring a Disability at an Advanced Age**

There are two distinct ways in which disability can affect older adults: acquiring a disability at an advanced age and aging with an early-onset disability. The effects of age and aging can differ in each case.

A. Factors Affecting Rehabilitation Potential

1. Age
   a. Scivoletto, Morganti, Ditunno, Ditunno, and Molinari (2003) found that adults older than age 50 with new spinal cord injury (SCI) have less favorable outcomes than younger people with the same injuries in regard to walking and bladder and bowel independence and tend to have more associated medical problems.
   b. Bagg, Pombo, and Hopman (2002) reported that the Functional Independence Measure (FIM™) score at admission is a better predictor than FIM™ score at discharge in older adults with stroke and recommended that age not be a factor in the decision to admit a client to rehabilitation.
   c. Yu (2005) found that an age of 80 or older and admission function affected functional gains and rehabilitation efficiency in an outpatient rehabilitation program.

2. Frailty
   a. One definition of frailty is unintentional weight loss, exhaustion, low energy expenditure, slow walking speed, and weakness in the older adult (Fried, Ferrucci, Darer, Williamson, & Anderson, 2004).
   b. Another research-based definition of frailty is an accumulation of deficits, which include symptoms, signs, diseases, and disabilities. The more deficits, the more frail (Rockwood, Mitniski, Song, Steen, & Skoog, 2006).
   c. Overall, frailty is the outcome of declines at the molecular, cellular, and physiologic system levels (Bandeen-Roche et al., 2006).
   d. Frail older adults are at higher risk for morbidity, disability, and mortality. Between 10% and 25% of people aged 65 and older are considered frail (Ostir, Ottenbacher, & Markides, 2004).
   e. Positive psychological factors, including positive affect, reduce the risk of frailty (Ostir et al., 2004).

3. Effects of normal aging: Reductions in endurance, strength, and function affect the speed of and potential for recovery
   a. Exercise tolerance: Pulmonary, cardiac, and muscle effects of aging affect exercise tolerance.
   b. Strength is reduced by a decrease in muscle mass and endurance.
   c. Balance is affected by comorbidities and the side effects of multiple medications.
   d. Mobility is changed by vision impairments, side effects of medications, weight changes, unsteady gait, foot problems.

4. Effects of chronic diseases: Chronic disease significantly compromises physical function and adversely affects the rehabilitation potential of the client after injury or trauma. In addition to the knowledge about the disease, an understanding of the client's functional expectations is essential during restorative management because rehabilitation depends on active participation in the program.
   a. Diabetes
      1) Glucose control: Poor glycemic control leads to deficits in cognitive function

(memory and processing) and increases the risk of vascular disease (Awad, Gagnon, & Messier, 2004).

    2) Peripheral neuropathy reduces sensations, increases risk of falls and injury, and also alters mobility if there are foot problems.

    3) Gastroparesis

    4) Blurred vision is common in clients with poor glycemic control. Glaucoma, blindness, and retinopathy are also noted. These can pose an extra challenge to rehabilitation efforts.

    5) Skin changes at the cellular level increase the risk of infection and lead to poor healing.

    6) Vascular disease: Loss of elasticity and hardening of arteries, risk of neuropathy

    7) Amputation after injury of lower extremities: More than 60% of nontraumatic amputation occurs in clients with diabetes (Centers for Disease Control and Prevention, 2011).

b. Heart disease: Severity of disease and comorbidity reduce the potential for rehabilitation.

    1) Exercise tolerance is reduced.

    2) Ejection fraction is affected by damaged heart muscle, reducing the client's ability to meet the demands of rehabilitation.

    3) Fluid balance: Overload may worsen functioning and increase dependency.

    4) Angina symptoms may be masked by reduced sensory perception.

    5) Edema affects the ability to participate in activity and build endurance.

c. Vascular disease

    1) Wounds heal poorly; risk is increased by poor circulation.

    2) Amputation is 15 times more common in people with diabetes.

    3) Pain sensation is reduced by neuropathy.

    4) Mobility is impaired in Charcot foot.

    5) Exercise tolerance is reduced.

d. Lung disease

    1) Exercise tolerance is reduced.

    2) Oxygenation is reduced.

e. Parkinson's disease

    1) Cognition: More time is needed to process information

    2) Mobility: Slow, stiff, poor coordination, shuffling gait

    3) Balance unsteady; tendency toward retropulsion

    4) Tremors: Increase in purposeful tremors

f. Dementia

    1) The ability to learn varies depending on the area affected and level of injury.

    2) Memory

    3) Behavior is unpredictable.

g. Depression: Prevalence is 1.8%–8.9% among older adults residing in the community and 25% among older adults residing in nursing homes (Menzel, 2008).

    1) Ability to learn

    2) Cognitive status

    3) Motivation

    4) Higher rate of suicide among older adults, particularly older White men

h. Anemia: A study conducted by Witkos, Uttaburanont, Lang, and Haddad (2009) showed that clients treated for anemia had better functional outcome on discharge than untreated clients. Anemia affects the blood supply to the body, which is directly correlated with the following:

    1) Exercise tolerance (affecting rehabilitation outcome)

    2) Healing of injury and recovery outcomes

    3) Postural hypotension (reduced oxygenation and volume)

i. Human immunodeficiency virus and acquired immune deficiency syndrome

    1) Exercise tolerance is reduced by a cachectic state.

    2) Healing is poor because of comorbidity and poor nutrition.

    3) Nutritional status is poor, leading to fatigue, muscle wasting, and higher risk of infection.

j. Cancer

    1) Pain varies.

    2) Exercise tolerance decreases.

    3) Mobility deteriorates with advancing stages.

k. Patrick, Knoefel, Gaskowsk, and Rexrath (2001) found that the severity of medical comorbidity was a significant predictor of rehabilitation efficiency (gains in functional independence divided by length of stay) in older adults with various disabilities.

l. Yu (2005) reported that the number of medical comorbidities and age affected length of stay in an outpatient rehabilitation program for older adults.

5. Baseline functional status: Yu (2005) found that age of 80 years or more and admission function affected functional gains and rehabilitation efficiency in an outpatient rehabilitation program.

6. Baseline cognitive status is needed to predict outcomes and develop a plan of care.
   a. Ability to learn
   b. Memory
   c. Motivation
   d. Mast, MacNeill, and Lichtenberg (1999) reported that 34.7% of people with stroke and 27.8% of those with lower-extremity fracture in their study met the criteria for dementia. Also, 33.3% of people with stroke and 25.1% of those with lower-extremity fracture scored as depressed on the Geriatric Depression Scale. They noted that older adults with stroke and lower-extremity fracture need treatment not only for the stroke or fracture but also for geriatric-specific problems such as depression, dementia, and multiple comorbidities.
   e. Hershkovitz, Kalandariov, Hermush, Weiss, and Brill (2007) reported that cognitive function, nutritional status, and depression were important prognostic factors affecting success of rehabilitation outcome in older adults with proximal hip fracture.
7. Polypharmacy
   a. Is defined as using two or more medicines to treat the same condition, using two or more drugs from the same chemical class, or using two or more drugs with similar actions to treat different conditions (Brager & Sloand, 2005). It is also defined as the prescription, administration, or use of more medications than are clinically indicated in a given client (Charles & Lehman, 2006).
   b. The risks of polypharmacy include increased likelihood of drug-drug or drug-disease interactions, adverse drug events, and client nonadherence to the medication plan (Charles & Lehman, 2006).
   c. Home health nurses in one study reported that up to 21% of older adults did not understand their medications on discharge from hospital, 78% took five or more drugs, 11% had limited cognitive ability, and 9% had medications ordered by more than one provider (Ellenbecker, Frazier, & Verney, 2004).
   d. Ostwald, Wasserman, and Davis (2006) reported that stroke survivors in their study were discharged home with an average of 11.3 medications from five different drug classifications. The number of medications prescribed was correlated with the number of stroke-related comorbidities. Receipt of medication from several different drug categories was also correlated with having more stroke-related comorbidities and more complications. The authors of this study reported that the average cost for a stroke survivor taking 10 commonly prescribed poststroke medications was $724.29 per month.

8. Social supports
   a. Family and significant others can have a positive impact on recovery time.
   b. Sources of income
      1) Social Security
      2) Pension
   c. Funding for health care
      1) Medicare
      2) Medicaid
      3) Private insurance
   d. Housing
      1) Members of the household can assist in care or provide moral support.
      2) The physical layout of the home environment determines the client's ability to be independent with activities of daily living (ADLs). Features such as stairs, ramps (if wheelchair use is warranted), safety devices (e.g., rails in shower), and countertops at a convenient work level influence discharge goals and length of stay.
   e. Transportation: Access to and availability of public and private transportation affect follow-up visits and health maintenance.
      1) Medical visits
      2) Grocery store
      3) Shopping
      4) Church and social groups
   f. Beaupre and colleagues (2005) demonstrated that functional status in a population age 65 and older was lower in clients with hip fracture and poor social supports than in those with good social supports. Subjects with poor social supports were also more likely to be living in an institution 6 months after discharge from rehabilitation than those with better social support.
   g. The Duke EPESE study (Mendes De Leon, Gold, Glass, Kaplan, & George, 2001) revealed that the larger the social network and the more interaction with that network, the less disability was present in study subjects (age 65 and older). Social interactions with friends were associated with lower disability, but interaction with children or relatives was not related to disability. The receipt of instrumental

support was correlated with disability: the higher the support, the more disability.

9. Commonly acquired disability in older adults
   a. Stroke
      1) Stroke is a leading cause of long-term disability in the United States.
      2) Onset is secondary to cardiovascular disease, high blood pressure, diabetes, smoking, high cholesterol, obesity, and family history.
      3) On average, one person in the United States has a stroke every 45 seconds.
      4) Eighty-eight percent of stroke deaths occur in people age 65 and older.
      5) More women than men die of stroke each year because of their longer life expectancy.
      6) Eighty-eight percent of strokes are ischemic, 9% intracranial hemorrhage, and 3% subarachnoid hemorrhage.
      7) In 2002, 71% of people discharged from short-stay hospitals with a primary diagnosis of stroke were older than 65 (American Heart Association [AHA], 2004; AHA/American Stroke Association, 2006).
   b. Head injury
      1) Falls are the second leading cause of traumatic brain injury (TBI) and the leading cause of TBI hospitalizations in people aged 65 and older.
      2) These injuries often result in death or impairment for older adults.
      3) TBIs in older adults account for 80,000 emergency department visits per year, 75% of which result in hospitalization (Menzel, 2008).
      4) Fifty-one percent of TBIs in older adults are caused by falls, 9% by motor vehicle accidents.
      5) Brenner, Homaifar, and Schultheis (2008) reported that 60% of brain injury survivors experience increased fatigue, especially mental fatigue and physical fatigue. Contributing factors are cognitive disturbances, sleeping problems, anxiety, depression, and alterations in endocrine neurotransmitters.
      6) Older women are more likely to be hospitalized after injury than older men.
      7) The rate of TBI in the general population is 60.6 per 100,000 people; after age 65, it increases to 155.9 per 100,000.
      8) Overall, in 2002 the U.S. rate of hospitalization after fall with TBI was 29.6 per 100,000 population; in people age 65–74, the rate increased to 58.6 per 100,000, and in those 75 years and older it was 203.9 per 100,000.
      9) Older age is recognized as an independent predictor for worse outcomes from TBI (Centers for Disease Control and Prevention [CDC], 2003; Thompson, McCormick, & Kagan, 2006).
      10) The risk of developing seizures after TBI increases after age 65 (LeBlanc, de Guise, Gosselin, & Feyz, 2006).
      11) Older adults have poor cognitive functioning after TBI, necessitating increased family involvement and increased use of community services or nursing homes.
   c. Falls with fracture
      1) Secondary to muscle weakness, impaired balance, osteoporosis, sensory loss, impaired gait, reduced muscle strength, poor vision, and use of psychoactive medication (Sherrington et al., 2008)
      2) One-third of falls in older adults are caused by environmental hazards in the home (**Figure 19-1**).
      3) Three to five percent of falls in U.S. older adults result in fracture, with 360,000–480,000 fall-related fractures per year in the United States.
      4) Hip fractures cause the most deaths and disability in older adults.
      5) Up to 25% of community-dwelling older adults experiencing hip fracture from falls remain institutionalized after 1 year (CDC, 2006a).
   d. Deconditioning: Often a result of the enforced immobility of acute hospitalization superimposed on the normal changes of aging. Between 25% and 60% of hospitalized older adults risk the loss of function during hospitalization. Prolonged hospitalization leads to nursing home placement and death (Francis, 2005).
      1) Loss of strength
      2) Reduction of muscle mass
      3) Weakness
      4) Increased risk of falls
   e. Contributing factors
      1) Lack of awareness by staff about importance of functional impairment on quality of life

Figure 19-1. Potential Environmental Risk Factors for Falls

- Flooring, such as throw rugs, high-pile carpeting, or slippery or wet tile
- Outdoor walkways that are wet or have leaves, snow, or ice on them
- Small children and pets
- Stairs and steps (especially those without handrails and those not clearly marked)
- Clutter in walkways and around the bedroom and bathroom areas
- Lack of handrails in the bathroom
- Adaptive equipment such as rolling walkers, canes, or splints
- Poor lighting in rooms or walkways
- Lack of a system to call for help (e.g., whistle, bell)
- Long cords such as those for phones or supplemental oxygen tanks
- Poor arrangement of living space, which requires a person to reach or move in ways that upset balance

    2) Organizational structure and process that limits knowledge about the client's baseline functional capacity

B. Geriatric Syndromes That Can Affect Rehabilitation
  1. Delirium
    a. Defined as acute onset of confusion; fluctuates during the course of the day; short attention span, impaired memory, and usually an identifiable and treatable cause
    b. Multiple causative factors and risk factors (Inouye, 2006; Tullmann, Mion, Fletcher, & Foreman, 2008)
      1) Advanced age
      2) Dementia
      3) Acute illness or infection
      4) Polypharmacy
      5) Substance abuse
      6) Untreated pain
      7) Electrolyte imbalance
      8) Change in surroundings
    c. Delirium has been found to predict poor outcomes in orthopedic surgery clients (Duppils & Wikblad, 2004; Segatore & Adams, 2001).
    d. Nurses often do not recognize the symptoms of delirium (Inouye, Foreman, Mion, Katz, & Cooney, 2001).
    e. General nursing interventions
      1) Identify and minimize risk factors when possible.
      2) Review medications.
      3) Provide a therapeutic environment.
      4) Monitor lab values.

      5) Treat signs and symptoms of delirium promptly.
      6) Work with the geriatric clinical nurse specialist (GCNS) or gerontological nurse practitioner (GNP) to monitor and treat.
  2. Falls
    a. More than one-third of older adults fall each year (Gray-Micelli, 2008).
    b. There are multiple causative factors.
    c. Falls are a leading cause of death and disability among older adults and the most common cause of nonfatal injuries.
    d. The highest fall incidence occurs in nursing homes, where 50%–75% of clients fall annually (Gray-Micelli, 2008).
    e. Of those who fall, 20%–30% sustain moderate to severe injuries that reduce independence and mobility.
    f. For people age 75 and older, those who fall are four to five times more likely to be admitted to a long-term care facility for a year or longer.
    g. Falls are a leading cause of TBI and fractures in older adults (CDC, 2006a).
    h. Risk factors
      1) Prior falls
      2) Advanced age
      3) Impaired gait
      4) Functional disability
      5) Physical restraints
      6) Polypharmacy
    i. General nursing interventions (Gray-Micelli, 2008)
      1) Assess fall risk upon admission and frequently thereafter (using a tool is recommended).
      2) Document and communicate findings with the rest of the team.
      3) Implement and monitor safety measures including general precautions.
      4) Incorporate fall prevention into the interdisciplinary plan of care.
  3. Dizziness
    a. Multiple causative factors (Mauk & Hanson, 2010)
    b. Four major types
      1) Vertigo
      2) Presyncope (lightheadedness)
      3) Disequilibrium (related to balance)
      4) Poorly defined (does not fit other categories)
    c. Tinetti, Williams, and Gill (2000) reported that 24% of people 72 years and older reported dizziness, 74% reported several triggering factors, and

56% of the dizzy subjects reported differing sensations. Associated factors included anxiety, depression, impaired hearing, polypharmacy, postural hypotension, impaired balance, and past myocardial infarction. The risk of dizziness increased with each added characteristic.

    d. General nursing interventions
       1) Determine the cause.
       2) Work with the GCNS, GNP, or physician to rule out benign paroxysmal positional vertigo if medications for vertigo are not effective.
       3) Educate the client and family regarding the type of vertigo and its treatment.

4. Urinary incontinence (UI)
    a. Multiple causative factors
    b. Risk factors
       1) Immobility
       2) Decreased fluid intake
       3) Cognitive impairment
       4) Medications
       5) Constipation
       6) Environmental barriers
       7) Urinary tract infections
       8) Diabetes
       9) Stroke
    c. Consequences include falls, depression, pressure ulcers, and social isolation (Cowley, Diebold, Gross, & Hardin-Fanning, 2006)
    d. General nursing interventions (Diebold, Hardin-Fanning, & Hanson, 2010; Dowling-Castronova & Bradway, 2008)
       1) Identify the type of UI.
       2) Implement interventions specific to the type of UI (for example, stress incontinence improves with pelvic-floor-muscle exercises).
       3) Monitor fluid intake and urine output.
       4) Keep an incontinence diary.
       5) Limit bladder irritants.
       6) Modify the environment to promote successful toileting.
       7) Avoid indwelling urinary catheters when possible.
       8) Evaluate for any contributing medications.
       9) Educate the client and family about prevention of UI episodes.

5. Malnutrition
    a. Multiple causative factors
    b. Major risk factor for complications and delayed recovery
    c. Often caused by disease or functional impairments
    d. Natural progression of end-stage dementia; supplemental, invasive feeding in clients with dementia is an ethical concern
    e. Includes both obese and underweight people
    f. Malnutrition increases risk of complications and death.
    g. Forty to sixty percent of hospitalized older adults have been found to be malnourished (Institute of Medicine, 2000).
    h. General nursing interventions (DiMaria-Ghalili, 2008)
       1) Check serum albumin or prealbumin.
       2) Consult with the dietitian.
       3) Alleviate dry mouth.
       4) Encourage oral intake.
       5) Make food appealing by controlling the environment.
       6) Provide oral supplements throughout the day.

6. Dehydration
    a. Multiple causative factors, including decreased thirst, reduced total body water in proportion to weight, body composition changes, impaired renal conservation of water, decreased effectiveness of vasopressin, and multiple comorbidities
    b. Risk factors for dehydration
       1) Age greater than 85
       2) Decreased mobility
       3) Decreased ability to perform ADLs
       4) More than four chronic conditions
       5) More than four medications
       6) Poor oral intake
       7) Communication difficulties
       8) Fever
       9) Few opportunities to drink
    c. Atypical presentation in older adults: Confusion, falls, change in level of consciousness, weakness, fatigue (Cowley et al., 2006)
    d. General nursing interventions are similar to those for malnutrition, particularly increasing fluid intake.

7. Functional loss
    a. Twenty-two percent of people 85 and older need assistance with personal care.
    b. Twenty to forty percent of older adults experience functional decline during hospitalization.
    c. Risk factors
       1) Acute illness
       2) Exacerbation of chronic illness
       3) Injuries
       4) Medications
       5) Depression

6) Malnutrition
7) Decreased mobility
8) Restraints
d. Complications include loss of independence, falls, incontinence, malnutrition, depression, decreased socialization, and increased risk for institutionalization (Geronurseonline, 2005a).
e. General nursing intervention are those for immobility, including physical and occupational therapy as needed. (Refer to Chapter 7 for more information.)
8. Polypharmacy
a. Twenty-five to forty percent of all prescriptions in the United States are written for older adults (Diebold et al., 2010).
b. Five to fifteen percent of all hospitalizations are medication related.
c. Forty to fifty percent of all over-the-counter medications are consumed by older adults.
d. In the United States 106,000 fatal adverse drug events occur annually.
e. Community-dwelling adults average four to six medications daily.
f. Symptoms of problems with medications include mental status changes, weight loss, dehydration, agitation, anorexia, urinary retention, and decline in functional status (Crowley et al., 2006).
g. General nursing interventions (Diebold et al., 2010)
1) Obtain a thorough history of medication use, including over-the-counter medications.
2) Be familiar with the medications that are problematic for older adults.
3) Participate in medication reconciliation within the hospital system.
4) Monitor clients' serum blood urea nitrogen and creatinine.
5) Understand and recognize normal aging changes and the effect on absorption, metabolism, and excretion of medications in the aging body.
6) Use the Crockroft-Gault formula for creatinine clearance as a more accurate measure than the serum creatinine alone (because it accounts for age, ideal body weight, and gender).
7) Be alert to recent dosage changes.
8) Educate clients and families about the side effects of medications.
9) Consider nonpharmacologic approaches to treatment.

C. Rehabilitation Nursing Interventions to Promote Successful Aging (**Figure 19-2**)
1. Primary prevention
a. Young age groups without disability: Prevention of chronic disease through promotion of healthy lifestyles
1) Nutrition: Maintaining balanced diet, healthy diet in moderation
2) Exercise: Daily exercise to maintain health and wellness
3) Weight management: To prevent side effects of obesity (hypertension, diabetes)
4) Smoking prevention or cessation
5) Safety awareness: Preventing avoidable injuries, driving within limits, wearing helmets, following safety recommendations at home and work
b. Early education about potential problems of aging and how to prevent them
1) In the rehabilitation setting, demonstrate cultural competency without language barriers. Teach the client, caregiver, and family. Provide adequate educational material in an understandable language, accommodating the needs of impaired clients and following priniciples of adult learning.
2) Provide education during the maintenance (stable) phase of disability, when perception and client readiness are hightest.
c. Older adults with or without disability: Prevent new chronic disease or disability through promotion of healthy lifestyles. Many aspects of mortality are modifiable through behavior change. Therefore, the U.S. Preventive Services Task Force and the Surgeon General have set some guidelines for screening and counseling for adults (Spalding & Sebesta, 2008).
1) Nutrition: Diets rich in healthy fats, fruits, and vegetables; nutrition counseling for clients with diabetes, hypertension, and risk for coronary heart disease (CHD)
2) Daily exercise reduces the risk of death and prevents osteoporosis and obesity. The U.S. Surgeon General recommends aerobic exercise 30 minutes three times per week and strengthening exercise twice a week.
3) Weight management reduces the risk of diabetes and CHD.
4) Smoking prevention or cessation: A 3-minute counseling session with or

Figure 19-2. Suggestions for Teaching Older Adults

Visual

Use bright, direct lighting unless contraindicated because of visual disturbances (such as recent cataract surgery).

Do not stand by a window; avoid glare.

When using visual aids, use large, well-spaced letters (black on white is best).

Keep clients close to the speaker, or, if in a large room, be certain that the audience can see and hear the speaker.

For individual teaching, make sure that the client's glasses are clean.

Auditory

Limit distractions: Eliminate extraneous noise, close doors, turn off television or radio, limit interruptions.

Face the audience; speak directly to the individual in a one-to-one setting.

Never cover your mouth when speaking (many older adults rely on lip reading to compensate for hearing deficits).

Speak slowly and clearly. If appropriate, wear bright lipstick to help elderly people who lip read.

Before proceeding, ask whether the client can hear you.

Use assistive devices as needed (make certain that hearing aids and microphones are turned on and that batteries are working) .

General Teaching and Learning Suggestions

Keep teaching sessions short and to the point.

Design handouts to be simple and clear.

Relate the relevance of the topic to adult experiences within the group.

Use the principles of adult learning when planning an educational session.

Pace the presentation to reflect the unique needs and understanding of the group or individual.

Avoid the temptation to overload with too much information.

Remember that adults need a motivation to learn.

Provide immediate feedback to questions and comments.

Give an overview of the material to be covered and explain its relevance.

Keep information simple and specific; avoid technical jargon.

Use a variety of teaching modalities such as videotapes, hands-on experiences, samples of products, group discussion, overheads, pamphlets, and handouts.

Emphasize the client's learning responsibility.

Be enthusiastic about the subject; if the teacher isn't, the learner will not be.

Summarize important points.

Teach a procedure close to the time it will take place.

When teaching skills, allow time for practice, return demonstrations, questions, and review sessions.

Stick to the essentials needed to maintain life and prevent complications but be prepared to address additional questions.

Keep the environment conducive to learning; for group sessions, the room temperature should be comfortable for the majority, potentially noxious stimuli (such as cigarette smoke) should be avoided, seats must be easily accessible.

Use a large enough room to accommodate those with wheelchairs, walkers, and other assistive devices. Make certain exits are not blocked. Have additional nursing personnel available should needs arise (such as toileting).

Be thoroughly familiar with resources available in the community and the individual facility.

From *Gerontological rehabilitation nursing* (p. 176), by K. L. Easton, 1999, Philadelphia: W.B. Saunders. Copyright 2011 by Kristen L. Mauk. Reprinted with permission.

without a pharmacological aid (Chantix, Wellbutrin, or nicotine patch) is recommended.

5) Safety awareness: Falls are a major cause of TBI and fractures. Maintaining a safe environment can reduce the risk of falls.
   a) Home environment: Keep the home free of barriers and obstacles that restrict mobility and increase risk of falls.
   b) Home safety evaluation: Identify unsafe conditions and measures to increase safety; educate family and caregivers on steps to prevent falls and injury.

6) Medication management
   a) Polypharmacy simulates symptoms produced by disease (delirium, hypotension, pseudoparkinsonism). A

national initiative is underway to reduce the number of medications used.

   b) Risk factors: Age, sex, living arrangements, number of medications taken (Farrell, Hill, Hawkins, Newman, & Learned, 2003)

   c) Psychoactive medications should not be used to control behavioral problems.

7) Driving skills must be reassessed because decline in cognition and visual and auditory changes can affect response time, decision making, and judgment.

8) Fall prevention: Addressing physical impairments leading to falls is the major goal (Muché & McCarty, 2009).

9) Vision correction is recommended because poor vision can lead to social isolation, decline in ability to perform ADLs, depression, and altered self-image (Muché & McCarty, 2009).

10) Hearing correction will prevent deterioration of social function, depression, and falls.

11) Seat belts: Seat belt use can reduce secondary injury.

12) Limit alcohol intake to two drinks per day for men, one drink per day for women.

13) Social supports

14) Aspirin therapy for clients at risk for CHD

15) Aggressive statin therapy for clients with high cholesterol levels and established cardiovascular disease or risk for CHD

16) Cancer screening: Depends on comorbidity, functional status, and life expectancy; colorectal screening is recommended for clients 50 years and older (Spalding & Sebesta, 2008).

17) Pneumonia vaccine for those older than 65 years and other high-risk clients; revaccinate every 5 years

18) Influenza vaccine yearly

19) Zoster: People age 60 and older (see CDC recommendations for adult vaccination)

20) Tetanus: After 5 years for wound management in clients older than age 65 (CDC, 2009); tetanus/diphtheria/pertussis once every 10 years

21) Varicella: Two doses for adults who have not had varicella

2. Secondary prevention for all age groups, with and without disability

   a. Smoking cessation: A 3-minute counseling session with or without pharmacological aid (Chantix, Wellbutrin, or nicotine patch) is recommended (Spalding & Sebesta, 2008).

   b. Pneumonia vaccine: Follow CDC recommendations.

   c. Flu vaccine yearly

   d. Zoster: People age 60 and older (see CDC recommendations for adult vaccination)

   e. Tetanus: After 5 years for wound management in clients older than age 65 (CDC, 2009); tetanus/diphtheria/pertussis once every 10 years

   f. Varicella: Two doses for adults who have not had varicella

3. Tertiary prevention in older adults without disability

   a. Chronic disease management

   b. Health maintenance

   c. Educating the older adult about

     1) The disease process

     2) How to prevent disease progression

     3) Recognition of complications and what to do

     4) Treatment compliance

4. Societal level

   a. Redesign of cars

   b. Redesign of roadways

   c. License renewal restrictions

   d. Special transportation services

5. CDC programs to promote healthy aging

   a. Web-based educational resources and tools related to aging issues

   b. Outreach services for older adults on disease prevention, advance directives, and end-of-life issues

6. Senior-friendly website to educate seniors: An easy-to-use website that reads content aloud to the viewer, developed by the National Institute on Aging and National Library of Medicine, is available at www.nihseniorhealth.gov.

IV. **Aging and Disability: Aging with an Early-Onset Disability**

A. Longevity: People with early-onset disability are living longer. An estimated 12 million people are currently living into middle and late life with an early-onset disability.

   1. Antibiotics and other medication advances

   2. Advances in technology

   3. Improvements in public health

   4. Improved medical care (Kemp & Mosqueda, 2004)

B. Aging as an Uncharted Course

1. Atypical aging seems to be the norm. Unanticipated changes occur in midlife (Kemp & Mosqueda, 2004).
2. Higher rates of medical and functional problems often occur 20–25 years earlier than in those without disability. Disability often occurs in those who have been most active and changes occur in the amount of assistance needed (Kailes, 2002; Kemp & Mosqueda, 2004).
3. This population has three to four times the number of secondary health problems as age-matched peers (Kailes, 2002).
4. Accelerated aging is aging related to the disability itself at the cellular or organ level (Kailes, 2002).
5. *Wear and tear* refers to increased stress on the body from living with disability over time (Kailes, 2002).
6. Results of rehabilitation depend on the era of onset: People disabled 30, 40, or 50 years ago received rehabilitation in a different era. Many factors have changed over time. People who are disabled today may not have the same outcomes in 20, 30, or 40 years (Kailes, 2002).
7. Latent illness: An impairment such as polio or cerebral palsy (CP) can start a cascade of events that cause illnesses in later life (Kailes, 2002).
8. Contributing factors
    a. Environment
        1) Limited accessibility exacerbates the effects of disability and aging.
        2) Modifications in the home and community can increase safety and accessibility and facilitate health maintenance.
    b. Nonaccommodating environments may increase stress on the body (Kailes, 2002).
    c. Equipment: Manual equipment may increase stress on joints and limbs over time.
    d. Medications: Long-term use of medications may affect the aging and health of body systems.
    e. Sedentary lifestyles increase the risk of cardiovascular disease and disuse syndromes.
    f. Preventive service use: Many people with disabilities do not maintain preventive services (e.g., vaccinations, cancer screening) because of a lack of knowledge, funding, or available and accessible services.
C. Unexpected Medical, Functional, and Psychosocial Problems (Kailes, 2002)
    1. Loss of strength, endurance, and range of motion
    2. Pain: Chronic pain, physical and emotional pain, limited coping strategies and training
    3. Employment difficulties: Ageism, changing work environment
    4. Decreased quality of life: Decreased income, unpredictable financial resources
    5. Family stress: Lack of support, loss of loved one, caregiver role, grandparenting role (Miyamoto, Tachimori, & Ito, 2010)
D. Late Life Syndrome: Disability-specific changes with aging are common, superimposed on normal changes of aging.
    1. Polio
        a. Postpolio syndrome (PPS)
            1) 440,000 people are at risk for PPS; 25%–60% of polio survivors may develop PPS.
            2) Signs and symptoms appear 30–40 years after original onset of polio.
            3) The exact cause is unknown, but it is thought to be a degeneration of overworked nerve terminals in motor units that remain after initial illness.
            4) Slow, stepwise, unpredictable course
            5) Decreased strength, fatigue
                a) In muscles previously affected by polio and in muscles not previously affected by polio
                b) Muscle atrophy occurs in some cases.
                c) PPS fatigue affects more than 1.63 million American polio survivors (Bruno, Cohen, Galski, & Frick, n.d.).
            6) Decreased respiratory efficiency: Pneumonia
            7) Dysphagia: Aspiration pneumonia
            8) Joint pain
            9) Muscle pain, cramping reported by 90% of clients
            10) Gait disturbance
            11) Autonomic dysfunction
            12) Sleep apnea
            13) Flat back syndrome (Muniz, 2011)
            14) Decreased function
            15) Depression
        b. The severity of PPS is predicted by the severity of initial residual disability after polio (Klingbiel, Baer, & Wilson, 2004; National Institute of Neurological Disorders and Stroke [NINDS], 2006b).
    2. CP
        a. Sixty-five to ninety percent of children with CP live into adulthood.
        b. Organ systems (heart, lungs) age prematurely.
        c. Postimpairment syndrome includes pain, weakness, and fatigue.
        d. Decline in functional status
            1) Walking
            2) Self-care

e. Increased falls
f. Contractures, especially lower extremities in nonambulators
g. Progressive deformity
h. Pulmonary changes impair breathing, making speech inaudible, and motor impairment in later life can cause difficulty in phonation and sentence production.
i. Kyphoscoliosis
   1) Pneumonia, right-sided heart failure, hypoxemia, decreased vital capacity
   2) Problems with positioning, seating
j. Increased bowel and bladder dysfunction
   1) Urinary tract infections
   2) Incontinence
k. Osteoporosis, osteopenia, and fractures
l. Oral motor and dental disorders
   1) Increased difficulty chewing, eating, and swallowing
   2) Increased risk of aspiration, malnutrition, and dental decay
   3) More common in those with dyskinesias or spastic CP
m. Arthritis: Association between presence of pain in weight-bearing joints and a cessation of ambulation around age 45
n. Spasticity is increased.
o. Pain
   1) Often related to musculoskeletal dysfunction, degenerative arthritis, and overuse syndromes
   2) Common sites include hip, knee, ankle, and lumbar and cervical spine
p. Spinal stenosis (Klingbiel et al., 2004; NINDS, 2006a)
q. Life expectancy is lower for those with severe impairment and poor mobility (De Vivo, 2004).
r. Strauss, Ojdana, Shavelle, and Rosenbloom (2004) found a marked decline in ambulation with aging for those with CP who were mobile when they became adults. There was a greater need for assistance with ADLs as age increased, greater need for residence in nursing facilities, and poorer survival among those who lost mobility. People with the most severe disability did not live to age 60.

3. Spina bifida
   a. Overuse syndrome
      1) Wheelchair users: Shoulders, wrists, hands; carpal tunnel syndrome; rotator cuff injuries
      2) Ambulators: Hip and knee pain
   b. Reduced muscle strength and endurance lead to decreased mobility and ability to ambulate and transfer.
   c. Reduced nerve function reduces sensations and circulation.
   d. Shunt malfunction
   e. Tethered cord syndrome (Brei & Merkens, 2003)
      1) Chiari problem: Apnea
      2) Syrinx
   f. Knee pain
   g. Osteoporosis: Increased risk for fractures; uneven pressure on joints causes arthritis and pain
   h. Kyphosis and scoliosis
   i. Charcot joints
   j. Skin changes: Pressure ulcers, abrasions
   k. Increased incidence and severity of latex allergy
   l Obesity from decreased mobility
   m. Renal system changes
      1) Renal damage leading to renal failure
      2) Bladder cancer associated with neurogenic bladder
      3) Changes in bladder control
   n. Increased risk of latex allergies (Klingbiel et al., 2004)
   o. Bowel function: Constipation, need for bowel evacuations and high-fiber diet
   p. Need for braces and equipment due to poor balance and increasing need for ADL assistance
   q. Reduced socialization leads to isolation
   r. Depression
   s. Different levels of need for ADL assistance depending on cognitive level (Brei & Merkens, 2003)

4. Down syndrome
   a. Fifty percent of infants who survive to age 1 can be expected to live past 50 years of age.
   b. Show signs of aging 20–30 years ahead of others in the general population
      1) Accelerated deterioration in later life after stressful event, depression, underactive thyroid; visual and hearing impairments are common
      2) Depression
      3) Hypothyroidism
      4) Hearing and visual impairment
      5) Vascular disease
      6) Graying hair
      7) Glucose intolerance and degenerative bone disease

8) High rates of cancer
9) Cognitive losses
c. Early-onset dementia
  1) Typically around age 40–50, as many as 75% of people with Down syndrome exhibit signs of Alzheimer's-type dementia.
  2) Atypical signs and symptoms
    a) Seizures
    b) Changes in ADL ability
d. Accelerated rate of functional losses after age 45
  1) Need the same health promotion programs at an earlier age as nondisabled people age 50–80 (Chen, 2006; Merck Manuals Online Medical Library, 2003)
  2) Menopause may occur 5–6 years earlier than in the general population (Holland & Benton, 2004).
e. Quality of life (Brown, Taylor, & Matthews, 2001)
  1) The majority report being happy.
  2) Privacy is important.
  3) Reminiscence may be helpful.
  4) Tidiness and cleanliness of surroundings are valued.

5. Spinal cord injury
a. Menter and Hudson's model of aging that develops functional decline identifies three post-SCI phases (Winkler, 2008).
  1) Acute restoration phase (first 2 years after SCI): Maximal function regained within limitations of SCI
  2) Maintenance phase
    a) Stable level of function over time
    b) Stable time varies
  3) Decline phase
    a) Degenerative effects of SCI
    b) Aging
b. Functional decline begins 10–20 years after injury.
  1) Depends on genetics, lifestyle, age at time of injury, current age, level of injury, weight, health history, comorbidities, available social support
  2) Children with SCI may have 20 years of stable functioning after injury, whereas adults older than age 50 may have just 5–7 years before decline begins.
c. Overuse syndrome
  1) Pain
    a) Incidence of pain increases from 41% 1 year after injury to about 80% more than 5 years after injury.
    b) More than 70% of people with SCI report upper-extremity pain.
    c) Nearly two-thirds of people with SCI have compressive neuropathies in the upper extremities.
  2) The most common overuse syndromes are degenerative joint disease, rotator cuff tears, rotator cuff tendinitis, subacromial bursitis, and capsulitis. (Winkler, 2008).
d. Osteoporosis and fractures
  1) Six percent of people with SCI have a lower-extremity fracture, most commonly femur; fracture potential is reached 1–9 years after SCI.
  2) As many as 10% of these fractures result in nonunion.
e. Scoliosis
  1) Nearly 97% of children and adolescents with SCI develop scoliosis.
  2) Nearly 50% of adults with SCI develop scoliosis.
f. Cardiovascular function
  1) Incidence of cardiovascular disease is more than 200% higher than in the non-injured population.
  2) Hypertension is twice as common in people with paraplegia as in the general population.
g. Gastrointestinal tract: Complications and dysfunction increase with age. Seventy-four percent develop hemorrhoids, 43% develop abdominal distention, and 20% develop difficulty in bowel evacuation.
h. Genitourinary tract: Incidence of bladder cancer increases from 0.2% in the first 10 years after injury to 9% after 30 years.
i. Skin: Soft-tissue changes and thinning of subcutaneous fat lead to risk of skin tears, breakdown, and poor healing.
  1) Susceptibility to pressure ulcers increases with age.
  2) Sitting tolerance may decrease with age because of the loss of adipose tissue.
  3) The incidence of pressure ulcers increases with age; 15%–30% of people with SCI develop pressure ulcers.
j. Decreased immunity
  1) Frequency of urinary tract infections, increased risk of falls.
  2) Pneumonia risk increases as a function of underlying comorbidities and decreased mobility.

k. Decreased pulmonary function; restrictive pulmonary disease can accelerate decline. There is a higher incidence of sleep apnea (Winkler, 2008).

l. Insulin resistance risk increases four times after SCI.

m. Hardware breakdown: Spinal rods

n. Social isolation (Menter, 1998; Winkler, 2008)

o. Bowel function: The ability to manage neurogenic bowel decreases after age 60 when the injury is 30 or more years old. There is an increased risk of colorectal cancer.

p. ADLs: The need for ADL assistance increases with age. Reasons for needing assistance include the following:
   1) Increased weakness
   2) Increased weight gain
   3) Increased pain

q. ADLs most affected are
   1) Bathing
   2) Transfer
   3) Dressing

r. Instrumental ADLs with which most SCI-injured people need assistance include the following:
   1) Household chores
   2) Shopping
   3) Meal preparation

6. TBI: Overwhelming behavioral changes and personality changes can make TBI frightening to the family and the client. A recent study of 286 survivors of moderate to severe TBI revealed the following chronic health conditions an average of 14.2 years after injury:
   a. Nervousness and tension
   b. Headaches
   c. Dizziness
   d. Sensitivity to noise and light
   e. Personality changes
   f. Arthritis
   g. Sleep disturbances
   h. Vision changes
   i. Hearing changes
   j. Allergies
   k. Potential for seizures
   l. Breathing problems (Colantonio, Ratcliff, Chase, & Vernich, 2004)
   m. Studies have shown an increased rate of social isolation.
   n. Memory problems, including slower processing, difficulty processing

7. Multiple sclerosis (MS)

a. People older than 65 years have greater disability.

b. Disease course and length of time after diagnosis are stronger predictors of current status than current age and other demographics (DeVivo, 2004).

c. Finlayson, Van Denend, and Hudson (2004) found that women aging with MS perceived that they had less freedom and needed more assistance than peers without MS. They shared concerns about unmet needs in the areas of personal care, housework, support groups, assistive technology, travel, and socialization.

E. Rehabilitation Nursing Interventions to Promote Successful Aging in Those with Early-Onset Disability (See p. 484 III.C for guidelines for primary prevention for young age groups and older adults and ongoing secondary prevention for all age groups with disability.)

V. Psychosocial Issues
   A. Grief and Loss
      1. Life changes with age
         a. Retirement
         b. Death of a spouse, children, friends
         c. Possible decline in health, including chronic illness and disability
         d. Menopause
         e. Possible change in economic status
         f. Possible social isolation
         g. Possible change in living arrangements
      2. Role changes with age
         a. Widowhood
         b. Caregiver role reversal (i.e., the person who has provided care becomes the person who is being cared for)
   B. Stress and Coping
      1. The ability to deal well with stress and adopt positive coping mechanisms is associated with successful aging (Vaillant, 2002).
      2. Assess coping strategies in relation to the amount of stress the person is experiencing and promote the use of positive coping strategies.
         a. Increased social support
         b. Activity and exercise
         c. Faith, hope, and spirituality
         d. Involvement in leisure activities the client enjoys
   C. Depression and Anxiety
      1. Depression

THE SPECIALTY PRACTICE OF REHABILITATION NURSING

a. It is estimated that 2 million older adults experience depression in some form (National Institute of Mental Health [NIMH], 2006).

b. Risk factors (Kurlowicz & Harvath, 2008)
  1) Incontinence
  2) History of substance abuse
  3) Social isolation
  4) Chronic pain or illness
  5) Being a caregiver
  6) Living alone (especially widow or widower)
  7) Functional disability
  8) Poor social support

c. Signs and symptoms
  1) Insomnia
  2) Memory impairment
  3) Feelings of worthlessness or powerlessness
  4) Fatigue
  5) Vague physical complaints

d. Results of depression (Diebold et al., 2010)
  1) Decreased quality of life
  2) Associated anxiety
  3) Higher mortality rates from other conditions
  4) Higher risk for cancer
  5) Poorer outcomes after surgery
  6) Higher rate of suicide

e. Nursing interventions (Butcher & McGonigal-Kenney, 2005)
  1) Psychotherapy or counseling
  2) Medications, especially tricyclic antidepressants, selective serotonin reuptake inhibitors, and antipsychotics (monoamine oxidase inhibitors used less because of side effects)
  3) Encourage participation in social activities.
  4) Promote a healthy lifestyle, including proper nutrition, good sleeping habits, and a daily routine.
  5) Enhance coping strategies.
  6) Connect to community resources.
  7) Enhance social support systems.
  8) Inspire hope.
  9) Be alert to suicidal ideations.

2. Anxiety
  a. It should be treated in conjunction with depression for best outcomes.
  b. Most older adults with major depression also have anxiety.
  c. It is not well understood or studied in older adults.
  d. Assess for risk factors such as certain medical conditions and medications that exacerbate anxiety (Diebold et al., 2010).

e. Selective serotonin reuptake inhibitors (used to treat depression) are medications of choice (Anxiety Disorders Association of America, 2006).

f. Also treated with cognitive-behavioral therapy

g. Nursing interventions are similar to those for depression; in addition, the rehabilitation nurse should develop a trusting relationship with the primary healthcare provider.

D. Life Review and Reminiscence
  1. Older adults may be undertaking an end-of-life review.
  2. They may experience anticipatory grieving.
  3. Erikson's development stage for older age, ego integrity versus despair, suggests that older adults need to feel that their life has purpose and meaning. (Refer to Chapter 17 for more information on developmental stages.)
  4. Rehabilitation nurses can use reminiscence therapy to help older adults recall positive memories that can be shared and discussed (Kart & Kinney, 2001).

E. Suicide
  1. Older White men are at highest risk for suicide.
  2. Older men tend to use more lethal means of suicide (e.g., firearms, hanging), whereas older women use less lethal means such as pills.
  3. Suicide is associated with alcoholism, diagnosis of a terminal disease, depression, presence of a chronic disease, being unmarried and living alone, having few support systems, drug abuse, bereavement, intractable pain, and social isolation; depression is the most notable associated condition.
  4. In 2000, 18% of suicide deaths were in older adults (NIMH, 2006).
  5. Up to 75% of those committing suicide visited their primary care physician within a month beforehand (NIMH, 2006).
  6. The risk can be lessened by strengthening social supports, treating depression, increasing involvement in social activities, and taking definitive action when suicidal ideations are expressed (Kart & Kinney, 2001).

F. Rehabilitation of Clients Who Are Terminally Ill
  1. Nurses should explore their own feelings about the rehabilitation of those who are at the end of life.
  2. There are many potential examples of situations that involve rehabilitating older adults with terminal illnesses.
    a. Late-stage cancer, including melanoma

b. Rapidly growing, inoperable tumors

c. End-stage renal disease

d. Last stages of AIDS

e. Other incurable diseases

3. Explore with the client and family the goals of rehabilitation therapy.

 a. Increase the quality of life.

 b. Increase independence enough to go home to die rather than remaining in a facility.

4. Discuss the purposes of palliative care and hospice (Krieger-Blake & Warring, 2010).

 a. Hospice helps clients "live until they die."

 b. Hospice provides bereavement services for the family after the death.

 c. Hospice provides pain management.

 d. Hospice provides symptom control at end of life.

 e. Palliative care can occur in many settings and clients do not have to be terminally ill to benefit from palliative care.

VI. General Aging Issues

 A. Preventive Services for Older Adults

 1. Primary

 a. Activities for health promotion and disease prevention.

 b. Immunizations to prevent illness; those recommended by the CDC for adults older than 65 years and those at high risk include the following (CDC, 2006b):

 1) Annual flu vaccine

 2) Pneumococcal vaccine once after age 65 and one-time revaccination for those older than age 75

 3) Tetanus and diphtheria vaccine every 10 years

 2. Secondary

 a. Follow recommendations of Healthy People 2010 (www.healthypeople.gov/).

 b. Screenings for clients at risk

 c. Screenings recommended by the U.S. Preventive Services Task Force with sufficient evidence to support (Nelson, 2006)

 1) Tobacco use

 2) Depression

 3) Hyperlipidemia

 4) Hypertension

 5) Osteoporosis for women older than 65 years

 6) Vision and hearing for older adults

 7) Mammography every 1–2 years for women

 8) Colorectal cancer screening by fecal occult blood test or sigmoidoscopy

 9) Physical and dental checkup (Lau & Kirby, 2009)

 3. Tertiary

 a. Rehabilitation of chronic health alterations as discussed throughout this core curriculum

 b. Focus on prevention of complications and maintenance of function

 B. End of Life

 1. Hospice or end-of-life care is focused on the dying process. It is prescribed by a physician for clients who are terminally ill and have fewer than 6 months to live (Pace, Burke, & Glass, 2006).

 a. More than 75% of hospice clients die at home (National Hospice and Palliative Care Organization, 2004).

 b. Hospice care provides support for people in the last phase of terminal illness.

 c. Promotes the concept of "living until you die."

 d. Hospice recognizes dying as a normal part of living.

 e. Focuses on maintaining quality of life until death.

 f. Grief and bereavement support for client and family

 g. Pain management is a priority.

 h. Services provided include the following:

 1) Nursing care

 2) Psychological counseling

 3) Spiritual care

 4) Grief counseling

 5) Social service support

 6) ADL care

 7) Household chores

 8) Respite services for caregivers (Pace, Burke, & Glass, 2006)]

 2. Palliative care

 a. Palliative care is comprehensive care of the discomfort, symptoms, and stress of serious illness. It also helps provide relief from pain, shortness of breath, fatigue, constipation, nausea, loss of appetite, and sleep disorders. It can help with the side effects of medical treatment. Palliative care has three operational components (Mahon, 2010).

 1) Aggressive symptom management

 2) Assistance with decision making

 3) End-of-life care when appropriate; this is comfort based, not curative

 b. Clients can receive treatment for conditions and still receive palliative care; pursuing treatment does not exclude clients from palliative care.

THE SPECIALTY PRACTICE OF REHABILITATION NURSING

c. Based on an interdisciplinary team model
d. Funded by Medicare, Medicaid, and private insurance
e. Provides emotional support for the client and family
f. Rehabilitation nurses can assist clients in the process of dying well because there is potential for self-growth even in the dying process (Byock, 1997).

3. Nursing interventions
   a. Advance directives
      1) Living will
         a) Is used in cases of terminal illness
         b) Makes the client's wishes known in advance when death is imminent, as certified by a physician
      2) Declaration document of life-prolonging procedures
         a) Describes steps to take to prolong life
         b) Is determined by the client
      3) Durable power of attorney for health care
         a) Allows another person to make decisions on behalf of the client
         b) Can encompass health, financial, property, and other issues
      4) Healthcare representative: Allows a healthcare professional to make decisions at the client's behest regarding health-related issues
      5) Five wishes (Aging with Dignity, 2011)
         a) Not legally recognized in all states
         b) In the states where this is recognized, people may complete the forms, available online, without the use of an attorney.
         c) Cost-effective and easy to use
         d) A nontraditional type of advanced directive that answers these five items according to a person's wishes
            i. Who makes healthcare decisions when the person is unable
            ii. What kind of medical treatment is wanted or not wanted
            iii. Comfort measures the person wants
            iv. How people should treat the person
            v. What he or she wants loved ones to know
      6) Allow natural death (Meyer, 2001; Warring & Krieger-Blake, 2006): More descriptive and positive than a do-not-resuscitate order

b. Intervening with common problems at the end of life
   1) Dyspnea
      a) Opioid therapy such as morphine can reduce shortness of breath.
      b) Elevate head of the bed 30–45 degrees.
      c) Provide a fan to move air in the room.
      d) Cool, humidified air
      e) Control oral secretions.
   2) Anxiety can be worsened by fear of suffering; antianxiety agents such as lorazepam given orally, sublingually, or rectally can help (McKinnis, 2002).
   3) Constipation
      a) Immobility, lack of exercise, decreased food and fluids, and use of pain medications contribute to constipation.
      b) Use a stool softener and stimulant combination.
   4) Nausea and vomiting
      a) Treatment depends on the cause.
      b) A combination of medications may be indicated.
      c) Prepare foods away from client's room.
      d) Eliminate noxious stimuli.
      e) Ice chips may help in eliminating aftertaste and dryness of mouth.
   5) Poor appetite
      a) Narcotic use reduces desire to eat.
      b) Eat as desired.
      c) Maintain a clean, tidy environment.
      d) There is a natural decrease in desire for food at the end of life.
      e) Artificial hydration may prolong suffering and increase edema through fluid overload (End of Life Nursing Education Consortium, 2004).
      f) Provide meticulous mouth care as fluid intake decreases.
   6) Pain
      a) Typically undertreated in older adults
      b) Identify and treat the type of pain.
      c) Fear of addiction should not be a factor.
      d) Cancer pain treatment generally follows a three-step ladder (World Health Organization, 1990) of nonsteroidal anti-inflammatory drugs, opioids, and analgesic adjuvants in combinations.

e) Be aware of cultural variations in tolerance to pain and expression of pain.
f) Offer effective pain interventions.
g) Use nonpharmacological methods such as music and aroma therapy.
c. Educating families about what to expect at the end of life
1) Signs of impending death (Marrone, 1997)
a) Decreased urine output
b) Changes in breathing patterns
c) Increasing periods of unresponsiveness
d) Mottling of extremities
e) Changes in vital signs
2) Ask about specific cultural or spiritual practices at end of life and death.
d. Ethical and moral dilemmas
1) Withholding treatment: Not beginning treatment (advance directives make the client's wishes explicit)
2) Withdrawing treatment: Removing life-sustaining interventions after they have been implemented (e.g., disconnecting a ventilator from a person who is unable to breathe independently, discontinuing nutritional interventions for a person who cannot otherwise eat or drink independently)
3) Assisted suicide
a) Defined as helping a person to terminate his or her own life
b) Illegal in most states
c) Legal in Oregon for a terminally ill client to be prescribed a lethal dose of medication by the physician; must be taken by the client
4) Euthanasia
a) Purposefully hastening the death of another person
b) An outside person may play a more active role in hastening the death of another with the purpose of ending his or her suffering.
C. Use of Physical and Chemical Restraints
1. Approximately 15% of nursing home residents are restrained for some portion of the day (Beers & Berkow, n.d.). Some side effects of restraint use include
a. Falls while attempting to free oneself from the restraint
b. Confusion caused by forceful restrictions of movement, inability to position, and reduced stimulation
c. Death from choking and entrapment
d. Pressure ulcers caused by immobility, damage to skin from friction and shear forces in attempts to free oneself
e. Pneumonia aspiration, fluid accumulation from reduced attempts to deep breathe and cough
f. Urinary tract infections, reduced fluid intake, withholding urge due to lack of access and immobility caused by restraints, incomplete emptying
2. The use of physical restraints must be assessed, justified, and documented every day and as recommended by regulatory agencies.
3. Physical restraints should be used only when the person is a danger to himself or herself or others.
4. The routine use of chemical restraints is inappropriate except in the most extreme circumstances for client safety.
5. Alternatives to restraints exist and should be explored (Cowley et al., 2006).
a. Companions or close supervision
b. Modifying the environment to reduce barriers and provide easy access
c. Reality orientation
d. Activities for diversion
e. Increasing physical activities
6. Restraint use increases the likelihood of injury in many instances.
7. A physician order is required for restraint use and must include documentation of the medical condition necessitating restraint, the type of restraint, the length of time for use, and guidelines for release and repositioning (according to Omnibus Budget Reconciliation Act 1987 guidelines). (Cowley et al., 2006).
D. Abuse or Mistreatment of Older Adults
1. May take many forms, including neglect; financial exploitation; and passive or active physical, emotional, and sexual abuse
2. Elder abuse is difficult to obtain statistics on and difficult to research (National Center on Elder Abuse, 2006).
a. Often not reported or is underreported by victims
b. As many as 5 million victims of financial abuse
c. Two to ten percent of older adults may be victims of abuse.
d. Between 1 and 2 million Americans may have been victimized in some way by those they depended on.
3. Characteristics of abusers

a. May have been victims of abuse themselves

b. May be men or women

c. May be family members or caregivers

d. May have social and emotional problems or a history of psychological problems

e. May abuse drugs or alcohol

f. May have a high level of stress or frustration, minimal coping abilities, and lack of knowledge

4. Characteristics of victims (DeCalmer & Glendenning, 1993; Pritchard, 1995, 1996): Many rehabilitation clients are at risk because of the following factors:

a. Social isolation

b. Advanced age

c. Poor health

d. Widowhood

e. Significant physical limitations

f. Gender (women are victims more often)

g. Dependence on others

h. History of family violence

5. Possible signs and symptoms of abuse or mistreatment

a. Poor physical hygiene

b. Dehydration or malnutrition

c. Multiple bruises of different colors (indicating different stages of healing)

d. A withdrawn, cowering, fearful, anxious, depressed, or hopeless demeanor

e. Presence of burns, skin tears, broken bones, or severe rashes that, when explained, do not fit the injury or trauma

f. Poor eye contact, communicates with short answers

6. Nursing interventions (**Figure 19-3**)

a. Perform a complete history and physical assessment.

b. Make certain the explanation fits the injury, realizing that rehabilitating older adults may experience falls as they increase their level of independence.

c. Be alert to possible signs and symptoms of abuse or neglect.

d. Interview the suspected abuser and the victim separately.

e. Consult with available resources as needed (e.g., psychologist, social worker).

f. Report any suspected case of abuse. This can be done anonymously to an adult protective services office.

g. Do not alienate the suspected perpetrator.

h. Take the necessary steps to protect the client.

Figure 19-3. Nursing Indications for the Prevention of Elder Abuse

- Establish a trusting relationship with the elderly person.
- Be able to refer families to resources available in the community.
- Strengthen social supports.
- Encourage regular respite for the caregiver.
- Identify caregivers who are at the highest risk of being abusers and target interventions to prevent stress from caregiver burden.
- Be aware of risk factors and contributing factors.
- Perform a thorough physical assessment and carefully document findings, including the client's appearance, nutritional state, skin condition, mental attitude and awareness, and the need for aids to enhance sensory perception.
- If abuse is suspected, interview the caregiver and other possible informants to confirm or refute suspicions.
- Know the laws governing the reporting of abuse.

From *Gerontological rehabilitation nursing* (p. 336), by K. L. Easton, 1999. Philadelphia: W. B. Saunders. Copyright 2011 by Kristen L. Mauk. Reprinted with permission.

i. Maintain confidentiality of conversation and develop client trust.

E. Polypharmacy

1. Polypharmacy is defined as the use of multiple medications, more than five medications, or inappropriate use of medication, using multiple medications to treat the same condition, simultaneous use of medications that cause drug interactions, inappropriate dosage, and medications used to counteract the side effects of other medications.

a. Older adults commonly take many medications, which can increase the risk of adverse reactions for many reasons.

1) Drugs are excreted more slowly by the kidneys.

2) Absorption in the intestines is slower.

3) Metabolism slows with age.

b. Older adults consume 34% of prescription medications and about 40% of nonprescription medications (American Society of Consultant Pharmacists, 2000).

c. The aforementioned factors cause the drugs to remain present in the body for a longer time.

d. Adverse drug reactions may occur at any time, or at a later time than expected with younger adults.

e. Older adults may use over-the-counter medications or herbal therapies they do not consider "drugs," but these substances may interact with other medications.

f. Incidence of polypharmacy is thought to increase with age.

g. Those older than age 85 are at higher risk because they typically take more medications.

h. Polypharmacy is associated with
  1) Number and severity of illnesses
  2) Hospitalization
  3) Number of physicians seen
  4) Number of pharmacies used
  5) Advanced client age

i. In long-term care facilities, psychotherapeutics are often misused.

j. Interventions to avoid polypharmacy have not been well researched or documented.

2. Nursing interventions

a. Avoid unnecessary polypharmacy.
  1) Teach clients and families to use a primary care provider to coordinate care.
  2) Obtain a list of all physicians and pharmacies used.
  3) Check for duplication of medications.
  4) Encourage use of one pharmacy.
  5) Be sure all physicians are informed of all medications prescribed by other physicians.
  6) Use Beer's criteria to review potentially inappropriate medication (Zwicker & Fulmer, 2008).
    a) List of medications to avoid for older adults
    b) Medications should not be taken under certain conditions.
    c) Review the medication list with every visit.
    d) Avoid duplications.
  7) Use the brown bag method of self-reporting to evaluate medication use.
  8) Encourage practitioners to assess the need for every medication. Consider a drug holiday if possible.
  9) Ask about alternative medications and over-the-counter medications.
  10) Encourage the client to use the same resource for refills.

b. Avoid negative effects of polypharmacy.
  1) Obtain a comprehensive medication history.
  2) Monitor blood urea nitrogen, creatinine, and creatinine clearance to check kidney function.
  3) Consider the possibility of adverse drug reactions when new symptoms appear (Cowley et al., 2006).
  4) Use or consider use of nonpharmacologic treatment when possible.
  5) Simplify the medication regimen.
  6) Review dietary habits.
  7) Consider effects and interactions of food and medication.
  8) Educate family and clients to be informed consumers.

c. Family and client education regarding medication errors
  1) Include the client and the family or caregiver.
  2) Follow the principles of teaching and learning with family members and with the client.
  3) Allow time for demonstration and return demonstration.
  4) Teach more than one family member whenever possible.
  5) Use medication boxes to assist with organization of medications and promote independence of the client when appropriate.
  6) Use large and simple medication lists that are readily accessible.
  7) Use pictures of medications on the list to assist with recognition.
  8) Be sure the client and family understand the purpose of the medication, time to be taken, amount, and route.
  9) Provide written discharge instructions in simple language (fourth-grade level).
  10) Encourage the client to carry a medication list with dosages in his or her wallet.
  11) Encourage the family and client to know medications by name and not by color or size of the medication.

d. Use of medication boxes
  1) Organizes the client's medications.
  2) Provides a system to decrease the risk of making medication errors at home.
  3) Allows family members to help monitor or set up the client's medications

e. Evaluate the client's ability to self-medicate using the Drug Regimen Unassisted Grading Scale (DRUGS) before discharge from the hospital and periodically.

F. Caregiver Issues
  1. Aging caregivers
    a. Many caregivers of older adults are older themselves.
    b. When the caregiver's health is poor, caregiver stress is likely to be higher; older caregivers are more likely to have more chronic illnesses by virtue of their age.

THE SPECIALTY PRACTICE OF REHABILITATION NURSING

c. Caregiving may also fill a need for the caregiver (Krieger-Blake, 2006).
2. Caregiver stress: A Japanese study revealed that behavioral, psychological, and functional symptoms of dementia in the form of aggression, screaming, and impaired ability to perform ADLs increase the burden of caregivers (Miyamoto, Tachimori, & Ito, 2010).
   a. Caregiver stress is defined as the emotional burden of caregiving.
   b. The level of dependency on the caregiver increases the amount of stress.
   c. Lack of family support adds to the burden of stress.
   d. The burden of caring can lead to depression, anxiety, difficulty coping, and problems with physical health of the caregiver.
   e. Women are more prone to this problem.
   f. Signs of caregiver stress include the following (U.S. Department of Health and Human Services, 2006):
      1) Sleeping problems
      2) Weight loss or gain
      3) Fatigue
      4) Irritability
      5) Withdrawal
      6) Headaches, stomach upset, or frequent vague physical symptoms
      7) Anxiety
   g. Interventions for reducing caregiver stress and improving quality of life
      1) Obtain respite care as needed.
      2) Get assistance in the home.
      3) Take care of one's own health through diet, daily exercise, and relaxation.
      4) Use community resources (e.g., National Family Caregiver Support Program).
      5) Use faith-based resources if possible.
      6) Attend support groups.
      7) Obtain caregiver training (McCullagh, Brigstocke, Donaldson, & Kalra, 2005).
      8) Caregiver resources: American Association of Retired Persons (AARP) caregiver website, Alzheimer's Association, Administration on Aging website, Red Cross.
G. Postrehabilitation Care
   1. Settings for care
      a. Long-term care facilities
         1) Provide a variety of levels of care
         2) May range from independent living to nursing home or skilled care
         3) Costs vary widely but depend largely on geographic location and nature of services needed.
      b. Independent living
         1) Senior living apartment
         2) Private home
         3) Apartment within a long-term care facility
      c. Assisted living
         1) Freestanding facilities
         2) Within a long-term care facility
         3) Group or foster homes
         4) Other community-based homes
         5) Adult day care services (for daytime only, not 24-hour supervision)
      d. Home health care
         1) Services vary according to the agency.
         2) Many agencies provide companion services that include light housekeeping and meal preparation or assistance with ADLs.
         3) If additional in-home therapy or nursing services are needed, investigate the exact nature of services that each agency will render and how expenses are billed.
   2. Assist clients and families with postrehabilitation placement
      a. Address cultural influences.
      b. Realize that people with some cultural backgrounds consider placement in a nursing home to be unacceptable and that other resources must be explored.
      c. Explore cultural norms and influences with the family and client.
   3. Help to select a facility
      a. Know the options available in the community.
      b. Obtain information through industry organizations such as the American Health Care Association.
      c. Access facilities' survey histories from the Centers for Medicare & Medicaid Services (formerly the Health Care Financing Administration) or from state health departments.
   4. Assist family members with placement decisions. Use appropriate resources such as social services to assist with placement, transfers, and finances.
      a. Provide the family with viable options and lists of community resources.
      b. Use mutual goal-setting techniques.
      c. Consult with the client's case manager or social worker for specific information on area facilities.
      d. Refer the family to information checklists available in the facility or through agencies such as the AARP or the United Way.

H. Funding: Public programs for long-term care needs.
 1. See Chapter 21 for a discussion of funding and insurance.
 2. Medicare Parts A and B (Beam & O'Hare, 2003)
    a. A social insurance program for people age 65 and older and certain younger people with disabilities and people of all ages with end-stage renal disease (www.longtermcare.gov/LTC/Main_Site/Paying_LTC/Public_Programs/Public_Programs.aspx)
    b. Part A
       1) Hospital insurance
       2) Funds hospital care, skilled nursing facility, hospice, and home health care, including mental healthcare (http://Medicare.gov)
    c. Part B
       1) Medical insurance
       2) Fees for physicians, surgeons, other healthcare providers
       3) Medical equipment rental
       4) Medical procedures, labs, diagnostics, X rays, radiation, certain screenings
       5) Monthly premium is paid; usually covers 80% of the Medicare-approved amount
    d. Medicare does not provide for custodial care unless skilled nursing or rehabilitation is also needed.
 3. Medicare Part D (Medicare.gov, 2006)
    a. Available to anyone with Medicare
    b. Income does not matter
    c. A prescription drug plan through the federal government
    d. Private companies issue plans through Medicare.
    e. Many different plans in each state
    f. Many different categories from which plans must offer at least two prescription drugs in each category, but plans do not cover all drugs
    g. Nurses can educate older adults to choose the best plan for them.
    h. A monthly premium is paid for the drug plan.
    i. Most plans have an annual deductible before Medicare pays.
    j. Costs to the person range from paying 100% out of pocket for those with low annual drug costs to 5% for those with high costs (e.g., more than $5,100, although this varies by plan).
    k. Financial assistance is available for those with low income; this is called "extra help."
    l. There is no cost containment for these drugs.
 4. Medicare Part C (Medicare.gov, 2010)
 5. Medicare Advantage Plan, purchased by individuals to get Medicare benefits through private companies or groups approved by Medicare; also includes prescription drug coverage
 6. Medicaid (Beam & O'Hare, 2003). Medicaid laws change frequently, so these are general guidelines.
    a. State-run program
    b. Largest source of medical care payments for low-income people
    c. Largest payer for nursing home services
    d. About 30 states offer optional personal care services for people to remain in the home.
    e. Individual income must be lower than a designated dollar amount to qualify.
    f. Applicants must pass an asset limitation test (i.e., assets must be spent down).
    g. State may adopt a medically needy program, which may include children younger than 18; pregnant women; or people who are elderly, blind, or disabled.
 7. Veteran's benefits (Beam & O'Hare, 2003)
    a. A potential source of long-term care benefits from a government source
    b. Veterans who satisfy a means test that looks at income and assets may be eligible.
    c. Care is generally provided in Veterans Administration facilities.
    d. Basic health benefits of the Veterans Administration
       1) Prevention and screenings
       2) Primary health care
       3) Diagnosis and treatment
       4) Surgery
       5) Mental health and substance abuse treatment
       6) Urgent care
       7) Medications
       8) Hospice and palliative care
       9) Limited other services such as certain nursing homes and adult day care in some programs
 8. Older Americans Act: The Older Americans Act is a federal program designed to organize, coordinate, and provide home- and community-based services to older adults and their families to help clients remain in the community as independently as possible.
 9. Long-term care insurance
    a. For cost coverage outside a hospital
    b. May cover any or all of the following services (Beam & O'Hare, 2003):

1) Nursing home
2) Assisted living
3) Hospice
4) Home health
5) Adult day care
6) Respite
7) Caregiver training
8) Home health coordinators

  c. Premiums (at age 65) range from $1,000 to $2,650 per year.

  d. Premiums increase with age.

  e. Benefits include peace of mind, more choices, and preservation of assets (Mauk & Mauk, 2010).

  f. Nurses should always ask whether clients have this type of coverage.

VII. Role of the Advanced Practice Nurse (APN)

A. Clinician

1. According to the American Nurses Credentialing Center (ANCC; ANCC, 2005), gerontological clinical nurse specialists

  a. Provide, direct, and influence care of older adults and their families.

  b. Work in a variety of settings.

  c. Have in-depth knowledge of aging.

  d. Have intervention skills focused on health promotion and management of health alterations.

  e. Provide comprehensive gerontological services.

  f. Engage in practice, research, theory use, collaboration, consultation, and administration.

  g. Certification through the ANCC (2010a) earns the clinical nurse specialist in gerontology (GCNS-BC) credential.

2. Gerontological nurse practitioners (ANCC, 2005)

  a. Are experts in healthcare provision to older adults

  b. Work in a variety of settings, particularly primary care

  c. Practice independently and collaboratively with other healthcare professionals.

  d. Maximize clients' functional abilities

  e. Promote, maintain, and restore health

  f. Prevent or minimize disabilities

  g. Promote death with dignity

  h. Engage in case management, education, consultation, research, administration, and advocacy for older adults

  i. Certification through the ANCC (2010b) earns the gerontological nurse practitioner (GNP-BC) credential.

B. Educator: The APN in the educator role may work in a variety of settings related to gerontological rehabilitation nursing.

1. Settings

  a. Rehabilitation unit in acute care hospital

  b. Freestanding rehabilitation facility

  c. Primary care practice in collaboration with physicians

  d. Outpatient clinic

  e. Academic setting or joint appointment collaborative agreement

  f. Private practice as consultant or seminar leader

2. Target audience

  a. Clients and families

  b. Interdisciplinary staff

  c. Physicians or other APNs

  d. Rehabilitation nurses

    1) Locally

    2) Regionally or nationally as an educational consultant

  e. Nursing students or other students in an academic setting

C. Leader

1. As a leader, the gerontological rehabilitation nurse may be involved in a variety of organizations relating to both specialties or in organizations dedicated to the advancement of the nursing profession through research.

  a. Association of Rehabilitation Nurses

  b. American Gerontological Society (interdisciplinary)

  c. The Gerontological Society of America

  d. Association for Geriatrics in Higher Education (interdisciplinary)

  e. National Gerontological Nursing Association

  f. John A. Hartford Institute for Geriatric Nursing (devoted to education of nurses in excellent care of older adults)

  g. Sigma Theta Tau International (international nursing honor society)

2. As a leader, the gerontological rehabilitation nurse in an advanced practice role may engage in the following activities:

  a. Membership in interdisciplinary care teams

  b. Developing standards of care for the specialty and professions

  c. Developing clinical guidelines

  d. Writing and advocating for certain healthcare policies

  e. Educating and mentoring colleagues in gerontological rehabilitation nursing

f. Participating in research related to gerontological rehabilitation
g. Membership in professional organizations
D. Consultant
1. Legal
a. Expert opinion
b. Expert testimony or expert witness
c. Types of cases commonly include the following:
1) Elder abuse or neglect
2) Wrongful death
3) Malpractice
4) Other cases related to practice below the appropriate standard of care
d. Employment as a regular part of a law office
e. Life care planning (Mauk & Mauk, 2010)
2. Educational
a. Through rehabilitation facilities, giving presentations in various locations
b. Self-employed
c. Working for others to develop online courses for continuing education, academic credit, or instructional materials for purchase
3. Clinical
a. May be combined with other types of consulting, including legal and educational
b. The expert clinician may be highly sought after as an educator in a variety of settings.
c. May develop subspecialty in other areas such as wound care or incontinence related to older adults with disabilities
4. Other (Mauk & Mauk, 2010)
a. Life care planning
b. Advocacy
c. Guardianship
E. Researcher (with example of evidence-based practice [EBP] related to APNs in palliative care)
1. EBP related to APNs in palliative care or hospice
a. Current trends suggest that APNs may play a significant role in the delivery of palliative care services to people at the end of life.
b. Educational programs for APNs should incorporate components of palliative and hospice care.
c. APNs caring for the dying client and his or her family should have a broad knowledge base related to the dying process and strategies to provide comfort to clients and families.
2. Clinical question: What is the role of APNs in care of clients receiving palliative care at end of life?

3. Appraisal of evidence
a. One level 1 article with good evidence (Skilbeck & Payne, 2003)
b. National guidelines: Level 1 with good evidence (*Clinical Practice Guidelines for Quality Palliative Care,* 2004). Although the practice guidelines are not specific to APNs, there is a strong recommendation to have an interdisciplinary team of advanced clinicians.
c. One level 4 article with good evidence (Froggatt & Hoult, 2002)
d. Two level 6 articles with good evidence (Volker, Kahn, & Penticuff, 2004a, 2004b)
e. Three level 7 sources in textbooks and article with good evidence (Ferrell & Coyle, 2001; Matzo & Sherman, 2001; Pitorak, 2003)
4. Recommendation for best rehabilitation nursing practice
a. The evidence generally demonstrates good support for APNs to play a significant role in palliative care at the end of life.
b. The evidence suggests that there are educational and direct care deficits in some settings for palliative or end-of-life care, including residential care and nursing homes, that can be directly addressed through APN interventions.
c. APNs can be instrumental in establishing links to health systems and resources.
d. APNs can provide a unique level of emotional support to clients and families through their expertise and effective communication skills.
e. APNs use advanced clinical skills to assess dying clients, provide comfort, and communicate essential information to the family.
f. More research is needed to explore strategies used by APNs to provide high-quality care to those at the end of life.
5. As researcher, the APN may also participate in the following activities:
a. Clinical expert on an interdisciplinary team
b. Link to clinical setting for collaborative research with academics
c. Advocate for using evidence-based practice in long-term care and rehabilitation facilities
d. Those prepared at the doctoral level
1) Design and conduct original research
2) Contribute to the development of nursing theory in gerontological rehabilitation
3) Obtain funding for research in the field
4) Publish findings to be used by others
5) Disseminate findings through presentations at conferences

References

Agahi, N., Ahacic, K., & Parker, M. S. (2006). Continuity of leisure participation from middle age to old age. *The Journal of Gerontology, 61B*(6), S340–S346.

Aging with Dignity. (2011). *Five wishes.* Retrieved August 18, 2011, from www.agingwithdignity.org/five-wishes.php.

American Heart Association. (2004). *Statistical fact sheet: Populations.* Retrieved November 3, 2006, from www.americanheart.org/downloadable/heart/1136584495498OlderAm06.pdf.

American Heart Association/American Stroke Association. (2006). *Heart disease and stroke: 2006 update.* Dallas, TX: American Heart Association.

American Nurses Credentialing Center. (2005). *Gerontological nurse: Application for ANCC.* Retrieved November 11, 2006, from www.nursingworld.org/ancc.

American Nurses Credentialing Center. (2010a). *Clinical nurse specialist in gerontology.* Retrieved August 18, 2011, from www.nursecredentialing.org/NurseSpecialties/GerontologicalCNS.aspx.

American Nurses Credentialing Center. (2010b). *Gerontological nurse practitioner.* Retrieved August 18, 2011, from www.nursecredentialing.org/NurseSpecialties/GerontologicalNP.aspx.

American Society of Consultant Pharmacists. (2000). Senior care pharmacy: The statistics. *Consultant Pharmacist, 15,* 310.

Anxiety Disorders Association of America. (2006). *Anxiety in the elderly.* Retrieved November 9, 2006, from www.adaa.org/GettingHelp/AnxietyDisorders/Elderly.asp.

Aptaker, R. L., Roth, E. J., Reichhardt, G., Duerden, M. E., & Levy, C. E. (1994). Serum albumin level as a predictor of geriatric stroke rehabilitation outcome. *Archives of Physical Medicine and Rehabilitation, 75*(1), 80–84.

Asplund, R. (2004). Nocturia, nocturnal polyuria, and sleep quality in the elderly. *Journal of Psychosomatic Research, 56*(5), 511–525.

Awad, N., Gagnon, M., & Messier, C. (2004). The relationship between impaired glucose tolerance, Type 2 diabetes and cognitive function. *Journal of Clinical and Experimental Neuropsychology, 8,* 1044–1080.

Bagg, S., Pombo, A. P., & Hopman, W. (2002). Effect of age on functional outcomes after stroke rehabilitation. *Stroke, 33,* 179–185.

Baltes, P. B. (1987). Theoretical propositions of life-span developmental psychology: On the dynamics between growth and decline. *Developmental Psychology, 23,* 611–626.

Baltes, P. B., & Baltes, M. M. (1990). Psychological perspectives on successful aging: The model of selective optimization with compensation. In P. B. Baltes & M. M. Baltes (Eds.), *Successful aging: Perspectives from the behavioral sciences* (pp. 1–34). New York: Cambridge University Press.

Bandeen-Roche, K., Xue, Q.-L., Ferrucci, L., Walston, J., Guralnik, J. M., Chaves, P., et al. (2006). Phenotype of frailty: Characterization in the Women's Health and Aging Studies. *Journals of Gerontology Series A: Biological Sciences and Medical Sciences, 61,* 262–266.

Beam, B. T., & O'Hare, T. P. (2003). *Meeting the financial need of long-term care.* Bryn Mawr, PA: The American College.

Beaupre, L. A., Cinats, J. G., Senthilselvan, A., Scharfenberger, A., Johnston, D. W., & Saunders, L. D. (2005). Does standardized rehabilitation and discharge planning improve functional recovery in elderly patients with hip fracture? *Archives of Physical Medicine and Rehabilitation, 86,* 2231–2239.

Beers, M., & Berkow, R. (Eds.). (n.d.). *The Merck manual of geriatrics* (Internet ed.), Merck & Company, Inc. and Medical Services USMEDSA, USHH. Retrieved January 20, 2005, from www.merck.com/mrkshared/mm_geriatrics/home.jsp.

Brager, R., & Sloand, E. (2005). The spectrum of polypharmacy. *Nurse Practitioner, 30,* 44–50.

Brei, T., & Merkens, M. (2003). *Challenging issues in care for adolescence and adults living with spina bifida.* Retrieved June 5, 2010, from www.spinabifidasupport.com/adultsbhealthcare.htm.

Brenner, L. A., Homaifar, B. Y., & Schultheis, M. (2008). Driving, aging and traumatic brain injury: Integrating findings from the literature. *Rehabilitation Psychology, 53*(1), 18–27.

Brown, R., Taylor, J., & Matthews, B. (2001). Quality of life: Ageing and Down syndrome. *Down Syndrome Research and Practices, 6*(3), 111–116.

Bruno, R. L., Cohen, J. M., Galski, T., & Frick, N. M. (n.d.). *The neuroanatomy of post-polio fatigue.* Retrieved October 28, 2006, from www.ott.zynet.co.uk/polio/lincolnshire/library.html.

Buhler, C. (1933). *Der menschliche Lebenslauf als psychologisches Problem* [Human life as a psychological problem]. Oxford, England: Hirzel.

Butcher, H. K., & McGonigal-Kenney, M. (2005). Depression and dispiritedness in later life. *American Journal of Nursing, 105*(12), 52–61.

Byock, I. (1997). *Dying well.* New York: Free Press.

Centers for Disease Control and Prevention. (2003). Public health and aging: Non-fatal fall-related traumatic brain injury among older adults: California 1996–1999. *MMWR Weekly, 52,* 276–278.

Centers for Disease Control and Prevention. (2006a). *Falls and hip fractures among older adults.* Retrieved November 3, 2006, from www.cdc.gov/ncipc/factsheets/falls.htm.

Centers for Disease Control and Prevention. (2006b). MMWR quick guide. Recommended adult immunization schedule: United States—October 2006–September 2007. *MMWR, 55*(40), 1–4.

Centers for Disease Control and Prevention. (2009). *Caregiving resources.* Retrieved August 18, 2011, from www.cdc.gov/aging/caregiving/resources.htm.

Centers for Disease Control and Prevention. (2011). *National diabetes fact sheet, 2011.* Retrieved August 18, 2011, from www.cdc.gov/diabetes/pubs/pdf/ndfs_2011.pdf.

Charles, C. V., & Lehman, C. A. (2006). Medications and laboratory values. In K. Mauk (Ed.), *Gerontological nursing: Competencies for care* (pp. 293–320). Sudbury, MA: Jones & Bartlett.

Chen, H. (2006). *Down syndrome.* Retrieved November 6, 2006, from www.emedicine.com/ped/topic615.htm.

Clinical practice guidelines for quality palliative care. (2004). Brooklyn, NY: National Consensus Project for Quality Palliative Care.

Colantonio, A., Ratcliff, G., Chase, S., & Vernich, L. (2004). Aging with traumatic brain injury: Long-term health conditions. *International Journal of Rehabilitation Research, 27*(3), 209–214.

Cowley, J. B., Diebold, C. M., Gross, J. C., & Hardin-Fanning, F. (2006). Management of common problems. In K. L. Mauk (Ed.), *Gerontological nursing: Competencies for care* (pp. 475–560). Sudbury, MA: Jones & Barlett.

Cumming, E., & Henry, W. (1961). *Growing old.* New York: Basic Books.

DeCalmer, P., & Glendenning, F. (Eds.). (1993). *The mistreatment of the elderly people.* London: Sage.

DeVivo, M. J. (2004). Aging with a neurodisability: Morbidity and life expectancy issues. *NeuroRehabilitation, 19,* 1–2.

Diebold, C., Hardin-Fanning, F., & Hanson, P. (2010). Management of common problems. In K. Mauk (Ed.), *Gerontological nursing: Competencies for care* (pp. 454–528). Sudbury, MA: Jones & Bartlett.

Digiovanna, A. G. (2000). *Human aging: Biological perspectives* (3rd ed.). Boston: McGraw-Hill.

DiMaria-Ghalili, R. A. (2008). *Nursing standard of practice protocol: Nutrition in aging.* Retrieved August 18, 2011, from http://consultgerirn.org/topics/nutrition_in_the_elderly/want_to_know_more.

Dowling-Castronovo, A., & Bradway, C. (2008). *Nursing standard of practice protocol: Urinary incontinence (UI) in older adults admitted to acute care.* Retrieved August 18, 2011, from http://consultgerirn.org/topics/urinary_incontinence/want_to_know_more.

Duppils, G., & Wikblad, K. (2004). Cognitive function and health related quality of life after delirium. *Orthopedic Nursing, 23,* 195–203.

Easton, K. L. (1999). *Gerontological rehabilitation nursing.* Philadelphia: W. B. Saunders.

Ellenbecker, C. H., Frazier, S. C., & Verney, S. (2004). Nurses' observations and experiences of problems and adverse effects of medication management in home care. *Geriatric Nursing, 25*(3), 164–170.

End of Life Nursing Education Consortium. (2004). *ELNEC curriculum.* Princeton, NJ: Robert Woods Johnson Foundation and City of Hope.

Farrell, V. M., Hill, V. L., Hawkins, J. B., Newman, L. M., & Learned Jr., R. E. (2003). Clinic for identifying and addressing polypharmacy. *American Journal of Health-System Pharmacy, 60*(18), 1834–1835.

Ferrari, A., Radaelli, A., & Centola, M. (2003). Invited review: Aging and the cardiovascular system. *Journal of Applied Physiology, 95*(6), 2591–2597.

Ferrell, B. R., & Coyle, N. (2001). *Textbook of palliative nursing.* New York: Oxford University Press.

Finlayson, M., Van Denend, T., & Hudson, E. (2004). Aging with multiple sclerosis. *Journal of Neuroscience Nursing, 26,* 245–248.

Fried, L. P., Ferrucci, L., Darer, J., Williamson, J. D., & Anderson, G. (2004). Untangling the concepts of disability, frailty, and comorbidity: Implications for improved targeting and care. *Journals of Gerontology. Series A, Biological Sciences and Medical Sciences, 59A,* 255–263.

Froggatt, K. A., & Hoult, L. (2002). Developing palliative care practice in nursing and residential care homes: The role of the clinical nurse specialist. *Journal of Clinical Nursing, 11,* 802–808.

Gray-Micelli, D. (2008). *Falls: Nursing standard of practice protocol: Fall prevention.* Retrieved August 18, 2011, from http://consultgerirn.org/topics/falls/want_to_know_more.

Greenberg, S. (2009). *A profile of older Americans: 2009.* Washington, DC: Administration on Aging, U.S. Department of Health and Human Services.

Hafez, B., & Hafez, E. (2004). Andropause: Endocrinology, erectile dysfunction, and prostate pathophysiology. *Archives of Andrology, 50,* 45–68.

Hall, J. (2004). Neuroendocrine physiology of the early and late menopause. *Endocrinology and Metabolism Clinics of North America, 33*(4), 637–659.

Hall, J. (2007). Neuroendocrine changes with reproductive aging in women. *Seminars in Reproductive Medicine, 25,* 344–356.

Harlow, R. E., & Cantor, N. (1996). Still participating after all these years: A study of life task participation in later life. Journal of Personality and Social Psychology, 71, 1235–1249.

Havighurst, R. J., Neugarten, B. L., & Tobin, S. S. (1963). Disengagement, personality and life satisfaction in the later years. In P. Hansen (Ed.), *Age with a future* (pp. 419–425). Copenhagen, Denmark: Munksgaard.

Havighurst, R. J., Neugarten, B. L., & Tobin, S. S. (1968). Disengagement and patterns of aging. In B. L. Neugarten (Ed.), *Middle age and aging* (pp. 67–71). Chicago: University Press.

Heineman, J. M., Hamrick-King, J., & Scaglione Sewell, B. (2010). Review of the aging of physiological systems. In K. Mauk (Ed.), *Gerontological nursing: Competencies for care* (pp. 128–231). Sudbury, MA: Jones & Bartlett.

Hershkovitz, A., Kalandariov, Z., Hermush, V., Weiss, R., & Brill, S. (2007). Factors affecting short-term rehabilitation outcomes of disabled elderly patients with proximal hip fracture. *Archives of Physical Medicine and Rehabilitation, 88*(7), 916–921.

Holland, T., & Benton, M. (2004). *Ageing and its consequences for people with Down's syndrome: A guide for parents and carers.* Retrieved November 6, 2006, from http://www.downs-syndrome.org.uk/component/content/article/28-medical-and-health/250-ageing-and-its-consequences-for-people-with-downs-syndrome.html.

Inouye, S. K. (2006). Delirium in older persons. *New England Journal of Medicine, 354,* 1157–1165.

Inouye, S. K., Foreman, M. D., Mion, L. C., Katz, K. H., & Cooney, L. M. (2001). Nurses' recognition of delirium and its symptoms: Comparison of nurse and researcher ratings. *Archives of Internal Medicine, 161*(20), 2467–2473.

Institute of Medicine. (2000). Overview: Nutritional health in the older person. In *The role of nutrition in maintaining health in the nation's elderly: Evaluating coverage of nutrition services for the Medicare population.* Retrieved November 6, 2006, from http://fermat.nap.edu/books/0309068460/html/46.html.

Ivey, F., Tracy, B., Lemmer, J., NessAiver, M., Metter, E., Fozard, J., et al. (2000). Effects of strength training and detraining on muscle quality: Age and gender comparisons. *Journals of Gerontology: Biological Sciences, 55A*(3), B152–B157.

Jackson, G., & Owsley, C. (2003). Visual dysfunction, neurodegenerative diseases, and aging. *Neurology Clinics of North America, 21,* 709–728.

Jung, C. G. (1960). *The structure and dynamics of the psyche. Collected works* (Vol. VIII). Oxford, England: Pantheon.

Kailes, J. I. (2002). *Aging with disability.* Retrieved November 7, 2006, from www.jik.com/awdrtcawd.html.

Kart, G. S., & Kinney, J. M. (2001). *The realities of aging.* Boston: Allyn & Bacon.

Kemp, B. J., & Mosqueda, L. (2004). Introduction. In *Aging with a disability: What the clinician needs to know.* Baltimore: Johns Hopkins University Press.

Klingbiel, H., Baer, H. R., & Wilson, P. E. (2004). Aging with a disability. *Archives of Physical Medicine and Rehabilitation, 85*(93), S68–S73.

Krauss Whitbourne, S. (2002). *The aging individual: Physical and psychological perspectives* (2nd ed.). New York: Springer.

THE SPECIALTY PRACTICE OF REHABILITATION NURSING

Kresevic, D. M. (2008). *Function: Nursing standard of practice protocol: Assessment of function in acute care.* Retrieved August 18, 2011, from http://consultgerirn.org/topics/function/want_to_know_more.

Krieger-Blake, L. S. (2006). Changes that affect independence in later life. In K. Mauk (Ed.), *Gerontological nursing: Competencies for care* (pp. 321–354). Sudbury, MA: Jones & Bartlett.

Krieger-Blake, L. S., & Warring, P. (2010). End of life care. In K. Mauk (Ed.), *Gerontological nursing: Competencies for care* (pp. 746–781). Sudbury, MA: Jones & Bartlett.

Kurlowicz, L. H., & Harvath, T. A. (2008). *Nursing standard of practice protocol: Depression.* Retrieved August 18, 2011, from http://consultgerirn.org/topics/depression/want_to_know_more.

Lange, J., & Grossman, S. (2010). Theories of aging. In K. L. Mauk (Ed.), *Gerontological nursing: Competencies for care* (pp. 50–73). Sudbury, MA: Jones & Bartlett.

Lau, D. T., & Kirby, J. B. (2009). The relation between living arrangement and preventive care among community dwelling elderly person. *American Journal of Public Health, 99*(7), 1315–1321.

LeBlanc, J., de Guise, E., Gosselin, N., & Feyz, M. (2006). Comparison of functional outcome following acute care in young, middle-aged and elderly patients with traumatic brain injury. *Brain Injury, 20*(8), 779–790.

Lemon, B. W., Bengston, V. L., & Peterson, J. A. (1972). An exploration of the activity theory of aging: Activity types and life satisfaction among in-movers to a retirement community. *Journal of Gerontology, 27,* 511–523.

Mahon, M. M. (2010). Advance care decision making: Asking the right people the right question. *Journal of Psychosocial Nursing, 48,* 7.

Marrone, R. (1997). *Death, mourning & caring.* Philadelphia: Wadsworth.

Maslow, A. H. (1954). *Motivation and personality.* New York: Harper & Row.

Mast, B. T., MacNeill, S. E., & Lichtenberg, P. A. (1999). Geropsychological problems in medical rehabilitation: Dementia and depression among stroke and lower extremity fracture patients. *Journals of Gerontology: Biological Sciences and Medical Sciences, 54,* M607–M612.

Matzo, M. L., & Sherman, D. W. (2001). *Palliative care nursing: Quality care to the end of life.* New York: Springer.

Mauk, J. M., & Mauk, K. L. (2010). Future trends in gerontological nursing. In K. Mauk (Ed.), *Gerontological nursing: Competencies for care* (pp. 782–795). Sudbury, MA: Jones & Bartlett.

Mauk, K. L., & Hanson, P. (2010). Management of common illnesses, diseases, and health conditions. In K. L. Mauk (Ed.), *Gerontological nursing: Competencie for care* (pp. 382–453). Sudbury, MA: Jones & Bartlett.

McCullagh, E., Brigstocke, G., Donaldson, N., & Kalra, L. (2005). Determinants of caregiving burden and quality of life in caregivers of stroke patients. *Stroke, 36,* 2181. Retrieved August 18, 2011, from http://stroke.ahajournals.org/cgi/content/abstract/strokeaha;36/10/2181.

McKinnis, E. A. (2002). Dyspnea and other respiratory symptoms. In B. M. Kingbrunner, J .J. Weinreb, & J. S. Pliczer (Eds.), *Twenty common problems in end-of-life care* (pp. 147–162). New York: McGraw-Hill.

Medicare.gov. (2006). *Medicare prescription drug coverage.* Retrieved November 7, 2006, from www.medicare.gov/publications/pub/pdf/11109.pdf.

Medicare.gov. (2010). *Mediare Advantage (Part C).* Retrieved August 18, 2011, from www.medicare.gov/navigation/medicare-basics/medicare-benefits/part-c.aspx.

Mendes De Leon, C. F., Gold, D. T., Glass, T. A., Kaplan, L., & George, L. K. (2001). Disability as a function of social networks and support in elderly African Americans and whites. *Journals of Gerontology: Psychological Sciences and Social Sciences, 56,* S179–S190.

Menter, R. (1998). *Aging with spinal cord injury.* Retrieved November 7, 2006, from www.thecni.org/reviews/09-1-p16-menter.htm.

Menzel, J. C. (2008). Depression in the elderly after traumatic brain injury: A systematic review. *Brain Injury, 22*(5), 375–380.

Merck Manuals Online Medical Library. (2003). *Aging body.* Retrieved November 6, 2006, from www.merckmanuals.com/home/sec26/ch327/ch327a.html.

Meyer, C. (2001). *Allow natural death: An alternative to DNR?* Retrieved November 4, 2005, from www.hospicepatients.org/and.html.

Minaker, K. (2004). Common clinical sequelae of aging. In L. Goldman & D. Ausiello (Eds.), *Cecil textbook of medicine* (22nd ed., pp. 105–111).Philadelphia: W. B. Saunders.

Miyamoto, Y., Tachimori, H., & Ito, H. (2010). Formal caregiver burden in dementia: Impact of behavior and psychological symptoms of dementia and activities of daily living. *Geriatric Nursing, 31*(4), 246–253.

Muché, J. A., & McCarty, S. (2009). *Geriatric rehabilitation.* Retrieved August 2, 2010, from http://emedicine.medscape.com/article/318521-overview.

Muñiz, F. M. (2011). *Postpolio syndrome.* Retrieved August 18, 2011, from http://emedicine.medscape.com/article/306920-overview#showall.

National Center on Elder Abuse. (2006). *Elder abuse prevalence and incidence. Fact sheet.* Washington, DC: Author.

National Hospice and Palliative Care Organization. (2004). *Keys to quality care.* Retrieved November 4, 2005, from http://nhpco.org/i4a/pages/index.cfm?pageid=3303.

National Institute of Mental Health. (2006). *Depression and suicide facts.* Retrieved November 9, 2006, from www.nimh.nih.gov/publicat/elderlydepsuicide.cfm.

National Institute of Neurological Disorders and Stroke. (2006a). *Cerebral palsy: Hope through research.* Retrieved November 6, 2006, from www.ninds.nih.gov/disorders/cerebral_palsy/detail_cerebral_palsy.htm.

National Institute of Neurological Disorders and Stroke. (2006b). *Post-polio syndrome fact sheet.* Retrieved November 6, 2006, from www.ninds.nih.gov/disorders/post_polio/detail_post_polio.htm.

Nelson, J. M. (2006). Identifying and preventing common risk factors in the elderly. In K. Mauk (Ed.), *Gerontological nursing: Competencies for care* (pp. 357–388). Sudbury, MA: Jones & Bartlett.

Nilsson-Ehle, H., Jagenburg, R., Landahl, S., & Svanborg, A. (2000). Blood haemoglobin declines in the elderly: Implications for reference intervals from age 70 to 88. *European Journal of Haematology, 65*(5), 297–305.

Ostir, G. V., Ottenbacher, K. J., & Markides, K. S. (2004). Onset of frailty in older adults and the protective role of positive affect. *Psychology and Aging.* Retrieved August 7, 2010, from www.apa.org/pubs/journals/releases/pag-193402.pdf.

Ostwald, S., Wasserman, J., & Davis, S. (2006). Medications, co-morbidities and complications in stroke survivors: The CAReS study. *Rehabilitation Nursing, 31,* 10–14.

Pace, B., Burke, A. E., & Glass, R. M. (2006). JAMA patient page. Hospice Care. *JAMA, 295*(6), 712.

Patrick, L., Knoefel, F., Gaskowsk, P., & Rexrath, D. (2001). Medical comorbidity and rehabilitation efficiency in geriatric patients. *Journal of the American Geriatrics Society, 49,* 1471–1477.

Peters, A. (2002). The effects of normal aging on myelin and nerve fibers: A review. *Journal of Neurocytology, 31,* 581–593.

Pitorak, E. F. (2003). Care at the time of death. *American Journal of Nursing, 103*(7), 42–52.

Plahuta, J. M., & Hamrick-King, J. (2006). Review of the aging of physiological systems. In K. Mauk (Ed.), *Gerontological nursing: Competencies for care* (pp. 143–264). Sudbury, MA: Jones & Bartlett.

Pritchard, J. (1995). *The abuse of older people: A training manual for detection and prevention.* London: Jessica Kingsley Publishers.

Pritchard, J. (1996). Darkness visible: Elder abuse. *Nursing Times, 92*(42), 26–31.

Pugh, K., & Wei, J. (2001). Clinical implications of physiological changes in the aging heart. *Drugs & Aging, 18*(4), 263–276.

Rees, T., Duckert, L., & Carey, J. (1999). Auditory and vestibular dysfunction. In W. Hazzard, J. Blass, W. Ettinger Jr., J. Halter, & J. Ouslander (Eds.), *Principles of geriatric medicine and gerontology* (4th ed., pp. 617–632). New York: McGraw-Hill.

Rockwood, K., Mitniski, A., Song, X., Steen, B., & Skoog, I. (2006). Long-term risks of death and institutionalization of elderly people in relation to deficit accumulation at age 70. *Journal of the American Geriatrics Society, 54,* 975–979.

Roubenoff, R. (2001). Origins and clinical relevance of sarcopenia. *Canadian Journal of Applied Physiology, 26*(1), 78–89.

Schroots, J. J. F. (1996). Theoretical developments in the psychology of aging. *Gerontologist, 36,* 742–748.

Scivoletto, G., Morganti, B., Ditunno, P., Ditunno, J. F., & Molinari, M. (2003). Effects of age on spinal cord lesion patients' rehabilitation. *Spinal Cord, 41,* 457–464.

Segatore, M., & Adams, D. (2001). Managing delirium and agitation in elderly hospitalized orthopaedic patients: Part 1: Theoretical aspects. *Orthopaedic Nursing, 20,* 31–46.

Seiberling, K., & Conley, D. (2004). Aging and olfactory and taste function. *Otolaryngologic Clinics of North America, 37*(6), 1209–1228.

Sherrington, C., Whitney, J. C., Lord, S. R., Herbert, P. D., Cummings, R. E., & Close, J. C. (2008). Effective exercise for the prevention of falls: A systematic review and meta-analysis. *Journal of the American Geriatrics Society, 56*(12), 2234–2243.

Skilbeck, J., & Payne, S. (2003). Emotional support and the role of clinical nurse specialists in palliative care. *Journal of Advanced Nursing, 43*(5), 521–530.

Spalding, M. C., & Sebesta, S. C. (2008). Geriatric screening and preventive care. *American Family Physician, 78*(2), 206–215.

Strauss, D., Ojdana, K., Shavelle, R., & Rosenbloom, L. (2004). Decline in function and life expectancy of older persons with cerebral palsy. *Neurorehabilitation, 19,* 69–78.

Thompson, H. J., McCormick, W. C., & Kagan, S. H. (2006). Traumatic brain injury in older adults: Epidemiology, outcomes and future implications. *Journal of the American Geriatrics Society, 54,* 1590–1595.

Tinetti, M. E., Williams, C. S., & Gill, T. M. (2000). Dizziness among older adults: A possible geriatric syndrome. *Annals of Internal Medicine, 132,* 337–344.

Tornstam, L. (1994). Gerotranscendence: A theoretical and empirical exploration. In L. E. Thomas & S. A. Eisenhandler (Eds.), *Aging and the religious dimension* (pp. 203–226). Westport, CT: Greenwood.

Tullmann, D. F., Mion, L. C., Fletcher, K., & Foreman, M. D. (2008). *Delirium nursing standard of practice protocol: Delirium: Prevention, early recognition, and treatment.* Retrieved August 18, 2011, from http://consultgerirn.org/topics/delirium/want_to_know_more.

U.S. Department of Health and Human Services. (2006). *Caregiver stress.* Retrieved November 9, 2006, from www.womenshealth.gov/publications/our-publications/fact-sheet/caregiver-stress.cfm.

Vaillant, G. (2002). *Aging well.* Boston: Little, Brown.

Volker, D. L., Kahn, D., & Penticuff, J. H. (2004a). Patient control and end-of-life care. Part I: The advanced practice nurse perspective. *Oncology Nursing Forum, 31*(5), 945–953.

Volker, D. L., Kahn, D., & Penticuff, J. H. (2004b). Patient control and end-of-life care. Part II: The patient perspective. *Oncology Nursing Forum, 31*(5), 954–960.

Wadensten, B., & Carlsson, M. (2001). A qualitative study of nursing staff members' interpretations of signs of gerotranscendence. *Journal of Advanced Nursing, 36,* 635–642.

Warring, P. A., & Krieger-Blake, L. S. (2006). End-of-life care. In K. Mauk (Ed.), *Gerontological nursing: Competencies for care* (pp. 779–814). Sudbury, MA: Jones & Bartlett.

Winkler, T. (2008). *Spinal cord injury and aging.* Retrieved November 7, 2008, from www.emedicine.com/pmr/topic185.htm.

Witkos, M., Uttaburanont, M., Lang, C., & Haddad, R. (2009). Effects of anemia on rehabilitation outcomes in elderly patients in the post-acute care setting. *Topics in Geriatric Rehabilitation, 25*(3), 222–230.

World Health Organization. (1990). *Cancer pain relief and palliative care.* Geneva, Switzerland: Author.

Yu, F. (2005). Factors affecting outpatient rehabilitation outcomes in elders. *Journal of Nursing Scholarship, 27*(3), 229–236.

Zwicker, D., & Fulmer, T. (2008). *Medication. Nursing standard of practice protocol: Reducing adverse drug events.* Hartford Institute of Geriatric Nursing. Retrieved July 28, 2010, from http://consultgerirn.org/topics/medication/want_to_know_more#Wrap.

The Environment of Care

CHAPTER 20
The Environment for Rehabilitation Nursing

Pamala D. Larsen, PhD CRRN FNGNA

Scientific and technological advances, an aging population, quantity and quality of life, and cost-conscious healthcare systems have influenced the delivery of rehabilitation services, the environments in which rehabilitation services are provided, and the role of rehabilitation nurses. The delivery and outcomes of rehabilitation services warrant oversight by expert rehabilitation nurses who serve as client advocates in maximizing services without jeopardizing outcomes and client safety. Although inpatient rehabilitation settings remain the cornerstone of providing services, an increased recognition of the community as a setting for care is apparent. Within the community, the infrastructure must be present to meet optimal outcomes for the client. The family provides the nucleus of the community support structure for the client (Parker & Neal-Boylan, 2007). Understanding family dynamics and relationships and the ways in which these affect the care and outcomes of the client are critical in providing services.

This chapter describes rehabilitation environments and demonstrates the role of the rehabilitation nurse and the rehabilitation process in the delivery of services. Rehabilitation nursing is an integral component of care delivery. The role of the rehabilitation nurse is to ensure that basic and advanced rehabilitation techniques are used and that specialized rehabilitation care is provided in the appropriate setting based on the client's medical stability and tolerance for rehabilitation efforts.

I. **Settings and Nursing Roles Where Rehabilitation Occurs**
   A. Overview
      1. The inclusion of the family unit is critical for rehabilitation services to be delivered successfully. The family may consist of the biological family of the client, friends, and significant others. The definition of *family* is individualized to each client.
      2. Care in any setting should be provided using the principles of rehabilitation.
      3. Patient-centered care (PCC) provides a framework for rehabilitation care (Lutz & Davis, 2008).
         a. Care is designed based on the specific needs of the client.
         b. PCC is an "approach that adopts the perspective of their patients and their families, with careful consideration of what is important to each and how care is likely to affect them" (Lutz & Davis, 2008, p. 22).

   4. Whatever the setting, rehabilitation is a partnership between the client, family, and care team. Often this is a long-term relationship.
   5. Goals for care should be developed with the client and family.
   6. Pryor's work (2010) described rehabilitative milieu therapy as the various strategies rehabilitation nurses use to create an environment conducive to rehabilitation. Pryor's work used inpatient rehabilitation facilities to identify data supporting nursing's contribution to the rehabilitation process.
   B. Acute Care
      1. Clients in this setting need medical management.
      2. This setting may or may not provide care based on rehabilitation principles.
      3. Clients in an acute care setting cannot tolerate intensive rehabilitation.
      4. The role of the nurse includes client and family teaching and care focusing on preventing complications to promote the client's ability to participate in rehabilitation at a later time.
      5. Acute care units for elders (ACE units)
         a. Because the majority of rehabilitation involves older adults, understanding how this segment of the population is cared for (in preparation for rehabilitation) is important.
         b. The ACE model of care specifically addresses the needs of older adults in a safe, homelike physical environment; it is client and family centered, with discharge planning for the least restrictive environment, and staff have expertise in aging and interdisciplinary teamwork (Amador, Reed, & Lehman, 2007). These units are located in acute care hospitals.
         c. These units are not rehabilitation units, but they provide age-appropriate care for older adults with a possible end result of transitioning to a rehabilitation setting.
         d. These units are not regulated like skilled nursing facilities and rehabilitation facilities; they are regulated and paid for like other acute care hospital units (Amador et al., 2007).

C. Inpatient Rehabilitation Facilities (IRFs)
   1. Overview
      a. Rehabilitation services may be provided through age-specific specialization (geriatric rehabilitation versus pediatric rehabilitation) or by diagnosis (e.g., stroke units, traumatic brain injury units, spinal cord injury units; Lutz & Davis, 2008).
      b. Specialized units use standardized guidelines from the Commission on Accreditation of Rehabilitation Facilities (CARF) or model programs from the National Institute on Disability and Rehabilitation Research to treat clients and their families.
      c. Cost-containment measures nationwide have resulted in shorter lengths of client stays and lowered reimbursement rates, resulting in shifting of care to less costly venues such as home health care and subacute or transition units.
      d. Nelson and colleagues' study on nurse staffing and client outcomes in IRFs revealed how staffing patterns affect client outcomes in IRFs. One pertinent finding of the study was that more certified rehabilitation registered nurses on staff correlated with better client outcomes as measured by FIM™ scores (Nelson et al., 2007).
   2. Acute rehabilitation may be provided in a specialized unit within a hospital setting or in a free-standing rehabilitation facility.
   3. Intensive inpatient rehabilitation with 24-hour nursing care is provided to address a range of issues including medication management, comorbidities, behavior, and the rehabilitative needs of the client and family.
   4. Clients are admitted to these facilities with a specific diagnosis.
   5. Much of the care provided in these settings focuses on the rehabilitation of older adults (Association of Rehabilitation Nurses, 2008).
   6. Medicare rules state that the need for intensive IRF services can be demonstrated by the need for at least 3 hours of skilled rehabilitative therapy a day for at least 5 days a week (Gage et al., 2009). There is also an expectation that these intensive services will yield significant improvement.
   7. Inpatient rehabilitation programs provide "coordinated and integrated medical and rehabilitation service that is provided 24 hours per day and endorses the active participation and choice of the persons served throughout the entire program" (CARF, 2006).
   8. If only therapy is needed, this can be performed on an outpatient basis (Mauk, 2009).
   9. Documenting 24-hour rehabilitation nursing is critical, especially for IRFs that care for Medicare clients. Hentschke (2009) provides guidance on how facilities can better document this care.
   10. Roles of the rehabilitation nurse
      a. The *Standards and Scope of Rehabilitation Nursing Practice* (ARN, 2008) provides the basis of practice for the rehabilitation nurse regardless of setting.
         1) Preventing medical and functional complications and readmission
         2) Engaging clients in care within medically indicated restrictions and precautions
         3) Promoting independence by increasing self-care actions
         4) Delegating and supervising aspects of rehabilitative and restorative care provided by licensed vocational nurses, technicians, and unlicensed assistive personnel
         5) Providing client and family education to support self-care and transitioning to home if feasible.
         6) Providing age and developmentally appropriate care
      b. Because much of the care provided in IRFs is for older adults, the rehabilitation nurse must be educated in geriatric principles to appropriately care for these clients and their families.

D. Subacute Care
   1. Subacute care emerged during the 1980s and 1990s as a lower-cost option for rehabilitative care (Lutz & Davis, 2008) for people who were not ready for intensive, acute rehabilitation or needed additional time to transition to the community (Quigley, 2007).
   2. The definition of such care is inconsistent across the literature, and the Centers for Medicare & Medicaid Services (CMS) does not define *subacute* in their payment categories for rehabilitative services.
   3. Subacute care units admit clients who cannot tolerate 3 hours of therapy per day and who need skilled medical and nursing care but not diagnostic or invasive procedures (Lutz & Davis, 2008).
   4. A professional organization supporting subacute care, the National Association of Subacute/Post Acute Care, was founded in the 1990s. However, this organization ceased to exist in 2010.
   5. Some hospitals may have subacute units called transition units.

6. Data demonstrate that clients receiving care in subacute rehabilitation programs have measurable functional improvement and that a high percentage of clients are discharged to community-based settings (Deutsch, Fiedler, Iwanenko, Granger, & Russell, 2003).

E. Skilled Nursing Facilities (SNFs)

1. SNFs are long-term care facilities commonly called nursing homes. These facilities may or may not provide rehabilitative services. Clients (called residents in long-term care) may need rehabilitation nursing and client and family education. Typically these clients are medically stable and can participate in some rehabilitation as appropriate. In a systematic review examining 41 randomized clinical trials (30 in the United States and 11 in Western Europe) and more than 3,000 clients in long-term care (nursing homes), physical rehabilitation was potentially effective when activity restriction was assessed as the primary outcome (Forster, Lambley, & Young, 2010).

2. Provide skilled postacute rehabilitation services in addition to skilled nursing services (Gage et al., 2009).

3. The goal of care remains the same: optimal client wellness.

4. Clients need less physician oversight than IRF clients because they are typically less severely impaired.

5. SNFs vary in the acuity of clients they accept and generally provide a lower intensity of service (Gage et al., 2007). However, it is noted that some specialized SNFs provide intensive postacute treatment such as ventilator monitoring (Gage et al., 2009).

6. Deutsch and colleagues (2006) found that for most clients, rehabilitation in IRFs results in higher functional outcomes than SNF-based rehabilitation programs.

F. Long-Term Care Hospitals (LTCHs)

1. LTCHs are certified as acute care hospitals but focus on clients who, on average, stay more than 25 days. Extended medical and rehabilitative care is provided to people whose needs are clinically complex and who have multiple acute or chronic conditions (American Hospital Association, n.d.).

2. Clients are transferred to such facilities from intensive or critical care units. Services provided typically include comprehensive rehabilitation, respiratory therapy, head trauma treatment, and pain management (CMS, 2009). These facilities are commonly referred to as long-term acute care.

G. Community Settings

1. For cost-containment purposes, more rehabilitative care is taking place in the community.

2. Home health care may provide a variety of rehabilitative services. Neal (1998) developed a home health nursing practice model for nurses based on rehabilitation principles.

II. **Community-Based Rehabilitation (CBR)**

A. Overview

1. Typically one thinks of CBR as services offered in a local community that may include home healthcare services, physical therapy, vocational rehabilitation, and the like. The rehabilitation client's community is characterized in terms of the wider environment and geographic location and the availability of housing, transportation, healthcare providers, community buildings, and other resources (Boylan & Buchanan, 2008).

2. CBR is population based, with a community focus (Boylan & Buchanan, 2008).

3. CBR services in one community will look different from those in another community because of the resources and services available.

4. Community-based rehabilitation nursing combines the expertise of the rehabilitation nurse with the skills of a community health nurse. A nurse in this role may conduct home visits, act as a case manager, coordinate care across settings, provide client and family education, and promote health. The ultimate goal of care is optimal health for the client and family (however that is defined). In community-based care, clients manage their care and daily activities independently, with assistance, or with supervision.

B. Types of Community-Based Care

1. Day treatment care programs and adult day services provide supervised care and therapeutic activities. This is a structured, comprehensive nonresidential program providing a variety of health, social, and related support services in a protective setting. The environmental design considers the impairments and limitations of the people served, promotes improvement and maintenance of their sense of control and self-determination, and provides them with a safe environment (CARF, 2006).

2. Independent living centers and congregate living facilities offer independent living and opportunities to share activities of daily living with other residents. Congregate facilities include retirement and life-care communities.

a. Shared activities in a congregate living setting may include meals, transportation, housekeeping, planned activities and outings, and religious services.

b. Health monitoring may or may not be included in the setting.

3. Community reentry programs and assisted care living facilities provide coordinated, personalized 24-hour assistance and support (both scheduled and unscheduled) in a congregate residential setting. The choices, privacy, independence, and rights of the people served are protected and promoted as an essential part of assisted living's core values and mission (CARF, 2006). The type of provider may vary.

C. Roles of the Nurse in the Community

1. Direct care provider: As the client's level of independence increases, the physical provision of care by the nurse decreases.

2. Educator: The nurse provides education to both the client and family.

3. Care or case manager: The nurse coordinates client care across settings, interacts with various care providers, and ensures the client's treatment plan is carried out (see Chapter 5).

4. Advocate: The nurse advocates for the client and family.

D. A Broader View of CBR

1. CBR is an international concept originated by the World Health Organization (WHO) Disability and Rehabilitation Team, whose vision is that all people with disabilities live in dignity, with equal rights and opportunities.

2. The focus of CBR, developed in the 1980s, is to enhance "the quality of life for people with disabilities and their families, meeting basic needs, and ensuring inclusion and participation. CBR is a multisectoral approach and has five major components: health, education, livelihood, social, and employment. CBR is implemented in more than 90 countries" (WHO, 2010a).

3. In 2004 a joint venture between the International Labour Organization (ILO), United Nations Educational, Scientific and Cultural Organization (UNESCO), and WHO repositioned CBR as a strategy for rehabilitation, equalization of opportunity, poverty reduction, and social inclusion of people with disabilities (WHO, 2010b). The goals of CBR are to ensure that the benefits of the Convention on Rights of Persons with Disabilities reach the majority by

a. Supporting people with disabilities to maximize their physical and mental abilities, to access regular services and opportunities, and to become active contributors to the community and society at large

b. Activating communities to promote and protect the human rights of people with disabilities, for example, by removing barriers to participation

c. Facilitating capacity building, empowerment, and community mobilization of people with disabilities and their families

4. CBR is a strategy with general community development. It is implemented through the combined efforts of people with disabilities themselves, their families, organizations and communities, and the relevant governmental and non-governmental health, education, vocational, social, and other services (WHO, 2010b).

III. Community Reentry and Integration

A. Focus: Transition to the community through a gradual acquisition of community skills, self-care, leisure and vocational activities, and psychosocial integration

B. Community-Based Barriers

1. Societal barriers such as reimbursement issues, ineligibility for services, cultural or attitudinal prejudices, and social stigma

2. Internal barriers within the individual such as negative attitude, poor self-esteem, lack of motivation, poor self-image, feelings of dependence, insecurity, an inability to plan and meet goals, and unrealistic expectations

3. Transportation problems that affect the client's environment and reintegration efforts

4. Housing barriers such as lack of accessible housing

5. Financial barriers

C. Conceptual Model for Nurses Working in Community Reentry and Independent Living Programs (Parker & Neal-Boylan, 2007, pp. 20–21).

1. The client serves as manager of his or her life and care in a community-based or independent living setting. The nurse's role is one of an active participant to help the client by providing education, coordinating resources, and understanding how the community's needs and resources affect the client's health.

2. The client's lifestyle and needs are considered in terms of his or her environment. The nurse's role is to promote health and the ability to meet self-care needs and to facilitate communication and collaboration with other healthcare professionals.

3. Client and family education is an ongoing process.

a. Education is focused and goal directed.

b. As the client reintegrates into the community, the focus of education changes to enhance the client's problem-solving skills.

c. Preventive care is emphasized.

4. The management of attendant care training and services facilitates independent living.

5. Equipment and supplies should be evaluated before the client is discharged from the acute rehabilitation setting (the nurse coordinates the assessment and monitoring of equipment needed in the community).

6. The client's and family's financial resources must be assessed in terms of the present and future.

7. The nurse identifies barriers and options in the community with the client and family.

References

Amador, L. F., Reed, D., & Lehman, C. (2007). The acute care for elders unit: Taking the rehabilitation model into the hospital setting. *Rehabilitation Nursing, 32*(3), 126–132.

American Hospital Association. (n.d.). *Long term acute care hospitals*. Retrieved July 27, 2011, from www.aha.org/aha_app/issues/Medicare/Long-Term-Care-Hospitals.

Association of Rehabilitation Nurses. (2008). *Standards and scope of rehabilitation nursing practice*. Glenview, IL: Author.

Boylan, L. N., & Buchanan, L. C. (2008). Community-based rehabilitation. In S. Hoeman (Ed.), *Rehabilitation nursing: Prevention, intervention and outcomes* (4th ed., pp. 178–191). St. Louis: Mosby Elsevier.

Centers for Medicare & Medicaid Services. (2009). *What are long term care hospitals?* CMS Publication No. 11347. Retrieved August 1, 2010, from www.medicare.gov/publications/pubs/pdf/11347.pdf.

Commission on Accreditation of Rehabilitation Facilities. (2006). *2006 CARF accreditation sourcebook*. Retrieved May 12, 2007, from www.carf.org.

Deutsch, A., Fiedler, R. C., Iwanenko, W., Granger, C. V., & Russell, C. F. (2003). The Uniform Data System for Medical Rehabilitation report: Patients discharged from subacute rehabilitation programs in 1999. *American Journal of Physical Medicine and Rehabilitation, 82*(9), 703–711.

Deutsch, A., Granger, C. V., Heinemann, A. W., Fiedler, R., DeJong, G., Kane, R. L., et al. (2006). Poststroke rehabilitation: Outcomes and reimbursement of inpatient rehabilitation facilities and subacute rehabilitation programs. *Stroke, 36,* 1477–1482.

Forster, A., Lambley, R., & Young, J. B. (2010). Is physical rehabilitation for older people in long-term care effective? Findings from a systematic review. *Age and Ageing, 39,* 169–175.

Gage, B., Pilkauskasm, N., Dalton, K., Constantine, R., Leung, M., Hoover, S., et al. (2007). *Long term care hospital (LTCH) payment system monitoring and evaluation*. Phase II Report. Research Triangle Park, NC: RTI International.

Gage, B., Smith, L., Coots, L., Macek, J., Manning, J., & Reilly, K. (2009, September). *Analysis of the classification criteria for inpatient rehabilitation facilities (IRFs)*. Research Triangle Park, NC: RTI International.

Hentschke, P. (2009). 24-hour rehabilitation nursing: The proof is in the documentation. *Rehabilitation Nursing, 34*(3), 128–132.

Lutz, B., & Davis, S. M. (2008). Theory and practice models for rehabilitation nursing. In S. Hoeman (Ed.), *Rehabilitation nursing: Prevention, intervention and outcomes* (4th ed., pp. 14–29). St. Louis: Mosby Elsevier.

Mauk, K. (2009). Rehabilitation. In P. Larsen & I. Lubkin (Eds.), *Chronic illness: Impact and intervention* (7th ed., pp. 577–617). Sudbury, MA: Jones & Bartlett.

Neal, L. (Ed.). (1998). *Rehabilitation nursing in the home health setting*. Glenview, IL: Association of Rehabilitation Nurses.

Nelson, A., Powell-Cope, G., Palacios, P., Luther, S. L., Black, R., Hillman, T., et al. (2007). Nurse staffing and patient outcomes in inpatient rehabilitation setting. *Rehabilitation Nursing, 32*(5), 179–202.

Parker, B. J., & Neal-Boylan, L. (2007). Community and family-centered rehabilitation nursing. In K. L. Mauk (Ed.), *The specialty practice of rehabilitation nursing: A core curriculum* (5th ed., pp. 13–26). Glenview, IL: Association of Rehabilitation Nurses.

Pryor, J. (2010). Nurses create a rehabilitative milieu. *Rehabilitation Nursing, 35*(3), 123–129.

Quigley, P. A. (2007). Environment of care and service delivery. In K. L. Mauk (Ed.), *The specialty practice of rehabilitation nursing: A core curriculum* (5th ed., pp. 386–394). Glenview, IL: Association of Rehabilitation Nurses.

World Health Organization. (2010a). *Community-based rehabilitation (CBR)*. Retrieved August 10, 2010, from www.who.int/disabilities/cbr/en/index.html.

World Health Organization. (2010b). *Community-based rehabilitation (CBR): What WHO is doing*. Retrieved August 10, 2010, from www.who.int/disabilities/cbr/activities/en/.

CHAPTER 21

Healthcare Financing and Health Policy in Rehabilitation

Anne Deutsch, PhD RN CRRN

This chapter provides an overview of healthcare financing and health policy making. The American healthcare system, including the delivery of rehabilitation services, is financed largely through federal and state programs and private health insurance. Rising healthcare costs have shifted the reimbursement of healthcare services by insurance companies and government agencies from a fee-for-service model to managed care and prospective payment models with shared financial risks. In addition to healthcare costs, healthcare quality is a key health policy issue that includes the development of standardized quality measures for public reporting of quality information, quality improvement, and pay-for-performance activities.

The processes of developing and modifying health policy provide opportunities for rehabilitation nurses to share their expertise with local, state, and federal government agencies and legislators. Rehabilitation nurses' unique knowledge and understanding of the needs of people with disabilities position them to advocate for health policy changes. A rehabilitation nurse's involvement may include a range of activities such as educating the public about health issues (e.g., at schools or senior centers) or promoting letter-writing campaigns to garner support for a proposed bill.

I. Economics: Financing the Delivery of Healthcare Services in the United States (Table 21-1)
  A. Public Programs
    1. Medicare: The federal health insurance program for people who are elderly or disabled under the authority of the U.S. Department of Health and Human Services (DHHS); began with the enactment of Title XVIII of the Social Security Act of 1965. In 2010 Medicare provided health insurance coverage to 47 million people, of whom 39 million were age 65 or older and 8 million had permanent disabilities and were younger than 65 years. With federal spending estimated at $3.6 trillion in 2010, the Medicare program accounted for 12% of the federal budget and 23% of national health expenditures (Henry J. Kaiser Family Foundation, 2010b; Medicare Payment Advisory Commission, 2010).
      a. Administration: Managed by the Centers for Medicare & Medicaid Services (CMS), which designates Medicare administrative contractors to process claims (CMS, 2011)
      b. Coverage
        1) Original Medicare plan

a) Medicare Part A: A hospital insurance plan that covers inpatient services provided by hospitals, home healthcare agencies (skilled care only), hospice care, and short-term stays in skilled nursing facilities (SNFs); most beneficiaries do not pay a monthly premium for Part A services but are responsible for a deductible ($1,100 in 2010) and coinsurance for extended hospital stays ($275 per day for days 61–90 in 2010) or extended SNF stays ($137.50 per day for days 21–100 in 2010); it is financed through the Hospital Insurance Trust Fund by taxes paid by employers and their employees.
b) Medicare Part B: Supplementary medical insurance program that covers physician, outpatient, home health, and preventive services; financed through the Supplementary Medical Insurance Trust Fund by federal taxes and monthly premiums from beneficiaries (typically $110.50 in 2010)
c) Medicare Part D: Outpatient prescription drug coverage offered through private companies. Coverage varies depending on the plan chosen. It is financed through taxes, beneficiary premiums, and state payments for people with both Medicare and Medicaid coverage.
d) Medicare beneficiaries in the original plan may buy private Medicare supplemental insurance (i.e., Medigap) to cover the costs not covered (e.g., deductibles, coinsurance, vision, and dental services). In 2007, 11% of Medicare beneficiaries did not have supplemental insurance coverage through private insurance or Medicaid (Henry J. Kaiser Family Foundation, 2010b).

	Programs			
	Medicare (Federal)	**Medicaid (State)**	**Workers' Compensation**	**Private Health Insurance**
Eligibility Requirements	Must be older than 65 years, have end-stage renal disease, or have been disabled for 2 years	For people with low income	Workers injured in the course of employment	Policyholders
Benefits	Part A—Hospital Part B—supplemental medical insurance Part C—Medicare Advantage plans Part D—Prescription drug coverage	Hospital costs and visits to a physician	Medical care for a work-related injury Income support during periods of disability	Hospital costs and outpatient treatment, as specified in policy Physician visits, as specified in policy May or may not cover rehabilitation care

From *The specialty practice of rehabilitation nursing: A core curriculum* (3rd ed., p. 227), by A. E. McCourt (Ed.), 1993, Skokie, IL: Association of Rehabilitation Nurses. Copyright 1993.

2) Medicare Part C: This Medicare Advantage program allows beneficiaries to enroll in private health plans. Plans include preferred provider organizations (PPOs), provider-sponsored organizations, private fee-for-service plans, high-deductible plans linked to medical savings accounts, and special needs programs for people who are dually eligible for Medicare and Medicaid. This program provides hospital and physician coverage and often includes prescription drug coverage and is an alternative to Part A, Part B, and Part D coverage. The plans receive payments from Medicare to provide Medicare-covered benefits. It is not separately financed from Parts A, B, and D. Medicare Advantage enrollees generally pay the monthly Part B premium and often pay an additional premium directly to their plan (average was $56 per month in 2010).

c. Eligibility

1) People age 65 and older qualify for Medicare Part A if they or their spouses are eligible for Social Security payments and have made payroll tax contributions for 10 or more years (40 quarters) and if they are U.S. citizens or permanent residents. People age 65 and older who are not entitled to Part A, such as those who did not pay enough Medicare taxes during their working years, can pay a monthly premium to receive Part A benefits. People entitled to Part A and others age 65 and older may elect to enroll in Part B. People are eligible for Part C (Medicare Advantage) if

they are entitled to Part A and enrolled in Part B. People are eligible for Part D (prescription drug coverage) if they are entitled to Part A or enrolled in Part B. Medicare is a secondary payer if the person also has private health insurance.

2) People younger than age 65 with permanent disabilities are eligible for Medicare Part A after receiving Social Security Disability Income (SSDI) for 24 months. People with end-stage renal disease or Lou Gehrig's disease are eligible for Medicare Part A as soon as they begin receiving SSDI payments, without the 24-month waiting period. People entitled to Part A and others age 65 and older may elect to enroll in Part B. People are eligible for Part C (Medicare Advantage) if they are entitled to Part A and enrolled in Part B. People are eligible for Part D (prescription drug coverage) if they are entitled to Part A or enrolled in Part B.

2. Medicaid: The health insurance program for certain individuals and families with low income and resources; began with the enactment of Title XIX of the Social Security Act of 1965 to provide medical assistance to people and families receiving cash assistance (welfare). Medicaid has expanded to cover health and long-term care services for specific categories of low-income people and will expand further in 2014 to include the majority of people younger than 65 years with income up to 133% of the poverty level (Henry J. Kaiser Family Foundation, 2010a). In 2007 Medicaid covered 59.4 million people (CMS, 2010), and Medicaid

THE SPECIALTY PRACTICE OF REHABILITATION NURSING

spending was approximately $339 billion in 2008. The Affordable Care Act is expected to mean coverage for an additional 16 million people by 2014 with eligibility reform, simplified enrollment, improved access to care, and changes in financing (Henry J. Kaiser Family Foundation, 2010a).

a. Administration: Managed by each state through a state agency with oversight from CMS; financed by a federal-state partnership in which the federal government matches state Medicaid spending.

b. Coverage: Medicaid covers a wide range of health and long-term care services, but covered services vary by state. Medicaid managed care and non-managed care options are available. Some states require enrollment in a managed care plan. Covered services include long-term care, mental health care, and services and supports needed by people with disabilities. Medicaid covers comprehensive services for children. It assists low-income Medicare beneficiaries, known as "dual eligibles." Medicaid is the largest funding source for coverage of long-term care, covering approximately 70% of all nursing home residents (Henry J. Kaiser Family Foundation, 2010a). The federal government requires states to provide the following: inpatient and outpatient hospital, physician, laboratory, X-ray, prenatal, and preventive-care services; federally qualified health center and rural health clinic services; family planning services and supplies; pediatric and nurse practitioner services; nurse midwife services; nursing facility services for people older than 21 years; home health care for people eligible for nursing facility services; and medically necessary transportation. States can add services to this list and can place certain limitations on the federally mandated services. States can get federal waivers to operate their Medicaid programs outside federal guidelines.

c. Eligibility

1) Under current law, people qualify for Medicaid if they meet the financial criteria and belong to one of the groups that are "categorically" eligible for the program. In addition, eligibility is limited to American citizens and certain lawfully residing immigrants. To be eligible for federal funds, states are required to provide Medicaid coverage for certain "mandatory" groups. The mandatory groups include the following:

a) Limited-income families with children who meet certain of the eligibility requirements in the state's Aid to Families with Dependent Children plan in effect on July 16, 1996

b) Most older adults and people with disabilities who receive Supplemental Security Income (SSI)

c) Children younger than age 6 and pregnant women whose family income is at or below 133% of the federal poverty level

d) Children ages 6–18 living below 100% of the federal poverty level

2) Under the Patient Protection and Affordable Care Act of 2010, most people younger than age 65 with income below a national "floor" will be eligible for Medicaid. Eligibility will remain limited to American citizens and certain lawfully residing immigrants.

3) States have the option to provide Medicaid coverage for other "categorically needy" groups. These optional groups share characteristics of the mandatory groups, but the eligibility criteria are somewhat more liberally defined. Examples of the optional groups that states may cover as categorically needy (and for which they will get federal matching funds) under the Medicaid program include the following:

a) Pregnant women, children, and parents with income exceeding the mandatory thresholds

b) Older adults and people who are disabled earning up to 100% of the federal poverty level

c) Working disabled people earning up to 250% of the federal poverty level

d) People residing in nursing facilities with income below 300% of the SSI standard

e) People who would be eligible if institutionalized but are receiving care under home- and community-based service waivers

f) "Medically needy" people who cannot meet the financial criteria but have high medical expenses relative to their income and who belong to one of the categorically eligible groups

3. State Children's Health Insurance Plan: Health insurance plan for children in families with incomes too high to qualify for Medicaid but too low to afford private health insurance. In 2010 the average monthly enrollment was 5.8 million children (CMS, 2010).
   a. Administration
      1) Jointly financed by the state and federal government. States are given broad flexibility in tailoring programs to meet their own circumstances.
      2) States can create or expand their own separate insurance programs, expand Medicaid, or combine both approaches.
   b. Eligibility: States have the opportunity to set eligibility criteria for age, income, resources, and residency within broad federal guidelines.
4. Workers' compensation: Government-sponsored and employee-financed systems for compensating employees who incur an injury or illness in connection with their employment. Benefits provided include medical care, disability payments, rehabilitation services, survivor benefits, and funeral expenses.
   a. Administration: Each state, the District of Columbia, Puerto Rico, and the U.S. Virgin Islands designates an agency that will administer the program (e.g., state department of labor, independent workers' compensation agency, court administration).
   b. Eligibility: Workers who are disabled by injury or families of a worker whose death arose out of and in the course of employment
   c. Coverage: Provides both medical care related to the compensable injury and income benefits through the following sources
      1) Private commercial insurance companies
      2) Self-insurance (corporations that are able to carry the risk)
      3) State funds
      4) State's second injury fund
   d. Medical care provisions
      1) Treatment and rehabilitative programs for work-related injury
      2) Reimbursement in full or, in certain states, according to a medical fee guide
   e. Vocational rehabilitation benefits: Most states provide job retraining, education, and job placement.
B. Private Health Insurance
   1. Purchasing private health insurance plans
      a. Employers and other organizations may purchase private health insurance on behalf of a group of individuals. Purchasing groups often negotiate coverage, so benefits often vary by group. Group members (e.g., employees) contribute to the insurance premium.
      b. An individual may purchase private health insurance and pay the full premium.
      c. Under the Affordable Care Act, health insurance coverage will be required by 2014.
   2. Types of health insurance and service plans
      a. Indemnity plans: Provide comprehensive coverage for medical and hospital services
         1) The employer or subscriber pays a premium, and the subscriber agrees to pay any required deductible, copayments, and amounts over the insurer's usual and customary rate for specific services.
         2) The subscriber may receive services from physicians, hospitals, or other qualified providers of his or her choice for services that are medically necessary and meet accepted standards of medical practice.
         3) Preapproval for coverage may be required.
         4) Experimental and other noncovered services may be negotiable under certain circumstances.
      b. Managed care plans (Kongstvedt, 2001)
         1) Overview
            a) Managed care plans provide an identified set of medical or hospital care services for a fixed, predetermined premium.
            b) The managed care organization (MCO) may restrict the subscriber's choice of providers and control subscriber access.
            c) Subscribers often choose or are assigned a primary care physician who is employed or under contract with the MCO. In many cases, the primary care physician acts as a gatekeeper for all other medical and hospital services.
            d) The different types of insurance plans were reasonably distinct until the late 1980s. Since that time, the differences between traditional forms of health insurance (e.g., indemnity plans) and managed care plans have decreased substantially.
            e) MCOs vary greatly in terms of their focus on controlling costs and quality (**Figure 21-1**).
               i. Less controlled: Managed indemnity plans that may include

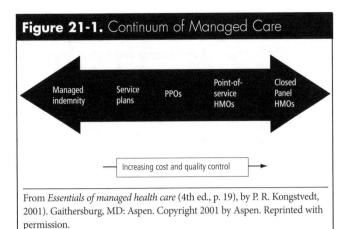

Figure 21-1. Continuum of Managed Care

Managed indemnity — Service plans — PPOs — Point-of-service HMOs — Closed Panel HMOs

Increasing cost and quality control →

From *Essentials of managed health care* (4th ed., p. 19), by P. R. Kongstvedt, 2001). Gaithersburg, MD: Aspen. Copyright 2001 by Aspen. Reprinted with permission.

precertification of elective admissions and case management of catastrophic cases

   ii. More controlled: Group and staff model health maintenance organizations (HMOs)

2) Types of managed care plans

  a) HMOs: Organized healthcare systems that are responsible for both the financing and delivery of a broad range of healthcare services to an enrolled population. The original definition of HMO also included financing health care for a prepaid fixed fee. HMOs must ensure their members have access to covered healthcare services and are responsible for the quality and appropriateness of these services.

  b) Preferred Provider Organizations (PPOs): Employer health benefit plans and insurance carriers contract with PPOs to purchase healthcare services for covered beneficiaries from a selected group of participating providers who typically agree to follow utilization management and other processes implemented by the PPO and agree to the reimbursement structure and payment models. PPOs offer incentives for enrollees to use participating providers. Enrollees are permitted to use non-PPO providers, but they typically must pay higher coinsurance or deductible amounts. Key attributes of a PPO include a selected provider panel, negotiated payment rates, rapid payment terms, utilization management, and consumer choice.

  c) Point-of-service (POS) plans: POS plans offer enrollees some indemnity-type coverage but typically have high deductibles and coinsurance to encourage members to use the HMO-type services.

  d) Consumer-driven healthcare programs: Many variations in these programs exist. Typically, employers provide employees with a personal care account of a fixed amount in the form of a voucher, refundable tax credit, higher wages, or some other transfer of funds. Employees choose their own services and providers and manage their own healthcare spending. Employees who use up all the funds in their account pay expenses up to a deductible, when catastrophic coverage begins. The employee can purchase health care through an intermediary.

c. Medicare supplemental benefits plan (Medigap): Purchased by Medicare beneficiaries to pay for expenses that are not covered by Medicare

d. Auto liability: Covers medical care needed as a result of a motor vehicle accident

C. Programs for Special Groups

1. Military personnel: TRICARE is the U.S. Department of Defense's health insurance program for military service members, retirees, and their families, formerly known as the Civilian Health and Medical Program of the Uniformed Services (CHAMPUS). TRICARE provides civilian health benefits for military personnel, military retirees, and their dependents, including some members of the reserves. It is managed by TRICARE Management Activity under the authority of the Assistant Secretary of Defense (Health Affairs). Veterans of any age, except those who have been dishonorably discharged, may apply for the Medical Benefits Package at the Department of Veterans Affairs (VA). To receive benefits from the VA Medical Benefits Package, the person must be a veteran, be enrolled in the VA health system, and go to VA facilities. People enrolled in the VA Medical Benefits Package may also have private health insurance or federally funded coverage through TRICARE or Medicare. The programs are independent and do not coordinate.

2. Indian Health Service (IHS): Administered by the U.S. DHHS to provide hospital care, dental and health benefits, substance abuse counseling,

public health nursing, and other services. IHS services are administered through 12 area offices and 161 IHS and tribally managed service units. Eligibility is limited to members of the 564 federally recognized Indian tribes and their descendants, and in 2010 the program included 1.9 million American Indians and Alaskan Natives living on or near reservations.

3. Railroad Retirement Act Program
4. Black Lung Benefits Act of 1972
5. Longshoremen and Harbor Workers' Compensation Act
6. Life care planning: The process of mapping out short- and long-term care needs, expenses, and resources for clients with a debilitating, chronic illness or injury. A life care plan is created to ensure the client receives consistent, comprehensive, cost-effective care from present and future caregivers (Barker, 1999).

II. **Reimbursement for Healthcare Services**
   A. Payment Terms
      1. Prospective payment system (PPS): The payment rate to the healthcare facility is predetermined based on the medical diagnosis, treatment, or other information, regardless of the cost for care for a specific client.
      2. Per discharge payment: The provider or hospital is paid one amount for all services delivered during one stay.
      3. Per diem payments: The healthcare facility is paid one amount for all services delivered to a client during one day.
   B. Medicare Payment Systems
      1. Acute care hospitals
         a. Inpatient hospital acute care
         b. Medicare implemented a per-discharge inpatient PPS in acute care hospitals in 1983. PPS payments are expected to cover all operating and capital costs. PPS payments are determined based on client and facility factors.
            1) The classification system for the inpatient PPS is Medicare Severity Diagnosis-Related Groups (MS DRGs). Data from the bill are used to assign each client into one of the MS DRGs (payment groups). There are 335 base DRGs, with many splitting into two or three MS DRGs based on the presence of a complication or comorbidity. Discharge destination and use of certain drugs are occasionally used with the principal diagnosis or procedure to assign the client into a base DRG.
            2) Adjustments are made for a rural location, indirect medical education, the proportion of low-income population, geographic differences in labor costs, and outlier cases.
            3) The base payment rate is updated each year.
      2. Critical access hospitals (CAHs)
         a. CAHs are small hospitals, limited to 25 beds, and operate primarily in rural areas. In addition to the 25 acute care beds, CAHs may have distinct skilled nursing facilities, 10-bed psychiatric units, 10-bed rehabilitation units, and home health agencies.
         b. Each CAH receives 101% of costs for outpatient, inpatient, laboratory, therapy, and post-acute care services in the hospital's swing beds.
      3. Skilled nursing facilities (SNFs)
         a. An SNF provides short-term skilled care (nursing or rehabilitation services) on an inpatient basis. Medicare beneficiaries must have a hospital stay of a least 3 days to be eligible for SNF services to be covered. The Medicare SNF benefit covers skilled nursing care, rehabilitation services, and other goods and services for up to 100 days if the client meets established criteria.
         b. The SNF client-assessment instrument is the Minimum Data Set (MDS 3.0). Data collected using the MDS 3.0, such as treatments provided and client characteristics, are used to categorize each client into a payment group and to calculate facility-level quality indicators.
         c. Medicare implemented a per diem SNF PPS in 1998. PPS payments are expected to cover all operating and capital costs, with certain high-cost, low-probability ancillary services paid separately. PPS payments are determined based on client and facility factors.
            1) The client classification system for the SNF PPS is Resource Utilization Groups (RUGs IV). Data from the MDS 3.0 are used to assign each client to 1 of the 66 RUGs (payment groups).
            2) Adjustments are made for rural or urban location and geographic differences in labor costs.
            3) The base payment rates are updated each year.

4. Home health agencies (HHAs)
   a. An HHA provides skilled care (from a nurse or physical or occupational therapist) on a part-time or intermittent basis in the person's home. To qualify for this benefit, Medicare beneficiaries generally are restricted to their homes.
   b. The home health agency client assessment instrument is the Outcome and Assessment Information Set (OASIS-C). Data collected using the OASIS-C, such as clinical characteristics, functional status, and service use rates, are used to categorize each client into a payment group and to calculate facility-level quality indicators.
   c. Medicare implemented a PPS for home health in 2000 that pays a predetermined rate to the agency for each 60-day episode. PPS payments are determined based on client and facility factors.
      1) The client classification system for the home health agency PPS is the Home Health Resource Groups (HHRGs). Data from the OASIS are used to assign each client to one of the 80 HHRGs (payment groups).
      2) Payments are adjusted if fewer than five visits are delivered during the 60-day episode and for other special circumstances, such as high-cost outliers.
      3) Adjustments are made for geographic differences in labor costs.
      4) The base payment rate is updated each year.
5. Inpatient rehabilitation facilities (IRFs)
   a. IRFs, which include freestanding rehabilitation hospitals and distinct rehabilitation units within general (acute care) hospitals, provide intensive rehabilitation services, such as physical, occupational, or speech therapy and hospital-level care to clients after an major illness, injury, or surgical care. Clients must be able to tolerate and benefit from 3 hours of daily therapy.
   b. The 60% rule (formerly known as the 75% rule) is a criterion used to define IRFs; it requires that 60% of clients admitted to an IRF have 1 of 13 qualifying medical conditions. The 13 conditions are stroke, spinal cord injury, congenital deformity, amputation, major multiple trauma, hip fracture, brain injury, neurological disorders (e.g., multiple sclerosis, Parkinson's disease), burns, three arthritis conditions for which aggressive and sustained outpatient therapy has not been effective, and joint replacement for both knees or both hips, when body mass index is 50 or higher or age is 85 years and older.
   c. The IRF standardized client assessment instrument is the Inpatient Rehabilitation Facility Patient Assessment Instrument (IRF-PAI). Data include demographic, diagnostic, and FIM™ instrument (functional status) data. Data are collected on admission and discharge, and admission data are used to categorize each client into payment groups.
   d. Medicare implemented a per-discharge IRF PPS in 2002 for Medicare fee-for-service clients. PPS payments are expected to cover all operating and capital costs, with certain high-cost ancillary services paid separately. PPS payments are determined based on client and facility factors.
      1) The client classification system for the IRF PPS is Case-Mix Groups (CMGs). In addition, payments are adjusted for the presence of a tiered comorbidity. Data from the IRF-PAI are used to assign each client into one of the CMG and comorbidity (payment) groups.
      2) A transfer rule aims to discourage IRFs from discharging clients to other institutional settings.
      3) Payments are adjusted for short-stay outliers and high-cost outliers.
      4) Adjustments are made for rural or urban location, treatment of low-income clients, teaching status, and geographic differences in labor costs.
      5) The base payment rate is updated each year.
6. Long-term care hospitals (LTCHs)
   a. An LTCH provides care to clients with clinically complex problems, such as multiple acute or chronic conditions, who need hospital care for extended periods of time. On average, LTCH clients must have a length of stay of 25 days. LTCHs are not distributed evenly across the United States.
   b. The 25% rule reduces payments for LTCHs that exceed the established percentage thresholds for clients admitted from certain referring hospitals during a cost reporting period. Less stringent thresholds are applied to hospitals within hospitals and satellites in rural areas or in urban areas where they are the sole

LTCH and there is a dominant acute care hospital.

   c. Medicare implemented a per-discharge LTCH PPS in 2002. PPS payments are expected to cover all operating and capital costs, with certain high-cost ancillary services paid separately. PPS payments are determined based on client and facility factors.

     1) The client classification system for the LTCH PPS is the Medicare Severity Long-Term Care Diagnosis-Related Groups (MS-LTC-DRGs). The MS-LTC-DRGs are the same groupings used in the acute care inpatient PPS, but the relative weights for each group are different. Data from the hospital bill (e.g., diagnosis, procedures, client characteristics) are used to assign each client into one of the MS-LTC-DRGs (payment groups).

     2) Payments are adjusted for short-stay outliers and high-cost outliers.

     3) Adjustments are made for indirect medical education and geographic differences in labor costs.

     4) Transfer policies aim to discourage transfers between an LTCH and a colocated acute care hospital and transfers to colocated SNFs, IRFs, and psychiatric facilities.

     5) The base payment rates are updated each year.

III. Economic Barriers to Care

  A. Lack of Health Insurance

    1. Overview: The majority of Americans younger than age 65 receive health insurance coverage through their employers, and almost all older adults receive coverage through Medicare. Medicaid and the State Children's Health Insurance Program provide insurance for millions of non-elderly low-income people, especially children. However, program limits and gaps in employer coverage have resulted in many people not having health insurance. The Affordable Care Act seeks to eliminate this increasing gap in health insurance coverage by making affordable coverage more accessible, including an expansion of the Medicaid program, and requiring people to obtain health insurance. In 2008, 37.6 million adults did not have health insurance (Holahan & Cook, 2009).

    2. Who does not have insurance?

     a. Low-income Americans (family incomes below 200% of the poverty level) are likely to be uninsured. More than one-third of the poor and 30% of the near-poor do not have health insurance.

     b. Approximately 81% of the uninsured are in working families. Low-wage workers are likely to be uninsured, as are people employed in small businesses, the service industries, and blue-collar jobs.

     c. Medicaid covers low-income children; coverage for adults is more limited. Parent income eligibility levels are much lower than the levels for children. There are also enrollment hurdles and lack of outreach.

     d. The rate of uninsured among older adults is low (less than 2%) as a result of the Medicare program; however, underinsurance can be an economic barrier for older adults who must supplement their insurance coverage with out-of-pocket money. Black and Hispanic older adults are disproportionately uninsured (Okara, Young, Strine, Balluz, & Mokdad, 2005).

  B. Underinsurance and Other Limitations of Access and Coverage

    1. Health insurance does not always ensure access to care. An estimated 16 million adults between 19 and 64 years of age are underinsured. There are often limitations on coverage for special services, such as behavioral health care, preventive care, long-term care, catastrophic illnesses or accidents, and psychiatric care. Also, exclusions or waiting periods for illnesses or conditions may exist at the time the person enrolls in the health plan.

    2. Most health insurance plans also include copayments or deductibles to discourage overuse of services and to reduce premium costs. Copayments and high deductibles can discourage some clients from seeking preventive care (e.g., immunizations, mammograms) and managing chronic conditions effectively. This is particularly a problem for people with low incomes.

    3. Substantial gaps in cost-sharing provisions and coverage exist in the traditional Medicare program. There are large deductibles and copayments for hospital care and restrictions on long-term care coverage.

    4. Low-income older adults may qualify for Medicaid in addition to Medicare. Although Medicaid is comprehensive, many physicians do not participate in the program because of its low level of payment. Therefore, barriers still exist for low-income older adults trying to access basic healthcare services.

C. Effects of a Lack of Adequate Health Insurance
   1. Lack of adequate health insurance creates substantial barriers to obtaining timely and appropriate health care.
      a. More than 40% of nonelderly uninsured adults have no regular source of health care, and many delay or go without needed care because of concerns about high medical bills.
      b. More than one-third of the uninsured have a serious problem paying medical bills, and one-quarter are contacted by collection agencies because of medical bills.
   2. Delaying or not receiving treatment can lead to more serious illness and avoidable health conditions.
      a. The uninsured are less likely to receive preventive care and are more likely to be admitted to a hospital for a preventable or avoidable condition than people with insurance.
      b. Researchers estimate that at least 18,000 Americans die prematurely each year because of lack of health insurance. A reduction in mortality of 5%–15% could be achieved if the uninsured had health insurance.
   3. Uninsured and underinsured clients typically receive care from a select group of providers (e.g., community clinics and public hospitals) that are willing to provide care regardless of a person's ability to pay, such as hospital-based outpatient departments, emergency rooms, and community-based clinics.
      a. Costs in these institutional settings often are high, increasing the total costs of delivering care.
      b. To cover the costs of caring for uninsured and underinsured people, providers must either shift fees to other payers or seek government or private subsidies.
      c. Current market forces, including managed care and fixed-fee schedules, make cost shifting difficult, resulting in decreasing services provided to underinsured and uninsured people.
   4. At a societal level, lack of adequate health insurance leads to more disability, lower productivity, and a greater burden on the healthcare system.
D. Responses to the Lack of Health Insurance
   1. The Health Insurance Portability and Accountability Act prohibits group insurance plans from including eligibility criteria related to health status, medical history, genetic information, or disability and reduces exclusions for preexisting conditions when the person was previously covered by a group insurance plan.
   2. The Consolidated Omnibus Budget Reconciliation Act gives people in specific categories the right to continued health plan coverage for up to 18 months after voluntary or involuntary termination of employment or reduction in work hours. The person must pay the entire premium.
   3. The Patient Protection and Affordable Care Act of 2010 seeks to eliminate this increasing gap in health insurance coverage by making affordable coverage more accessible, including an expansion of the Medicaid program, and requiring individuals to obtain health insurance.

IV. **Funding for Assistive Technology**
   A. Definition: *Assistive technology* refers to any item, piece of equipment, or product system—whether acquired commercially, off the shelf, modified, or customized—that is used to increase, maintain, or improve the functional capabilities of people with disabilities.
   B. Why Funding for Assistive Technology Is a Significant Problem
      1. Insurance and health programs do not pay for assistive devices if they are not considered medically necessary.
      2. The Technology Related Assistance for Individuals with Disabilities Act of 1988 (PL 100-407) provided grants to states
         a. To increase the availability of assistive technology
         b. To conduct need assessments
         c. To develop innovative programs
         d. To manage public awareness
         e. To identify policies that promote the availability of assistive technology
      3. In 1994 an amendment (PL 103-218) expanded and strengthened the 1988 act.

V. **Health Policy: Overview**
   A. Definition: *Policy* refers to the decisions that are made about goals and priorities and the ways in which resources are allocated to reach these goals. The choice of policies reflects the values, beliefs, and attitudes of those designing the policy. Health policy includes the decisions made to promote the health of individual citizens.
   B. Stakeholders: The healthcare industry has a variety of stakeholders who may have common or conflicting concerns about policies and policy changes.
      1. Clients tend to favor comprehensive coverage, high-quality health care, and low out-of-pocket expenses and tend to oppose limited access to care and increased client payments.

2. Providers (individual and entities) tend to favor income maintenance, autonomy, and comprehensive coverage and tend to oppose limits on provider payments.

3. Taxpayers tend to favor limits on provider payments and tend to oppose higher taxes.

4. Employers tend to favor cost containment, administrative simplification, and elimination of cost shifting and tend to oppose government regulation.

5. Regulators (government) tend to favor disclosure and reporting by providers, cost containment, access to care, and high-quality health care and tend to oppose provider autonomy.

6. Pharmaceutical manufacturers, biotech entities, assistive technology vendors, and suppliers tend to favor comprehensive coverage and tend to oppose limits on provider payments.

7. Private insurance companies tend to favor business autonomy.

8. Consumer organizations, such as the American Stroke Association and the Paralyzed Veterans' Association, favor securing money for research and public education.

C. Key Healthcare Policy Issues

1. The delivery of healthcare services

a. Access to care: Many people have limited ability to obtain necessary health services for two reasons.

1) Ability to pay: People have no health insurance or are underinsured.

2) Location: People may not have healthcare personnel and facilities that are close to where they live, accessible by transportation, culturally acceptable, or capable of providing appropriate care using the language with which the client is most familiar.

b. Costs of care

1) In 1960 national health expenditures represented 5.1% of the gross domestic product (GDP); expenditures per capita were $141.

2) In 2008 health care represented 16% of the GDP (i.e., 16 cents of every dollar was spent on health care).

3) As a result, various cost-containment strategies (e.g., PPS, managed care) are now used.

c. Quality of health care: Healthcare quality may be defined as the "degree to which patient care services increase the probability of desired patient outcomes and reduce the probability of undesired health outcomes given the current state of knowledge" (Institute of Medicine [IOM], 2006. p. 468). Although the United States offers advanced healthcare services, care is not always accessible, effective, safe, and efficient (IOM, 2006).

1) The IOM noted that the only way to know whether healthcare quality is improving is to document performance using standardized measures of quality. The term *quality measure* has been defined as the "quantification of the degree to which a desired healthcare process or outcome is achieved or the extent that a desirable structure to support healthcare delivery is in place. (IOM, 2006, p. 42).

2) Quality measures address several aspects of care, which have been defined by Donabedian (2005) as structure measures, process measures, and outcome measures. Structure measures track whether a particular mechanism or system is in place, and process measures track performance of a particular action (CMS, 2008). Outcome measures consider the end results of care, such as morbidity and mortality resulting from a disease.

3) The IOM identified the six aims of healthcare delivery as care that is safe, effective, patient centered, timely, efficient, and equitable. *Safe care* is care that does not injure the clients it is intended to help. *Effective care* means that services are based on scientific knowledge and provided to all who could benefit but not to those not likely to benefit. *Patient-centered care* refers to care that is respectful of and responsive to individual client preferences, needs, and values, and *timely care* is provided in a way that reduces wait times. *Efficient care* avoids waste, including waste of equipment, supplies, ideas, and energy, and *equitable care* refers to care that does not vary in quality because of personal characteristics (e.g., gender, ethnicity, geographic location, and socioeconomic status).

d. Health disparities: Disparities in healthcare use and outcomes for people from racial and ethnic minorities and low-income people result in significantly higher rates of chronic illness and disability.

2. Nursing services and workforce
   a. Reimbursement for nursing services, including rehabilitation nurses
   b. Scope of practice (e.g., for advanced practice nurses), as defined by state licensure laws and regulatory bodies
   c. Emerging critical shortage of nurses and nursing faculty
   d. Funding for nursing education and research
3. Social issues related to populations that rehabilitation nurses serve
   a. Community accessibility
   b. Discrimination against people with disabilities in hiring practices or in the workplace
   c. Disincentives for people with disabilities to return to work
   d. Availability of vocational rehabilitation services
4. Privacy and confidentiality
   a. Health Insurance Portability and Accountability Act privacy regulations on protected health information, effective April 2003
   b. Development and implementation of electronic medical records

VI. **Process of Making Health Policy**
   A. Phases of Healthcare Policy Making (**Figure 21-2**)
      1. Policy formulation (Longest, 2006)
         a. Agenda setting

1) This first stage of policy development refers to identifying problems and possible solutions proposed by diverse political interests.
2) Once issues become prominent in the political agenda, they can proceed to the next stage of policy formulation: the development of legislation. However, only a small percentage of issues reach that point.
   b. Development of legislation (**Figure 21-3**)
      1) The legislative process begins with proposals (bills), which may be drafted by senators or representatives and their staff members, by members of the executive branch, by political or special interest groups, and by individual citizens.
         a) Only members of Congress can officially sponsor a bill.
         b) Occasionally, identical bills are simultaneously introduced in the Senate and the House of Representatives for consideration.
      2) Each bill is assigned to the appropriate committee(s) based on its content and the jurisdiction of the committees and subcommittees. Hearings are held and the bill is marked up. Once it is approved by the full committee, the House or Senate receives the bill and places it on the legislative calendar for floor action. The bill may

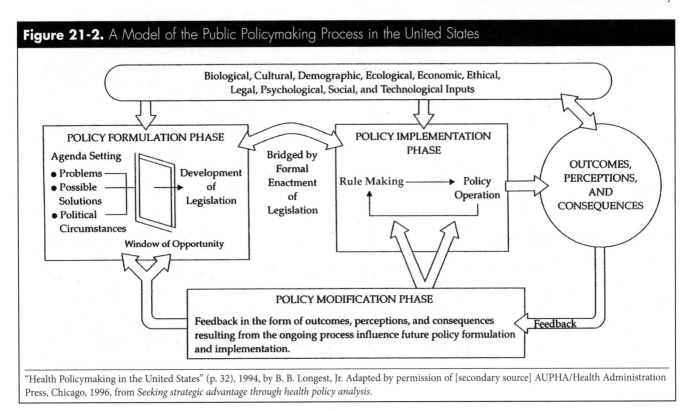

Figure 21-2. A Model of the Public Policymaking Process in the United States

"Health Policymaking in the United States" (p. 32), 1994, by B. B. Longest, Jr. Adapted by permission of [secondary source] AUPHA/Health Administration Press, Chicago, 1996, from *Seeking strategic advantage through health policy analysis.*

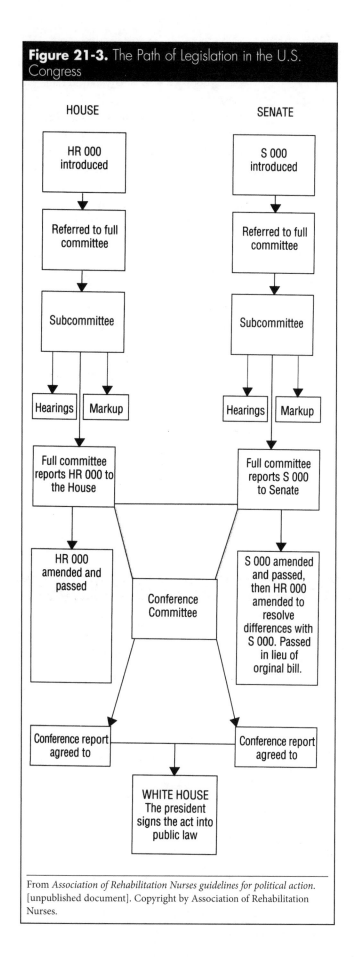

Figure 21-3. The Path of Legislation in the U.S. Congress

HOUSE

SENATE

HR 000 introduced

S 000 introduced

Referred to full committee

Referred to full committee

Subcommittee

Subcommittee

Hearings | Markup

Hearings | Markup

Full committee reports HR 000 to the House

Full committee reports S 000 to Senate

HR 000 amended and passed

Conference Committee

S 000 amended and passed, then HR 000 amended to resolve differences with S 000. Passed in lieu of orginal bill.

Conference report agreed to

Conference report agreed to

WHITE HOUSE The president signs the act into public law

From *Association of Rehabilitation Nurses guidelines for political action.* [unpublished document]. Copyright by Association of Rehabilitation Nurses.

be further amended during debate on the floor.

3) After the bill passes either the House or the Senate, it is sent to the other chamber of Congress, where the process is repeated. If the second chamber passes the bill, any differences between the House and Senate versions must be resolved before the bill is sent to the White House for presidential action.

4) The president has the option to sign the bill to make it a law or to veto the bill and return it to Congress with an explanation for the rejection. A presidential veto may be overridden by a two-thirds vote in both houses of Congress. If the president does not sign or veto the bill after 10 days, the bill automatically becomes law.

2. Policy implementation (includes rule making and policy operation)
   a. Once a law is enacted, implementation rests primarily with the executive branch of the government. Cabinet departments such as DHHS and agencies such as CMS and the Centers for Disease Control and Prevention oversee the implementation.
   b. Other agencies such as the Government Accountability Office, the Congressional Budget Office, the Congressional Research Office, and the Office of Technology and Assessment have oversight responsibility.
   c. Laws often are vague on implementation details, so the organization responsible for implementing the law publishes a "Notice of Proposed Rule Making" and "Final Rule" in the *Federal Register*.
   d. Policy implementation involves the actual operation of programs that are described in the enacted legislation.

3. Policy modification: This stage allows all prior decisions to be modified once the outcomes, perceptions, and consequences of existing policies are discovered. Modifications to any legislation must begin with the agenda-setting stage.

B. Opportunities for Rehabilitation Nurses to Influence Health Policy Making
   1. In policy formulation
      a. Agenda setting
         1) Define and document problems.
         2) Develop and evaluate solutions to problems.
         3) Shape political circumstances by lobbying and working through the legal system.

THE SPECIALTY PRACTICE OF REHABILITATION NURSING

b. Legislation development
   1) Participate in drafting legislation.
   2) Testify at legislative hearings.
2. In policy implementation or rule making
   a. Provide formal comments on proposed rules published in the *Federal Register*.
   b. Serve on and provide input to rule-making advisory bodies.
   c. Work on policy operation by interacting with policy operators.
3. In policy modification: Document cases for modification through operational experience and formal evaluations (i.e., research)

C. Reasons Why Nurses Should Get Involved in Developing Health Policy
1. Enables participation in decisions relating to the future of the profession and health care
2. Has a positive effect on the healthcare delivery system
3. Promotes the ability to provide input at policy-making and health-planning levels
4. Shows a commitment to maintaining healthcare standards

D. Guidelines for Taking Political Action
1. Register and vote for the candidates of your choice.
2. Be informed on issues.
3. Get involved in professional nursing associations and their health policy task forces.
4. Obtain lists of local, state, and national legislators (available from government offices, websites, or public libraries).
5. Join the Association of Rehabilitation Nurses (ARN) Health Policy Committee.
   a. Be informed about ARN's position on legislation by contacting the ARN office or the ARN Health Policy Committee Chair or by searching the ARN website (www.rehabnurse.org).
   b. Communicate with the ARN Health Policy Committee Chair about local and state issues and personal activities.
   c. Attend legislative conferences (e.g., Nurse-in-Washington Internship).
6. Do not act as a spokesperson for a national or local organization unless specifically authorized to do so.
7. Establish a relationship and communicate with federal, state, and local legislators to make them aware of positions on specific issues (**Figure 21-4**).
   a. Write letters.
   b. Make telephone calls.
   c. Send faxes.
   d. Send e-mail.
   e. Meet in person.
   f. Volunteer professional services or provide monetary support.
   g. Provide expert testimony.

VII. Healthcare System's Response to Health Policy (Nosse, Friberg, & Kovacek, 1999; Relman, 1988; Roper, Winkenwerder, Hackbarth, & Krakauer, 1988)
A. Growth and Development of the Healthcare Delivery System (1965–1980)
1. The structure of the delivery system included small independent physician group practices.
2. Larger multispecialty clinics were developing but were uncommon. Hospitals provided secondary and tertiary care.
3. The supply of and demand for healthcare services expanded in response to several factors
   a. Introduction of Medicare and Medicaid programs
   b. An increased need for the capacity, capabilities, and number and types of healthcare providers
   c. An increased number of people accessing the delivery system
   d. An increased amount of care provided
   e. New and improved treatments and technology
B. Cost Containment in the Delivery of Health Care (1981–1991)
1. Cost containment was a concern for physicians, hospitals, and public and private insurers.
2. Acute care PPS began in 1983 and helped reduce the costs of inpatient hospital care by
   a. Decreasing the average length of stay
   b. Decreasing the use of routine diagnostic tests during inpatient hospitalizations
   c. Shifting care to outpatient settings
   d. Increasing the use of postacute care services (e.g., home care, rehabilitation hospitals and units, SNFs)
3. The decrease in inpatient hospital use resulted in excess acute care bed capacity, decreased profits for hospitals and physicians, and imposed financial limits on purchasing new technologies and upgrading facilities.
4. These trends caused providers to compete for a larger share of the healthcare market and to react in many ways.
   a. Reduced costs through reorganization and staff layoffs
   b. Developed and modified alternative care options (e.g., rehabilitation services, home care, ambulatory care, long-term care)

c. Restructured the organization through vertical and horizontal integration with other providers so that hospital networks cover larger geographic areas and provide a full continuum of services

d. Focused new attention on marketing provider services

C. Value, Assessment, and Accountability (1990s to present)

1. Managed care enrollment increased dramatically in the early 1990s.

2. National, publicly traded, for-profit healthcare corporations became more common.

3. Small independent providers joined together to form specialty service networks to capture and hold market shares.

4. Large physician groups joined with hospitals or contracted with managed care organizations.

5. Interest in the quality of care and documenting the outcomes of health services, including publishing healthcare report cards, increased.

6. Consumerism increased.

7. Interest in evidence-based practice increased.

8. PPSs were developed for skilled nursing facilities, home health agencies, inpatient rehabilitation hospitals, and long-term care hospitals.

9. Quality measures were developed for public reporting, quality-improvement activities, and pay-for-performance activities.

VIII. Key Forces Shaping the Future of Healthcare Delivery in the United States (Kovner & Knickman, 2008; Sultz & Young, 2009)

A. Changing Demographics

1. Aging of the population: Healthcare resource use and costs increase significantly with advancing age.

2. Increasing ethnic diversity: Racial and ethnic minority groups in the United States have poorer health than the majority White population. If the current disparities continue, the burden of illness will increase as the minority population increases.

B. Reduced Spending for Medicare and Medicaid Programs: Changes to these programs will affect the entire healthcare marketplace because these two programs combined account for 36% of personal health expenditures, 48% of hospital expenditures, 33% of physician and professional expenditures, 61% of nursing home care, and 32% of home health care (Kovner & Knickman, 2008).

C. Public Belief That Our Own Behaviors Affect Our Health: There is increasing understanding that the determinants of health have little to do with the healthcare system and more to do with the way we lead our lives and the environment we live in.

D. Uninsured: The Affordable Care Act seeks to reduce the number of uninsured by 2014.

E. Adoption of Health Information Technology: Technology may facilitate accountability and increase productivity.

F. Genomics: The linking of human diseases with variations in specific genes

G. Technological Growth and Innovation: New diagnostic and treatment modalities are expected to further shift care into outpatient settings and prolong life.

H. Changing Professional Labor Supply: Shortages of key health professionals, redefinition of professional roles

I. Globalization of the Economy: Increased scrutiny of healthcare costs

References

Barker, E. (1999). Life care planning. *RN, 52*(3), 58–61.

Centers for Medicare and Medicaid Services. (2008). *Roadmap for quality measurement in the traditional fee-for-service program.* Washington, DC: Author.

Centers for Medicare & Medicaid Services. (2010). *CMS statistics.* Baltimore: Author.

Centers for Medicare and Medicaid Services. (2011). Medicare contracting reform overview. Retrieved August 17, 2011, from www.cms.gov/MedicareContractingReform.

Congress.org. (2011). Communicating with elected officials. Retrieved August 15, 2011, from www.congress.org/congress-org/issues/basics.

Donabedian, A. (2005). Evaluating the quality of medical care. 1966. *The Milbank Quarterly, 83*(4), 691–729.

The Henry J. Kaiser Family Foundation. (2010a). *Medicaid: A primer.* Menlo Park, CA: Author.

The Henry J. Kaiser Family Foundation. (2010b). *Medicare: A primer.* Menlo Park, CA: Author.

Holahan, J., & Cook, A. (2009, October). *Changes in health insurance coverage, 2007–2008: Early impact of the recession.* Menlo Park, CA: The Henry J. Kaiser Family Foundation.

Institute of Medicine. (2006). *Performance measurement: Accelerating improvement.* Washington, DC: The National Academies Press.

Kongstvedt, P. R. (2001). *Essentials of managed health care* (4th ed.). Gaithersburg, MD: Aspen.

Kovner, A. R., & Knickman, J. R. (2008). *Healthcare delivery in the United States.* New York: Springer.

Longest, B. B., Jr. (1996). *Health policymaking in the United States.* Chicago: Health Administration Press.

Longest, B. B. (2006). *Health policymaking in the United States* (4th ed.). Chicago: Health Administration Press.

McCourt, A. E. (Ed.). (1993). *The specialty practice of rehabilitation nursing: A core curriculum* (3rd ed.). Skokie, IL: Rehabilitation Nursing Foundation of the Association of Rehabilitation Nurses.

Medicare Payment Advisory Commission. (2010). *Data book: Healthcare spending and the Medicare program.* Washington, DC: Author.

Nosse, L. J., Friberg, D. G., & Kovacek, P. R. (1999). *Managerial and supervisory principles for physical therapists.* Baltimore: Williams & Wilkins.

Okara, C. A., Young, S. L., Strine, T. W., Balluz, L. S., & Mokdad, A. H. (2005). Uninsured adults aged 65 years and older. Is their health at risk? *Journal of Health Care for the Poor and Underserved, 16*(3), 453–463.

Relman, A. S. (1988). Assessment and accountability: The third revolution in medical care. *New England Journal of Medicine, 319*(18), 1220–1222.

Roper, W. L., Winkenwerder, W., Hackbarth, G. M., & Krakauer, H. (1988). Effectiveness in health care. An initiative to evaluate and improve medical practice. *New England Journal of Medicine, 319*(18), 1197–1202.

Sultz, H. A., & Young, K. M. (2009). *Health care USA* (6th ed.). Sudbury, MA: Jones & Bartlett.

Suggested Resources

Association of Rehabilitation Nurses. (2011). *Health policy and advocacy: Health policy tool kit.* Retrieved January 2, 2011, from www.rehabnurse.org/advocacy/content/toolkit.html.

Bodenheimer, T. S., & Grumbach, K. (2009). *Understanding health policy: A clinical approach* (5th ed.). Norwalk, CT: Appleton & Lange.

Center for Medicare & Medicaid Services: www.cms.gov

Dean-Baar, S. (2001). Health policy and legislation in rehabilitation. In J. B. Derstine & S. D. Hargrove (Eds.), *Comprehensive rehabilitation nursing* (pp. 42–49).Philadelphia: W. B. Saunders.

Edwards, P. A. (1999a). Financing health care. In P. A. Edwards, D. L. Hertzberg, S. R. Hays, & N. M. Youngblood (Eds.), *Pediatric rehabilitation nursing* (pp. 52–61). Philadelphia: W. B. Saunders.

Edwards, P. A. (1999b). Legislation and public policy. In P. A. Edwards, D. L. Hertzberg, S. R. Hays, & N. M. Youngblood (Eds.), *Pediatric rehabilitation nursing* (pp. 40–51). Philadelphia: W. B. Saunders.

Leavitt, J. K., Chaffee, M. K., & Vance, C. (2002). Learning the ropes of policy and politics. In D. J. Mason, J. K. Leavitt, & M. W. Chaffee (Eds.), *Policy & politics in nursing and health care* (pp. 31–43). St. Louis: Saunders.

Milstead, J. A. (2007). *Health policy and politics: A nurse's guide* (3rd ed.). Gaithersburg, MD: Aspen.

CHAPTER 22

Outcome Measurement and Performance Improvement

Terrie Black, MBA BSN RN BC CRRN • Michele Cournan, DNP RN CRRN ANP-BC FNP

Accountability and validation of value have become essential components of the healthcare delivery process. Today, outcomes of care are emphasized as never before (Black, 1999). Performance improvement focuses on the effectiveness of care or the results of services delivered by a clinician or team of clinicians. It is a key component that drives the quality and safety in an organization. Performance improvement and accountability depend on collaboration and shared goals by various stakeholders (Porter, 2010). Monitoring outcomes can help do the following:

- track efficiency and effectiveness
- identify trends
- facilitate communication between the client, family, treatment team, payers, referral source, and other stakeholders
- assess follow-up measures to determine whether progress is continuing after discharge
- identify areas for improvement
- measure access to programs.

Internal stakeholders interested in outcomes and quality of care may include a rehabilitation program's case managers, administrator, board of directors, clinicians, and parties such as researchers and quality-improvement practitioners who are interested in outcome data. Externally, stakeholders who often evaluate programs and services using outcome data include case managers, payers, referral sources, and direct consumers of healthcare services.

Outcomes can be benchmarked according to past trends within an organization or corporation, national and regional standards or norms, and best-practice standards. Corporations can identify outcomes and use various sites or regions as bases for comparison. Data can also be used to improve rehabilitation nursing care and serve as the basis for outcome research with the potential to influence health policy affecting rehabilitation.

This chapter examines outcomes of care in rehabilitation, describes the tools used by rehabilitation clinicians to collect information about outcomes, and profiles the agencies that accredit rehabilitation programs.

I. Overview

A. Primary Accreditation Agencies for Rehabilitation Providers

1. Centers for Medicare & Medicaid Services (CMS): Healthcare organizations that participate in and receive payment from either Medicare or Medicaid must comply with Conditions of Participation (CoP) set forth in federal regulations.

2. The Joint Commission (JC)

   a. May serve as deeming authority on behalf of CMS

   b. Enforces standards that meet the federal Conditions of Participation

3. The Commission on Accreditation of Rehabilitation Facilities (CARF)

4. State agencies

B. Benefits of Accreditation

1. Assists with the business, management, and quality strategies that organizations should have in place to meet consumer needs and maintain operations

2. Demonstrates to stakeholders that certain standards have been met, systems are in place to deliver high-quality services, results are as expected based on norms, and processes thought to be of expert consensus are followed

3. Assures consumers that an independent review process focuses on improving the quality of services

4. Provides organizations with a template for efficient and effective operations

5. Establishes a common level of program expectations and performance

6. Focuses on meeting the needs of people with disabilities and others who need rehabilitation

7. Offers a mechanism for purchasers, providers, and consumers to interact

8. Identifies organizations or programs that have met standards and reinforces and supports those organizations

9. May affect reimbursement ("deemed status")

II. Accrediting Agencies

A. The JC

1. General

   a. Mission: To continuously improve health care for the public, in collaboration with other stakeholders, by evaluating healthcare organizations and inspiring them to excel in providing safe and effective care of the highest quality and value (JC, 2009)

b. Vision: All people always experience the safest, highest quality, best-value health care across all settings (JC, 2009)
c. "Compliance": JC's term for referring to meeting standards
d. Organizational structure: Governed by a board of commissioners

2. Historical perspective
   a. 1910: Dr. Ernest Codman proposed a system of hospital standardization in which hospitals track every client to determine whether treatment is effective.
   b. 1918: The American College of Surgeons began on-site inspections of hospitals.
   c. 1926: The first 18-page standard manual was published.
   d. 1951: The American College of Physicians, the American Hospital Association, the American Medical Association, and the Canadian Medical Association joined to create the Joint Commission on Accreditation of Hospitals (JCAH), whose primary purpose was to provide voluntary accreditation.
   e. 1953: JCAH publishes standards for hospital accreditation.
   f. 1966: Long-term care accreditation began.
   g. 1970: Registered nurses joined physicians in conducting surveys.
   h. 1982: The first public member began serving on the JCAH Board of Commissioners.
   i. 1987: The organization changes its name to the Joint Commission on Accreditation of Healthcare Organizations (JCAHO) to reflect its expanded scope of activities.
   j. 1988: Accreditation for home care organizations began.
   k. 1993
      1) The *Accreditation Manual for Hospitals* is reorganized around important patient care and organization functions from standards that measure an organization's capability to perform to those that look at actual performance.
      2) The number and nature of Type 1 recommendations against an organization became public information.
      3) JCAHO began making random, unannounced surveys of accredited organizations.
   l. 1996: The sentinel event policy is established.

m. 1997: The JCAHO ORYX initiative was launched to integrate outcomes and other performance measures into the accreditation process.
n. 2002
   1) In June the 2002 National Patient Safety Goals were announced. The purpose of the National Patient Safety Goals is to improve safety. The goals focus on problems in healthcare safety and how to solve them.
   2) The JCAHO launches the Disease-Specific Care (DSC) certification program.
o. 2007: The Joint Commission (JC) introduces its refreshed brand identity (name and logo) in support of its continuing efforsts to improve the value of accreditation.
p. 2009: The JC launched its Center for Transforming Healthcare in September, which develops solutions through the application of robust process improvement methods and tools.
q. 2009: CMS approved the continuation of deeming authority for the JC's hospital accreditation program through July 2014.
r. 2010: The JC launches its Leading Practices Library.

3. Accreditation process
   a. An organization submits an application to the JC.
   b. The organization prepares for the survey using the Survey Activity Guide.
   c. An initial conference with the organization's leaders is held on the first day of the survey to finalize the survey schedule.
   d. The survey includes a tour of the facility, reviews of medical records and documentation, observation of staff, and interviews with clients and staff.
   e. The major focus is on direct input from care providers, with the surveyors providing education while measuring compliance with standards.
   f. Elements of performance (EP) are the performance expectations for determining whether a standard is in compliance. EPs are scored on a 3-point scale.
      1) 0 = insufficient compliance
      2) 1 = partial compliance
      3) 2 = satisfactory compliance

4. Accreditation decisions or outcomes
   a. Preliminary accreditation: The organization demonstrates compliance with selected

standards used in the surveys conducted under the Early Survey Policy.

    b. Accreditation: An organization that is in compliance with all standards at the time of the on-site survey or has successfully addressed all requirements for improvement in an Evidence of Standards Compliance submission within 45 or 60 days after the posting of the Accreditation Survey Findings Report and does not meet any other rules for other accreditation decisions

    c. Accreditation with follow-up survey: The healthcare organization is not in compliance with specific standards that require a follow-up survey within 30 days to 6 months.

    d. Contingent accreditation: The healthcare organization fails to successfully address all requirements of the accreditation with a follow-up survey decision.

    e. Preliminary denial of accreditation results when there is justification to deny accreditation to a healthcare organization for one or more of the following reasons: an immediate threat to health or safety for clients or the public, failure to resolve the requirements of an accreditation with follow-up survey status after two opportunities to do so, failure to resolve the requirements of a contingent accreditation status, or significant noncompliance with JC standards.

    f. Denial of accreditation results when a healthcare organization has been denied accreditation.

5. The ORYX initiative

    a. Introduced in 1997

    b. Designed to help organizations strengthen their quality improvement efforts and to identify issues that warrant attention

    c. Uses data from organizations to monitor performance between on-site survey visits

    d. Supports the JC's mission and is a critical link between accreditation and client care outcomes

6. Benefits of JC accreditation and certification

    a. Strengthens community confidence in the quality and safety of care, treatment, and services

    b. Provides a competitive edge in the marketplace

    c. Improves risk management and risk reduction

    d. Helps organize and strengthen client safety effort

    e. Provides education on good practices to improve business operations

    f. Provides professional advice and counsel, thereby enhancing staff education

    g. Provides deeming authority for Medicare certification

    h. Recognized by insurers and other third parties

    i. May reduce liability insurance costs (JC, 2006)

7. Tracer method: The Tracer method is an evaluation method in which surveyors select a client, resident, or client and use that person's record as a roadmap to move through an organization to assess and evaluate the organization's compliance with selected standards and the organization's systems of providing care and services.

8. Unannounced surveys: The JC conducts unannounced surveys

    a. To help healthcare organizations focus on providing safe, high-quality care at all times, not just when preparing for a survey

    b. To affirm the expectation of continuous standard compliance both by the JC of its accredited organizations and by these organizations of themselves

    c. To increase the credibility of the accreditation process by ensuring that surveyors observe organization performance under normal circumstances

    d. To reduce the unnecessary costs healthcare organizations incur to prepare for surveys

    e. To address public concerns that the JC receives an accurate impression of the quality and safety of care

9. Sentinel events: In support of its mission to continuously improve the safety and quality of health care provided to the public, the JC reviews organizations' activities in response to sentinel events in its accreditation process. A sentinel event is an unexpected occurrence involving death or serious physical or psychological injury or the risk thereof. Such events are called "sentinel" because they signal the need for immediate investigation and response.

B. CARF

1. General

    a. Mission: The mission of CARF is to promote the quality, value, and optimal outcomes of services through a consultative accreditation process that centers on enhancing the lives of the people served (CARF, 2011).

b. "Conformance": CARF's term referring to meeting standards

c. Organizational structure
1) Six divisions
    a) Medical Rehabilitation: Accredits programs such as comprehensive integrated inpatient rehabilitation, brain injury, stroke specialty, spinal cord injury systems of care, pain programs, outpatient programs, health enhancement, occupational rehabilitation, case management, and home- and community-based rehabilitation programs
    b) Behavioral Health: Accredits providers of behavioral health programs (e.g., alcohol and drugs, mental health, psychosocial rehabilitation, integrated behavioral health)
    c) Employment and Community Services: Accredits organizations that provide employment services, community services, and psychosocial rehabilitation programs
    d) Aging Services: Accredits programs that provide services to older adults and other adults in residential or community-based group settings
    e) Child and Youth Services: Accredits programs that provide child welfare, protection, and well-being services to children, youth, and their families
    f) Durable medical equipment, prothesis, orthotics and supplies (OMEPOS) suppliers
2) Board of Trustees: Approves standards, awards accreditation, and oversees policies and financial matters (CARF, 1999)

2. Historical perspective
a. 1966: Founded as a nonprofit organization
b. 1993: Accredited its first program in Canada
c. 1995: Enacted new standards for occupational rehabilitation and comprehensive pain-management programs in the medical rehabilitation division
d. 1996: Accredited its first program in Europe
e. 1999: Published standards for adult day services
f. 2000: Published standards for assisted living programs
g. 2001: Recognized by the Substance Abuse & Mental Health Services Administration as an approved accrediting organization for opioid treatment programs
h. 2003: Acquired the Continuing Care Accreditation Commission
i. 2005: Accredited first program in South America
j. 2008: CARF's ASPIRE to Excellence framework is introduced.

3. Development and creation of standards
a. National Advisory Committees (NACs): Each year, NACs are formed to review existing standards and create new standards. This is usually the starting point in the development of new standards. In years when there are no NACs, CARF solicits informal feedback from surveyors, consumers, other purchasers, and interested stakeholders.
b. Field review: Proposed standards are sent to the rehabilitation field for review by national professional groups, third-party purchasers, consumers, surveyors, and advocacy groups. Feedback, suggestions, and requests are evaluated by CARF.
c. Vote by Board of Trustees: New or revised standards are approved by the board before they go into effect (CARF, 1999).

4. Accreditation process
a. Contact a CARF office to verify which standard manual to use. Each standard manual year runs from July 1–June 30.
b. Perform a self-study. A facility may opt to complete a self-study and evaluation before and in preparation for the survey. CARF publishes numerous resources to help organizations in this process.
c. Submit an application at least 3 months before the requested survey.
d. Schedule the survey date. Surveyors are selected based on their expertise and knowledge of the programs being surveyed. Generally, there is an administrative surveyor and at least one program surveyor for medical rehabilitation programs.
e. Have an orientation conference. This is done on the first day of the survey to allow surveyors to give an overview of the survey process and the organization to describe itself to the survey team.
f. Have an exit conference. This provides immediate feedback to the organization about strengths, areas for improvement, suggestions, and any recommendations made by the survey team.

THE SPECIALTY PRACTICE OF REHABILITATION NURSING

g. The surveyor's report is edited by CARF and sent to the Board of Trustees for an accreditation decision.

h. The survey report with accreditation outcome is sent to the organization.

i. The organization submits a quality-improvement plan that addresses any recommendations in the survey report.

j. Submit an annual conformance-to-quality report (CARF, 2006).

5. Key terminology related to CARF's survey process

   a. Standard conformance rating scale

      1) 0 = *Nonconformance*: The program does not even partially conform to a standard.

      2) 1 = *Partial conformance*: The program or service has achieved some components of a standard or made progress toward conformance yet does not meet expectations for full conformance.

      3) 2 = *Conformance*: The program or service fully meets the intent of a standard.

      4) 3 = *Exemplary conformance*: The program or service significantly exceeds the level of practice necessary to achieve conformance to a standard.

   b. Consultation: Suggestions from the survey team for improving services in the organization based on experience in the rehabilitation field. Suggestions are not linked to conformance to the standards in that an organization is not required to implement or act on them (CARF, 2006).

6. Accreditation decisions, ultimately made by the Board of Trustees

   a. 3-year accreditation: Demonstrates substantial conformance to the standards.

   b. 1-year accreditation: Indicates that the organization is basically meeting the standards, but there are some significant areas of deficiency.

   c. Provisional accreditation: Indicates that an organization received a 1-year accreditation on its immediately preceding survey, and although the organization is basically meeting the standards, there continue to be significant problem areas. Upon resurvey, an organization that has a provisional accreditation must achieve a 3-year accreditation or it will be nonaccredited.

   d. Nonaccreditation: Major deficits exist in meeting standards, and concerns exist about whether the organization meets the needs of the people it serves.

   e. Preliminary accreditation is awarded to allow new programs to establish demonstrated use and implementation of the standards (CARF, 2006).

C. National Council on Quality Assurance

   1. Oversees managed care companies

   2. Uses the Health Employment Data Information Set as its dataset

III. **Key Concepts in Rehabilitation**

   A. World Health Organization (2001) Model: International Classification of Functioning, Disability, and Health (ICF) is a classification of health and health-related domains that describe body functions and structures, activities, and participation. It is a conceptual framework, not an assessment instrument. The domains are classified from body, individual, and societal perspectives. Because a person's functioning and disability occur in a context, ICF also includes a list of environmental factors.

   B. Body Functions and Structures: An abnormality of body structure, appearance, and organ or system function resulting from any cause. Impairments occur at the organ level (e.g., dysphagia, hemiparesis).

   C. Activities and Participation: The consequences of impairment in terms of a person's functional performance and activity; the nature and extent of function at the individual level. There may be activity disturbances at the level of the person (e.g., bathing, dressing, communication, walking, grooming). Participation: The disadvantages in work, family, and social roles experienced as a result of impairments; the nature and extent of a person's involvement in life and various activities. Participation reflects interaction with and adaptation to one's surroundings.

   D. Environmental Factors: Barriers and Facilitators

IV. **Tools for Monitoring Rehabilitation Outcomes**

   A. Global Adult Scales (which measure motor, physical, and cognitive elements)

      1. Functional Independence Measure (FIM™) instrument (**Figure 22-1**)

         a. Looks at severity of disability and the need for assistance (burden of care)

         b. Designed to promote a uniform language among the rehabilitation team and to describe the severity of disability

         c. Is included as part of the Inpatient Rehabilitation Facility Patient Assessment Instrument (IRF-PAI), which includes demographic, diagnostic, financial, and functional information about rehabilitation clients

         d. Includes 18 items (13 motor, 5 cognitive)

Figure 22-1. Functional Independence Measure (FIM™) Instrument

FIM™ Instrument

LEVELS		
	7 Complete Independence (timely, safely) 6 Modified Independence (device)	**NO HELPER**
	Modified Dependence 5 Supervision (subject = 100%) 4 Minimal Assistance (subject = 75%+) 3 Moderate Assistance (subject = 50%+) **Complete Dependence** 2 Maximal Assistance (subject =25%+) 1 Total Assistance (subject = less than 25%)	**HELPER**

	ADMISSION	**DISCHARGE**	**FOLLOW-UP**
Self-Care			
A. Eating			
B. Grooming			
C. Bathing			
D. Dressing - Upper Body			
E. Dressing - Lower Body			
F. Toileting			
Sphincter Control			
G. Bladder Management			
H. Bowel Management			
Transfers			
I. Bed, Chair, Wheelchair			
J. Toilet			
K. Tub, Shower			
Locomotion			
L. Walk/Wheelchair	W Walk C Wheelchair B Both	W Walk C Wheelchair B Both	W Walk C Wheelchair B Both
M. Stairs			
Motor Subtotal Rating			
Communication			
N. Comprehension	A Auditory V Visual B Both	A Auditory V Visual B Both	A Auditory V Visual B Both
O. Expression	A Auditory V Visual B Both	A Auditory V Visual B Both	A Auditory V Visual B Both
Social Cognition			
P. Social Interaction			
Q. Problem Solving			
R. Memory			
Cognitive Subtotal Rating			
TOTAL FIM™ RATING			

NOTE: Leave no blanks. Enter 1 if patient is not testable due to risk.

e. Involves a hierarchy of motor items that progress from eating (easiest) to using stairs (most difficult)

f. Uses a 7-level scale in which 1 = *total assistance* (client performs less than 25% of an activity) and 7 = *total independence* (client performs an activity without an assistive device or a helper in a safe and timely manner)

g. Is used internationally and considered to be the gold standard in assessing functional status

h. Can be used by trained members of any discipline

i. Provides the basis for predicting outcomes for various client populations

j. Is the foundation for establishing case mix groups (CMGs)

k. Can be used to estimate the burden of care for activities of daily living (ADLs; based on the FIM™ "Rule of Thumb Burden of Care" chart; Deutsch, Braun, & Granger, 1997; Uniform Data System for Medical Rehabilitation, 1996)

2. Inpatient Rehabilitation Facility Patient Assessment Instrument (**Figure 22-2**)

a. Is the data collection instrument for the Inpatient Rehabilitation Facility Prospective Payment System

b. Required by the CMS to be completed for all Medicare Part A clients admitted to inpatient rehabilitation facilities

c. Has the FIM™ instrument as a core component for rating clients (12 motor items, 5 cognitive items; tub and shower transfer is excluded in determining the CMG)

d. Completed on admission and discharge; admission rating determines the CMG to which the client is assigned, thereby affecting the payment and projected length of stay

e. CMG then determines unadjusted federal prospective payment; additional facility adjusters include the wage index, rural versus urban setting, teaching adjuster, and the low-income client rate.

f. Code 0 (*activity does not occur*) is used for admission only for items not occurring during the 3-day admission assessment timeframe.

g. Can be uploaded into a database to allow facilities to examine factors such as demographic data, diagnoses, and financial information. These databases also allow comparison of FIM™ data over time and with the data of other subscribers.

h. Specific guidelines exist for correctly rating the IRF-PAI. Validity and reliability of raters are critical because they can affect payment.

3. Patient Evaluation and Conference System (**Figure 22-3**)

a. Comprehensive, lengthy interdisciplinary tool that examines 76 distinct functional areas

b. Uses a 7-level scale in which 1 = *most dependent* and 7 = *independent*; 0 = a functional area that is not tested or is unmeasurable

4. PULSES: Represents the initial letters of the categories it measures (Moskowitz, 1957)

a. Physical condition

b. Upper extremities

c. Lower extremities

d. Sensory components

e. Excretory function

f. Social and mental status

5. Functional Assessment Measure (Hall, 1997)

a. Developed to serve as an adjunct to the FIM™ instrument to address some functional items that are essential to brain-injury rehabilitation

b. Measures 12 items including cognitive, behavioral, communication, and community functioning

c. Uses a 7-level scoring method similar to that of the FIM™ instrument

B. ADL Scales (which measure motor and physical elements; Dittmar & Gresham, 1997; **Figure 22-4**)

1. Barthel Index (Mahoney & Barthel, 1965)

a. Uses a 0–100 scoring system (100 = *total independence*, 0 = *dependence*) that assesses 10 domains

b. Is popular in European rehabilitation facilities

c. One of the oldest developed measures of ADLs

2. Kenny Self-Care Evaluation

a. Examines six domains: Transfers, bed activity, feeding, personal hygiene, dressing, and locomotion

b. Uses a 5-level scale in which 0 = *completely dependent* and 4 = *independent*

3. Katz Index of Independence in Activities of Daily Living (Katz, Lord, Moskowitz, Jackson, & Jaffe, 1963): Uses letters (e.g., A = *independent*, G = *dependent*) to score various functional areas

4. Klein-Bell Activity of Daily Living Scale

a. Designed to assess the client's current level of function

b. Includes 170 items in six functional areas: Dressing, elimination, mobility, eating,

Figure 22-2. Patient Assessment Instrument

DEPARTMENT OF HEALTH AND HUMAN SERVICES
CENTERS FOR MEDICARE & MEDICAID SERVICES

Form Approved
OMB No. 0938-0842

INPATIENT REHABILITATION FACILITY – PATIENT ASSESSMENT INSTRUMENT

Identification Information*

1. Facility Information
   A. Facility Name

   _____
   _____
   _____

   B. Facility Medicare
      Provider Number _____

2. Patient Medicare Number _____

3. Patient Medicaid Number _____

4. Patient First Name _____

5A. Patient Last Name _____

5B. Patient Identification Number _____

6. Birth Date _____/_____/_____
                MM / DD / YYYY

7. Social Security Number _____

8. Gender (1 - Male; 2 - Female) _____

9. Race/Ethnicity (Check all that apply)
   American Indian or Alaska Native   A. _____
                             Asian   B. _____
             Black or African American C. _____
                   Hispanic or Latino D. _____
   Native Hawaiian or Other Pacific Islander E. _____
                             White   F. _____

10. Marital Status   _____
    (1 - Never Married; 2 - Married; 3 - Widowed;
    4 - Separated; 5 - Divorced)

11. Zip Code of Patient's Pre-Hospital Residence _____

Admission Information*

12. Admission Date _____/_____/_____
                    MM / DD / YYYY

13. Assessment Reference Date _____/_____/_____
                              MM / DD / YYYY

14. Admission Class   _____
    (1 - Initial Rehab; 2 - Evaluation; 3 - Readmission;
    4 - Unplanned Discharge; 5 - Continuing Rehabilitation)

15. Admit From   _____
    (01 - Home; 02 - Board & Care; 03 - Transitional Living;
    04 - Intermediate Care; 05 - Skilled Nursing Facility;
    06 - Acute Unit of Own Facility; 07 - Acute Unit of Another
    Facility; 08 - Chronic Hospital; 09 - Rehabilitation Facility;
    10 - Other; 12 - Alternate Level of Care Unit; 13 – Subacute
    Setting; 14 - Assisted Living Residence)

16. Pre-Hospital Living Setting   _____
    (Use codes from item 15 above)

17. Pre-Hospital Living With   _____
    (Code only if item 16 is 01 - Home;
    Code using 1 - Alone; 2 - Family/Relatives;
    3 - Friends; 4 - Attendant; 5 - Other)

18. Pre-Hospital Vocational Category   _____
    (1 - Employed; 2 - Sheltered; 3 - Student;
    4 - Homemaker; 5 - Not Working; 6 - Retired for
    Age; 7 - Retired for Disability)

19. Pre-Hospital Vocational Effort   _____
    (Code only if item 18 is coded 1 - 4; Code using
    1 - Full-time; 2 - Part-time; 3 - Adjusted Workload)

Payer Information*

20. Payment Source
    A. Primary Source   _____

    B. Secondary Source   _____

    (01 - Blue Cross; 02 - Medicare non-MCO;
    03 - Medicaid non-MCO; 04 - Commercial Insurance;
    05 - MCO HMO; 06 - Workers' Compensation;
    07 - Crippled Children's Services; 08 – Developmental
    Disabilities Services; 09 - State Vocational Rehabilitation;
    10 - Private Pay; 11 - Employee Courtesy;
    12 - Unreimbursed; 13 - CHAMPUS; 14 - Other;
    15 - None; 16 – No-Fault Auto Insurance;
    51 – Medicare MCO; 52 - Medicaid MCO)

Medical Information*

21. Impairment Group
                              _____   _____
                              Admission   Discharge
    Condition requiring admission to rehabilitation; code
    according to Appendix A, attached.

22. Etiologic Diagnosis   _____
    (Use an ICD-9-CM code to indicate the etiologic problem
    that led to the condition for which the patient is receiving
    rehabilitation)

23. Date of Onset of Impairment _____/_____/_____
                                 MM / DD / YYYY

24. Comorbid Conditions; Use ICD-9-CM codes to enter up to
    ten medical conditions

    A. _____   B. _____

    C. _____   D. _____

    E. _____   F. _____

    G. _____   H. _____

    I. _____   J. _____

Medical Needs

25. Is patient comatose at admission?   _____
                                           0 - No, 1 - Yes

26. Is patient delirious at admission?   _____
                                           0 - No, 1 - Yes

27. Swallowing Status   _____   _____
                                 Admission   Discharge

    3 - Regular Food: solids and liquids swallowed safely
          without supervision or modified food consistency
    2 - Modified Food Consistency/ Supervision: subject
          requires modified food consistency and/or needs
          supervision for safety
    1 - Tube /Parenteral Feeding: tube / parenteral feeding
          used wholly or partially as a means of sustenance

28. Clinical signs of dehydration _____   _____
                                  Admission   Discharge

    (Code 0 – No; 1 – Yes) e.g., evidence of oliguria, dry
    skin, orthostatic hypotension, somnolence, agitation

*The FIM data set, measurement scale and impairment
codes incorporated or referenced herein are the property of
U B Foundation Activities, Inc. ©1993, 2001 U B Foundation
Activities. Inc. The FIM mark is owned by UBFA. Inc.

Form CMS-10036 (01/06)

1
continued

Figure 22-2. Patient Assessment Instrument *continued*

DEPARTMENT OF HEALTH AND HUMAN SERVICES
CENTERS FOR MEDICARE & MEDICAID SERVICES

INPATIENT REHABILITATION FACILITY – PATIENT ASSESSMENT INSTRUMENT

Function Modifiers*

Complete the following specific functional items prior to scoring the FIM™ Instrument:

	ADMISSION	DISCHARGE
29. Bladder Level of Assistance (Score using FIM Levels 1 - 7)	☐	☐
30. Bladder Frequency of Accidents (Score as below)	☐	☐

7 - No accidents
6 - No accidents; uses device such as a catheter
5 - One accident in the past 7 days
4 - Two accidents in the past 7 days
3 - Three accidents in the past 7 days
2 - Four accidents in the past 7 days
1 - Five or more accidents in the past 7 days

Enter in Item 39G (Bladder) the lower (more dependent) score from Items 29 and 30 above.

	ADMISSION	DISCHARGE
31. Bowel Level of Assistance (Score using FIM Levels 1 - 7)	☐	☐
32. Bowel Frequency of Accidents (Score as below)	☐	☐

7 - No accidents
6 - No accidents; uses device such as an ostomy
5 - One accident in the past 7 days
4 - Two accidents in the past 7 days
3 - Three accidents in the past 7 days
2 - Four accidents in the past 7 days
1 - Five or more accidents in the past 7 days

Enter in Item 39H (Bowel) the lower (more dependent) score of Items 31 and 32 above.

	ADMISSION	DISCHARGE
33. Tub Transfer	☐	☐
34. Shower Transfer	☐	☐

(Score Items 33 and 34 using FIM Levels 1 - 7; use 0 if activity does not occur) See training manual for scoring of Item 39K (Tub/Shower Transfer)

	ADMISSION	DISCHARGE
35. Distance Walked	☐	☐
36. Distance Traveled in Wheelchair	☐	☐

(Code items 35 and 36 using: 3 - 150 feet; 2 - 50 to 149 feet; 1 - Less than 50 feet; 0 – activity does not occur)

	ADMISSION	DISCHARGE
37. Walk	☐	☐
38. Wheelchair	☐	☐

(Score Items 37 and 38 using FIM Levels 1 - 7; 0 if activity does not occur) See training manual for scoring of Item 39L (Walk/Wheelchair)

*The FIM data set, measurement scale and impairment codes incorporated or referenced herein are the property of U B Foundation Activities, Inc. ©1993, 2001 U B Foundation Activities, Inc. The FIM mark is owned by UBFA, Inc.

39. FIM™ Instrument*

	ADMISSION	DISCHARGE	GOAL
SELF-CARE			
A. Eating	☐	☐	☐
B. Grooming	☐	☐	☐
C. Bathing	☐	☐	☐
D. Dressing - Upper	☐	☐	☐
E. Dressing - Lower	☐	☐	☐
F. Toileting	☐	☐	☐
SPHINCTER CONTROL			
G. Bladder	☐	☐	☐
H. Bowel	☐	☐	☐
TRANSFERS			
I. Bed, Chair, Wheelchair	☐	☐	☐
J. Toilet	☐	☐	☐
K. Tub, Shower	☐	☐	☐

W - Walk
C - wheelChair
B - Both

LOCOMOTION	ADMISSION	DISCHARGE	GOAL
L. Walk/Wheelchair	☐☐	☐☐	☐
M. Stairs	☐	☐	☐

A - Auditory
V - Visual
B - Both

COMMUNICATION	ADMISSION	DISCHARGE	GOAL
N. Comprehension	☐☐	☐☐	☐
O. Expression	☐☐	☐☐	☐

V - Vocal
N - Nonvocal
B - Both

SOCIAL COGNITION	ADMISSION	DISCHARGE	GOAL
P. Social Interaction	☐	☐	☐
Q. Problem Solving	☐	☐	☐
R. Memory	☐	☐	☐

FIM LEVELS

No Helper
7 Complete Independence (Timely, Safely)

6 Modified Independence (Device)

Helper - Modified Dependence
5 Supervision (Subject = 100%)

4 Minimal Assistance (Subject = 75% or more)

3 Moderate Assistance (Subject = 50% or more)

Helper - Complete Dependence
2 Maximal Assistance (Subject = 25% or more)

1 Total Assistance (Subject less than 25%)

0 Activity does not occur; Use this code only at admission

Form CMS-10036 (01/06)

2

continued

Figure 22-2. Patient Assessment Instrument *continued*

DEPARTMENT OF HEALTH AND HUMAN SERVICES
CENTERS FOR MEDICARE & MEDICAID SERVICES

INPATIENT REHABILITATION FACILITY – PATIENT ASSESSMENT INSTRUMENT

Discharge Information*

40. Discharge Date   ____/____/____
MM / DD / YYYY

41. Patient discharged against medical advice? _____
(0 - No, 1 -Yes)

42. Program Interruption(s) _____
(0 - No; 1 - Yes)

43. Program Interruption Dates
(Code only if Item 42 is 1 - Yes)

A. 1st Interruption Date
[_____]
MM / DD / YYYY

B. 1st Return Date
[_____]
MM / DD / YYYY

C. 2nd Interruption Date
[_____]
MM / DD / YYYY

D. 2nd Return Date
[_____]
MM / DD / YYYY

E. 3rd Interruption Date
[_____]
MM / DD / YYYY

F. 3rd Return Date
[_____]
MM / DD / YYYY

44A. Discharge to Living Setting _____
(01 - Home; 02 - Board and Care; 03 - Transitional Living; 04 - Intermediate Care; 05 - Skilled Nursing Facility; 06 - Acute Unit of Own Facility; 07 - Acute Unit of Another Facility; 08 - Chronic Hospital; 09 - Rehabilitation Facility; 10 - Other; 11 - Died; 12 - Alternate Level of Care Unit; 13 - Subacute Setting; 14 - Assisted Living Residence)

44B. Was patient discharged with Home Health Services? _____
(0 - No; 1 - Yes)
(Code only if Item 44A is 01 - Home, 02 - Board and Care, 03 - Transitional Living, or 14 - Assisted Living Residence)

45. Discharge to Living With _____
(Code only if Item 44A is 01 - Home; Code using 1 - Alone; 2 - Family / Relatives; 3 - Friends; 4 - Attendant; 5 - Other

46. Diagnosis for Interruption or Death _____
(Code using ICD-9-CM code)

47. Complications during rehabilitation stay
(Use ICD-9-CM codes to specify up to six conditions that began with this rehabilitation stay)

A. _____   B. _____

C. _____   D. _____

E. _____   F. _____

Quality Indicators

RESPIRATORY STATUS
(Score items 48 to 50 as 0 - No; 1 - Yes)

	Admission	Discharge
48. Shortness of breath with exertion	_____	_____
49. Shortness of breath at rest	_____	_____
50. Weak cough and difficulty clearing airway secretions	_____	_____

* The FIM data set, measurement scale and impairment codes incorporated or referenced herein are the property of U B Foundation Activities, Inc. ©1993, 2001 U B Foundation Activities, Inc. The FIM mark is owned by UBFA, Inc.

Quality Indicators

PAIN
51. Rate the highest level of pain reported by the patient within the assessment period:
Admission: _____ Discharge: _____

(Score using the scale below; report whole numbers only)

0   1   2   3   4   5   6   7   8   9   10
No Pain   Moderate Pain   Worst Possible Pain

Pressure Ulcers

52A. Highest current pressure ulcer stage
Admission _____ Discharge _____

(0 - No pressure ulcer; 1 - Any area of persistent skin redness (Stage 1); 2 - Partial loss of skin layers (Stage 2); 3 - Deep craters in the skin (Stage 3); 4 - Breaks in skin exposing muscle or bone (Stage 4); 5 - Not stageable (necrotic eschar predominant; no prior staging available)

52B. Number of current pressure ulcers
Admission _____ Discharge _____

PUSH Tool v. 3.0 ©

SELECT THE CURRENT LARGEST PRESSURE ULCER TO CODE THE FOLLOWING. Calculate three components (C through E) and code total score in F.

52C. Length multiplied by width (open wound surface area)
Admission _____ Discharge _____

(Score as   0 - 0 cm²; 1 - < 0.3 cm²; 2 - 0.3 to 0.6 cm²; 3 - 0.7 to 1.0 cm²; 4 - 1.1 to 2.0 cm²; 5 - 2.1 to 3.0 cm²; 6 - 3.1 to 4.0 cm²; 7 - 4.1 to 8.0 cm²; 8 - 8.1 to 12.0 cm²; 9 - 12.1 to 24.0 cm²; 10 - > 24 cm²)

52D. Exudate amount
Admission _____ Discharge _____
0 - None; 1 - Light; 2 - Moderate; 3 - Heavy

52E. Tissue type
Admission _____ Discharge _____
0 - Closed/resurfaced: The wound is completely covered with epithelium (new skin); 1 - Epithelial tissue: For superficial ulcers, new pink or shiny tissue (skin) that grows in from the edges or as islands on the ulcer surface. 2 - Granulation tissue: Pink or beefy red tissue with a shiny, moist, granular appearance. 3- Slough: Yellow or white tissue that adheres to the ulcer bed in strings or thick clumps or is mucinous. 4 - Necrotic tissue (eschar): Black, brown, or tan tissue that adheres firmly to the wound bed or ulcer edges.

52F. TOTAL PUSH SCORE (Sum of above three items -- C, D and E)
Admission _____ Discharge _____

SAFETY   Admission   Discharge

53. Balance problem   _____   _____
(0 - No; 1 - Yes)
e.g., dizziness, vertigo, or light-headedness
                                              Discharge
54. Total number of falls during the rehabilitation stay   _____

Figure 22-3. Listing of Patient Evaluation and Conference System Items and Item Groupings

I. **Rehabilitation Medicine (MED)**
1. Motor Loss
2. Spasticity/Involuntary Movement
3. Joint Limitations
4. Autonomic Disturbance
5. Sensory Deficiency
6. Perceptual & Cognitive Deficits
7. Associated Medical Problems
8. Postural Deviations

II. **Rehabilitation Nursing (NSG)**
1. Performance of Bowel Program
2. Performance of Urinary Program
3. Performance of Skin Care Program
4. Assumes Responsibility for Self-care
5. Performs Assigned Interdisciplinary Activities
6. Patient Education
7. Safety Awareness

III. **Physical Mobility (PHY)**
1. Performance of Transfers
2. Performance of Ambulation
3. Performance of Wheelchair Mobility
4. Ability to Handle Environmental Barriers (e.g., stairs, rugs, elevators)
5. Performance of Car Transfer
6. Driving Mobility
7. Assumes Responsibility for Mobility
8. Position Changes
9. Endurance
10. Balance

IV. **Activities of Daily Living (ADL)**
1. Performance in Feeding
2. Performance in Hygiene/Grooming
3. Performance in Dressing
4. Performance in Home Management
5. Performance of Mobility in the Home Environment (including utilization of environmental adaptations for communication)
6. Bathroom Transfers

V. **Communication (COM)**
1. Ability to Comprehend Spoken Language
2. Ability to Produce Language
3. Ability to Read
4. Ability to Produce Written Language
5. Ability to Hear
6. Ability to Comprehend and Use Gesture
7. Ability to Produce Speech
8. Ability to Swallow
9. Impairment in Thought (Verbal Linguistic) Processing (NP4)

VI. **Medications (DRG)**
1. Knowledge of Medications

VII. **Nutrition (NUT)**
1. Nutritional Status—Body Weight
2. Nutritional Status—Lab Values
3. Knowledge of Nutrition and/or Modified Diet
4. Skill with Nutrition & Diet (Adherence to Nutritional Plan)
5. Utilization of Nutrition & Diet (Nutritional Health)

VIII. **Assistive Devices (DEV)**
1. Knowledge of Assistive Mobility Devices

2. Skill with Assuming Operating Position of Assistive Mobility Devices
3. Utilization of Assistive Mobility Devices

IX. **Psychology (PSY)**
1. Distress/comfort
2. Helplessness/self-efficacy
3. Self-directed Learning Skills
4. Skill in Self-management of Behavior and Emotions
5. Skill in Interpersonal Relations
6. Ability to Participate in the Rehabilitation Program
7. Acceptance/understanding of Disability

X. **Neuropsychology (NP)**
1. Impairment of Short-term Memory
2. Impairment of Long-term Memory
3. Impairment in Attention-concentration Skills
4. Impairment in Verbal Linguistic Processing
5. Impairment in Visual Spatial Processing
6. Impairment in Basic Intellectual Skills
7. Orientation
8. Alertness/Coma State

XI. **Social Issues (SOC)**
1. Ability to Problem Solve and Utilize Resources
2. Family: Communication/Resources
3. Family: Understanding of Disability
4. Economic Resources
5. Ability to Live Independently
6. Living Arrangements

XII. **Vocational/Educational Activity (V/E)**
1. Active Participation in realistic Voc/Ed Planning
2. Realistic Perception of Work-related activity
3. Ability to Tolerate Planned Number of Hours of Voc/Ed
4. Vocational/Educational Placement
5. Physical Capacity for Work

XIII. **Therapeutic Recreation (REC)**
1. Participation in Group Activities
2. Participation in Community Activities
3. Interaction with Others
4. Participation and Satisfaction with Individual Leisure Activities
5. Active Participation in Sports

XIV. **Pain (PAI)**
1. Pain Behavior
2. Physical Activity
3. Social Interaction
4. Pacing
5. Sitting Tolerance
6. Standing Tolerance
7. Walking Tolerance
8. Use of Body Mechanics
9. Use of Relaxation Techniques
10. Performance of Medication Program

XVI. **Pastoral Care (PC)**
1. Awareness of Spiritual Dimensions of Illness/Disability
2. Knowledge of Spiritual Resources
3. Skill in Self-management of Spirituality
4. Utilization of Spiritual Resources

Figure 22-4. Characteristics of Selected Activity of Daily Living (ADL) Scales

Scale	Items Included	Type of Scale	Evaluation
Katz Index of ADL	Bathing, dressing, toileting, transferring, continence, feeding; order of items reflects natural progression in loss and acquisition of function	Dichotomous rating of independence or dependence on each item; forms a six-level Guttman Scale	By professional raters
Kenny Self-Care Evaluation	Seventeen activities in six categories: bed activities, transfers, locomotion, personal hygiene, dressing, and feeding	Each activity rated on a four-point scale (0= complete dependence, 4= complete independence); an average score is created for each of six categories, allowing a possible total score of 24	By rehabilitation staff; scores constructed on the basis of observations
Barthel Index	Feeding, transferring, grooming, toileting, bathing, walking, or propelling a wheelchair; climbing stairs, bladder control, bowel control	Partial scores for performing ADLs with help, full score for independent performance; items weighted; full score of 100 signifies ability to do all tasks independently	By rehabilitation staff

Jacelon, C. S. (1986). The Barthel Index: A review of the literature. *Rehabilitation Nursing, 11*(4), 9–11.

bathing and hygiene, and emergency telephone communication

    5. Quadriplegia Index Function
      a. Is specific to people with quadriplegia
      b. Involves the domains of transfers, grooming, bathing, feeding, dressing, wheelchair mobility, bed activity, bladder program, bowel program, and understanding of personal care for a total of 37 items
      c. Uses a 5-level scale in which 4 = *independent* and 0 = *dependent*; 9 = *not applicable*

C. Instrumental Activities of Daily Living (IADLs) Scale (Dittmar & Gresham, 1997)
    1. Encompasses activities that go beyond basic ADLs
    2. IADLs include doing laundry, shopping, preparing meals, using a phone, and managing finances.

D. Scales That Measure the Effects of Primary and Secondary Handicaps
    1. Community Integration Questionnaire, a 15-item tool that assesses home integration, social integration, and productive activity (Willer, Ottenbacher, & Coad, 1994)

    2. Craig Handicap Assessment Reporting Technique (Hall, Dukers, Whiteneck, Brooks, & Krause, 1998)
      a. Designed to assess the reintegration of people with spinal cord injury
      b. Includes 32 items categorized into six dimensions (physical independence, cognitive independence, mobility, occupation, social integration, and economic self-sufficiency)
      c. Has a maximum score of 100 for each dimension

E. Pediatric Tools
    1. WeeFIM™ instrument (**Figure 22-5**; Braun, 1998)
      a. Designed for children age 6 months–7 years and older
      b. Derived from the FIM™ instrument
      c. Can be used by members of any discipline
      d. Measures actual performance across various settings
      e. The 0–3 Module (optional) of the WeeFIM™ instrument is designed to measure precursors to function in children ages 0–3 years who have a variety of disabilities.
        1) Intended to complement the WeeFIM™ instrument by measuring early functional performance and changes in performance over time
        2) Used across many settings, including early intervention and preschool
    2. Pediatric Evaluation of Disability Inventory (Haley, 1999)
      a. Provides an assessment of key functional areas in children between the ages of 6 months and 7 years
      b. Examines performance in three domains: self-care, mobility, and social function
    3. Home Observation for Measurement of the Environment (Caldwell & Bradley, 1977)
      a. Initial version consists of 45 items
      b. Designed to measure the quality and quantity of stimulation and support available to a child in the home environment
      c. Bases data collection on actual observation

F. Outpatient Tools
    1. LIFEware℠ assessment tools (Granger, 1999)
      a. Designed for outpatient medical rehabilitation programs
      b. Examines physical function, pain, affective well-being, and cognitive functioning
      c. Customized for various client populations
    2. Focus on Therapeutic Outcomes (Dobrzykowski & Nance, 1997)
      a. Created in 1992 as an outcome measurement system for outpatient orthopedic rehabilitation

b. Monitors the efficiency and effectiveness in the outpatient orthopedic population

3. Short Form 36, developed to assess a client's well-being and perception of overall health (Ware & Sherbourne, 1992)

G. Home Environment Tools: Outcome and Assessment Information Set

1. Mandated by the CMS for use in home care

2. Has 100 questions covering 14 categories of care (e.g., ambulation, management of medication, psychological and emotional behavior, living arrangements)

3. Involves data information being sent to state agencies

4. Is a standardized measurement for monitoring outcomes of adults in the home setting

5. Serves as the data collection instrument for prospective payment systems

6. Monitors the quality of home health care

H. Other Tools

1. Minimum Data Set (MDS) assessment (Refer to Chapter 21.)

a. Mandated by CMS for use in long-term care and subacute or postacute settings

b. Serves as the data collection instrument for prospective payment systems

c. Uses Resource Utilization Groups, Version IV, a 66-group client classification system in which periodic assessments are done

d. Involves client information being sent to the fiscal intermediaries for reimbursement and MDS information being sent to state survey and certification agencies (Medicare Payment Advisory Commission, 1999)

Figure 22-5. WeeFIM™ Instrument

WeeFIM™ Instrument

L E V E L S	7 Complete Independence (timely, safely) 6 Modified Independence (device)	**NO HELPER**
	Modified Dependence 5 Supervision (subject = 100%) 4 Minimal Assistance (subject = 75%+) 3 Moderate Assistance (subject = 50%+) **Complete Dependence** 2 Maximal Assistance (subject =25%+) 1 Total Assistance (subject = less than 25%)	**HELPER**

Self-Care   ASSESSMENT   GOAL
A. Eating
B. Grooming
C. Bathing
D. Dressing - Upper Body
E. Dressing - Lower Body
F. Toileting
G. Bladder
H. Bowel

Self-Care Total

Mobility
I. Chair, Wheelchair
J. Toilet
K. Tub, Shower   W Walk
L. Walk, Wheelchair   C Wheelchair
M. Stairs   L Crawl   B Combination

Mobility Total

MOTOR SUBTOTAL RATING

Cognition   A Auditory   V Visual   B Both
N. Comprehension
O. Expression   V Vocal
P. Social Interaction   N Nonvocal
Q. Problem Solving   B Both
R. Memory

Cognition Total

WEEFIM® TOTAL RATING

NOTE: Leave no blanks. Enter 1 if patient is not testable due to risk.

2. Nursing home quality measures: The nursing home quality measures come from resident assessment data that nursing homes routinely collect on residents at specified intervals during their stay. These measures assess the resident's physical and clinical conditions and abilities, preferences, and life-care wishes. These assessment data have been converted to develop quality measures that give consumers another source of information about how well nursing homes are caring for their residents' physical and clinical needs. The quality measures have four intended purposes:
    a. To give information about the care at nursing homes to help people choose a nursing home for themselves or others
    b. To give information about the care at nursing homes where people already live
    c. To get people to talk to nursing home staff about the quality of care
    d. To give data to the nursing home to help them with their quality-improvement efforts

V. Program Evaluation
A. Overview
1. Program evaluation is a systematic method for collecting, analyzing, and using information to evaluate and improve a particular program.
2. Performance indicators play a key role in the development of a successful outcome system.
3. Performance indicators are quantitative values that can be collected by providers and reported to various stakeholders.

B. General Considerations
1. When assessing the efficiency, effectiveness, and other critical outcomes of rehabilitation, an organization must use a system for evaluation that has demonstrated reliability and validity.
    a. Reliability: Reproducibility of an instrument's findings
    b. Validity: Ability of the tool to measure what it was designed or intended to measure
2. Data collection instruments and systems used by rehabilitation programs should be valid and reliable so accurate performance can be identified.
3. Development of a successful program evaluation and outcome system with an emphasis on rehabilitation nursing interventions should include specific critical design elements.
    a. Functional status: Documents the rehabilitation gains of physical function
    b. Discharge destination: Determines whether discharge to the community or to the least restrictive environment has been achieved

c. Efficiency: The extent to which a specific intervention, procedure, regimen, or service, when applied in routine circumstances, does what it is intended to do for a specific population (Last, 1995)
d. Client perception: Satisfaction of the client, family, and other stakeholders
e. Effectiveness: The end results achieved in relation to the resources (e.g., money, time) expended (Last, 1995)
f. Follow-up: Determines whether progress was made or maintained after discharge from a rehabilitation program

VI. Quality and Performance Improvement in Health Care
A. Overview
1. Definition of quality improvement: "A management process or approach to continuous study and improvement of the processes of providing healthcare services to meet the needs of individuals and others" (JCAHO, 1999)
2. To Err Is Human: Building a Safer Health System (Institute of Medicine [IOM], 2000)
    a. IOM report that was intended to be a roadmap to a safer healthcare system
    b. Reports that thousands of Americans die each year from preventable medical errors
    c. Belief that with adequate leadership, attention, and resources improvement can be made
3. Crossing the Quality Chasm: A New Health System for the 21st Century (IOM, 2001)
    a. Presents a comprehensive plan to reinvent the healthcare system to foster innovation and improve delivery of care
    b. Health care needs to be safe, effective, client centered, timely, efficient, and equitable
    c. Ten rules for redesign
        1) Care is based on continuous healing relationships.
        2) Care is customized according to client needs and values.
        3) The client is the source of control.
        4) Knowledge is shared, and information flows freely.
        5) Decision making is evidence based.
        6) Safety is a system property.
        7) Transparency is necessary.
        8) Needs are anticipated.
        9) Waste is continuously decreased.
        10) Cooperation between clinicians is a priority.

B. Tools for Quality Improvement (Brassard & Ritter, 1994)
   1. Brainstorming allows team members to create as many creative ideas and solutions as possible; all suggestions are recorded to be evaluated at a later time.
   2. A cause-and-effect diagram (fishbone diagram) allows team members to visually and graphically explore the relationship between the effects and possible causes of identified problems.
   3. An affinity diagram gathers large amounts of data and helps organize the information into groupings based on the relationships between the items.
   4. A check sheet allows team members to record and collect data from various sources so patterns and trends may be identified.
   5. A run chart is used to visually display data and to identify any changes that occur.
   6. A histogram displays the distribution of data and reveals the amount of variation within a process.
   7. A scatter diagram is used to study the possible cause-and-effect relationship between two variables.
   8. A control chart is used to monitor, control, and improve variances in performance by identifying the source; it is similar to a run chart but with statistical upper and lower limits.
   9. A flowchart is a pictorial representation of various steps of a process that allows team members to easily identify the flow of events.
   10. A force field analysis identifies the forces in place that affect an issue or problem; ideally, it reinforces positives and eliminates negatives.
   11. A pareto chart is a display of bar graphs that can help focus on and determine which problems to solve and in which order so that efforts are directed to the problems that have the greatest improvement potential.
C. Models for Performance Improvement
   1. Plan, Do, Check, Act approach
      a. Plan what you want to accomplish.
      b. Do what you planned to do.
      c. Check the results.
      d. Act on the information.
   2. Failure Mode Effects Analysis: Systematic, proactive approach to evaluating a process
      a. Identify all steps of a process.
      b. Identify when and how the steps might fail.
      c. Assess the impact of each potential failure.
      d. Identify which steps are in most in need of change.
   3. Six Sigma
      a. The focus is on reducing variation, then improving process capability.
      b. Certification is available through the Institute of Industrial Engineers and the American Society for Quality.
   4. Lean Approach
      a. A Toyota production system model designed to improve efficiency and effectiveness though process redesign
      b. Rules of Lean
         1) Structure every activity.
         2) Clearly connect every customer or supplier.
         3) Specify every flow path.
         4) Improve through experimentation toward the ideal state.
      c. Lean requires that participants in the process come to high-level agreement.
      d. Tools
         1) Waste elimination: Identify potential wastes (multiple handoffs, many people doing the same thing, paper versus automated processes).
         2) Five Ss: Separate, sweep, sort, sanitize, sustain
         3) Standardized work: Everyone does the process the same way.
         4) Process mapping (*kaizen*): A way of looking at a process by identifying every step of the process, then identifying wastes, and coming to high-level agreement on a new process
         5) Visual management: The use of signage to label spaces so that objects are put back in the same place every time
         6) Problem solving
D. National Quality Forum (NQF)
   1. The NQF is a voluntary consensus standard-setting organization.
   2. The mission of the NQF is to improve the quality of American health care by setting national priorities and goals for performance improvement, endorsing national consensus standards for measuring and publicly reporting on performance, and promoting the attainment of national goals through education and outreach programs.
   3. The National Data Base of Nursing Quality Indicators contains data for the following indicators:
      a. Nursing staff skill mix
      b. Nursing hours per client day
      c. Assault and injury rates
      d. Catheter-associated urinary tract infection rate

e. Central line–associated bloodstream infection rate

f. Fall and injury rates

g. Hospital- or unit-acquired pressure ulcer rates

h. Nurse turnover rate

i. Pain assessment-intervention-reassessment cycles completed

j. Peripheral intravenous line infiltration rate

k. Physical restraint prevalence

l. Registered nurse education and certification

m. Registered nurse survey

n. Practice environment scale

o. Job satisfaction

p. Ventilator-associated pneumonia rate

VII. Theories of Outcome Evaluation

Interventions to affect outcomes operate at different levels (e.g., individual, team, organization, and system or environment of care). Depending on the level at which the intervention is focused, different theories may be relevant (Eccles, Grimshaw, Walker, Johnston, & Pitts, 2005).

Interventions at the individual and team levels are best served by theories of individual behavior, such as behavior change theory (Schulte, 2007) and Rogers's diffusion theory (Rogers, 1983).

Interventions at the organization or system levels are best served by theories of organizational change (Eccles et al., 2005) such as Lewin's change theory (Yukl, 2006) or the ecological theory of organizational change (Hannan & Freeman, 1984).

A. Quality Health Outcomes Model (Mitchell, Ferketich, & Jennings, 1998)

1. Components: system, outcomes, client, interventions

2. Interventions must act through the system and client to affect the outcome.

3. Five categories of outcomes: achievement of appropriate self-care, demonstration of health-promoting behaviors, health-related quality of life, perception of being well cared for, and symptom management

B. Outcomes Theory (Duignan, 2005)

1. Components: Outcome hierarchies, outcome systems.

2. Outcome hierarchies are a cascading set of causes and effects, viewed as elements that can be caused by other elements and can cause other elements to occur or not occur.

3. Outcome systems attempt to provide frameworks within which interventions occur. They are directed toward maximizing the achievement of outcomes. Evidence-based practice is an example of an outcome system.

4. Outcomes can differ based on their characteristics.

a. Influencibility: Extent to which an intervention can influence the outcome

b. Controllability: Extent to which the intervention is the only major factor influencing the outcome

c. Measurability: Extent to which the outcome can be measured

d. Attributability: Extent to which changes in the outcome can be attributed to the intervention

e. Accountability: Extent to which the organization is sanctioned (positively or negatively) based on the change or lack of change in the outcome

f. Response consistency: Extent to which the outcome varies in a consistent manner in response to its causes

g. Lag: Time delay between the cause and the outcome

VIII. The Future of Outcome Management

A. Increasing Importance of Outcomes

1. Outcomes across the continuum will continue to have greater importance.

2. CMS has proposed quality measures for rehabilitation facilities (CMS, 2011).

3. Computer adaptive testing is a potential alternative to traditional assessment instruments.

4. The emphasis of satisfaction will move from provider to payer to client or consumer (Jones & Evans, 1998).

a. Satisfaction is evidenced by disclosure statements, which have a great influence in rehabilitation.

b. Example: CARF's medical rehabilitation division maintains a public disclosure policy in which a person may request an organization's survey summary and CARF provides the summary to the person at no charge. This meets the "need to know" element for various stakeholders (e.g., consumers).

B. Greater Accountability to Stakeholders

1. Rehabilitation providers are experiencing an increase in accountability to demonstrate positive outcomes.

2. Rehabilitation providers are increasingly expected to share information about programs and outcomes.

C. Increased Focus on Measuring and Monitoring Outcomes

1. Measuring and monitoring outcomes and the quality and durability of outcomes will become an even larger component of rehabilitation nursing practice.
2. Management of clients' needs across the continuum will be critical for successful chronic disease management.
3. Rehabilitation nurses have the skills and knowledge to improve outcomes for clients.

References

Black, T. M. (1999). Outcomes: What's all the fuss about? *Rehabilitation Nursing, 24*(5), 188–189, 191.

Brassard, M., & Ritter, D. (1994). *The Memory Jogger IITM: A pocket guide of tools for continuous improvement and effective planning.* Methuen, MA: Goal/QPC.

Braun, S. (1998). The Functional Independence Measure for children (WeeFIM^SM instrument): Gateway to the WeeFIM™ system. *Journal of Rehabilitation Outcomes Measurement, 2*(4), 63–68.

Caldwell, B., & Bradley, R. (1977). Home observation for measurement of the environment: A validation study of screening efficiency. *American Journal of Mental Deficiency, 84,* 235–244.

Centers for Medicare & Medicaid Services. (2011, April). Medicare program; Inpatient rehabilitation facility prospective payment system for federal year 2012: A proposed rule.

Commission on Accreditation of Rehabilitation Facilities. (2006). *Standards manual for medical rehabilitation.* Tucson, AZ: Author.

Commission on Accreditation of Rehabilitation Facilities. (2011). CARF's mission, vision, core values, and purposes. Retrieved July 27, 2011, from www.carf.org/about/mission/.

Deutsch, A., Braun, S., & Granger, C. V. (1997). The Functional Independence Measure (FIM™) instrument. *Journal of Rehabilitation Outcomes, 1*(2), 67–71.

Dittmar, S., & Gresham, G. (1997). Appendix A: Description and display of selected functional assessment and outcome measures in physical rehabilitation. In *Functional assessment and outcome measurement for the rehabilitation healthcare professional* (pp. 90–138). Gaithersburg, MD: Aspen.

Dobrzykowski, E., & Nance, T. (1997). The Focus on Therapeutic Outcomes (FOTO) outpatient orthopedic rehabilitation database: Results of 1994–1996. *Journal of Rehabilitation Outcomes Measurement, 1*(1), 56–60.

Duignan, P. (2005). *Outcomes theory knowledge base* (Organizational; pp. 1–3). Retrieved December 10, 2010, from http://knol.google.com/k/introduction-to-outcomes-theory.

Eccles, M., Grimshaw, J., Walker, A., Johnston, M., & Pitts, N. (2005). Changing the behaviour of healthcare professionals: The use of theory in promoting the uptake of research findings. *Journal of Clinical Epidemiology, 58,* 107–112.

Granger, C. (1999). The LIFEware system. *Journal of Rehabilitation Outcomes Measurement, 3*(2), 63–69.

Haley, S. (1999). The Pediatric Evaluation of Disability Inventory (PEDI). *Journal of Rehabilitation Outcomes, 1*(1), 61–69.

Hall, K. (1997). The Functional Assessment Measure (FAM). *Journal of Rehabilitation Outcomes Measurement, 1*(3), 63–65.

Hall, K., Dukers, M., Whiteneck, G., Brooks, C.A., & Krause, J. (1998). The Craig Handicap Assessment and Reporting Technique (CHART): Metric properties and scoring. *Journal of Rehabilitation Outcomes Measurement, 2*(5), 39–49.

Hannan, M., & Freeman, J. (1984). Structural inertia and organizational change. *American Sociological Review, 49,* 149–164.

Institute of Medicine. (2000). *To err is human: Building a safer health system.* Washington, DC: National Academy Press.

Institute of Medicine. (2001). *Crossing the quality chasm: A new health system for the 21st century.* Washington, DC: National Academy Press.

Jacelon, C. S. (1986). The Barthel Index: A review of the literature. *Rehabilitation Nursing, 11*(4), 9–11.

The Joint Commission. (2009). Mission statement. Retrieved from July 27, 2011, from www.jointcommission.org/assets/1/18/mission_statement_8_09.pdf.

Joint Commission on Accreditation of Healthcare Organizations. (1999). *1999 accreditation manual for hospitals.* Oakbrook Terrace, IL: Author.

Jones, M., & Evans, R. (1998). Outcomes in a managed care environment. *Topics in Spinal Cord Injury Rehabilitation, 3*(4), 61–73.

Katz, S., Lord, A. B., Moskowitz, R. W., Jackson, B. A., & Jaffe, M. W. (1963). Studies of illness in the aged. The index of ADL: A standardized measure of biological and psychological function. *Journal of the American Medical Association, 185,* 914–919.

Last, J. M. (1995). *Dictionary of epidemiology* (3rd ed.). New York: Oxford University Press.

Mahoney, F. I., & Barthel, D. (1965). Functional evaluation: The Barthel Index. *Maryland State Medical Journal, 14,* 56–61.

Medicare Payment Advisory Commission. (1999, March). Post acute care providers: Moving toward prospective payment. In *Report to Congress: Medicare payment policy* (pp. 81–98). Washington, DC: Author.

Mitchell, P. H., Ferketich, S., & Jennings, B. M. (1998). Quality health outcomes model. *Journal of Nursing Scholarship, 1*(30), 43–46.

Moskowitz, E., & McCann, C. B. (1957). Classification of disability in the chronically ill and aging. *Journal of Chronic Disease, 5,* 342–346.

Porter, M. (2010). What is value in healthcare? *New England Journal of Medicine* (pp. 1–5). Retrieved December 8, 2010, from www.nejm.org/doi/pdf/10.1056/NEJMc1101108.

Ransom, S. B., Joshi, M. S., & Nash, D. B. (Eds.). (2005). *The healthcare quality book.* Chicago: Health Administration Press.

Rogers, E. (1983). *Diffusion of innovations.* New York: Free Press.

Schulte, S. K. (2007). Avoiding culture shock: Using behavior change theory to implement quality improvement programs. *Journal of AHIMA, 78*(4), 52–56.

Uniform Data System for Medical Rehabilitation. (1996). *Guide for the Uniform Data Set for Medical Rehabilitation.* Buffalo: State University of New York.

Ware, J. E., & Sherbourne, C. D. (1992). The MOS 36-item short health survey (SF-36): Conceptual framework and item selection. *Medical Care, 30,* 472–480.

Willer, B., Ottenbacher, K., & Coad, M. L. (1994). The Community Integration Questionnaire. *American Journal of Physical Medicine and Rehabilitation, 73*(2), 103–111.

World Health Organization. (2001). *International classification of functioning, disability and health (ICF).* Geneva, Switzerland: Author.

Yukl, G. (2006). *Leadership in organizations* (6th ed.). Albany, NY: Prentice Hall.

Suggested Resources

Agency for Healthcare Research and Quality: www.ahrq.gov

American Nurses Association Nursing World: www.nursingworld.org

Hoeman, S. (Ed.). (1996). *Rehabilitation nursing: Process and application* (2nd ed.). St. Louis: Mosby.

Institute for Healthcare Improvement: www.IHI.org

National Database of Nursing Quality Indicators: www.nursingquality.org

Roberts, S., Wells, R., Brown, I., Bryant, J., Hutchinson, H. T., Kurushima, C., et al. (1999). The FRESNO: A pediatric functional outcome measurement system. *Journal of Rehabilitation Outcomes, 3*(1), 11–19.

WeeFIM™ Guide: Uniform Data System for Medical Rehabilitation. (2005). *The WeeFIM™ II system clinical guide* (version 6.0). Buffalo, NY: UDSMR.

Wilkerson, D. (1997, Winter). On the language and classification of disablement and a new ICIDH. *American Congress of Rehabilitation Medicine Newsletter,* 5–7.

Copies of *Crossing the Quality Chasm: A New Health System for the 21st Century* are available for sale from the National Academies Press; call 800.624.6242 or 202.334.3313 (in the Washington, DC, metropolitan area), or visit the NAP home page at www.nap.edu. The full text of this report is available at www.nap.edu/books/0309072808/html/.

Copies of *To Err Is Human: Building a Safer Health System* are available for sale from the National Academies Press; call 800.624.6242 or 202.334.3313 (in the Washington, DC, metropolitan area), or visit the NAP home page at www.nap.edu. The full text of this report is available at www.nap.edu/books/0309068371/html/.

Index

globalization and, 526
of healthcare, 513–527, 514*t*
Edema, 479
Education. *See also* Caregivers; Client
education
assessment of, 238
disability laws, 45*f*
nursing shortages and, 26
prevalence of disability and, 77
Edwards, Patricia, 21
Efavirenz (Sustiva), 411
Effectiveness, ethics, 47
Effort syndrome, 348
Ego, 434
Egyptians, 15
Elastin, production of, 111
Elder abuse. *See also* Older clients
abusers, 494–495
nursing interventions, 495
prevention of, 495*f*
signs of, 495
victims, 495
Electrical burns, 339, 342
Electronic medical records, 25
Electrotherapy, 17
Elimination. *See also* Bladder function;
Bowel function
in ALS, 207–208
assessment of, 237, 272–273
overview, 117–120
pediatric burn injuries, 455
sexual relationships and, 141*f*
Embolic stroke, 221
Emotional support, 454
Emphysema, 374–375
Employers, ADA and, 4
Employment
aging and, 487
case managers and, 66–67
disabilities and, 87
disability laws, 45*f*
prevalence of disability and, 77
Employment agencies, 4
Emtricitabine (Emtriva), 411
End-of-life decision making
for children with disabilities, 467
issues related to, 26
nursing interventions, 493–494
for older adults, 492
End-of-life ethical issues, 47
Endocrine disorders, 290, 293–294
Endocrine system, aging and, 477
Enfuvirtide (T-20, Fuzeon), 411
Engle, Dagny, 19
Entry landing safety checklist, 91*t*
Entryway safety checklist, 91*t*
Environment

aging and, 475, 487
cancers and, 415
fall risk factors, 482*f*
in Parkinson's disease, 200
for rehabilitation nursing, 507–511
Environmental consequences of
behavior theory, 436
Epidermis, 110–111. *See also* Skin
Epidural hematoma, 251–252
Epidural space, 172
Equal Employment Opportunity
Commission, 44, 87
Equipment, nursing interventions, 241
Erectile dysfunction, 141*f*
ERIC database, 59*t*
Erikson, Erik, 435–436
Erikson, Joan, 436
Erikson's social learning theory,
145–146
Estate planning, 44
Esteem needs, 439
Estrogen replacement therapy, 300
Estrogens, osteoporosis and, 293–294
Etanercept (Enbrel), 310
Ethical issues
case management and, 70–71
concepts, 71–72
conflicts, 39–40
decision making and, 32*f*, 33*f*,
34–36
dilemmas, 25, 40
end-of-life decisions and, 494
rehabilitation nurses and, 31–44
relativism, 34
rights and, 40
steps in, 37*t*
Ethical principles, 40, 41*t*
European Pressure Ulcer Advisory
Panel, 110
Euthanasia, 494
Evidence
generation of, 53
levels of, 58
locating, 58–60
searching for, 58–59
synthesis of, 53
Evidence-based practice
adoption of, 63
cultural competency and, 394*f*
evolution toward, 103
implementation of, 63
importance of, 53
rehabilitation and, 51–64
research and, 25
seven critical steps, 58
in stroke care, 245–246

theory of, 53
Evidence-Based Rehabilitation (ARN),
22, 25
Ewing's family tumors, 420–421
Excitotoxicity, 201
Exenatide, 402
Exercise
counseling, 484
tolerance for, 478, 479
Expand Medicaid and Child Health
Plan, 467
Experimental research, 53, 55*t*
Exterior door safety checklist, 91*t*
Exubera, 403
Eye movements, desentization of, 325,
349

F

Facioscapulohumeral muscular
dystrophy, 460
Failure Mode Effects Analysis, 543
Falls
after amputations, 335
aging and, 269
environmental risk factors, 482*f*
in older adults, 481
osteoporosis and, 290
prevention of, 98*f*, 486
rehabilitation potential and, 482
risk of, 89–100
Families. *See also* Caregivers
aging and stress on, 487
basic tasks of, 440
coping after amputations, 338–339
education of, 110, 232–233, 334
effect of disability on, 158
end-of-life decisions and, 494
involvement of, 81
pediatric care interventions, 450
resources for, 233–234
support for stroke clients, 232
types of, 158–159
Family-centered care, 158, 449
Family development and function
theories, 440–441, 442*t*–443*t*
Family life cycle theory, 441
Family room safety checklist, 92*t*
Family Stress and Adaptation Model,
78
Fascia, 110
Fat, normal aging and, 478
Fatigue
after amputations, 337
cancer therapy and, 419
in SCI, 279
Febuxostat, 319
Federal Board for Vocational

Inhalation burns, 339
Initiative *versus* guilt, 436
Inpatient rehabilitation facilities
    (IRFs), 508, 519
Inpatient Rehabilitation Facility
    Patient Assessment Instrument, 7,
    25, 535, 536f–538f
Insomnia, 130, 131. *See also* Sleep
Institute for Crippled and Disabled, 17
Institute of Medicine (IOM), 28
Instrumental Activities of Daily Living
    (IADLs), 540
Insulin pump therapy, 404
Insulin resistance, 399, 423
Insulins, types of, 402–404, 403t
Insurance. *See* Health insurance
Insurance Company of North
    America, 65
Integra, 342
Integrase inhibitors, 411
Integrating Rehabilitation and
    Restorative Nursing Concepts into
    the MDS (ARN), 21
Integrity, ethics and, 47
Integrity *versus* despair, 436
Integumentary system. *See also* Skin
    assessment in SCI, 273
    assessment in TBI, 261
    normal aging and, 478
Intellectualization, 434
Interactional model, 436–437
Interagency communication, 81
Intercourse, positions, 142f
Interdisciplinary team model, 6
    for children with disabilities, 467
    for clients with dysphagia, 108
    effectiveness of, 71
    ethics committee and, 43–44, 71
    pediatric care interventions, 450
Interferon-beta, 193
Internal carotid arteries, 177–178, 219
International Academy of Life Care
    Planners, 66
International Classification of
    Impairment, Disability and
    Handicap, 5
International Code of Ethics, 42
International Year of the Disabled
    Person, 20
Interstitial lung disease, 377–378
Interstitial pulmonary fibrosis (IPF),
    378
Interventions, managed care plans, 71.
    See also specific conditions
Intervertebral discs, 183
Intestinal obstruction, 377
Intimacy *versus* isolation, 436

Intracerebral hemorrhage, 252
Intrapsychic theories, 431–437
Iowa Model of Evidence-Based
    Practice, 58
Irritability, sleep-related, 131
Ischemic stroke, 219–222
Isoniazid, 290

J
Job Accommodation Network, 87
Johnson, Dorothy, 78, 444t
Joint Commission (JC)
    accreditation by, 529–531
    quality improvement and, 529
    on stroke care, 231
    surveys, 531
Joint replacement, 301, 315–316
Josephson Institute of Ethics, 35
Judgment, definition of, 150
Jung, Carl, 435
Juvenile idiopathic arthritis (JIA), 305,
    306t
Juvenile rheumatoid arthritis, 462

K
Kant's moral law, 33
Kaplan's Stages and Descriptions of
    Human Sexual Response Cycle, 138,
    139t
Kaposi's sarcoma, 412
Katz Index of Independence in
    Activities of Daily Living, 535, 540f
Keloid scars, 341
Kenny, Elizabeth, 15, 444t
Kenny Self-Care Evaluation, 535, 540f
Kidneys, aging and, 478
Kinesthetic sense, 477
King, Imogene, 78, 445
Kitchen safety checklist, 94t, 96t
Klein-Bell Activity of Daily Living
    Scale, 535, 540
Knee replacement, 301
Knowledge deficits
    amputations and, 338–339
    assessment in blast injuries, 346
    in coronary heart disease, 373
Knowledge transfer, 53
Kohlberg, Lawrence, 438–439
Kohlbert's theory of moral
    development, 438t
Korean War, 19
Krusen, Frank H., 15, 17–18
Kugelberg-Welander syndrome, 460
Kyphoplasty, 301
Kyphoscoliosis, 488
Kyphosis, 488

L
Labor unions, 4
Lacunar infarcts, 221
Laminectomy, 311
Lamivudine (3TC), 411
Langerhans cells, 111
Language difficulties, 225–226
Large cell carcinoma, 378
Late life syndrome, 487–490
Latent phase, 434
Lateral corticospinal tract, 183
Lateral spinothalamic tract, 183
Latex allergy, 459
Latex sensitivity, 453–454
Laundry rooms, 94t
Leadership, 245
Lean Approach, 543
Leflunomide (Arava), 310
Leg length discrepancy, 461–462
Legg-Calvé-Perthes disease, 461
Legislation
    ethics and, 47t
    paths in the U.S., 524f
    prevalence of disability and, 77–78
    rehabilitation-related, 3–4
Leininger, Madeleine, 444t, 445
Leisure, nursing interventions, 241
Leukemias, 414
Leukodystrophy, 461
Levels of care, ethics, 46
Levels of consciousness, 107, 251
Levels of evidence (LOE), 103
Levine, Myra, 444t
Liberty Mutual, 16, 18, 65
Licensed practical nurses (LPNs), 10
Licensure, 10
Life care plans
    advanced practice nurses and, 245
    case management and, 69–70
Life expectancy, 488
Life review, aging and, 491
Life satisfaction, 279
Life Satisfaction Index, 159
Lifelong care, 21
Lifespan development paradigm, 475
Lifestyle factors
    aging and, 487
    osteoarthritis and, 311
    osteoporosis and, 290
LIFEware^SM, 540
Ligaments, spinal, 183
Lighting, safety checklist, 90t
Limb deficiencies, 455–457, 456. *See
    also* Amputations
Limb girdle muscular dystrophy, 460
Limb loss, incidence of, 289. *See also*
    Amputations

THE SPECIALTY PRACTICE OF REHABILITATION NURSING

Muscle wasting, 104
Muscular dystrophy, 459–461
Musculoskeletal system
    assessment in SCI, 273, 275
    assessment in TBI, 260–261
    blast injury, 345
    diagnosis of disorders, 329–339
    normal aging, 476
Myasthenia Gravis Foundation of
    America, 209, 210
Myasthenia gravis (MG), 208–212
    classification, 209
    epidemiology, 208
    etiology, 208
    management, 209–211
    manifestations, 209
    nursing interventions, 211
    nursing process, 211
    pathophysiology, 208
    plans of care, 211
Myasthenic crisis, 209, 211
Myelodysplasia, 458–463
Myelomeningocele, 458–463
Myers-Briggs Type Indicator, 439
Myocardial infarction (MI), 366
Myoclonus, 414
Myotonic dystrophy, 460

N

Nails, aging and, 478
NANDA, on risk, 88
Naproxen, 318
National AgrAbility Project, 87
National Alliance for Caregiving, 233
National Amputation Foundation, 457
National Association of State Head
    Injury Administrators, 262
National Center for Medical
    Rehabilitation Research, 262
National Council on Quality
    Assurance, 533
National Database of Nursing Quality
    Indicators, 27, 543–544
National Dysphagia Diet (NDD), 108
National Family Caregivers
    Association, 233
National Guideline Clearinghouse, 60
National Institute of Child Health and
    Human Development, 262
National Institute on Disability and
    Rehabilitation Research, 44
National Institutes of Health, 43
National Institutes of Health Stroke
    Scale, 229, 235f–236f
National Park Service, U.S., 87
National Pressure Ulcer Advisory
    Panel, 110

National Quality Forum (NQF),
    543–544
Nausea, cancer therapy and, 418
Nausea and vomiting, 493
Necrosis, 188–189
Nelfinavir (Viracept), 411
Neonatal intensive care units (NICUs),
    450
Nerve supply, skin function and, 110
Nervous system
    assessment, 346
    blast injury, 345
Neuman, Betty, 444t
Neural recovery, 188–190
Neuroanatomy, 171–190
Neurobehavioral Functioning
    Inventory, 256
Neurogenic bladder, 122–125
    classifications, 123
    hydrocephalus and, 458
    management strategies, 123–124
    pediatric TBIs and, 453
Neurogenic bowel, 127, 128, 458
Neurogenic function, 188
Neurogenic osteoporosis, 292
Neurogenic shock, 270
Neurologic function
    assessment in SCI, 272, 275
    assessment in TBI, 256, 260
    classification of, 188
    normal aging, 477
Neurological assessment, 187–188
Neurological diseases, 191–216
Neurological injuries, 112
Neuromatrix theory, 385–386
Neurons
    bipolar, 172
    composition of, 172
    differentiation of, 189–190
    multipolar, 172
    pseudounipolar, 172
    types of, 172
Neuropathic pain, 383
Neuropathies, 401
Neuroprotective agents, 230
Neuropsychological testing, 256
Neurostimulants, 229
Neurotic anxiety, 434
Nevirapine (Viramune), 411
New Freedom Initiative, 44
Newman, Margaret, 445
Night terrors, 131
Nightingale, Florence, 15, 16
Nightmares, 131, 347
Nitrogen balance, 275
Nitrogen wasting, 109
No Child Left Behind Program, 44

Non-small-cell lung cancer (NSCLC),
    378
Nonexperimental research, 55t
Nonmaleficence, 41t
Nonnucleoside reverse transcriptase
    inhibitors (NNRTIs), 411
Nonsteroidal anti-inflammatory drugs
    (NSAIDs)
    for gout, 318
    for osteoarthritis, 314
    in pain management, 389
    for rheumatoid arthritis, 309, 309t
Normative ethics, 31
North American Brain Injury Society,
    262
North American Nursing Diagnosis
    Association International
    (NANDA-I), 103
North American Nursing Diagnosis
    Association (NANDA), 82, 83,
    89–100
Norton Scale, 113
Nothing-by-mouth, 105–106
Novak, Susan, 19
Nucleoside analog reverse
    transcriptase inhibitors (NRTIs),
    411
Nucleus pulposus, 183
Nuremberg Code, 43, 44f
Nurse Case Managers, 70
Nurse-in-Washington program, 20
Nurse practitioners, 469
Nurses, role responsibilities, 11–12
Nursing beliefs and values, 7–8, 442
Nursing diagnoses
    for bowel impairments, 127–128
    care planning and, 103
    multiple sclerosis, 195–196
    nutrition status-related, 103–109
    skin integrity-related, 113
    sleep-related, 130
    in urinary incontinence, 121
Nursing homes
    quality measures, 542
    restraint use in, 494
Nursing interventions. *See also specific
    conditions*
    in ALS, 207–208
    ALS and, 203
    bowel impairment, 128
    cognitive maturation and, 146–
    149
    for dysphagia, 107–108
    immobility, 136
    for incontinence, 122
    mobility issues and, 134–135
    multiple sclerosis, 196–197